Perioperative Pediatric Patient Blood Management and Transfusion Safety

Norma J. Klein
Editor

Perioperative Pediatric Patient Blood Management and Transfusion Safety

A Case-Based Review

Springer

Editor
Norma J. Klein
Department of Anesthesiology and Pain Medicine
University of California, Davis
Sacramento, CA, USA

ISBN 978-3-031-81665-9 ISBN 978-3-031-81666-6 (eBook)
https://doi.org/10.1007/978-3-031-81666-6

This Springer imprint is published by the registered company Springer Nature Switzerland AG
The registered company address is: Gewerbestrasse 11, 6330 Cham, Switzerland

Contents

Introduction

1

Norma J. Klein

1.1 Introduction

The definition of patient blood management (PBM) has undergone several revisions since initial characterization almost 20 years ago. Pediatric PBM is recognized but has advanced little since then, with most published evidence arising from adult-based research. Ethical and practical limitations impacting pediatric medical science investigations in general further hamper pediatric PBM development and data acquisition [1]. Pediatric blood management outcomes and benchmarks are unknown, save for large registries that often rely on laborious self-reporting. A general lack of transfusion medicine knowledge within the ranks of anesthesiology, surgery, and general medicine trainees creates additional clinical knowledge gaps [2, 3]. Medical students and residents often work in settings that offer little education on rational and safe transfusion decision-making. However, the future is not entirely dim, as the electronification of health record is increasingly tied to our transfusion behaviors which supports an ability to regularly update outcome data and evidence-based standards.

Primum non nocera: First, do no harm. Adherence to this basic patient care principle requires critical thinking and the ability to know what we do not know. A blood transfusion is an organ transplant and, by any other organ system name, would be subject to highly regulated protocol before reaching the hands of well-intended practitioners. Furthermore, transfusionists must have the knowledge and tools to preserve the donated blood that they order and handle. Select chapters in this book discuss tasks crucial to optimal blood stewardship, including the patient verification process, blood handling requirements, and blood conservation solutions.

The recommendation summaries in the various chapters of this book derive from the limited evidence available in the literature on how to apply PBM principles in

N. J. Klein (✉)
Department of Anesthesiology and Pain Medicine, University of California, Davis, Sacramento, CA, USA
e-mail: nklein@ucdavis.edu

N. J. Klein (ed.), *Perioperative Pediatric Patient Blood Management and Transfusion Safety*, https://doi.org/10.1007/978-3-031-81666-6_1

children undergoing surgery. The discussions and management suggestions are case-based, and the chapter authors have selected key learning objectives based on common gaps in transfusion medicine and PBM knowledge. The "what" has been refocused as "how to" for many of the included topics. The case scenario challenges will be familiar to readers who manage blood loss in children undergoing surgery.

Clinical education for pediatric perioperative PBM can only undergo improvement. Successive writings and research results will be scraped and scoured through artificial intelligence (AI) algorithms, potentially providing enhanced guidance for rational pediatric PBM practices. An initial (and free) ChatGPT (version 3.5) query in late 2022 under the search term "pediatric perioperative patient blood management" produced a brief description that included identification of preoperative anemia and bleeding disorders, intraoperative cell salvage, postoperative hemoglobin monitoring, and pain management to "reduce the need for opioids, which can lead to anemia." A specific chatbot query as to how opioids can lead to anemia stated that opioids may suppress erythropoietin production, decrease gastrointestinal motility (and subsequent iron absorption), and increase histamine production leading to vasodilation and subsequent blood loss, "in some cases." A later ChatGPT query in early 2024 lacked the opioid-anemia association. However, it included additional PBM strategies such as autologous transfusion, multidisciplinary team development, patient and family education (including risks and alternatives to selected PBM strategies), and a need for more clinical trials. The evolution (or, learning) of this AI generated PBM guidance illustrates the importance of practical experience and keeping an eye open for conjured information that may be untrue or misrepresent the patient at hand [4]. In the meantime, this scoping review of pediatric PBM will hopefully serve to answer many practical questions that arise when managing an anemic or bleeding child in the perioperative period.

References

1. Furth SL. Trials and tribulations—the challenges of clinical trials in children. NEJM Evid. 2023;2(12):EVIDe2300280.
2. Connelly NR, Adler AC, Vanderberg LE, Conlin F, Mitchell JD, Goldstein S, et al. Anesthesiology resident knowledge of transfusion medicine: results from the anesthesiology transfusion education study. Anesth Analg. 2024;138(3):655–63.
3. Haspel RL, Lin Y, Mallick R, Tinmouth A, Cid J, Eichler H, et al. Internal medicine resident knowledge of transfusion medicine: results from the BEST-TEST international education needs assessment. Transfusion. 2015;55(6):1355–61.
4. Chen RJ, Wang JJ, Williamson DFK, Chen TY, Lipkova J, Lu MY, et al. Algorithmic fairness in artificial intelligence for medicine and healthcare. Nat Biomed Eng. 2023;7(6):719–42.

Establishing a Patient Blood Management Program in Your Hospital

2

Jonathan H. Waters

Case Scenario

You are an anesthesiologist at a large community hospital and recently appointed as chairperson of the hospital transfusion committee. The hospital CEO has contacted you to say that the hospital is spending hundreds of thousands of dollars on blood products, and she would like to see a cost savings. She also heard about patient blood management programs at a recent meeting of hospital administrators and has asked you to develop a program for the hospital. You are new to administration work and have not been given a budget.

Key Learning Objectives

- What is PBM?
- What is a PBM "program"?
- What are the elements of a PBM program?
- What are the benefits of a PBM program?
- Is a PBM program a regulatory requirement?
- Can my hospital certify in PBM?
- What are some of the known obstacles to establishing and maintaining a PBM program?

J. H. Waters (✉)
Anesthesiology and Bioengineering, UPMC Patient Blood Management Program, University of Pittsburgh Medical Center, Magee Womens Hospital, Pittsburgh, PA, USA
e-mail: watejh@upmc.edu

N. J. Klein (ed.), *Perioperative Pediatric Patient Blood Management and Transfusion Safety*, https://doi.org/10.1007/978-3-031-81666-6_2

2.1 Discussion

2.1.1 What Is PBM?

Patient blood management (PBM) has been defined by the Society for the Advancement of Patient Blood Management (SABM) as "…a patient-centered, systematic, evidence-based approach to improve patient outcomes by managing and preserving the patient's own blood, while promoting patient safety and empowerment" [1]. The American Association for Blood and Biotherapies (AABB) defines it a little more broadly as "an evidence-based, multidisciplinary approach to caring for patients who might need a blood transfusion" [2]. The international foundation for patient blood management (IFPBM) defines it as a patient-centered, systematic, evidence-based approach to improve patient outcomes by managing and preserving a patient's own blood, while promoting patient safety and empowerment [3].

The concept of PBM arose from the development of bloodless medicine programs in the 1980s. The concept of a bloodless medicine program was developed to protect patients for whom blood transfusion is not an option. This tends to be two groups: Jehovah's Witnesses or those patients who have received repetitive transfusions and are alloimmunized to the point that there is no compatible blood for them. This second category generally includes sickle cell disease patients and others with a hemoglobinopathy.

With the creation of these bloodless programs, it was realized that the bloodless patients had outcomes which were equivalent or better than those patients with whom allogeneic transfusion was acceptable [4–6]. This led to the terminology being changed to "blood conservation." This term did not resonate with the blood banking community, so the term morphed into "blood management." This term was also confusing in that it didn't differentiate from the management of patients to what is done in the blood bank every day which is "inventory blood management," where blood is moved from place to place to minimize wastage. Thus, the term "patient blood management" arose to distinguish what is done for the patient versus what is done behind the walls of the blood bank.

2.1.2 What Is a PBM "Program"?

A PBM program is an organized, multidisciplinary approach to minimize or eliminate the need for allogeneic transfusion. In the context of perioperative care, PBM includes, but is not limited to [7]:

- Preoperative phase of care: anemia screening and management, consideration of autologous blood donation, optimization of coagulation status, multidisciplinary planning.
- Intraoperative phase of care: cell salvage; maintenance of normothermia, normotension, and acid base status; antifibrinolytics; consideration of noninvasive surgical techniques; hemostatic agents; noninvasive physiologic monitoring.

- Postoperative phase of care: minimizing iatrogenic blood loss, vigilant monitoring for bleeding and coagulopathy development, consideration of cell salvage from wound and drains, anemia treatment.

2.1.3 What Are the Elements of a PBM Program?

Each organization, which touches upon the domain of PBM, will define the elements differently. At the University of Pittsburgh, a 6-step strategy is used, which is outlined in Table 2.1.

Below is a short explanation for what each of these elements mean.

2.1.3.1 Leverage Computerized Physician Order Entry (CPOE) Systems to Guide Evidence-Based Transfusions

Probably the easiest of the PBM elements to implement is leveraging CPOE systems to encourage compliance with prevailing evidence associated with when a transfusion might be indicated. For instance, all studies to date seem to indicate that an RBC transfusion is not indicated in stable, hospitalized adult patients until a hemoglobin is in the 7–8 gm/dL range [8]. Historically, a transfusion trigger of 10 gm/dL was used. Many clinicians still hang on to this historical teaching. Electronic tools to educate as to where the evidence base lies help move transfusion practice towards the evidence base. In addition, these tools can be used to identify departments or hospitals that in need of education as to where the current evidence lies.

Likewise, a plasma transfusion has traditionally been performed any time an INR/PT (international normalized ratio/prothrombin time) is elevated outside the normal limit of 1.2. However, there appears to be significant data to suggest that plasma transfusion has little effect until the INR is above 1.6 [9]. In addition, classic plasma dosing has occurred with two-unit doses, which is inadequate to correct an elevated INR. Doses of 15–20 mL/kg should be used to give any meaningful increase in coagulation factor concentration. Coagulation factor levels measured in vivo that are 20% of normal provide adequate hemostasis in the absence of concomitant coagulation deficiencies.

Table 2.1 Six point patient blood management strategy at the University of Pittsburgh Medical Center

Six point patient blood management strategy
Leverage computerized physician order entry (CPOE) systems to guide evidence-based transfusions
Reduce all forms of waste related to blood transfusion practices
Promote alternative blood transfusion methods and systems
Promote anemia management strategies
Limit iatrogenic blood loss
Provide blood management education, awareness and auditing for clinicians; application of patient-centered shared decision-making tools

The ease of implementation of these electronic tools is dependent on having an efficient CPOE. This is dependent upon having the programmers to implement these tools, as well as the institutional will to support the ongoing software and program support necessary to maintain pace with practitioners' clinical needs.

2.1.3.2 Reduce All Forms of Waste Related to Blood Transfusion Practices

Waste reduction is one of the more interesting areas of work associated with transfusion. Waste in the health care system has been identified as a huge opportunity to reduce health care costs [10]. Waste comes in many forms, starting with anemia caused by overly aggressive phlebotomy to mishandling of blood (Table 2.2).

Waste related to mishandling leads to the disposal of a unit of blood. This typically relates to temperature noncompliance. A little device is placed in each cooler of blood that changes color when the temperature in the cooler rises above 6^0 C. If the temperature becomes too high, then the blood is discarded. In the current environment of blood shortages, wasting blood that has been donated is something that should not happen. Figuring out where waste is occurring and stopping it is key to eliminate waste of donated blood. Frequently, this simply relates to an educational effort, following by ongoing monitoring of compliance measures.

Other waste that occurs with transfusion is associated with too many typing and crossmatches of blood. Depending upon the contract that a hospital may have with their blood provider, the hospital may pay $12 for a blood type screening and a similar price for a crossmatch. A metric that is commonly used is the crossmatch to transfusion (C:T) ratio. The industry standard is that the C:T ratio should be less than 2, with an ideal ratio of 1:1. In other words, no more than two crossmatches should be associated with one transfusion. There is usually variability across specialties in the C:T ratio which helps educate departments as to their actual use. Historically, over crossmatching was performed from a perception that the crossmatching process was a timely activity that would interfere with blood being obtained. In most hospitals, electronic crossmatching is performed which takes less than 5 min, whereas a serologic crossmatch (e.g., mixing the patient's blood with reagent cells or antibodies) would take more than 45 min. An electronic crossmatch is generally done if the initial screening or the patient's medical history reveals no unusual antibodies. Hospitals may not allow electronic crossmatching in certain

Table 2.2

Sources of blood waste
Preoperative autologous donation (PAD)
Inappropriate transfusions
Excessive phlebotomy
Elevated crossmatch to transfusion ratio (C:T)
Wasted blood products
Dispensing of blood to the OR before it is needed

patient populations, such as bone marrow and stem cell transplant patients, and infants <4 months.

Another opportunity to reduce waste related to transfusion is to have an up-to-date, maximum surgical blood order system (MSBOS). A MSBOS is an institution specific, data-based list of blood administered in the past according to surgery type. It improves the efficiency of preoperative blood ordering, including requests to crossmatch and "hold" blood units which is often unnecessary [11].

Many patients and practitioners believe that preoperative autologous donation (PAD) preserves the community blood supply, but poor preoperative communication and rescheduled surgeries places a significant portion of this donated blood at risk of unnecessary waste.

2.1.3.3 Promote Alternative Blood Transfusion Methods and Systems

Alternative blood transfusion methods primarily involve autotransfusion where the patient's shed surgical blood is collected, filtered, washed, and readministered. Classically, this has been called "cell salvage"; however, this terminology stems from the name of the original machine, which was the "cell saver." This is a brand name for a machine manufactured by Haemonetics. There are several other machines (CATS®, Autolog®, XTRA) that do the same thing but manufactured by other companies. The latest generation of the cell saver is called the "Elite®." The CATS® is often used in pediatric surgeries because of a continuous spin mode. When using autotransfusion, there should be quality assurance associated with its implementation. This means making sure that the machine is working like it should, e.g., it is concentrating and washing in a fashion that is safe for the recipient of the blood, and that the operators of the machine are well-trained and know the hazards of mismanaging the equipment.

2.1.3.4 Promote Anemia Management Strategies

Anemia management seems like something that should be intuitive; however, anemia is frequently ignored. This probably stems from the ease of ordering a transfusion. Optimizing a patient's hemoglobin preoperatively and during any hospitalization requires extra time (several weeks in most cases), extra effort on the part of the clinical team, and extra expense. Generally, this involves identifying the cause of the anemia and then fixing it. Anemia can be caused by gastrointestinal blood loss, folate deficiency, iron deficiency, or chronic disease. The most common cause of a perioperative transfusion is a preoperative anemia. Solutions to this spectrum of causes ranges from stopping the GI blood loss, iron or folate supplementation, or erythropoietin use.

2.1.3.5 Limit Iatrogenic Blood Loss

Avoidable blood loss that results from excessive phlebotomy is the first place to start to reduce iatrogenic blood loss. In the current era, noninvasive surgical techniques also avoid excessive blood loss.

Phlebotomy loss in the ICU has been estimated to be responsible for 30% of the ICU transfusions [12]. Phlebotomy waste can be minimized by eliminating orders for routine blood draws, use of low-fill (e.g., pediatric-sized) vacutainers, and using closed blood sampling systems (VAMP systems) [13]. Additionally, using point-of-care (POC) testing devices allows for microliters of blood to be used to gather information regarding coagulation function, hemoglobin concentration, and electrolyte concentrations.

2.1.3.6 Provide Blood Management Education and Ongoing Audits of Clinician Practices as Well as Patient-Centered Shared Decision-Making Tools

This is one of the more exciting elements of PBM. Auditing creates awareness: reporting is done for high volume procedures where there is large variability between providers. Examples are shown in Figs. 2.1 and 2.2. These figures illustrate blood product data for total hip replacement by provider and by hospital. The variability is an opportunity for process improvement. Early in the development of this reporting, the variability was much larger than it is currently as shown in these figures. The data is shown in two different formats. The first (Fig. 2.1) is a “bullet” graph, where each dot represents either a surgeon or hospital. The size of the bullet represents the number of cases done in a reporting period. The “x” axis shows the percentage of patients who were transfused with RBCs. The “y” axis shows the number of RBC units that were transfused during a transfusion episode. The second way of showing this data is through a tabular form (Fig. 2.2). Figure 2.2 illustrates data associated with the cost of taking care of the patients and the average length of stay. Tranexamic acid (TXA) use is also shown which has become the gold standard in minimizing blood loss during orthopedic surgery.

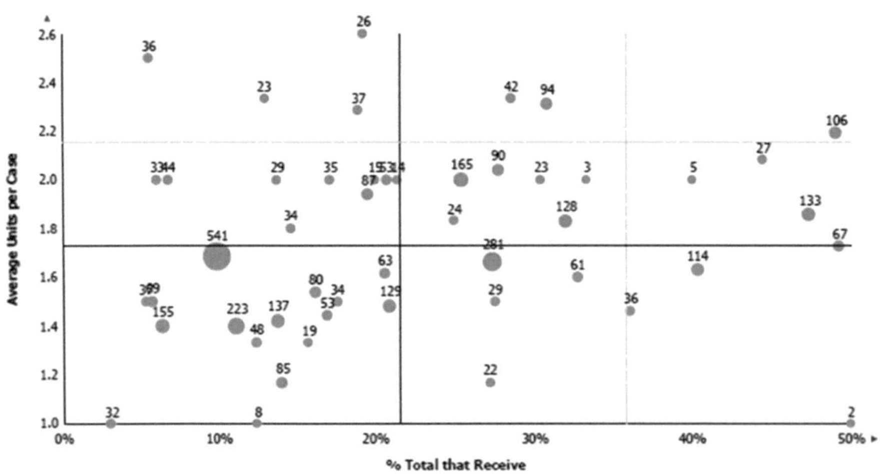

Fig. 2.1 RBC blood use by surgeon for primary total hip replacement at one medical complex

1 2 %Units	Physician	Discharges	Total Receiving Blood (1)	Average Units per Case (2)	ALOS w/	ALOS w/o	Ave Charges w Blood w/	Ave Charges w Blood w/o	% Autologous
		386	86.8%	2.2	1.9	1.9	$82,961	$78,596	3.3%
		350	4.3%	1.5	3.3	2.4	$54,309	$49,840	
		189	29.6%	1.3	4.7	4.0	$111,934	$103,235	3.6%
		123	36.6%	1.5	3.4	2.8	$71,220	$76,212	42.2%
		86	36.0%	1.8	4.3	3.3	$56,221	$49,339	
		82	42.7%	2.0	4.6	2.4	$106,666	$74,389	5.7%
		68	16.2%	1.8	5.1	4.3	$55,418	$41,696	
		57	35.1%	1.4	6.2	4.4	$135,311	$121,190	
		51	23.5%	2.5	4.6	4.2	$56,386	$54,757	66.7%
		50	16.0%	1.9	4.2	3.7	$81,000	$70,393	
		46	41.3%	1.7	4.3	4.0	$54,480	$49,625	47.4%
		45	20.0%	1.8	3.8	3.9	$48,475	$45,170	66.7%
		44	15.9%	1.4	2.9	2.1	$71,095	$64,127	14.3%
		40	40.0%	2.1	5.3	3.5	$39,866	$35,703	
		32	78.1%	2.4	3.2	3.4	$105,314	$89,677	
		29	27.6%	1.1	3.9	3.4	$70,340	$64,517	37.5%
		27	11.1%	5.0	9.3	3.9	$88,742	$52,354	
		26	11.5%	1.3	3.3	3.7	$36,732	$37,561	33.3%
		25	48.0%	1.2	4.9	5.1	$78,875	$71,438	66.7%

Fig. 2.2 RBC blood use by surgeon for primary total hip replacement at one medical complex. The green color represents surgeons that are 1 standard deviation (SD) above average with respect to blood use compared to peers; yellow color is the average use ±1 SD; red is 1 SD below average for blood use. "2 units" represents multiple RBC unit administration rather than a single unit which is often sufficient and should be followed up with a hemoglobin assessment before administering the second unit

The second part of clinical education and monitoring in a PBM program is building patient-centered clinical decision support (CDS) tools. For instance, Jehovah's witnesses are identified upon hospital admission which triggers a cascade of events, starting with identifying these patients for the blood bank so that blood is not cross-matched and "held" for these patients. Henceforth, clinicians are alerted through electronic and other channels of the patient's blood management choices early during care.

2.1.4 What Are the Benefits of a PBM Program?

Ideally, outcome benefits such as shorter length of stay and decreased post-operative infections would be measured; however, these benefits can be mixed in that there are a lot of co-factors which can alter the length of stay [5, 14–19]. The least debatable outcome is the cost of caring for these patients; US Medicare reimbursement in 2013 numbers is less than 12% of the direct cost per RBC unit [5, 14, 20]. In a 2024 report of cost savings related to blood acquisition in an academic, multidisciplinary PBM program, the return on investment (ROI) was 9.6-fold over a 10-year period, or $2.9 million per year [21]. When the PBM program savings were combined with a well-structured bloodless medicine program, the cost savings was an additional $5 million per year, for a combined 7.5-fold ROI. Patient outcomes were unchanged throughout the reporting period. Full support from hospital administration was noted to be a crucial component of the program success [21].

2.1.5 Is a PBM Program a Regulatory Requirement?

There is no regulatory requirement to create a PBM program in the USA. The primary drivers for creating a PBM program should be resultant cost reductions and better patient outcomes.

2.1.6 Can My Hospital Certify in PBM?

There is one route for achieving accreditation which is through the Association for the Advancement of Blood & Biotherapies (AABB; United States) in conjunction with the US Joint Commission (TJC). This accreditation doesn't necessarily assure the quality of a program, but it is a good step toward doing so. It can also be useful when defending malpractice cases against a hospital or provider [22]. Part of the accreditation process is a survey of a hospital and its quality program. There are also provider certificate courses. SABM has a certification process. SABM's certificate course is done by an exam and its audience is focused on physicians, nurses and other allied health professionals. The American Society of Extracorporeal Technology (AmSECT) has a certificate course aimed at perfusionists and autotransfusionists [23]. This exam is administered three times a year. To sit for the exam, the applicant needs to provide a case log and a college or high school diploma.

2.1.7 What Are Some of the Known Obstacles to Establishing and Maintaining a PBM Program? [19, 24, 25]

- Lack of knowledge or awareness about PBM
- Lack of information access
- Preconceptions or cultural inertia
- Lack of validated data on the most effective PBM modality(s)
- Staff shortages
- Inability to support an ongoing clinician monitoring program
- Funding

Finally, it is important to point out that PBM is a multidisciplinary accomplishment, and a program cannot be successful without interdepartmental collaboration, support, and information sharing. In an effective program, clinicians that order or administer blood have an obligation to their patients and to the institution to become involved in being part of the PBM solution. Participating in hospital committees, including the local transfusion committee, is a good start.

2.2 Summary of Key Learning Objectives

The scenario presented—a new administrative position with no funding—is typical of US hospital employment. As chair of the hospital transfusion committee, one goal is to convince colleagues and the administration that PBM can improve patient outcomes and advance institutional priorities. The following is a practical toolkit to begin your assignment:

- Establish a "team" of colleagues who are passionate about PBM and blood banking. These are sometimes called "champions."
- Obtain a seat on several hospital committees for interdisciplinary information gathering and outreach.
- Locate a source of "free" information about transfusion practices, organizational improvements, and patient outcomes in your hospital:
  - The electronic medical record.
  - Blood bank.
  - Hospital quality improvement (QI) and incident report database.
  - The American College of Surgeons (ACS) National Surgical Quality Improvement Program (NSQIP) database.
- Develop QI projects to get colleagues involved in your mission and to make it clear that you are intent on setting outcomes benchmarks.
- Become an active member of PBM societies:
  - Society for the Advancement of Patient Blood Management (SABM).
  - American Association for Blood and Biotherapies (AABB).
  - International Foundation for Patient Blood Management (IFPBM).
  - Network for the Advancement of Patient Blood Management (NATA).
  - The International Society of Blood Transfusion (ISBT).
- Start a PBM subcommittee within your own professional organization(s).

Hospital-wide education is essential to a successful PBM program but can be very difficult to accomplish. In addition to standard grand rounds and hospital-wide announcements from the administration, information about PBM practices can be disseminated through protocol-based electronic order entry, a "blood school" continuing education program, or orchestrating a hospital-wide "PBM Day." No one educational approach has been shown to be most successful. Ongoing clinical practice monitoring is the other essential feature of a successful PBM program, although what the best form of monitoring is remains unclear.

Key Points

- Patient blood management (PBM) is, by one definition, a patient-centered, systematic, evidence-based approach to improve patient outcomes by managing and preserving a patient's own blood while promoting patient safety and empowerment.
- A PBM program is an organized, multidisciplinary approach to minimize or eliminate the need for allogeneic transfusion. All phases of perioperative

care—pre-, intra-, and postoperative—offer opportunity to improve patient outcomes through PBM.
- Each organization or hospital will define the elements of their PBM program differently, depending on resources and institutional will.
- PBM benefits found in published research studies include improvements in hospital length of stay (LOS), overall RBC transfusions, institutional costs, hospital mortality rates, infections, and single-unit transfusions. PBM programs also offer an alternative to patients who refuse blood transfusions.
- There is no regulatory requirement to create a PBM program.
- Hospital PBM certification is possible. In the USA, the AABB offers a program in conjunction with The Joint Commission (TJC).
- Obstacles to PBM implementation include staff shortages, a lack of knowledge or awareness about PBM, and costs.

References

1. SABM Standards, quality guide and executive guide. What is patient blood management (PBM)? 2023. http://sabm.org. Accessed 2 Mar 2024.
2. Patient blood management. American Association for Blood and Biotherapies (AABB). 2023. https://www.aabb.org/news-resources/resources/patient-blood-management. Accessed 4 June 2023.
3. What is patient blood management? International Foundation for Patient Blood Management (IFPBM). 2023. https://www.ifpbm.org/knowledge/what-is-patient-blood-management. Accessed 4 June 2023.
4. Lo BD, Pippa A, Sherd I, Scott AV, Thomas AJ, Hendricks EA, et al. Clinical outcomes, blood utilization, and ethical considerations for pediatric patients in a bloodless medicine and surgery program. Anesth Analg. 2024;138(2):465–74.
5. Frank SM, Pippa A, Sherd I, Scott AV, Lo BD, Cruz NC, et al. Methods of bloodless care, clinical outcomes, and costs for adult patients who decline allogeneic transfusions. Anesth Analg. 2022;135(3):576–85.
6. Kayoum AA, Rivera Flores E, Reyes M, Almasarweh SI, Ojito J, Burke RP, Sasaki J. Safety of bloodless open-heart surgery on cardiopulmonary bypass in selected children: a single center experience with minimal invasive extracorporeal circulation. Perfusion. 2024;39(2):391–8.
7. Warner MA, Shore-Lesserson L, Shander A, Patel SY, Perelman SI, Guinn NR. Perioperative anemia: prevention, diagnosis, and management throughout the spectrum of perioperative care. Anesth Analg. 2020;130(5):1364–80.
8. Carson JL, Triulzi DJ, Ness PM. Indications for and adverse effects of red-cell transfusion. N Engl J Med. 2017;377(13):1261–72.
9. Waters JH, Yazer MH. The mythology of plasma transfusion. Anesth Analg. 2018;127(2):338–9.
10. Berwick DM, Hackbarth AD. Eliminating waste in US health care. JAMA. 2012;307(14):1513–6.
11. Frank SM, Oleyar MJ, Ness PM, Tobian AA. Reducing unnecessary preoperative blood orders and costs by implementing an updated institution-specific maximum surgical blood order schedule and a remote electronic blood release system. Anesthesiology. 2014;121(3):501–9.
12. Corwin HL, Parsonnet KC, Gettinger A. RBC transfusion in the ICU. Is there a reason? Chest. 1995;108(3):767–71.
13. O'Hare D, Chilvers RJ. Arterial blood sampling practices in intensive care units in England and Wales. Anaesthesia. 2001;56(6):568–71.

14. Leahy MF, Hofmann A, Towler S, Trentino KM, Burrows SA, Swain SG, et al. Improved outcomes and reduced costs associated with a health-system-wide patient blood management program: a retrospective observational study in four major adult tertiary-care hospitals. Transfusion. 2017;57(6):1347–58.
15. Drabinski T, Zacharowski K, Meybohm P, Rüger AM, Ramirez de Arellano A. Estimating the epidemiological and economic impact of implementing preoperative anaemia measures in the German healthcare system: the health economic footprint of patient blood management. Adv Ther. 2020;37(8):3515–36.
16. Trentino KM, Mace HS, Symons K, Sanfilippo FM, Leahy MF, Farmer SL, et al. Screening and treating pre-operative anaemia and suboptimal iron stores in elective colorectal surgery: a cost effectiveness analysis. Anaesthesia. 2021;76(3):357–65.
17. Wan S, Sparring V, Cabrales DA, Jansson K, Wikman A. Clinical and budget impact of treating preoperative anemia in major orthopedic surgery-a retrospective observational study. J Arthroplast. 2020;35(11):3084–8.
18. World Health Organization (WHO). Policy brief: the urgent need to implement patient blood management. 2021. https://www.who.int/publications/i/item/9789240035744. Accessed 3 Aug 2023.
19. Ozawa S, Ozawa-Morriello J, Perelman S, Thorpe E, Rock R, Pearse BL. Improving patient blood management programs: an implementation science approach. Anesth Analg. 2023;136(2):397–407.
20. Frank SM, Waters JH, editors. Patient blood management: multidisciplinary approaches to optimizing care. Bethesda: AABB Press; 2016. p. 41.
21. Frank SM, Hensley NB, Thomas AJ, Dawson CG, Resar LMS, Ulatowski JA, Crowe EP. Greater than sevenfold return on investment for a comprehensive patient blood management program with equivalent or improved outcomes. Anesth Analg. 2024;138(6):1345–8. https://doi.org/10.1213/ANE.0000000000006862.
22. The Joint Commission (TJC). Certification through the joint commission and AABB. 2023. https://www.amsect.org/Certification/PBMT-Exam. Accessed 4 June 2023.
23. American Society of Extracorporeal Technology. Perioperative Blood Management Technologist (PBMT) Exam. 2023. https://www.amsect.org/Certification/PBMT-Exam. Accessed 4 Jun 2023.
24. Delaforce A, Duff J, Munday J, Hardy J. Overcoming barriers to evidence-based patient blood management: a restricted review. Implement Sci. 2020;15(1):6.
25. An AABB White Paper: Building a Better Patient Blood Management Program. American Associat ion of Blood and Biotherapies (AABB). 2015. https://www.aabb.org/docs/default-source/default-document-library/resources/aabb-pbm-whitepaper.pdf?sfvrsn=4578189_0. Accessed 15 Feb 2023.

Part I

Preoperative Phase of Care

3 Pretransfusion Testing

Justin Genziano, Michelle Banas, Lisa Eisler, and Eldad Hod

3.1 Case Scenario

An 8-month-old male with a history of anemia and complex craniosynostosis presents for open cranial vault remodeling (OCVRS). He was born full-term, with no prior history of hospitalization or blood transfusion. His hemoglobin is currently 10 g/dL (normal for age, 11–14 g/dL). The surgical team has ordered red blood cells (RBCs) on hold, at a volume supported by the local maximum surgical blood order schedule (MSBOS). The patient was a difficult phlebotomy in the preoperative clinic, so a blood sample has not been sent to the hospital's blood bank for pretransfusion testing. The parents and surgeon ask whether a sample can be sent from the operating room after the induction of anesthesia, to prevent additional venipuncture attempts on an awake child. You consult a senior anesthesiology colleague who suggests it is best to wait a few extra minutes for a type and screen (T&S) result.

J. Genziano
UCSF Department of Anesthesia and Perioperative Care, San Francisco, CA, USA
e-mail: justin.genziano@ucsf.edu

M. Banas
Department of Anesthesiology, Perioperative Care, and Pain Medicine at NYU Grossman School of Medicine, New York, NY, USA
e-mail: Michelle.Banas@nyulangone.org

L. Eisler (✉)
Department of Anesthesiology, Columbia University Irving Medical Center, New York, NY, USA
e-mail: ldl2113@cumc.columbia.edu

E. Hod
Department of Pathology and Cell Biology, Columbia University Irving Medical Center, New York, NY, USA
e-mail: eh2217@cumc.columbia.edu

N. J. Klein (ed.), *Perioperative Pediatric Patient Blood Management and Transfusion Safety*, https://doi.org/10.1007/978-3-031-81666-6_3

Key Learning Objectives

- What is the basis of testing requirements before a blood transfusion?
- Why should a T&S and a crossmatch be performed before the blood bank releases blood to the operating room?
- Why is patient verification a crucial step in the pretransfusion process?
- What is a "Maximum Surgical Blood Order Schedule" (MSBOS) and what are its advantages?
- What type of blood is released for emergency transfusion in an infant with incomplete pretransfusion testing?

3.2 Discussion

3.2.1 Pretransfusion Testing Regulations

Regulatory standards for pretransfusion testing are designed to promote patient transfusion safety, specifically, to prevent transfusion of ABO-incompatible blood components due to incorrect identification of a patient during specimen collection or other errors made in the pretransfusion testing process [1]. In the United States (US), the Food and Drug Administration (FDA) sets the baseline regulatory standards for blood compatibility testing. The FDA requires standard procedures for collecting and identifying recipient blood samples, protocols for the age of the sample, the ability to demonstrate incompatibility between donor and recipient, and a process to expedite transfusion in life-threatening emergencies [2]. Additionally, the Association for the Advancement of Blood & Biotherapies (AABB) and the College of American Pathology (CAP) set guidelines including the timing of the sample blood draw, the need for two determinations of the recipient's ABO type, as well as the requirements for pretransfusion testing results prior to blood product release. Hospital accreditation in the USA is not possible without adherence to these standards. Resource-rich countries follow similar procedures, and the World Health Organization (WHO) recommends that nations that collect and distribute blood products prioritize the promotion of patient safety through organized national oversight and standardization [3, 4].

3.2.2 The Basis for Required Pretransfusion Testing

Before blood can be distributed to the operating room, the recipient patient's blood type and the presence of any unexpected plasma alloantibodies must be determined through a blood type and screen (T&S). Blood typing determines which ABO- and Rhesus-(Rh) antigens are expressed on erythrocytes (there are no ABO- or Rh-antigens on the surface of type O, Rh-negative RBCs.) A blood typing involves two steps. The first step, also known as forward (cell) typing, involves mixing patient RBCs with serum containing antibodies against A and B antigens. The RhD antigen is tested in the same manner. The second step, also known as reverse (serum) typing, mixes patient plasma with type A and B RBCs.

The "screen" component of a T&S determines if the patient has formed alloantibodies other than those suggested by their ABO blood typing. The screen, also known as an indirect antiglobulin or indirect Coombs test, is aimed at detecting common, clinically significant RBC alloantibodies that are associated with hemolysis. These include, among others, anti-D, -E, -K, and Fy^a [5]. The antibody screen typically involves testing the patient's plasma against a reagent panel of RBCs (type O) with known antigen specificities [6]. The US FDA requires that antigen reagent panels include the ability to test for at least 18 alloantibodies, although many more are known to exist and may be associated with extravascular or delayed hemolysis [7]. Umbilical cord or neonatal blood may react differently to standardized testing, compared to adult blood samples. Furthermore, certain autoimmune diseases (e.g., Raynaud's), viral infections, transplant history, and medications, such as intravenous or Rh-immunoglobulin or daratumumab, may produce false-positive antibody screen results, prolonging the antibody screening process by several hours or even days [7]. For these reasons, the importance of a timely pre-procedure T&S performed before the day of surgery cannot be overstated. Furthermore, if the patient has no prior blood bank history, the presence of a second, separately collected, "confirmatory" sample for testing should also be ensured.

When preparing blood to be "held" for a patient, a crossmatch is performed to identify available blood units that are compatible with the patient's blood. This can be done either through serologic testing, in which the donor RBCs are physically mixed with the patient serum and observed for hemolysis, or through a much more efficient process known as computer (or, "electronic") crossmatch [8, 9]. A computer crossmatch involves matching recipient blood with fully pretested ABO-and Rh-compatible donor blood through an electronic system. In many protocols, an electronic match is employed in patients that have a 90-day history that is *negative* for pregnancy or transfusion, a history of intravenous (IV) drug abuse, or a history for RBC alloantibodies. The computer crossmatch process also requires a record of two matching ABO-and Rh-type results [8, 9]. The first ABO-and Rh-determination must come from a current blood sample and the second determination by one of the following methods:

1. Comparison with previous records that the blood bank accepts.
2. Testing a second sample collected at a time different from the first sample, including a new verification of patient identification.
3. Retesting the same sample if patient identification was initially verified using a validated electronic identification (ID) system.

Extensive serologic crossmatching (i.e., actual mixing of recipient serum with donor RBCs) was used in the past for all patients. A "positive" result is visualized agglutination or cloudiness in the admixture. It is a time- and resource-consuming procedure; however, serologic testing may reduce the risk of an acute hemolytic transfusion reaction because it ensures the detection of low-incidence recipient alloantibodies reactive to antigens that may not be present on reagent panel screening RBCs [10]. Today, with improvements in the antibody screening techniques using reagent panel cells, outcomes following a negative antibody screen are rarely enhanced through additional serologic crossmatch testing [6, 11, 12]. Serologic crossmatching, therefore, is most useful for patients with a history of or currently positive antibody screen to confirm donor unit is correctly phenotyped and as a double check of full compatibility prior to transfusion [10].

Pretransfusion screening for infants is more nuanced than it is in adults, primarily because of immunologic immaturity and placental transfer of antibodies. Alloimmunization in infants is rare, particularly in premature infants and neonates, and this has been well-documented in a number of studies [13–15]. In the first few months of life, maternal antibodies and antigens are present in the newborn's circulation until passively cleared between 4 and 6 months. If an antibody screen is positive, those antibodies are likely maternal in origin; therefore, maternal blood should accompany infant blood in pretransfusion testing for the first few months of life [16].

A child who is old enough to have cleared maternal antibodies, between 4 and 6 months of age, and has never had a previous blood transfusion is unlikely to have developed clinically significant atypical RBC alloantibodies [14, 17]. The rate of alloimmunization or "unexpected antibodies" in adults reported in prior studies is 1% to as high as 10% in individuals who have received multiple transfusions [6]. Other patient populations with higher rates of unexpected antibodies include those with sickle cell disease and those who have undergone cardiac or other major surgeries, multiple transfusions, exchange transfusion, or massive transfusion [18]. If these exposures occurred before the maturation of an infant's immune system (i.e., before 4–6 months of age), it is conceivable that the risk of alloimmunization would be mitigated by the lack of immune response. However, pretransfusion testing is still required in these patients.

Some institutions may use maternal blood in lieu of neonatal blood for crossmatching to help prevent phlebotomy blood losses that may result in iatrogenic anemia. Additionally, if maternal or placental blood is not available for antibody screening, type O, Rh-negative RBC's will be issued until the infant blood type can be confirmed [19]. This latter practice is common in pediatric cardiac surgery centers that perform surgery on affected newborns from other hospitals; the maternal blood samples are often unavailable before the infant goes to the operating room. Unfortunately, this practice can lead to significant overutilization of a community's type O, Rh-negative RBC blood supply. In a recent study of 78 newborns ≥35 weeks gestation, placental blood samples were tested for ABO and Rhesus type, antibodies, and direct antiglobulin (DAT) [20]. Results indicated a high degree of concordance with heel stick samples, suggesting that blood of placenta or heel stick origin may be used for pretransfusion testing in neonates when type O, Rh-negative RBC blood is scarce.

In general, pretransfusion testing can be completed up to 45 days in advance if the patient has not been pregnant or transfused in the preceding 90 days. Some blood banks have shorter pretesting interval cutoffs (e.g., 7 or 30 days). If the patient has been transfused or is pregnant within those preceding 90 days, testing is valid for only 72 h, although there is controversy over whether an even shorter window would be safer from the standpoint of preventing acute or delayed hemolytic transfusion reactions in patients who were very recently transfused [21, 22]. A history of IV drug use may also trigger the 72-h restriction, as well.

An exception is made for neonates, since they do not have the immunologic maturity to produce new antibodies until 4–6 months of age [16]. This means that even if they had previously been transfused, they would be unable to develop new antibodies in response to those transfusions. Therefore, their initial pretransfusion tests do not need to be repeated until after they are 4 months old, even if they were transfused in the interim. If the initial type and screen is positive for antibodies, the recommended strategy is to screen every 7 days to determine when the maternal antibodies have cleared [16]. Some blood banks may require more restrictive pretransfusion testing requirements in young infants than those mentioned above.

3.2.3 Patient Verification

The pathway to transfusion contains multiple steps, each of which is a potential source of patient harm. The critical safety steps are outlined below (Fig. 3.1) [24]:

A transfusion safety checklist, based on years of cumulative hemovigilance data from the United Kingdom Serious Hazards of Transfusion (SHOT) registry, highlights the importance of proper bedside specimen labeling. All specimen labels should be printed at bedside, and specimens should be labeled and matched to the patient's ID band at bedside with patient participation [25]. A problem particular to busy operating rooms and other critical care areas is that old labels belonging to prior patients are often left in the work area and are then applied to the current operative patient's specimens. Thus, dual verification using two providers, a wristband barcode, or a conscious patient who can identify herself is as a top safety priority. Verification for infants and nonverbal patients is discussed in Chap. 19, entitled, "Patient Verification".

Patient verification using electronic barcode scanning at the bedside is considered a safer option for correct patient identification and prevention of transfusion to the wrong patient. Barcode scanning has been shown to reduce the rate of wrong-blood-in-tube (WBIT) from 1:3000 to 1:15,000 transfusions [5]. WBIT events occur when the correct patient's blood tube is stamped with another patient's identification label, or vice versa. However, the barcode scanning process is not perfect, and studies have found it vulnerable to the same human error (or negligence) as other patient identification techniques. In one multicenter study, 43 out of 331 reported WBIT errors were associated with incorrect or negligent use of an available electronic verification system [26, 27]. In a recent review of over 6000 blood samples, only one-third were scanned for both patient and specimen as required per protocol [28]. Strict adherence to patient identification protocol and procedural redundancy are critical to avoid fatal hemolysis secondary to ABO-incompatibility, particularly in the case of nonverbal children, anesthetized patients, and unconscious patients who are unable to identify themselves.

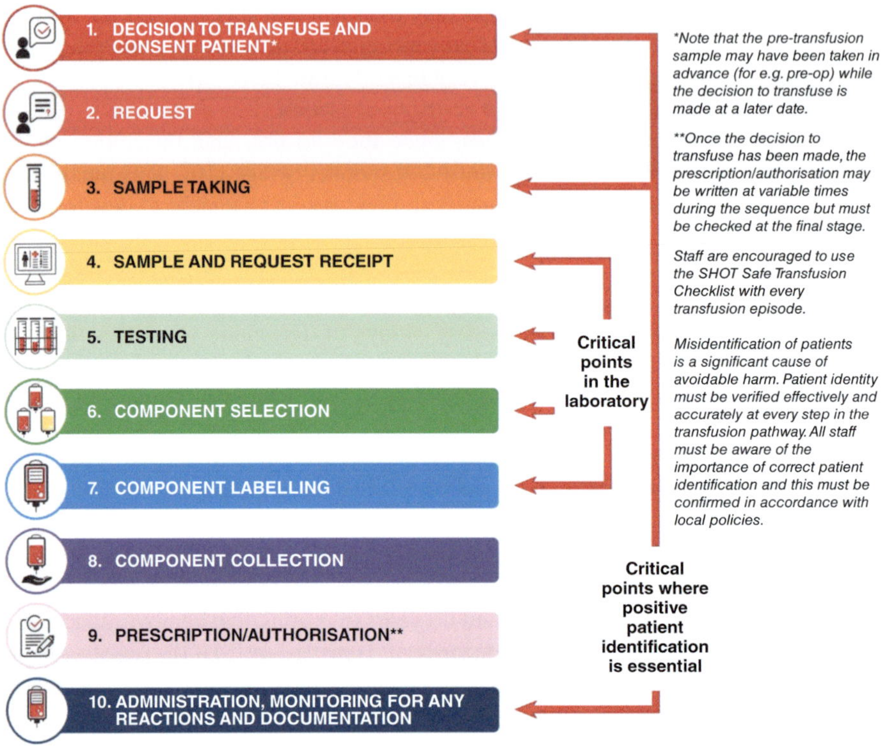

Fig. 3.1 Ten steps in transfusion safety. (Reprinted with permission from S. Narayan [23])

WBIT errors comprised the majority of reported "near miss" events in the 2020 SHOT annual report (n = 1130), of which 44 occurred in children [25]. In that report, the blood type of approximately one-half of the near miss patients was found to be incompatible with the intended transfusion, creating the potential for fatal hemolysis. Because most WBIT events occur at the point of care (although mislabeling also occurs inside the blood bank where multiple specimens may be processed simultaneously), both the AABB and SHOT recommend that all patients actively participate in their own identification before a pretransfusion sample is drawn and that the correct patient label on the blood tube is verified before leaving the patient's bedside [5, 29]. In the case of nonverbal or unconscious patients, this involves asking a parent, guardian, or another licensed provider to double check that the patient's identification (ID) band corresponds with the patient label. All facilities that are licensed to perform blood transfusion have specific policies outlining the pretransfusion patient verification process.

3.2.4 The Maximum Surgical Blood Order Schedule (MSBOS)

The Maximum Surgical Blood Ordering Schedule (MSBOS) is a data-driven predictor of transfusions, based on historical data from operative and anesthesia records. An MSBOS is institution-specific and can objectively guide physician ordering practices on appropriate blood product quantities to be requested for pending procedures [30]. The MSBOS can also provide guidance on the necessity of preoperative pre-transfusion testing, based on surgeon- or procedure-associated transfusion rates, in order to prevent a testing delay on the day of surgery. Patients with a >5% probability of transfusion, determined by historical data on the scheduled procedure and/or surgeon, are considered to be at sufficient risk for an intraoperative transfusion; pretransfusion testing should be completed no later than the day before surgery [31].

Because not all procedures require a T&S, a MSBOS can also function to reduce arbitrary blood tests that may lead to iatrogenic anemia. Unnecessary pretransfusion testing has been shown to be further reduced, while maintaining sensitivity, through artificial intelligence (AI) and machine learning algorithms that include patient-specific factors [32]. In one multicenter study, variables predicting appropriate pretransfusion testing included the patient's preoperative hemoglobin, age, and coagulation status [32].

An open cranial vault remodeling surgery (OCVRS) requires the surgeon to retract the majority of the scalp off of the cranium followed by large osteotomies. This typically results in significant blood loss. In a review of the Pediatric Craniofacial Surgery Perioperative Registry, 95% of children less than or equal to 24 months and 79% of children older than 24 months received at least one transfusion [33]. Most of these transfusions occurred intraoperatively. The anesthesiologist must communicate with the surgical team during the pre-incision "time-out" procedure whether crossmatched blood is immediately available or whether there will be a delay in the preparation of blood products before incision. Ideally, there is a debrief to discuss the factors contributing to blood loss. When blood is not available in a high blood loss procedure, particularly when the patient is an infant or small, the blood bank may have to release valuable, universal donor blood products. In the worst case scenario, significant patient morbidity or death may result from a delayed response to hemorrhage, including coagulopathy and adverse events related to rapid blood transfusion (e.g., hypotension and hyperkalemia) [25, 34].

3.2.5 Active Bleeding in the Face of Incomplete Pretransfusion Testing

Pretransfusion testing or "turnaround" times vary between institutions. Under ideal conditions, ABO and Rh-D typing takes approximately 15 min. Screening for atypical or unexpected alloantibodies will add an additional 30 min, translating into approximately 45 min total needed for a T&S. Completing a crossmatch will add 15 more minutes, if it is a computerized crossmatch (1 hour total), and at least an additional hour, if a serologic crossmatch is required (>2 h total) [6]. These times reflect ideal conditions with dedicated staffing, but at certain times of day, obtaining T&S results may take longer due to other staff demands. Certain patient populations, including chronically transfused sickle cell patients, may be highly alloimmunized. In those cases, the blood bank may have to seek outside sources of rare blood types, including distant blood banks or the American Rare Donor Program [35, 36]. This process can take many hours to days, jeopardizing the timely procurement of a reliable blood supply for a high blood loss surgery. For this reason, a preoperative T&S should always be performed at least 1 day before any high blood loss procedure.

In an emergency when there is no pretransfusion testing available for an infant, type O Rh-negative RBC's and type AB or type A Rh-negative plasma are typically released for administration. Although beyond the scope of this discussion, type A plasma has demonstrated relative safety in massively transfused adult trauma patients despite the fact that it may contain anti-A and -AB antibodies [37]. This is the same blood that is typically provided for all patients requiring blood emergently when recipient blood type is unknown or when there is no pretransfusion testing.

Infants who are 4–6 months old, with a current T&S, and have not had a crossmatch order completed can receive ABO- and Rh-compatible blood that has not yet been crossmatched. Thereafter, all distributed, emergency release blood is crossmatched as soon as possible following release to the operating room. Administration of compatible blood using this process also preserves emergency units of type O Rh-negative RBCs and type AB Rh-negative plasma for other critically ill patients. It is important to understand that "compatibility" does not necessarily mean that the patient and the donor blood types are identical in phenotype. Table 3.1 illustrates "compatible" blood products for a particular patient blood type.

ABO *compatibility* is required for RBC's, plasma, and cryoprecipitate. Ideally, platelets are ABO compatible or identical, the latter being most desirable in infants; "incompatible" platelets may be distributed in times of inventory shortage. A crossmatch is only required for RBCs [5, 6].

Proceeding to the operating room without the necessary quantity of blood available will be based on the acuity of a case, as assessed by anesthesiologist and

Table 3.1 Blood compatibility. Type O, RhD-negative RBCs and type AB plasma are "universal donor" product

Patient blood type	Compatible RBC type	Compatible plasma and cryoprecipitate type[a]
A	A, O	A, AB
B	B, O	B, AB
O	O	AB, A, B, O
AB	AB, A, B, O	AB
RhD positive	RhD positive or negative	RhD positive or negative
RhD negative	RhD negative[b]	RhD positive or negative

[a]Type A donor plasma may be substituted for Type AB in massively transfused patients with unknown blood type [37]

[b]Only required in females of childbearing age, or if patient is already alloimmunized to RhD

surgeon. An elective, high blood loss case can proceed in several ways in the absence of pretransfusion testing. One option is to wait to proceed to the operating room until the required blood is available. This means the patient completes the required pretransfusion testing and awaits results while in preoperative holding. Another option is proceeding to the OR, inducing general anesthesia, obtaining the appropriate pretransfusion samples, and requesting the minimum blood products. This option hinges on the fact that the flow of the surgical case is predictable and requires tight collaboration and communication to meet the expectation that the most surgically invasive components of the operation will not take place until the minimum blood products are readily available.

There is limited evidence on the safety of emergency release of uncrossmatched blood in children during the perioperative period. A study by Bahr et al. showed no clear evidence of transfusion reactions in a retrospective review of transfusions with emergency released blood products in young infants [38]. Leeper et al. demonstrated the early safety of low antibody titer group O whole blood (LTOWB, which contains anti-A and -B antibodies) in a sample of 18 traumatized civilian children [39]. The reported incidence of alloimmunization to non-ABO RBC antigens following receipt of emergency release type O RBCs ranges from 0% to over 10%; however, this data is based on relatively small studies in complex patient populations with likely survival bias [40]. Goodell et al. reported 1 hemolytic transfusion reaction in over 1000 transfusions in emergency room patients [41]. In general, the risk of acute intravascular hemolysis secondary to emergency release, universal donor blood products is currently considered to be minimal to none [42]. On the other hand, the incidence of *delayed* hemolysis following receipt of emergency release blood, which can be indolent, difficult to diagnose, and sometimes fatal, is unknown. In its 2019 annual summary, the US FDA cited an increase in the number of hemolytic, non-ABO-related deaths compared to prior years: 11 deaths were secondary to non-ABO hemolytic transfusion reactions (compared to 4 ABO-related fatal reactions), two of which were traceable to emergency release blood products [29]. Another controversy regarding the administration of uncrossmatched emergency blood products and alloimmunization is the use of Rhesus-D positive blood products in Rhesus-D antigen patients. Rh-D alloimmunization rates in Rh-negative patients may be as high as 35% in hospitalized patients who receive at least 1 unit of Rh-positive RBCs [43]. This may increase the risk of hemolytic disease in the fetus of future pregnancies and, uncommonly, acute or delayed hemolysis in the recipient. McCoy et al. found no difference in hemolysis labs at 3 days posttransfusion in a small cohort of adult, Rh-negative trauma patients who received Rh-positive blood [44]. The rate of anti-RhD formation in traumatized children is unknown, but the overall rate was approximately 35% in one study of 335 RhD-negative adult patients, and 7.8% in another [45, 46]. The alloimmunization rate is known to increase with age, approximating 0% in neonates, increasing to over 1.8% in adolescents [15]. In a recent survey of American trauma centers, more than 90% report distributing only Rh-negative blood for females under 18 years of age, and approximately one-half do so for males ≤18 [47].

3.3 Summary of Key Learning Points

3.3.1 What Is the Basis of Testing Requirements for a Blood Transfusion?

In the USA, pretransfusion testing is standardized and is a requirement for hospital accreditation, as directed by the US FDA, the AABB, and the CAP. The basis for this regulation is to promote patient transfusion safety, as well as the rational use of a precious and potentially life-saving resource, the blood supply.

3.3.2 Why Must a T&S and a Crossmatch Be Performed Before the Blood Bank Releases Blood to the Operating Room?

Patient blood management (PBM) is a "patient-centered, systematic, evidence-based approach to improve patient outcomes by managing and preserving a patient's own blood, while promoting patient safety and empowerment" [48]. In this case, the patient is an anemic, nonverbal child going into an elective high blood loss surgery, with incomplete pretransfusion testing to enable timely blood product preparation. Assuming that this child has not been previously transfused, it is unlikely that this patient will have alloantibodies necessitating prolonged T&S and crossmatch testing. However, this all-too-common clinical presentation—and the pressure to proceed with a high blood loss surgery despite the fact that crossmatched blood is not immediately available—sets the stage for escalation of care in the event the patient does have an unexpected alloantibody. Furthermore, a special consideration in this population is whether the patient has syndromic craniosynostosis, in whom early intraoperative transfusion within the first 30 min of surgery has been shown to be associated with improved postoperative outcomes and a higher hemoglobin nadir [49]. To obtain this benefit, all pretransfusion testing would need to be performed prior to arrival in the operating room. A blood sample obtained within 45 days of surgery could have been used to prepare blood products for this patient. In this case, the risk of proceeding without proper pretransfusion testing, which can lead to unpredictable wait times for product availability and overuse of universal donor blood, outweighs a benefit based on concerns over patient comfort or operating schedule convenience. In addition, this patient is anemic, a demonstrated risk factor for transfusion in patients undergoing OCVRS [50].

3.3.3 Why Is Patient Verification a Crucial Step in Pretransfusion Process?

Strict adherence to patient identification protocol and procedural redundancy are critical to avoid fatal hemolysis secondary to ABO-incompatibility, particularly in the case of nonverbal children, anesthetized patients, and unconscious patients who are unable to identify themselves. Because most WBIT events occur at the point of care, both the AABB and SHOT recommend that all patients actively participate in their own identification before a pretransfusion sample is drawn (when feasible) and that the correct specimen label is verified before leaving the patient's bedside. This situation not only places a great deal of production pressure on the blood bank—which is likely processing many other blood product orders at the same time this patient's specimen becomes available—but it also distracts the anesthesiologist with a demand for two separate blood draws (and proper patient identification) and specimen labeling early in a complex surgical case. Adding to the potential chaos of the operating room atmosphere is the potential for a rushed receipt of the prepared blood products, again, at a time when the operating room personnel and the anesthesiologist are predictably distracted. Dual verification using a second person or a standardized, validated barcode scanning procedure at the point of care is always necessary to prevent a WBIT or hemolytic transfusion reaction.

3.3.4 What Is a "Maximum Surgical Blood Order Schedule" (MSBOS) and What Are Its Advantages?

Recent evidence suggests that over three-quarters of OCVRS patients require a perioperative transfusion [33]. Reference to the hospital's data driven MSBOS when this child was scheduled for surgery would have indicated the need for full pretransfusion testing and immediate blood availability.

3.3.5 What Blood Is Released for Emergency Transfusion in an Infant with Incomplete Pretransfusion Testing?

Emergency release of universal donor blood from the blood bank for an *elective* surgery is an all-too-common event. ABO- and Rh-compatible, uncrossmatched blood can often be released to a patient with suspected (though not confirmed) negative antibody screen within 15 min. A best practice advisory of the American College of Surgeons (ACS) calls for availability of balanced ratio blood product for exsanguinating patients within 15 min [51]. The surgical field must be closely monitored because blood loss in OCVRS cases is difficult to assess. Falling behind on blood replacement, particularly in infants, can lead to a fatal outcome [52, 53]. It is usually less likely for patients to be transfused early in the course of surgery, and the data suggests that the overall likelihood of a hemolytic transfusion reaction as a result of having unexpected, atypical antibodies is minimal in this population. However, the benevolence of the blood bank must be counterbalanced by the unnecessary utilization of precious community resources, specifically, the critical and persistent global shortage of ABO- and Rh-compatible "universal donor" blood [54].

Key Points

- The regulations for pretransfusion testing are based in part on concerns for patient safety.

- In the interest of patient safety as well as preservation of the precious universal donor blood supply, full pretransfusion testing (e.g., a T&S and a crossmatch) should be performed before the blood bank releases blood products to the operating room.
- Patient verification a critical step in the pretransfusion process to prevent a potentially fatal hemolytic transfusion reaction.
- The Maximum Surgical Blood Order Schedule (MSBOS) is an institution specific, data-driven prediction tool of pretransfusion testing and transfusion requirements.
- Alloimmunization in infants is a rare occurrence. Patient populations with higher rates of unexpected antibodies include those with sickle cell disease, and those who have undergone cardiac or other major surgeries, multiple transfusions, exchange transfusion, or massive transfusion. Pretransfusion testing is required in these infants.
- Emergency release of universal donor blood for an elective, high blood loss surgical procedure because pretransfusion testing was not performed is inappropriate blood utilization.

References

1. Standards for blood banks and transfusion services. 32nd edition. Bethesda: AABB Press; 2020.
2. Title 21. Food and drugs subchapter F: biologics. Code of Federal Regulations: Food and Drug Administration; 2001. https://www.ecfr.gov/current/title-21/chapter-I/subchapter-F. Accessed 25 May 2023.
3. Milkins C, Berryman J, Cantwell C, Elliott C, Haggas R, Jones J, et al. Guidelines for pretransfusion compatibility procedures in blood transfusion laboratories. British Committee for Standards in Haematology. Transfus Med. 2013;23(1):3–35.
4. Blood safety and availability. World Health Organization (WHO) 2023. https://www.who.int/news-room/fact-sheets/detail/blood-safety-and-availability. Accessed 17 Feb 2023.
5. Alquist C, Harm SK. Transfusion service related activities. In: Cohn C, Delaney M, Johnson ST, Katz LM, editors. Technical manual. 20th ed. Bethesda: AABB; 2020. p. 504.
6. Yazer MH. The blood bank "black box" debunked: pretransfusion testing explained. CMAJ. 2006;174(1):29–32.
7. Ev LS, Bailey DJ. Identification of antibodies to red cell antigens. Chapter 13. In: In: Cohn CS, Delaney M, Johnson ST, Katz LM. 20th edition Technical Manual. Bethesda: AABB. 2020. p. 389–425.
8. Hendrickson JE, Tormey CA. Red blood cell antibodies in hematology/oncology patients: interpretation of immunohematologic tests and clinical significance of detected antibodies. Hematol Oncol Clin North Am. 2016;30(3):635–51.
9. Butch SH, Judd WJ, Steiner EA, Stoe M, Oberman HA. Electronic verification of donor-recipient compatibility: the computer crossmatch. Transfusion. 1994;34(2):105–9.
10. Wallis JP. Is it time to give up the crossmatch? J Clin Pathol. 2000;53(9):673–5.
11. Tormey CA, Hendrickson JE. Transfusion-related red blood cell alloantibodies: induction and consequences. Blood. 2019;133(17):1821–30.
12. Alquist CR, Helander L. Transfusion blood bank (recipient) testing. Clin Lab Med. 2021;41(4):599–610.

13. Strauss RG, Cordle DG, Quijana J, Goeken NE. Comparing alloimmunization in preterm infants after transfusion of fresh unmodified versus stored leukocyte-reduced red blood cells. J Pediatr Hematol Oncol. 1999;21(3):224–30.
14. Türkmen T, Qiu D, Cooper N, Sachs UJ, Wößmann W, Schranz D, et al. Red blood cell alloimmunization in neonates and children up to 3 years of age. Transfusion. 2017;57(11):2720–6.
15. Tamai Y, Ohto H, Takahashi H, Kitazawa J, Consortium PRA. Transfusion-related alloimmunization to red blood cell antigens in Japanese pediatric recipients. Transfus Med Rev. 2021;35(1):29–36.
16. Wong ECCP, RC. Neonatal and pediatric transfusion practice. In: Cohn CDM, Johnson S, Katz L, editors. AABB Technical manual. 20th ed. Bethesda: AABB; 2020.
17. Floss AM, Strauss RG, Goeken N, Knox L. Multiple transfusion fail to provoke antibodies against blood cell antigens in human infants. Transfusion. 1986;26(5):419–22.
18. Rankin A, Darbari D, Campbell A, Webb J, Mo YD, Jacquot C, et al. Screening for new red blood cell alloantibodies after transfusion in patients with sickle cell disease. Transfusion. 2021;61(8):2255–64.
19. Barcelona SL, Thompson AA, Coté CJ. Intraoperative pediatric blood transfusion therapy: a review of common issues. Part II: transfusion therapy, special considerations, and reduction of allogenic blood transfusions. Paediatr Anaesth. 2005;15(10):814–30.
20. Alissa R, Williams PD, Baker EL, Hipp JA, Saremian J, Aysola AE. Suitability of placental blood samples of newborns for pre-transfusion testing. Front Pediatr. 2021;9:661321.
21. Boisen ML, Collins RA, Yazer MH, Waters JH. Pretransfusion testing and transfusion of uncrossmatched erythrocytes. Anesthesiology. 2015;122(1):191–5.
22. Shulman IA, Nelson JM, Nakayama R. When should antibody screening tests be done for recently transfused patients? Transfusion. 1990;30(1):39–41.
23. Narayan S (ed) D Poles et al. on behalf of the Serious Hazards of Transfusion (SHOT) Steering Group. The 2021 Annual SHOT Report. 2022
24. Serious Hazards of Transfusion (SHOT). Safe transfusion practice: fig. 4.1. Transfusion Checklist 2020. https://www.shotuk.org/wp-content/uploads/myimages/SHOT-REPORT-2020.pdf. Accessed 23 April 2022.
25. Serious Hazards of Transfusion and Medicines and Healthcare Products Regulatory Agency (SHOT).. https://www.shotuk.org/shot-reports/(2020). United Kingdom 2020. Accessed 25 May 2023.
26. Dunbar NM, Kaufman RM, WBIT Study Investigators TeBEfSTBC. Factors associated with wrong blood in tube errors: an international case series—the BEST collaborative study. Transfusion. 2022;62(1):44–50.
27. Murphy MF, Jayne Addison J, Poles D, Dhiman P, Bolton-Maggs P. Electronic identification systems reduce the number of wrong components transfused. Transfusion. 2019;59(12):3601–7.
28. Al-Eshaq DH, Bradley RT, McBride ERA, Ford JC. Patient and specimen identification in a tertiary care pediatric hospital: barcodes do not scan themselves. Transfusion. 2023;63:1310.
29. US FDA. Fatalities Reported to the FDA Following Blood Collection and Transfusion Annual Summary for FY2019. 2020.. https://www.fda.gov/media/147628/download#:~:text=During%20FY2019%2C%20we%20received%20a, were%20potentially%20associated%20with%20donation. Accessed 6 Sept 2022.
30. Woodrum CL, Wisniewski M, Triulzi DJ, Waters JH, Alarcon LH, Yazer MH. The effects of a data driven maximum surgical blood ordering schedule on preoperative blood ordering practices. Hematology. 2017;22(9):571–7.
31. Frank SM, Oleyar MJ, Ness PM, Tobian AA. Reducing unnecessary preoperative blood orders and costs by implementing an updated institution-specific maximum surgical blood order schedule and a remote electronic blood release system. Anesthesiology. 2014;121(3):501–9.
32. Lou SS, Liu H, Lu C, Wildes TS, Hall BL, Kannampallil T. Personalized surgical transfusion risk prediction using machine learning to guide preoperative type and screen orders. Anesthesiology. 2022;137(1):55–66.

33. Stricker PA, Shaw TL, Desouza DG, Hernandez SV, Bartlett SP, Friedman DF, et al. Blood loss, replacement, and associated morbidity in infants and children undergoing craniofacial surgery. Paediatr Anaesth. 2010;20(2):150–9.
34. Bhananker SM, Ramamoorthy C, Geiduschek JM, Posner KL, Domino KB, Haberkern CM, et al. Anesthesia-related cardiac arrest in children: update from the pediatric perioperative cardiac arrest registry. Anesth Analg. 2007;105(2):344–50.
35. Flickinger C. REGGI and the American rare donor program. Transfus Med Hemother. 2014;41(5):342–5.
36. Laureano M, Clarke G, Yan MTS. How do I provide rare red cells to patients? Transfusion. 2023;63(4):670–8.
37. Dunbar NM, Yazer MH. Investigators BEfSTBCatSS. Safety of the use of group a plasma in trauma: the STAT study. Transfusion. 2017;57(8):1879–84.
38. Bahr TM, DuPont TL, Christensen TR, Rees T, O'Brien EA, Ilstrup SJ, et al. Evaluating emergency-release blood transfusion of newborn infants at the Intermountain Healthcare hospitals. Transfusion. 2019;59(10):3113–9.
39. Leeper CM, Yazer MH, Cladis FP, Saladino R, Triulzi DJ, Gaines BA. Use of uncrossmatched cold-stored whole blood in injured children with hemorrhagic shock. JAMA Pediatr. 2018;172(5):491–2.
40. Mulay SB, Jaben EA, Johnson P, Badjie K, Stubbs JR. Risks and adverse outcomes associated with emergency-release red blood cell transfusion. Transfusion. 2013;53(7):1416–20.
41. Goodell PP, Uhl L, Mohammed M, Powers AA. Risk of hemolytic transfusion reactions following emergency-release RBC transfusion. Am J Clin Pathol. 2010;134(2):202–6.
42. Yazer MH, Waters JH, Spinella PC. AABB (formerly known as the American Association of Blood Banks)/Trauma H, Oygenation Resuscitation Network (THOR) working party. Use of uncrossmatched erythrocytes in emergency bleeding situations. Anesthesiology. 2018;128(3):650–6.
43. Yazer MH, Freeman A, Harrold IM, Anto V, Neal MD, Triulzi DJ, et al. Injured recipients of low-titer group O whole blood have similar clinical outcomes compared to recipients of conventional component therapy: a single-center, retrospective study. Transfusion. 2021;61(6):1710–20.
44. McCoy CC, Montgomery K, Cotton ME, Meyer DE, Wade CE, Cotton BA. Can RH+ whole blood be safely used as an alternative to RH- product? An analysis of efforts to improve the sustainability of a hospital's low titer group O whole blood program. J Trauma Acute Care Surg. 2021;91(4):627–33.
45. Yazer MH, Triulzi DJ, Sperry JL, Seheult JN. Rate of RhD-alloimmunization after the transfusion of multiple RhD-positive primary red blood cell-containing products. Transfusion. 2021;61(Suppl 1):S150–S8.
46. Raval JS, Madden KM, Neal MD, Moore SA. Anti-D alloimmunization in Rh(D) negative adults with severe traumatic injury. Transfusion. 2021;61(Suppl 1):S144–S9.
47. Yazer MH, Dunbar NM, Delaney M, Collaborative BEfST. Survey of the RhD selection and issuing practices for uncrossmatched blood products at pediatric trauma hospitals in the United States: the BEST collaborative study. Transfusion. 2021;61(12):3328–34.
48. Shander A, Hardy JF, Ozawa S, Farmer SL, Hofmann A, Frank SM, et al. A global definition of patient blood management. Anesth Analg. 2022;135(3):476–88.
49. Kurnik NM, Bristol R, Maneri C, Singhal R, Singh DJ. Open craniosynostosis surgery: effect of early intraoperative blood transfusion on postoperative course. J Craniofac Surg. 2017;28(5):e505–e10.
50. Fernandez PG, Taicher BM, Goobie SM, Gangadharan M, Homi HM, Kugler JA, et al. Predictors of transfusion outcomes in pediatric complex cranial vault reconstruction: a multicentre observational study from the Pediatric Craniofacial Collaborative Group. Can J Anaesth. 2019;66(5):512–26.
51. Meyer DE, Vincent LE, Fox EE, O'Keeffe T, Inaba K, Bulger E, et al. Every minute counts: time to delivery of initial massive transfusion cooler and its impact on mortality. J Trauma Acute Care Surg. 2017;83(1):19–24.

52. Ramamoorthy C, Haberkern CM, Bhananker SM, Domino KB, Posner KL, Campos JS, et al. Anesthesia-related cardiac arrest in children with heart disease: data from the Pediatric Perioperative Cardiac Arrest (POCA) registry. Anesth Analg. 2010;110(5):1376–82.
53. Lee AC, Reduque LL, Luban NL, Ness PM, Anton B, Heitmiller ES. Transfusion-associated hyperkalemic cardiac arrest in pediatric patients receiving massive transfusion. Transfusion. 2014;54(1):244–54.
54. BloodBankGuy Podcast. 096CE: navigating blood shortages with Claudia Cohn. 2022.. https://www.bbguy.org/2022/03/30/096/. Accessed 2 June 2023.

Preoperative Anemia

4

Alyssa Brzenski, Brian Frugoni, Claire Soria, and Susanna Shaw

4.1 Case Scenario

A 2-year-old, ex-28-week premature child presents for elective open resection of a large liver cyst. The cyst was found incidentally when the patient's mother reported the patient had decreased appetite and, on routine checkup, the pediatrician palpated an enlarged liver on physical exam. The patient underwent an abdominal ultrasound and subsequent CT abdomen, which revealed a large mass encircling the portal vein, suspected to be a cyst. The patient has otherwise been asymptomatic, growing well, and meeting all developmental milestones.

One week prior to surgery, the patient is noted to have a hemoglobin (Hgb) of 8.6 g/dL.

Key Learning Objectives

- What Hgb value indicates anemia in children?
- Does perioperative anemia influence postoperative morbidity and mortality in pediatric patients?
- What is an acceptable, minimum preoperative Hgb value for a child?
- What are the most common types of anemia in the different pediatric age groups?
- What preoperative testing should be performed if a child is anemic prior to a blood loss surgery?
- What is a suggested approach to the preoperative management of the anemic child?

A. Brzenski (✉) · B. Frugoni · C. Soria · S. Shaw
University of California San Diego School of Medicine, San Diego, CA, USA
e-mail: abrzenski@health.ucsd.edu; bfrugoni@health.ucsd.edu; cssoria@health.ucsd.edu; s1shaw@health.ucsd.edu

N. J. Klein (ed.), *Perioperative Pediatric Patient Blood Management and Transfusion Safety*, https://doi.org/10.1007/978-3-031-81666-6_4

4.2 General

Anemia is a common health condition that affects a large portion of pediatric surgery patients [1]. Historically, perioperative anemia management has relied heavily on the administration of blood transfusions based on laboratory values [2, 3]. However, blood transfusions carry risks and community supplies of allogenic blood are tenuous on a global scale [4, 5]. Patient blood management (PBM) shifts the focus away from reactively transfusing red blood cells (RBCs) and toward proactively optimizing the individual patient factors. There are three essential measures to achieve this goal [6]:

- Optimizing native hematologic status, including red cells and coagulation factors.
- Reducing blood loss.
- Optimizing tolerance of anemia.

Identifying, evaluating, and treating the underlying cause of anemia achieves the first tenet of PBM by optimizing an individual patient's red cell mass. Ideal optimization is heavily dependent on an individual patient's ability to tolerate anemia. Preoperative planning also entails consideration of patient and procedure-specific factors that influence perioperative blood loss. The following discussion will address preoperative anemia evaluation, anemia tolerance, and Hgb optimization necessary to improve perioperative outcomes in anemic children.

4.2.1 What Hgb Value Indicates Anemia in Children?

Establishing normal hematologic values in children is challenging. A broad representation requires obtaining potentially unnecessary blood samples in healthy infants and children for study purposes. As a result, historical and current data often lack adequate sampling to be truly representative [7].

Multiple groups have attempted to determine modern reference ranges for Hgb and hematocrit (Hct) in children. Fulgoni et al. mined data from the National Health and Nutrition Examination Survey (NHANES), a large population-based, cross-sectional survey on Americans' health and dietary status conducted by the United States (US) Centers for Disease Control and Prevention (CDC) [8]. Their findings support a lower limit "normal" Hgb of 11 g/dL for both males and females aged 12–35 months. Other population-based studies in noninfants found a normal Hgb range of 10–11 g/dL, with lower levels in children <4 years [7, 9, 10].

Neonates and premature infants are the groups with the least available data to validate normal Hgb reference ranges. The Intermountain Health Care study has provided the largest group of values to date [11, 12]. A convenience cohort from

Table 4.1 Normal RBC reference ranges for premature neonates and infants less than 3 months

Age	Hemoglobin (g/dL)	Hematocrit (%)	Mean corpuscular volume (Fl)	Red blood cell distribution (%)
Extremely preterm (<28 weeks)	8–17	40–47	80–125	
Very preterm (28–32 weeks)	9–21	47–50	90–122	
Moderate to late preterm (32–37 weeks)	9.8–23	50–53	90–118	
<4 days	12–23	37–56	93–118	15–20
4–7 days	10–22	36–56	86–118	15–19
8–14 days	9–21	32–53	82–118	14–17
14–90 days	8–15	26–45	80–110	13–16

Adapted from Christensen et al. [11]

nine clinical laboratories was gathered from 6632 samples taken from ex-premature infants 0–90 days old. Neonates were found to have relatively high Hgb values with wide reference ranges. Premature neonates had lower initial Hgb values compared to term neonates, with very premature neonates (born <28 weeks) having the lowest Hgb values. The results for infants less than 3 months are summarized in Table 4.1 [11].

Studies have described lower values for African Americans of all ages, suggesting a "normal" Hgb reference range 0.5–0.73 g/dL lower than Whites [13]. Many healthcare organizations are abandoning race-based protocols, arguing that these differences reflect health disparities related to social determinants and that all patients should be treated based on the same lower limit of normal [14]. The National Institutes of Health (NIH) reports that 12% of Hispanic toddlers are anemic, compared to 6% of their White and Black counterparts [15]. Based on data from the American College of Surgeons National Surgical Quality Improvement Program (ACS NSQIP) database for the years 2012–2019, children belonging to an underrepresented minority were more likely than White children to receive a blood transfusion for femur fracture surgery [16].

Lower- and middle-income countries are particularly affected with the burden of anemia. The World Health Organization (WHO) estimates that almost one-half of preschool children across the globe are anemic [17]. Data from North America indicates that the prevalence of anemia in patients presenting for noncardiac surgery is 24% in children >1 year and 21.7% in the neonatal surgical population [18, 19]. In a recent South African study, nearly 50% of the patients presenting for noncardiac surgery were anemic [20]. The median hemoglobin in this latter group was 10.2 g/dL.

Aggregate data from these studies suggest that normal Hgb levels vary based on age and sex. However, generalizations can be made among broad categories of age ranges. Notable differences between sexes become pronounced at approximately 14 years (Table 4.2).

Table 4.2 Red blood cell (RBC) normal values in children and adults

Age	Hemoglobin (g/dL)	Hematocrit (%)	Mean corpuscular volume (Fl)	RBC distribution (%)
90 days–2 years	10–14	25–41	68–90	11.5–20
2–5 years	11–14	28–40	74–90	11.5–18
6–12 years	11.5–15	30–44	70–90	11.5–20
12–18 years	11–17	34–45	74–94	11.5–16.5
Male adult	12–17	36–50	78–95	11.5–14
Female adult	11–15	34–45	75–95	11.5–18

Adapted from Wong [115]

4.2.2 Does Perioperative Anemia Influence Postoperative Morbidity and Mortality in Pediatric Patients?

There is a strong association between preoperative anemia and postoperative morbidity in adults undergoing noncardiac surgery [21, 22]. Recent studies in the pediatric surgical population have established similar findings. For example, a 2016 analysis of pediatric NSQIP data found that preoperative anemia was associated with a higher risk of in-hospital mortality for both non-transfused (0.43% anemic versus 0.10% nonanemic; $P < 0.001$) and transfused (1.45% anemia versus 0.40% nonanemic vs. $P < 0.001$) children [19]. The anemic children in this study were younger and had greater comorbidity, including hematologic or neurologic disease, immune disorders, and a need for mechanical ventilation. The same study group looked at neonatal NSQIP data. Thirty-two percent of neonates were anemic preoperatively, with an increased risk of in-hospital mortality after adjusting for other mortality-related factors when the preoperative Hct level was <40% (3.5%; 95% CI, 1.3–9.0%) compared to those with a Hct > 40% in the preoperative phase of care (1.3%; 95% CI, 0.4–4.1%) [18].

It is difficult to determine the effects of preoperative anemia on postoperative outcomes if anemia alone is analyzed. Because anemia is usually associated with underlying disease states, it is important to consider socioeconomic, environmental, and other factors when examining its perioperative effects [20]. In another analysis of NSQIP data, this time focusing on term infants, preoperative anemia did not impose increased perioperative risk [23]. Kedir et al. retrospectively examined over 2900 infants undergoing pyloromyotomy, a common and low-risk surgical procedure with minimal associated blood loss. Anemia was defined as ≤40% in infants 0–30 days old and ≤30% in infants >30 days old. The median age was 35 days; patients who were premature or had comorbidities were excluded from analysis. The investigators found that preoperative anemia conferred no increased risk of any complication in otherwise healthy, term infants, including postoperative mortality or readmission (adjusted OR 1.2; 95% CI, 0.8–1.7).

In contrast, other studies have found that preoperative anemia is independently associated with postoperative complications in patients undergoing noncardiac surgery [24]. For example, an observational South African study of 1094 children (of which 46.2% were anemic) found that 9.9% of patients experienced complications postoperatively, with patients who were anemic having an increased risk of all post-operative complications (OR of 1.99; 95% CI 1.28–3.10, $P = 0.002$) [20]. Anemic patients in this study also had an increased risk of intraoperative blood transfusion (OR 3.60, 95% CI 1.83–7.05, $P < 0.001$). In a database study of 36,335 adolescents undergoing spinal surgery, patients with preoperative anemia were twice as likely to have at least one in-hospital complication (OR 2.1; 95% CI, 1.5–2.94, $p < 0.0001$) [25].[1]

4.2.2.1 To Transfuse or to Not Transfuse?

If preoperative anemia is associated with an increased risk of postoperative complications, a question arises as to whether an RBC transfusion is indicated before surgery. Best practice in surgery and anesthesia includes adherence to the tenants of patient blood management (PBM), the first of which is optimizing the patient's RBC mass prior to surgery [6]. This includes evaluating the patient for treatable forms of anemia. The Choosing Wisely Campaign (Campaign), a task force and quality improvement program that functions in collaboration with leading medical societies, including the American Society of Pediatric Hematology/Oncology (ASPHO), found no evidence that a preoperative RBC transfusion is beneficial in patients with the most common type of anemia: iron deficiency (ID) [26]. The Campaign has identified hematologic-related practices in children that should be avoided because they are not supported by evidence or because they involve medical risk (Table 4.3).

The Campaign also emphasizes that transfusion does not appropriately treat ID anemia in the absence of hemodynamic instability or active bleeding. Furthermore, the iron from transfused RBCs is not immediately available for erythropoiesis and does not replete iron stores. Instead, an unnecessary RBC transfusion exposes patients to transfusion-related risk.

Intraoperative blood loss may lead to intraoperative RBC transfusion and must be closely monitored. Underappreciated or a delayed response to blood loss was identified in the Pediatric Perioperative Cardiac Arrest Registry (POCA) as the number-one identifiable cause of anesthesia-related cardiac arrest [27]. An

Table 4.3 Hematologic tests and treatments to question in children

Choosing Wisely Campaign 2019
Do not:
Treat iron deficiency in hemodynamically stable children with an RBC transfusion
Perform preoperative coagulation testing in healthy children with no personal or family history of a bleeding diathesis
Administer platelets to children >1 year old with hypoproliferative thrombocytopenia who have a platelet count >10 × $10^3/\mu L$ unless actively bleeding or an invasive procedure is anticipated
Perform thrombophilia testing for venous access-associated thrombosis if there is no family history of a clotting disorder

Adapted from O'Brien et al. [26]

[1] For further discussion on anemia outcomes, see the Chap. 17.

intraoperative blood transfusion is not without risks, particularly if given rapidly and in large volumes to small children who may face an additional burden of hyperkalemic arrest and volume overload [28, 29]. Data from a 2016 NSQIP study showed that anemic patients who received a blood transfusion intraoperatively had an increased mortality risk compared to anemic patients that were not transfused [19]. Of note, the NSQIP investigators considered that their study was unable to identify the indications for intraoperative transfusion, specifically, if RBCs were administered for active bleeding or otherwise. The investigators note that concomitant anemia, transfusion, and bleeding increases mortality and speculate that transfusion for anemia alone (without additional bleeding) may modify this mortality rate. In a 2016, retrospective review of over 3000 adult patients undergoing orthopedic surgery, long-term mortality risk was increased in nonanemic patients who received an intraoperative RBC transfusion (95% CI adjusted HR; 4.39, 2.14–8.98; $P < 0.001$), but it was not increased in severely anemic patients (Hgb < 9 g/dL) who were transfused (95% CI; 0.81, 0.24–2.73; $p = 0.73$). This finding suggests that administering an RBC transfusion for severe anemia may mitigate perioperative risk in some clinical situations [30]. However, the role of RBC transfusions on surgical outcomes when a patient has preoperative anemia is not entirely clear. In a retrospective review of over 4000 adults undergoing cardiac surgery, of which 30% were anemic beforehand, acute kidney injury (AKI) was directly associated with preoperative anemia but not transfusion [31]. The investigators concluded thru mediation analysis that the effect of an RBC transfusion in the presence of anemia depends on the outcome sought; in this study, prolonged hospital length of stay was directly attributed to anemia and was mitigated by RBC transfusion [31].

The anesthesiologist who participates in the care of children will encounter preoperative anemia and thus has some responsibility to initiate evaluation of all preoperative patients for modifiable disease. While the weight of the literature suggests an anemia diagnosis increases postoperatively morbidity and mortality, treatment with an RBC transfusion also contributes to postoperative complications and thus should be avoided unless a patient is hemodynamically unstable or actively bleeding. A question thus arises as to what an acceptable preoperative Hgb should be in a child going to surgery.

4.2.3 What Is an Acceptable Minimum Preoperative Hgb Level for a Child?

The optimal Hgb value in pediatric patients before an elective surgical procedure is unknown [32]. It is crucial to gauge whether oxygen delivery to the tissues can match required uptake at the tissues level when evaluating a patient's Hgb before surgery [33]. Assessment of an individual patient's ability to tolerate anemia, the blood loss history associated with a particular procedure, and the ability to assess ongoing blood loss must be considered when making a blood management decision in anemic patients.

4.2.3.1 Perioperative Anemia Tolerance

Most data addressing optimal preoperative Hgb levels comes from adult literature [34, 35]. Pediatric patients present unique considerations compared to adults. Studies examining pediatric anemia tolerance have not typically included the perioperative period but are generally extrapolated from pediatric intensive care unit (PICU) or neonatal intensive care unit (NICU) data. The TRIPICU study explored a liberal versus restrictive transfusion trigger in PICU patients (3 days to 14 years) [36]. There was no difference in outcomes between these two groups, suggesting that a restrictive transfusion trigger of 7.0 g/dL is safe in stable, critically ill pediatric patients. Premature neonates were not included in this study. The PINT and ETTNO studies explored liberal versus restrictive transfusion practices within the NICU [37, 38]. These studies demonstrated no difference in liberal versus restrictive transfusion practices on outcomes. Of note, the transfusion triggers in the PINT study differed by postnatal age and the need for baseline oxygen support. However, a post hoc analysis of the PINT study showed a difference in cognitive delay at 18–21 months corrected age favoring the liberal threshold group [39]. Longitudinal follow-up of longer-term neurologic outcomes, including cerebral palsy, cognitive delay by Bayley Scales of Infant Development- II Mental Development Index, and visual and hearing difficulties were determined via this later PINT study group [40]. An increased rate of cognitive delay was found in this study group when the Mental Development Index < 85 (1 standard deviation; SD) was used. No other neurologic differences were noted. The more recent ETTNO study examined the same neurologic outcomes in extremely premature neonates who were transfused under liberal versus restrictive transfusion thresholds [38]. The ETTNO study did not find any difference in cognitive outcomes (Mental Development Index <85) at 24 months corrected age. The transfusion thresholds for each group were different in the PINT and ETTNO studies, with the ETTNO study having a higher transfusion threshold than the PINT for all groups which may have contributed to the difference in observed neurologic outcomes [40, 41].

Physicians often seek individualized, age-based transfusion triggers when attempting to manage perioperative anemia. Individual patients tolerate different levels of anemia based on their underlying physiology. As stated, otherwise healthy children without significant comorbidities, as well as stable, critically ill children, may be able to tolerate a considerable degree of anemia (e.g., Hbg 7 g/dL) without short-term complications. This is particularly relevant when the anemia is chronic and physiologic compensation has occurred [42]. A 2018 consensus statement by the Transfusion and Anemia Expertise Initiative (TAXI) consortium recommends RBC thresholds as low as 5 g/dL in stable, sick children more than 6 months old [43]. It is important to consider that these patients are hospitalized and under observation, setting them apart from the perioperative child who is about to undergo the physiologic stress of surgery, blood loss, and discharge to home.

Certain patient populations require special consideration when evaluating anemia tolerance. Children undergoing cardiac surgery may require a higher baseline Hgb level for a satisfactory outcome. In a 2016 retrospective study, Park SK et al.

found that preoperative anemia was associated with an increased risk of postoperative acute kidney injury (AKI; OR 2.4, 95% CI, 1.07–5.4) within the first week after surgery in 220 children with congenital heart disease [44]. In a later, retrospective, propensity-matched review of 141 children with cyanotic heart disease, Zhou et al. demonstrated that children with congenital heart disease and Hgb values below the age-adjusted lower limit of normal before cardiac surgery had an increased risk of in-hospital mortality and hospital length of stay [45].

Neonatal patients and infants also have different tolerance for anemia. Neonates, especially preterm neonates, are often transfused at a higher Hgb level than older children and adults [46]. Most premature and low-birth-weight neonates receive a blood transfusion within the first month of life [38]. There are various reasons for this practice, including apnea prevention and the thinking that an increase in Hgb will promote improved end-organ oxygenation and weight gain. RBC transfusions have been associated with a decrease in the rate of apnea events in very low-weight (≤1500 g) preterm infants independent of extraneous oxygen requirement [47]. Other studies have found that neonates compensate for anemia by increasing their cardiac output (CO) (primarily through an increase in heart rate) to support improved oxygen delivery (DO_2). When compensatory physiologic mechanisms are maximized, a transfusion may decrease CO, reduce overall anemia-related stress, and potentially reduce lactate levels produced through anaerobic metabolism [48, 49].

Theoretically, DO_2 at the tissue level is a function of oxygen content of the blood (CaO2) and CO according to the oxygen delivery equation:

$$DO_2 = CO \times CaO_2$$

$$DO_2 = CO \times \left[1.34(\text{ml}/\text{g}) \times \text{Hgb}(\text{g}/\text{dl}) \times SpO_2(\%)\right] + \left(PaO_2 \times 0.003\right);$$

when ($PaO_2 \times 0.003$) represents the quantity of dissolved oxygen in the arterial circulation and SpO_2 is peripheral oxygen saturation. In children with cyanotic heart or pulmonary disease, a physiologic compensation takes place in response to low baseline SpO2. Erythropoietin production increases in response to hypoxemia which increases Hgb concentration and consequently DO_2 [50]. However, tissue extraction can differ between subclasses of patients. A recent study performed mathematical modeling to quantify the physiologic Hgb level in patients with single ventricle physiology [51]. This in vitro model found that Hgb greater than 13 g/dL was required to maintain arterial oxygen saturation > 70% when CO is maintained at 6 L/m^2/min; a Hgb 9 g/dL (a transfusion threshold considered "liberal" in healthier patients) was associated with significant arterial desaturation. However, this is only a mathematical model without clinical correlation testing and assumes that increased RBC mass will consistently increase oxygen-carrying capacity. A patient's microcirculation as well as the nature of transfused RBCs also impact attempts to improve global oxygenation through an RBC transfusion [33].

Assessment of anemia tolerance is complex and best achieved by assessing an individual patient's DO_2, end-organ perfusion, oxygen extraction, and compensatory physiology. Currently, there is no consistent standard to evaluate the effects of an RBC transfusion on anemia or one that can determine the optimal preoperative Hgb in different pediatric patient populations.

Objective assessment tools are usually available in only in the sickest, hospitalized patients. In the future, newer technologies to monitor the optimal thresholds for perioperative RBC transfusions may become routine, including regional tissue oxygenation, hemoglobin oxygen content, and tissue oxygen extraction [52–56].

4.2.3.2 Procedure-Specific Blood Loss History

The three pillars of PBM should be applied in all procedures or patients at risk for surgical blood loss through optimizing the patient's RBC mass. If the procedure or patient factors create a risk of surgical bleeding, assessment for preoperative anemia as well as the impact of treatment should be assessed. Anemia treatment is an inconvenience and potential monetary expense to the patient, with doctor visits, new medications that may not be well tolerated, and a delay in surgery. Surgical procedures, such as liver transplantation, craniosynostosis, neurosurgery, major orthopedic surgery, thoracic, and abdominal surgeries, are associated with the potential for significant blood loss and the need for blood transfusion [57]. A Maximum Surgical Blood Order Schedule (MSBOS) is available at many hospital blood banks [58]. The MSBOS is a data-based model indicating the likelihood of blood transfusion during specific surgeries (and at times, specific surgeons) at a particular institution. It typically indicates the need for a pretransfusion crossmatch in those cases that require a transfusion 5–10% of the time, and it also indicates which cases require only a type-and-screen. The predictive value of a MSBOS can be increased through incorporation of patient factors associated with an intraoperative transfusion by incorporating an artificial intelligence (AI) algorithm [59].

4.2.3.3 Assessing Ongoing Blood Loss

The practical challenges in assessing blood loss in the intraoperative setting underscore the critical importance of optimizing a child's Hgb in the preoperative period. The ability to assess present or ongoing intraoperative bleeding in a small child is hampered by several pediatric-specific factors, including physiologic compensatory mechanisms, monitoring equipment limitations, and environmental constraints. Neonatal tachycardia occurs in response to volume loss (rather than increased stroke volume which remains fixed secondary to a relatively noncompliant myocardium) and may be confused with a pain reflex or a response to the anesthetic. Peripheral blood pressure measurements may remain normal despite significant blood loss (e.g., ≥20% of estimated blood volume; EBL) [60, 61]. Compensatory vasoconstriction may produce decreased SpO_2 values or blunting of the waveform, which are often interpreted as artifact. As a result, the use of physiologic parameters alone to estimate intraoperative blood loss is not accurate and is not recommended to assess the need for RBC replacement in actively bleeding children [62]. The intraoperative availability of other physiologic monitors such as invasive arterial lines and cerebral oximetry are not always present or necessary, nor have they been validated in children to indicate a need for RBC transfusion during active bleeding. Serum lactate or pH values obtained through blood gas analysis may guide volume replacement but not specifically an RBC transfusion. A Hgb value alone does not reflect a child's present or ongoing blood loss and is not reflective of future intraoperative blood loss. Assessment of intraoperative blood loss is further complicated by the fact that a child's allowable blood loss (ABL) is calculated on a weight-based standard using EBV: a neonate may have an EBV of 90 ml/kg and a toddler, 70 ml/kg. Visual assessment of ongoing blood loss is challenging in a setting where the surgical field can camouflage a small quantity of blood loss that may be clinically significant in an infant. In an in vitro study measuring the capacity of saline-soaked surgical gauze, a 2″ × 2″ gauze was estimated to contain 3.25 ml ± 1.25 ml of blood when 100% soaked [63]. Thus, two, 2″ × 2″ gauze alone can constitute 5% of a 2 kg neonate's blood volume.

Current assessment tools for clinically relevant blood loss in critically ill children are found in the intensive care literature. Despite reported inter-rater reliability of 0.74 (95% CI, 0.6–0.9), a recent tool to assess clinically relevant bleeding in sick children was based on parameters or observations summarized from expert consensus, but not validated through higher level evidence [64]. Based on a 2021 review of clinically significant bleeding in sick children (but not under anesthesia), "severe" bleeding indicating that a future RBC transfusion should be urgently addressed includes signs of organ dysfunction, a Hgb decrease >20% in 24 h, or bleeding ≥5 ml/kg/h for ≥1 h [65]. Enhanced scrutiny is indicated for bleeding in potentially closed spaces such as the spine and cranium.

Performing prospective, randomized, controlled experiments to ascertain when a bleeding child should be transfused is a real-world impracticality, if not an impossibility. To avoid the critical trap of getting behind on blood loss in a small child, some experts recommend "topping up" during ongoing blood loss or going into surgery with a slightly higher Hgb than the restrictive 7 gm/dL in the stable, hospitalized patient [66–68]. In the 2007 update to the POCA registry, Bhananker et al. found that almost one-half of anesthesia-related cardiac arrests due to blood loss were attributable to a failure to diagnose [27]. Late-stage assessments of intraoperative blood loss, such as hypotension resistant to 40 ml/kg of crystalloid or administration of vasopressors, can have critical consequences.

4.2.4 What Are the Most Common Types of Anemia in the Different Pediatric Age Groups?

The etiology of an anemia diagnosis can often be narrowed down through readily available data already present in the medical record: the patient's age and, in cases of nonacute blood loss, the RBC mean corpuscular volume (MCV). The following is a discussion of age- and MCV-related diagnoses that may be evident in the pre-anesthesia clinic.

4.2.4.1 Age-Related Anemia Diagnoses

Term Newborns

A "physiologic anemia of infancy" is common in term infants under 3 months of age, with a nadir (i.e., Hgb 10–11 g/dL) occurring at 6–9 weeks of extrauterine life. This anemia is the result of decreased erythropoietin production due to increased tissue oxygenation associated with transitional circulation at birth [69]. During the first weeks of life, a more severe decrease in Hgb (e.g., Hgb < 9 g/dL) or symptomatic anemia (e.g., tachypnea, growth delay, irritability) point to a pathologic process such as blood loss or hemolysis [70]. Inborn errors of metabolism may also present with anemia in the first 30 days of life. Although rare, over 50% of patients with inborn errors of metabolism will have hematologic manifestations [71].

Preterm Infants

Because a large portion (80%) of maternal-fetal iron transfer occurs throughout the third trimester of pregnancy, premature infants are at increased risk for iron deficiency anemia (IDA) [15]. Term infants of anemic mothers are also at risk. Preterm infants are born with lower Hgb levels and develop an earlier, more severe anemia termed "anemia of prematurity." An immature liver with inadequate erythropoietin response to tissue hypoxia, reduced iron stores, and RBCs with reduced circulating lifespan contribute anemia of prematurity [72, 73]. Furthermore, these small patients are also often subject to repeated phlebotomy, leading to insidious blood loss.

Older Infants and Children

Term infants older than 3–6 months begin to manifest acquired causes of anemia, including iron and micronutrient deficiency, systemic disease (e.g., microangiopathic processes such as hemolytic uremic syndrome, disseminated intravascular coagulation (DIC)), toxins or drugs (e.g., antibiotics, lead poisoning), and immune mediated hemolysis [74]. Anemias of chronic disease and autoimmune disorders emerge during adolescence, and teen aged females are particularly susceptible to iron deficiency secondary to inadequate dietary iron intake.

Figure 4.1 illustrates the etiologies of pediatric anemia by age.

4.2.4.2 Red Blood Cell Volumes

IDA may be differentiated initially based on the MCV taken from a peripheral blood smear (Fig. 4.2). An abnormal MCV is described as micro-, normo-, or macrocytic.

Microcytosis

The most common form of microcytic anemia is iron deficiency. Thalassemia also present with a small red cell MCV or microcytosis. Thalassemia may go undiagnosed, as the severity of the anemia is directly related to the number of affected genes and can present from asymptomatic, mild anemia to severe, symptomatic anemia. Thalassemia affects either alpha-globin or beta-globin production and may be found in patients of Mediterranean, African, or Southeast Asian descent. Hemoglobin F (HgbF) comprises up to 80% of fetal Hgb in the third trimester of

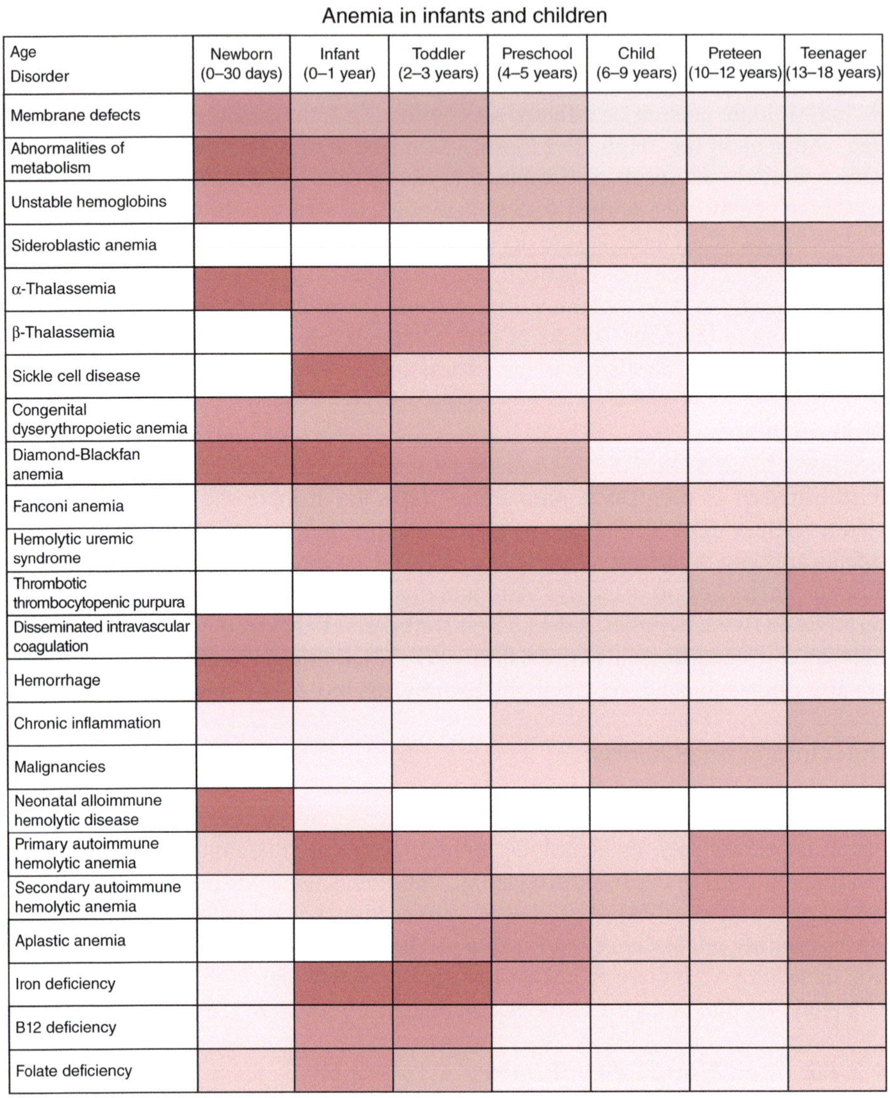

Fig. 4.1 Anemia etiologies by age. Reprinted with permission from Gallagher [74]

gestation, and Hgb production switches to adult HgbA and $HgbA_2$ by 6–12 months postnatal age. By that age, HgbF is only 2% of total Hgb levels in patients with normal alpha-globin or beta-globin production. As a result, thalassemia typically does not present until 3–6 months of life when this switch to HgbA production should begin. Four alpha-globin variants are usually lethal while patients with one to three alpha-globin variants have surivable, but varied clinical presentations. The American Academy of Pediatrics (AAP) recommends regular screening for lead

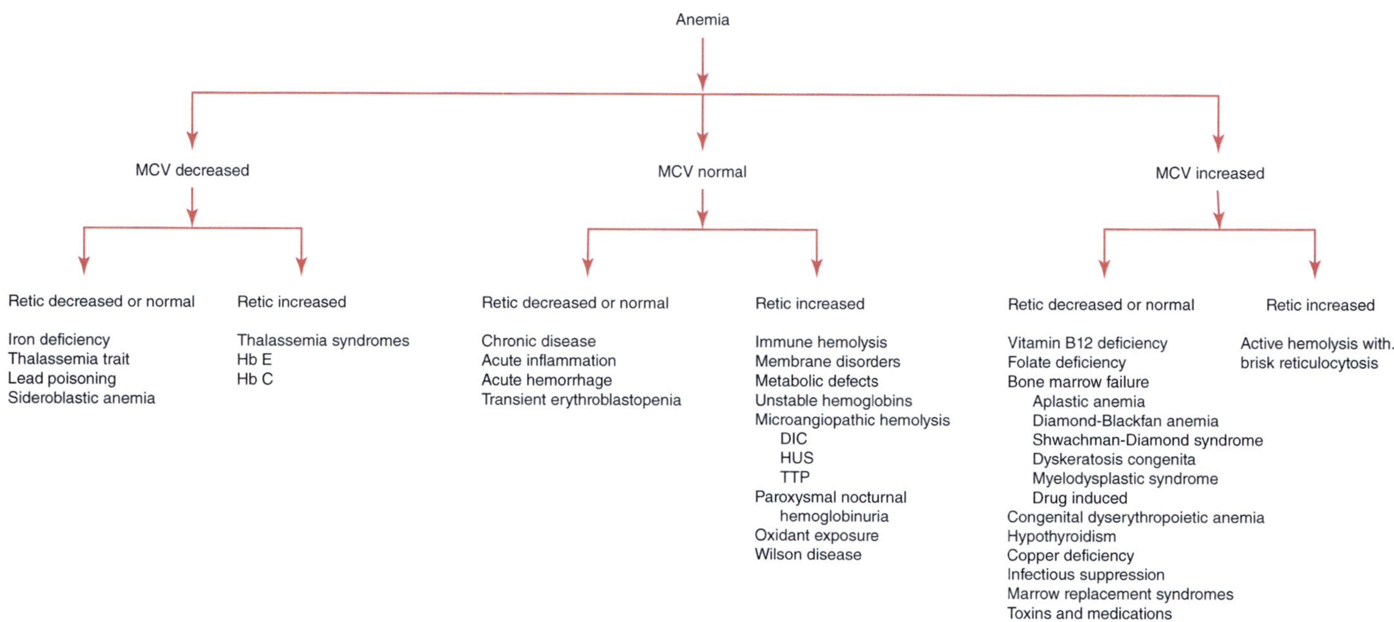

Fig. 4.2 Anemia diagnosed using RBC MCV indices. Reprinted with permission from Gallagher [74]

levels in high-risk patient populations (e.g., family housing built before 1960, residence in a smelter community, or a food insecure household) at early as 6 months [76, 77].

Iron Deficiency Anemia (IDA)

Iron deficiency anemia (IDA) classically presents as microcytosis or a reduced MCV on blood smear. Globally, IDA is the most common type of acquired anemia in children, affecting at least 20% and 40% of children in the USA and in nonindustrialized countries worldwide, respectively [77]. Although worldwide estimates of IDA showed a decrease between 1990 and 2010, children under 4–5 years continue to suffer disproportionately. IDA begins to manifest in term infants by 4–6 months as iron stores and breastfeeding declines [78]. ID continues to affect toddlers who experience rapid growth and may consume large amounts of iron-poor cow's milk (>24 ounces per day). A second peak in IDA is seen in postmenarchal females, also related to dietary requirements out of step with iron losses [74] [Fig. 4.2].

Iron Deficiency (ID)

IDA is a symptom of late-stage ID. As a child's iron stores become depleted, the ID progresses from subclinical disease to what is seen as anemia as measured by Hgb or Hct.

ID alone is thought to affect one-half of children worldwide but the true incidence is unknown [79]. Most persons in the US consume the minimally recommend amounts of iron through a mixed diet [15]. Exceptions include premature infants, children 6 months to 5 years, and pregnant women, all of whom have increased requirements secondary to increased growth. The WHO estimates that approximately 40% of those with ID develop IDA, which suggests that the other one-half with ID may go undiagnosed when Hgb or Hct laboratory values are normal and are used in isolation to diagnose ID [17]. ID adversely affects physical and neurologic development and has been associated with growth retardation, chronic fatigue, attention deficit hyperactivity disorder (ADHD), immune dysfunction, gastric atrophy, and even increased blood lead levels [15, 77]. Recommended dietary allowances (RDA; the healthy daily intake recommended for most persons) for elemental iron are listed in Table 4.4 [15, 80, 81]. These recommendations vary according to age, sex, and vegetarian status.

Normocytosis

Most anemias begin as normocytic before folate and iron stores are consumed, including ID and the anemia of acute blood loss. Normocytic anemia in childhood can classified into several categories: decreased production of RBCs, increased destruction of RBCs, hemodilution, or acute blood loss. Decreased RBC production is seen in chronic inflammatory conditions, endocrine disorders (hypothyroidism, hypogonadism, adrenal insufficiency), bone marrow disorders, or renal failure [82]. Bone marrow suppression due to various infectious processes is a common cause of a reduction in all blood cell lines. Several medications can also lead to bone marrow suppression: sulfa drugs, phenytoin, and azathioprine [74]. Increased destruction of

Table 4.4 The US recommended daily allowances (RDA) for iron in different age groups. RDA is different than supplementation, which varies with age and risk group

Patient age	Male	Female	Vegetarian diet
0–4 months & breastfed[a]	0.27 mg	0.27 mg	Double the RDA
7–12 months	11 mg	11 mg	
1–3 years	7 mg	7 mg	
4–8 years	10 mg	10 mg	
9–13 years	8 mg	8 mg	
14–18 years	11 mg	15 mg	
19–50 years	8 mg	18 mg	
Pregnancy		30 mg early in pregnancy; 60–120 mg/day if Hgb < 9 g/dL	

Adapted from NIH Office of Dietary Supplement [15]
Infants who are not exclusively breast fed and are at risk for IDA should receive iron supplementation after 4 months as iron stores become depleted
[a]Premature infants <6 months require up to 2–4 mg/kg of elemental iron per day

RBCs may be seen with hemolytic disorders (hereditary spherocytosis, G6PD deficiency) or mechanical destruction (hemolytic uremic syndrome, prosthetic heart valves). Increased plasma volume (e.g., hemodilution) occurs with excessive hydration seen in hospitalized children with an IV line in place or those undergoing surgery [83]. Normocytic anemia is also seen in acute blood loss, including that associated with surgery and repeat phlebotomy. Hemoglobinopathies, such as sickle cell disease, may also present as normocytic anemia after 6 months when HgbF production decreases.

Macrocytosis

Macrocytic anemia is uncommon in pediatrics but may be seen with nutritional deficiencies or congenital causes of anemia. Folate or vitamin B12 deficiency classically presents with macrocytosis. In the perioperative setting, macrocytosis is seen in healthy children several days after acute blood loss secondary to a reticulocyte response: reticulocytes are large, immature RBCs. Congenital causes include Diamond-Blackfan anemia, Fanconi Anemia, and Shwachman-Diamond syndrome [74]. A 2023 retrospective review of over 40,000 anemic adult patients found that patients with macrocytosis (vs. micro- or normocytosis) had prolonged operative recovery times, although all three MCV groups had poorer outcomes than their nonanemic counterparts [84].

Due to the large number and potential complexity of pediatric anemias, the pediatric anesthesiologist should remain vigilant for potential hemoglobinopathies, chronic inflammation, infectious processes, and congenital disease in their anemic preoperative patients. A definitive diagnosis, if sought, should always be made by a hematology specialist.

4.2.5 What Preoperative Testing Should Be Performed if a Child is Anemic Prior to Blood Loss Surgery?

It is not uncommon to encounter an anemic or iron-deficient patient in the perioperative setting. The WHO estimates that one-third of the world's patients who present for surgery are anemic [17]. A cross-sectional analysis of a French database covering 16 centers found that of 2345 adult preoperative patients, 34.2% were anemic and one-third of those patients had iron deficiency [85]. Up to one-quarter of infants presenting for noncardiac surgery may be anemic [18, 19].

Preoperative testing is determined by the patient's general medical condition and the planned surgery. The AAP and WHO recommend routine screening for anemia as early as 1 year of age and selective screening earlier in patients with risk factors for iron deficiency [81, 86]. Table 4.5 is a summary of patients at risk for preoperative anemia:

Under expert consensus guidelines, routine preoperative laboratory testing is not recommended if a planned surgery has a low risk for bleeding or does not present a significant risk for associated cardiopulmonary or neurologic complications [87]. Baseline anemia screening should be performed for cases with the potential for

Table 4.5 Causes of ID in children

Iron deficiency (ID) etiology	At-risk patients and factors
Iron-deficient diet	Infants on: Single food, unfortified Excessive cow's milk (>24 oz./day) Associated with the following: Non-white ethnicity Household income below poverty line
Increased growth & metabolism	Menstruation Infants >4 months & exclusively breastfed Ex-premature infant Infants of diabetic mother Ages 13–17 years
Increased acquired requirements	Athletes Obesity Regular blood donors
Decreased adsorption	Inflammatory bowel disease Gastritis Disease of chronic inflammation *H. Pylori* infection Celiac disease Hereditary iron-resistance; defect of iron transport
Increased losses	Frequent or excessive phlebotomy Gastrointestinal bleeding Parasitic infection Hemosiderosis Menorrhagia Excessive exercise

Adapted from Tong and Vichinsky [77]; Baker et al. [81]

significant blood loss to plan for Hgb optimization and to calculate the patient's allowable blood loss (ABL) during the surgery. Former premature infants should also be evaluated for anemia in the preoperative period, in advance of even low-risk procedures, because the risk of postoperative apnea has been shown to increase with a hematocrit less than 30% [88–90].

If ID is suspected based on risk factors, or if a low hemoglobin is identified on preoperative evaluation, further workup may be required. As stated, the patient's age may offer insight into possible etiologies. Nutritional deficiency, excess cow milk intake, or other risk factors may be apparent from history alone. A review of the birth course, including a history of jaundice requiring phototherapy, may be elicited. Other medical issues, medications, or an active infectious process should be identified. A family history of anemia may point to congenital disease. Physical exam findings can reflect the acuity and severity of the anemia. However, a diagnosis of anemia based on a physical finding of pallor has uncertain sensitivity and specificity [91]. Physical findings may not be present until the patient's Hgb is less than 7–8 g/dL [92]. Subtle signs of anemia include restlessness, irritability, and decreased exercise tolerance; severe anemia may manifest as high output congestive heart failure. Other potential physical findings include a systolic ejection murmur, hepatosplenomegaly, and petechiae [93]. Craniofacial or limb dysmorphism may also suggest a congenital hematologic syndrome.

If an etiology for anemia is not apparent on initial H&P, a complete blood count (CBC) to evaluate MCV and other RBC indices is the first step [74]. A CBC will also identify if the anemia is isolated or is associated with other cytopenias that may suggest additional disease. However, a Hgb or Hct alone are insufficiently specific or sensitive to evaluate iron status. Serum ferritin is the most sensitive and cost-effective test available to diagnose ID [77, 80]. Ferritin is the primary intracellular storage protein for iron, and levels are reduced before RBC anemia is apparent [77]. A serum level <100 ug/L indicates iron deficiency; <30 ug/L is consistent with IDA [80]. It is important to note that serum ferritin levels are increased during inflammation. A reticulocyte count reflects the robustness of any anemia response. Other blood iron chemistries (e.g., total iron binding capacity (TIBC), transferrin saturation, and hepcidin) should be ordered after consulting with the patient's pediatrician or a hematologist. Transferrin is the major transporter of ferric iron throughout the body [94]. However, the transferring saturation test is expensive and not often used clinically. If the serum ferritin level is equivocal (e.g., 30–100 μg/L), the transferrin saturation (<20%) may indicate anemia of inflammation. Hepcidin, an important regulator of iron in the body, is decreased in IDA but increased in cases of "functional" ID whereby iron stores are unavailable for erythropoiesis (such as in inflammatory conditions). If an RBC destructive process is suspected, a bilirubin, direct antibody test (DAT), and peripheral blood smear are in order [74].

Diagnosis and management of preoperative anemia can be challenging. A simplified algorithm of initial laboratory tests and selected treatment is illustrated in Fig. 4.3:

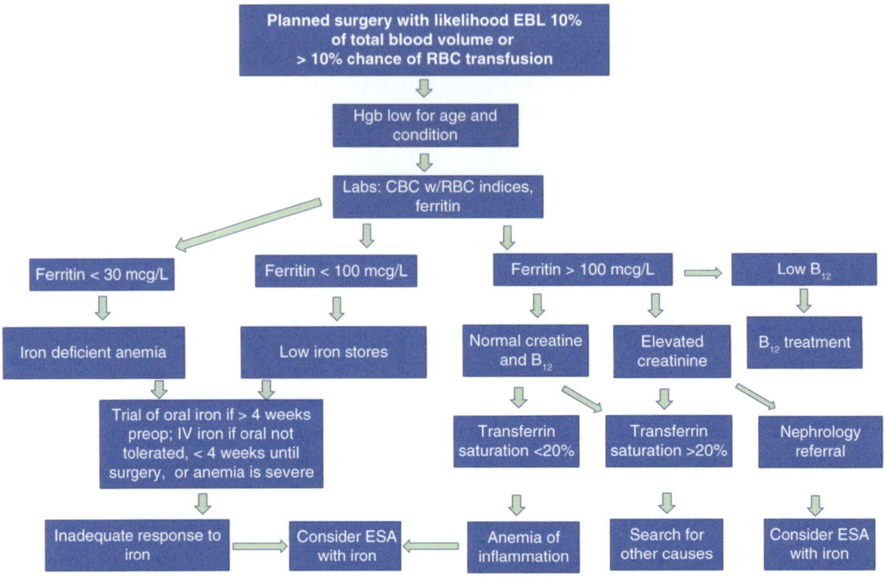

Fig. 4.3 Preoperative anemia evaluation and treatment. (Adapted from Lin [94])

4.2.6 What Is a Suggested Approach to the Preoperative Management of the Anemic Child?

Once anemia is diagnosed, it should be managed to optimize the patient's surgical outcome and to avoid unnecessary allogeneic transfusions. An essential consideration in preoperative anemia management is that *anemia is a symptom*, not a diagnosis per se. Appropriate anemia treatment will likely depend on the underlying cause. Both diagnosis and treatment, if any, are best overseen by a pediatric hematologist or primary care physician who can provide continuity of care.

Anemic pediatric patients are likely to be iron deficient. Traditionally, children with microcytic anemia were often assumed to be iron-deficient and administered a trial of iron supplementation [77]. In children with IDA, iron supplementation improves hemoglobin levels significantly (3.4–7.6 g/L depending on intermittent or frequent dosing regimen) [95]. However, poor compliance with medication regimens, undesirable side effects (particularly gastrointestinal (GI) distress and constipation), and failure to follow up treatment is a common sequelae to oral iron therapy [77]. A recent meta-analysis of iron dosing regimens found similar improvements in anemia when oral iron was administered weekly (versus daily dosing), revealing an option when treatment compliance is a concern [95]. Dietary counseling and iron therapy ideally occur under the care of a pediatrician who can provide continuity with appropriate follow up [86]. If there is no improvement after 4–8 weeks of therapy, further testing for an underlying condition may be required[2] [77].

[2] For further discussion of perioperative anemia evaluation, refer to Chap. 17.

If a child is determined to have IDA, parents should be counseled about increasing iron consumption naturally through diet. The body absorbs less than 30–40% of dietary iron, depending on the patient's existing iron stores. Heme iron present in meats is absorbed twice as efficiently as nonheme iron (which is absent in meats), prompting a recommended daily allowance (RDA) of elemental iron for those who do not eat meat that is almost double the daily iron recommendation for meat eaters [77]. Iron-rich foods include red meat, pork, legumes, dried fruits, and iron-fortified cereals. Coffee and tea reduce iron absorption; foods high in ascorbic acid facilitate iron absorption. In developing countries, iron fortification of foods (e.g., corn flour, soy sauce, fish sauce, and rice) is used to meet elemental iron requirements for older infants and toddlers [81]. In the USA, fortification of infant formula and infant cereal has been associated with a decrease in the incidence of IDA. Food iron fortification in ex-premature infants and toddlers is problematic because both age groups have additional growth-related iron requirements, with typical diets that do not supply necessary quantities [81]. A recent study found that premature infants fed only iron-fortified formula did not achieve adequate iron stores or the recommended daily dose of 2 mg/kg/day elemental iron [96]. Iron stores accumulated in the last months of gestation are depleted in term infants by 4–6 months. Exclusively breastfed infants should receive iron supplementation after 6 months of life, as breast milk has low iron concentrations (albeit with high bioavailability) [97]. The US Centers for Disease Control (CDC) recommends that infants who are not exclusively breastfed receive iron-fortified formula (standardized at 12 mg/L in the USA) or fortified cereals when they begin to eat solids [81].

There are many oral and intravenous (IV) iron formulations available to treat preoperative anemia in children [81]. Ferrous fumarate and gluconate are available in tablet form, and ferrous sulfate is available as drops and oral solutions (elixir, syrup, and extended-release tablets) [86]. However, these preparations are often associated with significant adverse GI effects. A polysaccharide-iron complex, which is ferric iron mixed with water and saccharide, may be better tolerated but with reduced absorption. The different iron preparations vary with respect to available iron content: fumarate 33%, sulfate 20%, and gluconate 12% elemental iron by weight [15]. The daily recommended iron dosing for treating IDA are listed in Table 4.6 [15, 80, 81].

Supplemental iron therapy should not be administered in a vacuum before the patient's iron status is examined. Overtreatment or accidental overdose is a potential complication of iron therapy, particularly when it is packaged as a sweet or

Table 4.6 Supplemental oral iron therapy dosing for patients with IDA

Age	Dosing regimen	Iron preparations
All children	Initial: 3 mg/kg/day. Advance to 6 mg/kg/day if tolerated and no improvement in 4–8 weeks	0–23 months: Drops or syrup 24–59 months: Drops, syrup, spansule beads, tablet >5 years: Capsules, tablets
6–23 months and living in community with 40% prevalence anemia or gross undernutrition	2 mg/kg/day for 3 months per year	

"gummy," is not secured in a child-resistant container, or is administered to patients with hemochromatosis. Premature infants are susceptible to iron overload secondary to repeated RBC transfusions [81]. An "upper limit" of 40 mg iron is established as the highest daily dose that can be administered without adverse systemic effect in the average individual [15]. However, accidental ingestion of doses >36 mg/kg can be fatal in children [15]. Iron administration may increase lead absorption and decrease zinc absorption; coadministration with calcium supplements can inhibit iron absorption [15, 81]. Furthermore, iron therapy in patients with chronic disease is controversial as it may be associated with untoward infectious and cardiovascular side effects and should be initiated by a hematology specialist. Anemia of chronic disease is best managed by treating the underlying disease.

IV iron should be considered as a treatment option for IDA when oral iron is ineffective or poorly tolerated [77, 94, 98]. Other indications for IV iron therapy (versus oral therapy) include:

- An urgent surgery that cannot be postponed for anemia treatment.
- No change in ID after several months of oral iron therapy.
- Absorption defect (celiac disease, gastrectomy, ulcerative colitis, Chron's disease).
- Concomitant with erythropoiesis-stimulating agent (ESA) therapy.
- Ongoing blood losses.
- Postoperatively when gastric or intestinal absorption is reduced due to stress or altered anatomy.

New IV iron preparations are associated with few side effects, without the anaphylaxis reputation of the older, high-molecular-weight dextran formulation [77]. Current preparations include iron sucrose (the most commonly used), low-molecular-weight dextran, and ferric gluconate, with an adverse event rate of 1%, including a serious event rate of 1:200,000. The newer dextran preparation may require a test dose prior to initiation [99, 100].

An erythropoiesis stimulating agent (ESA) is administered to treat perioperative anemia in specific patient populations: multiple alloantibodies leading to difficult crossmatch, objection to blood transfusions, or patients who are very anemic after autologous blood donation [94, 101–103]. In the past, the most common indication for ESA use in children has been chronic disease, including renal failure, epidermolysis bullosa, and cancer, all long-term diseases that are typically transfusion dependent [102]. Most research regarding pediatric ESA administration has been in the premature neonate population, which suffers from anemia of prematurity and a high rate of RBC transfusions [101]. Pediatric data on the preoperative administration of ESAs, however, is limited. ESAs have been used with success prior to pediatric craniofacial and cardiac surgery, citing reduced rates and volumes of allogeneic RBC transfusions [104–107]. Consensus guidelines support preoperative administration of ESA's only in select patient populations, mentioned above [108]. Reports of thromboembolism in adults (but not children), combined with limited prospective data in the pediatric surgical population, has led to a general hesitancy to administer ESAs to anemic children outside of special situations [105, 109, 110]. Additional obstacles to routine ESA administration in anemic children is uncertainty over treatment regimens (e.g., dosing, duration, and appropriate patient selection), expense, inconvenience of serial injections, and a lack of compelling risk-benefit outcome data. It is prudent to consider preoperative ESA administration only in cases of certain and significant blood loss when the patient has a Hgb level close to the restrictive transfusion threshold or has reduced ability for endogenous erythropoietin production. Although ESA administration is an important consideration in patient blood management, it is best to refer the patient to a pediatric hematologist when ESA therapy is considered to ensure follow-up [86].

In major surgery where large volume blood loss is expected, patients should be informed of the higher risk of morbidity and mortality associated with preoperative anemia, educated about alternatives, and encouraged to postpone nonurgent surgery for anemia management when feasible. Various adult guidelines, including the Network for Advancement of Transfusion Alternatives (NATA), the Seville Document (from a multidiscipline group of Spanish experts), and the British Committee for Standards in Hematology, recommend postponing surgery for 4 weeks of anemia treatment [34, 111–114].

4.3 Summary of Key Learning Objectives

4.3.1 What Hgb Value Indicates Anemia in Children?

Population based data suggest that "normal" Hgb values vary by age and sex. Neonates tend to have relatively higher Hgb values (up to 23 g/dL) with wide reference ranges. Premature neonates have lower initial Hgb values compared to term neonates (8–9 gm/dL), with the very premature neonates (born <28 weeks gestation) having the lowest Hgb value of all age groups. The lower limit of the normal Hgb value for infants and older children is 10–11 g/dL. Notable differences between sexes become pronounced at about age 14 years when females reach menarche.

4.3.2 Does Perioperative Anemia Influence Postoperative Morbidity and Mortality in Pediatric Patients?

There is evidence of a strong association between preoperative anemia and postoperative morbidity in adults undergoing surgery. Two recent database analyses from NSQIP found that a relatively high percentage—over one quarter—of neonates and older children in the USA are anemic prior to surgery, with significantly worse outcomes and increased mortality, compared to nonanemic children. Isolated anemia in the absence of other comorbidities may not affect mortality in nonblood loss procedures. However, preoperative anemia is associated with perioperative allogeneic transfusions which carry their own risks.

4.3.3 What Is an Acceptable, Minimum Preoperative Hgb Value for a Child?

The optimal Hgb value in pediatric patients before an elective surgical procedure is unknown. Assessment of anemia tolerance is complex and best achieved by assessing an individual patient's oxygen delivery, end-organ perfusion, oxygen extraction, and compensatory physiology. Certain patient populations require special consideration when evaluating anemia tolerance. Children with cyanotic heart disease require a relatively higher Hgb to maintain aerobic metabolism, and neonates may have limited oxygen delivery secondary to fixed stroke volumes in the face to maximized heart rate. In addition, the volume of blood loss associated with a particular procedure as well as the practitioner's ability to assess ongoing blood loss (which can be challenging in small patients) have bearing on the optimal preoperative Hgb value.

4.3.4 What Are the Most Common Types of Anemia in the Different Pediatric Age Groups?

Iron deficiency anemia (IDA) is the most common type of anemia in children. At-risk populations include premature neonates, toddlers, and pregnant women. Infants less than 3 months normally experience a physiologic anemia, but premature infants have reduced iron stores at birth and suffer from anemia of prematurity. Congenital hemoglobinopathies and inborn errors of metabolism manifest in infancy, whereas acquired etiologies such as hemolytic uremic syndrome are more common in the 2–5-year age groups. Anemias of chronic disease and autoimmune disorders emerge during adolescence, and teen aged females are often iron-deficient secondary to inadequate dietary intake.

4.3.5 What Preoperative Testing Should Be Performed if a Child Is Anemic Prior to Blood Loss Surgery?

Routine preoperative laboratory testing is not recommended if a planned surgery has a low risk for bleeding or does not present a significant risk for associated cardiopulmonary or neurologic complications. If a planned surgery has a likelihood of blood loss equal to 10% of the child's estimated blood volume or is known to have a > 10% chance of an RBC transfusion *and* the child's Hgb is low for age, the following preliminary tests may be performed:

- A CBC with indices
- Serum ferritin
- Reticulocyte count

Blood iron chemistries may be warranted but should done be at the discretion of a hematology specialist:

- Total iron binding capacity
- Transferrin saturation
- Hepcidin

4.3.6 What Is a Suggested Approach to the Preoperative Management of the Anemic Child?

Once anemia is diagnosed it should be managed to optimize the patient's surgical outcome and to avoid unnecessary allogeneic transfusions. Patients should be informed of the higher risk of morbidity and mortality associated with preoperative anemia and available alternatives, including surgery postponement when feasible. Anemic preoperative pediatric patients are most likely to be iron deficient. Initially, dietary counseling about iron rich food is offered to the family. Consider delaying elective and nonurgent *blood loss* procedures for 4–8 weeks so that iron therapy can be instituted, under the direction of the patient's pediatrician to ensure continuity and follow up. If the patient does not tolerate oral iron, IV preparations which now have improved safety profiles may be an option. Erythropoiesis stimulating agents may be used in special groups of patients (e.g., chronic renal disease, ex-premature neonates, difficult crossmatching, refusal of all blood transfusions) but should be managed by a hematologist or the patient's pediatrician.

Key Points

- Normal Hgb reference ranges for children vary by age, with the lowest "normal" values in premature newborns (8 g/dL for the fifth percentile), and 11 g/dL for infants and older children according to population-based studies.
- There is a strong association between preoperative anemia and postoperative morbidity in both children and adults undergoing noncardiac surgery.
- The optimal Hgb value in pediatric patients for elective surgical procedures is unknown. Critically ill but stable children may tolerate a Hgb as low as 7 g/dL, but life threatening, active bleeding should be treated independent of Hgb value.
- An RBC transfusion decision should never be made based on a solitary Hgb value.
- Iron deficiency anemia is the most common type of acquired anemia in children, affecting 20–50% of populations worldwide.
- If anemia is suspected in a preoperative patient because of history, physical exam, or inclusion in an at-risk population, a Hgb level should be tested and, if below normal for age, should be following by a complete blood count with RBC indices, a serum ferritin, and a reticulocyte count.
- If a preoperative patient is anemic, blood loss surgeries and procedures should be delayed 4–8 weeks, when feasible, to evaluate the anemia and optimize the patient's RBC mass.

Bibliography

1. Kassebaum NJ, Collaborators GA. The global burden of anemia. Hematol Oncol Clin North Am. 2016;30(2):247–308.
2. Mazine A, Rached-D'Astous S, Ducruet T, Lacroix J, Poirier N, Network PALIaSI. Blood transfusions after pediatric cardiac operations: a north American multicenter prospective study. Ann Thorac Surg. 2015;100(2):671–7.
3. New HV, Grant-Casey J, Lowe D, Kelleher A, Hennem S, Stanworth SJ. Red blood cell transfusion practice in children: current status and areas for improvement? A study of the use of red blood cell transfusions in children and infants. Transfusion. 2014;54(1):119–27.
4. Lavoie J. Blood transfusion risks and alternative strategies in pediatric patients. Paediatr Anaesth. 2011;21(1):14–24.
5. BloodBankGuy Podcast. 096CE: navigating blood shortages with Claudia Cohn. 2022. https://www.bbguy.org/2022/03/30/096/. Accessed 2 June 2023..
6. Gombotz H, Hofman A, Rehak P, Kurz J. Patient blood management (part 2). Practice: the 3 pillars. Anasthesiol Intensivmed Notfallmed Schmerzther. 2011;46(7–8):466–74.
7. Staffa SJ, Joerger JD, Henry E, Christensen RD, Brugnara C, Zurakowski D. Pediatric hematology normal ranges derived from pediatric primary care patients. Am J Hematol. 2020;95:E255.
8. Fulgoni VL, Agarwal S, Kellogg MD, Lieberman HR. Establishing pediatric and adult RBC reference intervals with NHANES data using piecewise regression. Am J Clin Pathol. 2019;151(2):128–42.
9. Adeli K, Raizman JE, Chen Y, Higgins V, Nieuwesteeg M, Abdelhaleem M, et al. Complex biological profile of hematologic markers across pediatric, adult, and geriatric ages: establishment of robust pediatric and adult reference intervals on the basis of the Canadian Health Measures Survey. Clin Chem. 2015;61(8):1075–86.
10. Tahmasebi H, Higgins V, Bohn MK, Hall A, Adeli K. CALIPER hematology reference standards (I). Am J Clin Pathol. 2020;154(3):330–41.
11. Christensen RD, Henry E, Jopling J, Wiedmeier SE. The CBC: reference ranges for neonates. Semin Perinatol. 2009;33(1):3–11.
12. Christensen RD, Henry E, Bennett ST, Yaish HM. Reference intervals for reticulocyte parameters of infants during their first 90 days after birth. J Perinatol. 2016;36(1):61–6.
13. Robins EB, Blum S. Hematologic reference values for African American children and adolescents. Am J Hematol. 2007;82(7):611–4.
14. Bulletins—Obstetrics ACoOaGCoP. Anemia in pregnancy: ACOG Practice Bulletin, Number 233. Obstet Gynecol. 2021;138(2):e55–64.
15. NIH Office of Dietary Supplement. Iron: fact sheet for health professionals. National Institutes of Health. 2022. https://ods.od.nih.gov/factsheets/Iron-HealthProfessional/. Accessed 17 Jan 2023.
16. Malyavko A, Quan T, Kraft D, Mathur A, Ramamurti P, Tabaie S. Racial disparities in outcomes following open treatment of pediatric femoral shaft fractures. Cureus. 2022;14(12):e33149.
17. WHO. The urgent need to implement patient blood management: policy brief. 2021. https://www.who.int/publications/i/item/9789240035744. Accessed 17 Jan 2023.
18. Goobie SM, Faraoni D, Zurakowski D, DiNardo JA. Association of preoperative anemia with postoperative mortality in neonates. JAMA Pediatr. 2016;170(9):855–62.
19. Faraoni D, DiNardo JA, Goobie SM. Relationship between preoperative anemia and in-hospital mortality in children undergoing noncardiac surgery. Anesth Analg. 2016;123(6):1582–7.
20. Meyer HM, Torborg A, Cronje L, Thomas J, Bhettay A, Diedericks J, et al. The association between preoperative anemia and postoperative morbidity in pediatric surgical patients: a secondary analysis of a prospective observational cohort study. Paediatr Anaesth. 2020;30(7):759–65.
21. Musallam KM, Tamim HM, Richards T, Spahn DR, Rosendaal FR, Habbal A, et al. Preoperative anaemia and postoperative outcomes in non-cardiac surgery: a retrospective cohort study. Lancet. 2011;378(9800):1396–407.

22. Baron DM, Hochrieser H, Posch M, Metnitz B, Rhodes A, Moreno RP, et al. Preoperative anaemia is associated with poor clinical outcome in non-cardiac surgery patients. Br J Anaesth. 2014;113(3):416–23.
23. Kedir H, Miller R, Syed F, Hakim M, Walia H, Tumin D, et al. Association between anemia and postoperative complications in infants undergoing pyloromyotomy. J Pediatr Surg. 2019;54(10):2075–9.
24. Policy brief: the urgent need to implement patient blood management. World Health Organization. 2021. https://www.who.int/publications/i/item/9789240035744. Accessed 3 Jan 2023.
25. De la Garza RR, Goodwin CR, Abu-Bonsrah N, Jain A, Miller EK, Huang N, et al. Patient and operative factors associated with complications following adolescent idiopathic scoliosis surgery: an analysis of 36,335 patients from the Nationwide Inpatient Sample. J Neurosurg Pediatr. 2016;25(6):730–6.
26. O'Brien SH, Badawy SM, Rotz SJ, Shah MD, Makarski J, Bercovitz RS, et al. The ASH-ASPHO Choosing Wisely Campaign: 5 hematologic tests and treatments to question. Pediatr Blood Cancer. 2021;68(8):e28967.
27. Bhananker SM, Ramamoorthy C, Geiduschek JM, Posner KL, Domino KB, Haberkern CM, et al. Anesthesia-related cardiac arrest in children: update from the Pediatric Perioperative Cardiac Arrest Registry. Anesth Analg. 2007;105(2):344–50.
28. Yamada C, Edelson M, Lee A, Saifee NH, Bahar B, Delaney M. Transfusion-associated hyperkalemia in pediatric population: prevalence, risk factors, survival, infusion rate, and RBC unit features. Transfusion. 2021;61(4):1093–101.
29. Serious Hazards of Transfusion (SHOT) Annual Report. 2021. https://www.shotuk.org/wp-content/uploads/myimages/SHOT-REPORT-2021-FINAL-bookmarked-V3-November.pdf. Accessed 2 June 2023.
30. Smilowitz NR, Oberweis BS, Nukala S, Rosenberg A, Zhao S, Xu J, et al. Association between anemia, bleeding, and transfusion with long-term mortality following noncardiac surgery. Am J Med. 2016;129(3):315–23.e2.
31. Warner MA, Hanson AC, Schulte PJ, Sanz JR, Smith MM, Kauss ML, et al. Preoperative anemia and postoperative outcomes in cardiac surgery: a mediation analysis evaluating intraoperative transfusion exposures. Anesth Analg. 2024;138(4):728–37.
32. Downey LA, Goobie SM. Perioperative pediatric erythrocyte transfusions: incorporating hemoglobin thresholds and physiologic parameters in decision-making. Anesthesiology. 2022;137(5):604–19.
33. Faraoni D, DiNardo JA. Commentary: red blood cells transfusion in patients undergoing congenital cardiac surgery: still far from physiology-based practice. J Thorac Cardiovasc Surg. 2022;
34. Munoz M, Acheson AG, Auerbach M, Besser M, Habler O, Kehlet H, et al. International consensus statement on the peri-operative management of anaemia and iron deficiency. Anaesthesia. 2017;72(2):233–47.
35. Munoz M, Gomez-Ramirez S, Campos A, Ruiz J, Liumbruno GM. Pre-operative anaemia: prevalence, consequences and approaches to management. Blood Transfus. 2015;13(3):370–9.
36. Lacroix J, Hébert PC, Hutchison JS, Hume HA, Tucci M, Ducruet T, et al. Transfusion strategies for patients in pediatric intensive care units. N Engl J Med. 2007;356(16):1609–19.
37. Kirpalani H, Whyte RK, Andersen C, Asztalos EV, Heddle N, Blajchman MA, et al. The Premature Infants in Need of Transfusion (PINT) study: a randomized, controlled trial of a restrictive (low) versus liberal (high) transfusion threshold for extremely low birth weight infants. J Pediatr. 2006;149(3):301–7.
38. Franz AR, Engel C, Bassler D, Rüdiger M, Thome UH, Maier RF, et al. Effects of liberal vs restrictive transfusion thresholds on survival and neurocognitive outcomes in extremely low-birth-weight infants: the ETTNO Randomized Clinical Trial. JAMA. 2020;324(6):560–70.
39. Whyte RK, Kirpalani H, Asztalos EV, Andersen C, Blajchman M, Heddle N, et al. Neurodevelopmental outcome of extremely low birth weight infants randomly assigned to restrictive or liberal hemoglobin thresholds for blood transfusion. Pediatrics. 2009;123(1):207–13.

40. Whyte RK. Neurodevelopmental outcome of extremely low-birth-weight infants randomly assigned to restrictive or liberal hemoglobin thresholds for blood transfusion. Semin Perinatol. 2012;36(4):290–3.
41. Whyte R, Kirpalani H. Low versus high haemoglobin concentration threshold for blood transfusion for preventing morbidity and mortality in very low birth weight infants. Cochrane Database Syst Rev. 2011;(11):CD000512.
42. Charuvila S, Aziz TT, Davidson SE, Naznin U, Sinha S, Ahmed S, et al. An observational study of paediatric preoperative transfusion practice in a resource-limited setting. World J Surg. 2022;46(3):709–17.
43. Doctor A, Cholette JM, Remy KE, Argent A, Carson JL, Valentine SL, et al. Recommendations on RBC transfusion in general critically ill children based on hemoglobin and/or physiologic thresholds from the pediatric critical care transfusion and anemia expertise initiative. Pediatr Crit Care Med. 2018;19(9S Suppl 1):S98-S113:S98.
44. Park SK, Hur M, Kim E, Kim WH, Park JB, Kim Y, et al. Risk factors for acute kidney injury after congenital cardiac surgery in infants and children: a retrospective observational study. PLoS One. 2016;11(11):e0166328.
45. Zhou D, Deng LJ, Ling YF, Tang ML. Preoperative hemoglobin level, oxygen saturation and postoperative outcomes in children with cyanotic congenital heart disease: a propensity-score matching analysis. Front Pediatr. 2021;9:762241.
46. Guillén U, Cummings JJ, Bell EF, Hosono S, Frantz AR, Maier RF, et al. International survey of transfusion practices for extremely premature infants. Semin Perinatol. 2012;36(4):244–7.
47. Zagol K, Lake DE, Vergales B, Moorman ME, Paget-Brown A, Lee H, et al. Anemia, apnea of prematurity, and blood transfusions. J Pediatr. 2012;161(3):417–21.e1.
48. Lachance C, Chessex P, Fouron JC, Widness JA, Bard H. Myocardial, erythropoietic, and metabolic adaptations to anemia of prematurity. J Pediatr. 1994;125(2):278–82.
49. Bard H, Fouron JC, Chessex P, Widness JA. Myocardial, erythropoietic, and metabolic adaptations to anemia of prematurity in infants with bronchopulmonary dysplasia. J Pediatr. 1998;132(4):630–4.
50. Gidding SS, Stockman JA. Erythropoietin in cyanotic heart disease. Am Heart J. 1988;116(1 Pt 1):128–32.
51. Ahmed M, Acosta SI, Hoffman GM, Tweddell JS, Ghanayem NS. Mathematical analysis of hemoglobin target in univentricular parallel circulation. J Thorac Cardiovasc Surg. 2023;166(1):214–20.
52. Liu L, Qiang Z, Zhang J, Ren Y, Zhao X, Fu W, et al. Effect of hemoglobin content on cerebral oxygen saturation during surgery for scoliosis in pediatric patients. BMC Anesthesiol. 2021;21(1):165.
53. Mintzer JP, Parvez B, Chelala M, Alpan G, LaGamma EF. Monitoring regional tissue oxygen extraction in neonates <1250 g helps identify transfusion thresholds independent of hematocrit. J Neonatal Perinatal Med. 2014;7(2):89–100.
54. Balegar VKK, Low GK, Nanan RK. Regional tissue oxygenation and conventional indicators of red blood cell transfusion in anaemic preterm infants. EClinicalMedicine. 2022;46:101365.
55. Chock VY, Smith E, Tan S, Ball MB, Das A, Hintz SR, et al. Early brain and abdominal oxygenation in extremely low birth weight infants. Pediatr Res. 2022;92(4):1034–41.
56. Özakın E, Özcan Yazlamaz N, Baloğlu Kaya F, Çanakçı ME, Bilgin M. Lactate and base deficit combination score for predicting blood transfusion need in blunt multi-trauma patients. Ulus Travma Acil Cerrahi Derg. 2022;28(5):599–606.
57. Keung CY, Smith KR, Savoia HF, Davidson AJ. An audit of transfusion of red blood cell units in pediatric anesthesia. Paediatr Anaesth. 2009;19(4):320–8.
58. Frank SM, Oleyar MJ, Ness PM, Tobian AA. Reducing unnecessary preoperative blood orders and costs by implementing an updated institution-specific maximum surgical blood order schedule and a remote electronic blood release system. Anesthesiology. 2014;121(3):501–9.
59. Lou SS, Liu H, Lu C, Wildes TS, Hall BL, Kannampallil T. Personalized surgical transfusion risk prediction using machine learning to guide preoperative type and screen orders. Anesthesiology. 2022;137(1):55–66.

60. Special Patient Populations. Wong ECC, Roseff SD, editors. In: Pediatric transfusion: a handbook. Bethesda: AABB; 2020. p. 241.
61. Barcelona SL, Thompson AA, Coté CJ. Intraoperative pediatric blood transfusion therapy: a review of common issues. Part II: transfusion therapy, special considerations, and reduction of allogenic blood transfusions. Paediatr Anaesth. 2005;15(10):814–30.
62. Valentine SL, Bembea MM, Muszynski JA, Cholette JM, Doctor A, Spinella PC, et al. Consensus recommendations for RBC transfusion practice in critically ill children from the pediatric critical care transfusion and anemia expertise initiative. Pediatr Crit Care Med. 2018;19(9):884–98.
63. Hughes K, Chang YC, Sedrak J, Torres A. A clinically practical way to estimate surgical blood loss. Dermatol Online J. 2007;13(4):17.
64. Aran AA, Karam O, Nellis ME. Bleeding in critically ill children-review of literature, knowledge gaps, and suggestions for future investigation. Front Pediatr. 2021;9:611680.
65. Karam O, Nellis ME, Zantek ND, Lacroix J, Faustino EVS, BatPALIaSIP N. Criteria for clinically relevant bleeding in critically ill children: an international survey. Pediatr Crit Care Med. 2019;20(3):e137–e44.
66. Cote CJ, Grabowski EF, Stowell CP. Chapter 12: strategies for blood product management, reducing transfusions, and massive blood transfusion. In: Cote CJ, Lehman J, Anderson BJ, editors. Cote and Lerman's a practice of anesthesia for infants and children. 5th ed. Elsevier; 2019. p. 208–10, 259–80, 307, 317.
67. Sheth MM, Gangadharan M, Chau DF, Klein NJ. Pediatric blood management. In: Scher CS, Kaye AD, Liu H, Perelman S, editors. Essentials of blood product management in anesthesia. Springer; 2021. p. 243.
68. Josephson CD, Strauss RG. Chapter 497: Red blood cell transfusions and erythropoietin therapy. In: Kliegman RM, Geme JS, editors. Nelson textbook of pediatrics e-book. 21. 2019. Elsevier-OHCE; p. 2581–2587.
69. Kling PJ, Schmidt RL, Roberts RA, Widness JA. Serum erythropoietin levels during infancy: associations with erythropoiesis. J Pediatr. 1996;128(6):791–6.
70. Gallagher PG. The neonatal erythrocyte and its disorders. Nathan and Oski's Hematology and Oncology of Infancy and Childhood, 8th ed, Orkin SH, Fisher DE, Look T. Lux SE. Nathan DG (Eds), WB Saunders, Philadelphia: Ginsburg D; 2015. p. 52.
71. Evangeliou A, Dafnis E, Perdikoyanni C, Spilioti M, Lionis C, Kalmanti M. Hematological abnormalities in inborn errors of metabolism--how frequent are they? The Cretan experience Pediatr Hematol Oncol 2002;19(8):581–585.
72. Brown MS, Phibbs RH, Garcia JF, Dallman PR. Postnatal changes in erythropoietin levels in untransfused premature infants. J Pediatr. 1983;103(4):612–7.
73. Kaplan E, Hsu KS. Determination of erythrocyte survival in newborn infants by means of Cr51-labelled erythrocytes. Pediatrics. 1961;27:354–61.
74. Gallagher PG. Anemia in the pediatric patient. Blood. 2022;140(6):571–93.
75. Muncie HL, Campbell J. Alpha and beta thalassemia. Am Fam Physician. 2009;80(4):339–44.
76. Lanphear BP, Lowry JA, Ahoot S. Prevention of childhood lead toxicity. Pediatrics. 2016;138(1):e20161493. https://doi.org/10.1542/peds.2016-1493.
77. Tong S, Vichinsky E. Iron deficiency: implications before anemia. Pediatr Rev. 2021;42(1):11–20.
78. Chaparro CM, Suchdev PS. Anemia epidemiology, pathophysiology, and etiology in low- and middle-income countries. Ann N Y Acad Sci. 2019;1450(1):15–31.
79. Ning S, Zeller MP. Management of iron deficiency. Hematology Am Soc Hematol Educ Program. 2019;2019(1):315–22.
80. WHO. Guideline Daily Iron Supplementation in Infants and Children. 2016. https://apps.who.int/iris/bitstream/handle/10665/204712/9789241549523_eng.pdf. Accessed 17 Jan 2023.
81. Baker RD, Greer FR, Committee on Nutrition American Academy of P. Diagnosis and prevention of iron deficiency and iron-deficiency anemia in infants and young children (0-3 years of age). Pediatrics. 2010;126(5):1040–50.
82. Brill JR, Baumgardner DJ. Normocytic anemia. Am Fam Physician. 2000;62(10):2255–64.

83. Alobaidi R, Morgan C, Basu RK, Stenson E, Featherstone R, Majumdar SR, Bagshaw SM. Association between fluid balance and outcomes in critically ill children: a systematic review and meta-analysis. JAMA Pediatr. 2018;172(3):257–68.
84. Benediktsson SB, Karason S, Sigurdsson MI. Haemoglobin levels and outcomes of subgroups of patients with pre-operative anaemia based on red cell size: a retrospective cohort study. Acta Anaesthesiol Scand. 2023;67(4):422–31.
85. Lasocki S, Belbachir A, Mertes PM, Pelley EL, Capdevila X, study attiotP. Evaluation of anemia and iron deficiency in French surgical departments: The National Multicenter Observational PERIOPES Study. Anesth Analg. 2023.
86. Wang M. Iron deficiency and other types of anemia in infants and children. Am Fam Physician. 2016;93(4):270–8.
87. Basel A, Bajic D. Preoperative evaluation of the pediatric patient. Anesthesiol Clin. 2018;36(4):689–700.
88. Welborn LG, Hannallah RS, Luban NL, Fink R, Ruttimann UE. Anemia and postoperative apnea in former preterm infants. Anesthesiology. 1991;74(6):1003–6.
89. Bishara N, Ohls RK. Current controversies in the management of the anemia of prematurity. Semin Perinatol. 2009;33(1):29–34.
90. Eichenwald EC, Committee on Fetus and Newborn AeAoP. Apnea of prematurity. Pediatrics. 2016;137(1)
91. Vyas N, Hendren S, Tushar Sehgal DM, Monga C, Ranjan R, Chaturvedi H, et al. The accuracy of physical examination to diagnose anemia among patients five years or older: a systematic review. Indian J Hematol Blood Transfus. 2023;39(1):90–101.
92. Thornburg CD. The anemias. In: Kliegman RM, Geme JS, editors. Nelson Textbook of Pediatrics E-book. 21 2019. Elsevier-OHCE. p. 2505–2506.
93. Irwin JJ, Kirchner JT. Anemia in children. Am Fam Physician. 2001;64(8):1379–86.
94. Lin Y. Preoperative anemia-screening clinics. Hematology Am Soc Hematol Educ Program. 2019;2019(1):570–6.
95. Andersen CT, Marsden DM, Duggan CP, Liu E, Mozaffarian D, Fawzi WW. Oral iron supplementation and anaemia in children according to schedule, duration, dose and cosupplementation: a systematic review and meta-analysis of 129 randomised trials. BMJ Glob Health. 2023;8(2)
96. Fuerst ML. Formula-fed preterm infants more likely to have iron deficiency. Oncology Times. 2023;45(S4):22.
97. Pizarro F, Yip R, Dallman PR, Olivares M, Hertrampf E, Walter T. Iron status with different infant feeding regimens: relevance to screening and prevention of iron deficiency. J Pediatr. 1991;118(5):687–92.
98. Powers JM, Daniel CL, McCavit TL, Buchanan GR. Deficiencies in the management of iron deficiency anemia during childhood. Pediatr Blood Cancer. 2016;63(4):743–5.
99. Warner MA, Shore-Lesserson L, Shander A, Patel SY, Perelman SI, Guinn NR. Perioperative anemia: prevention, diagnosis, and management throughout the Spectrum of perioperative care. Anesth Analg. 2020;130(5):1364–80.
100. Cohen CT, Powers JM. Intravenous iron therapy in pediatrics: who should get it and when is the right time? Hematology Am Soc Hematol Educ Program. 2023;2023(1):630–5.
101. Saito-Benz M, Flanagan P, Berry MJ. Management of anaemia in pre-term infants. Br J Haematol. 2020;188(3):354–66.
102. Killian A. Pediatric use of recombinant erythropoietin. Pediatric. Pharmacotherapy. 2002:8. https://med.virginia.edu/pediatrics/wp-content/uploads/sites/237/2015/12/200211.pdf. Accessed 28 Jan 2023
103. Ali SME, Hafeez MH, Nisar O, Fatima S, Ghous H, Rehman M. Role of preoperative erythropoietin in the optimization of preoperative anemia among surgical patients—a systematic review and meta-analysis. Hematol Transfus Cell Ther. 2022;44(1):76–84.
104. Aljaaly HA, Aldekhayel SA, Diaz-Abele J, Karunanayka M, Gilardino MS. Effect of erythropoietin on transfusion requirements for Craniosynostosis surgery in children. J Craniofac Surg. 2017;28(5):1315–9.

105. Naran S, Cladis F, Fearon J, Bradley J, Michelotti B, Cooper G, et al. Safety of preoperative erythropoietin in surgical calvarial remodeling: an 8-year retrospective review and analysis. Plast Reconstr Surg. 2012;130(2):305e–10e.
106. Meneghini L, Zadra N, Aneloni V, Metrangolo S, Faggin R, Giusti F. Erythropoietin therapy and acute preoperative normovolaemic haemodilution in infants undergoing craniosynostosis surgery. Paediatr Anaesth. 2003;13(5):392–6.
107. Shimpo H, Mizumoto T, Onoda K, Yuasa H, Yada I. Erythropoietin in pediatric cardiac surgery: clinical efficacy and effective dose. Chest. 1997;111(6):1565–70.
108. Faraoni D, Meier J, New HV, Van der Linden PJ, Hunt BJ. Patient blood Management for Neonates and Children Undergoing Cardiac Surgery: 2019 NATA guidelines. J Cardiothorac Vasc Anesth. 2019;33(12):3249–63.
109. Smith KJ, Bleyer AJ, Little WC, Sane DC. The cardiovascular effects of erythropoietin. Cardiovasc Res. 2003;59(3):538–48.
110. Stowell CP, Jones SC, Enny C, Langholff W, Leitz G. An open-label, randomized, parallel-group study of perioperative epoetin alfa versus standard of care for blood conservation in major elective spinal surgery: safety analysis. Spine (Phila Pa 1976). 2009;34(23):2479–85.
111. Beris P, Munoz M, Garcia-Erce JA, Thomas D, Maniatis A, Van der Linden P. Perioperative anaemia management: consensus statement on the role of intravenous iron. Br J Anaesth. 2008;100(5):599–604.
112. Leal-Noval SR, Munoz M, Asuero M, Contreras E, Garcia-Erce JA, Llau JV, et al. [The 2013 Seville Consensus Document on alternatives to allogenic blood transfusion. An update on the Seville Document]. Rev Esp Anestesiol Reanim. 2013;60(5):263 e1- e25.
113. Kotze A, Harris A, Baker C, Iqbal T, Lavies N, Richards T, et al. British Committee for Standards in Haematology guidelines on the identification and management of pre-operative anaemia. Br J Haematol. 2015;171(3):322–31.
114. Shander A, Corwin HL, Meier J, Auerbach M, Bisbe E, Blitz J, et al. Recommendations from the International Consensus Conference on Anemia Management in Surgical Patients (ICCAMS). Ann Surg. 2023;277(4):581–90.
115. Wong ECC. Hematology tests. In: Wong ECC, Brugnara C, Straseski JA, editors. Pediatric reference intervals. London: Academic Press; 2020. p. 215–52.

Informed Consent for Blood Transfusion

5

Norma J. Klein

Case Scenario

A 12-year-old boy with a hemoglobinopathy is admitted for central line placement. He requires chronic transfusion and chelation therapy, and his peripheral venous access is very limited. During the preoperative interview, the surgeon asks you to order an RBC transfusion because his hemoglobin is 6 g/dL. When you ask the surgeon if the boy and his family have given informed consent for the transfusion, he replies that a separate informed consent is unnecessary because the general surgical consent form includes the possibility of transfusion. Both the patient and his parents question the indication for transfusion. He has a history of frequent transfusion reactions, including fevers and alloantibody formation. He is asymptomatic, his vital signs are normal for age, and he is hemodynamically stable.

Key Learning Objectives

- Does a blood transfusion require a separate informed consent?
- May a 13-year-old boy refuse a blood transfusion?

5.1 General

5.1.1 Introduction

The following case scenario highlights two important aspects of pediatric informed consent for blood transfusion. The first is whether a separate transfusion-related informed consent is necessary. The second important issue is patient refusal. The following discussion with review the necessity for a separate informed consent for

N. J. Klein (✉)
Department of Anesthesiology and Pain Medicine, University of California, Davis, Sacramento, CA, USA
e-mail: nklein@ucdavis.edu

N. J. Klein (ed.), *Perioperative Pediatric Patient Blood Management and Transfusion Safety*, https://doi.org/10.1007/978-3-031-81666-6_5

blood transfusion as well as the legal, regulatory, and ethical background supporting pediatric patient refusal of transfusion.

5.2 Discussion

Informed consent is the result of a shared agreement between patient or surrogate and the physician to undergo a treatment following disclosure of relevant risks, benefits, and alternatives [1]. The principle of informed consent is grounded in a history of legal precedents and ethical principles. As early as the eighteenth century, a British court recognized that performing a procedure on a person without prior permission is akin to battery [2]. Later legal proceedings in the United States (US) recognized the importance of patient autonomy or self-determination, which became a springboard for the term, "informed consent" [3, 4]. The elements of informed consent and the practitioner's duty of disclosure were later described in US Supreme Court cases during the 1960s [5, 6]. The bioethical underpinnings of informed consent include recognition of patients' right to self-determination or autonomy, maximization of benefits, minimization of harm, preservation of privacy, and equitable treatment [7]. Recently, the Institute of Medicine, the American Medical Association (AMA), and the AABB (Association for the Advancement of Blood & Biotherapeutics) have prioritized patient-centered care, defined as, "providing care that is respectful of and responsive to individual patient preferences, needs, and values and ensuring that patient values guide all clinical decisions" [1, 8–10]. Given that a blood transfusion is a clinical decision, a properly executed informed consent entails a shared and patient-centered decision-making process, including pediatric patients when possible [10–12].

5.2.1 Informed Consent for Blood Transfusion

Many practitioners consider a transfusion to be a minor or noninvasive event when, in fact, it is a form of organ transplantation with many associated risks [13–15]. Heightened public concern over transfusion risks arose during the HIV epidemic of the 1980s, when hemophilia patients developed unusual symptoms from a yet unidentified disease. When that disease was described in 1984 and a donor screening test for HIV was developed a year later, it became apparent that HIV transmission could occur through the donor blood supply [13]. Other transfusion transmitted infections (TTI) of concern included hepatitis B and C in the hemophiliac patient population in the 1960s and hepatitis C in the 1990s. Creutzfeldt-Jacob disease (CJD), for which there is still no serologic testing and which may be impossible to trace to a specific transfusion event, creates a dilemma over the content of an informed consent risk discussion [16].

The US Centers for Disease Control (CDC) and other outcome-related surveillance programs have identified patterns in transfusion-related adverse reactions and events as a result of systemic monitoring programs developed in the early part of this century [17, 18]. These organized monitoring efforts have resulted in process and education improvements, including a recommendation that a separate and focused informed consent procedure occur prior to all blood transfusions [1, 18]. Although many hospital consent forms list the possibility of blood transfusion, this fact is often glossed over, or only found in the fine print of the consent form [19]. The International Society of Blood Transfusion (ISBT) first recommended that a procedure specific consent process occur prior to transfusion in 1980 [1]. The AABB, a gold standard for US blood bank certification in blood product quality and patient transfusion safety, followed with a similar recommendation in 1986 [1, 20, 21]. In some settings, a transfusion-specific informed consent process is required by law: California's Paul Gann Act was passed in 1990 after political activist, Paul Gann, contracted HIV from a blood transfusion received during surgery [20]. The Gann Act requires discussion of risks, benefit, alternatives, as well as the potential for autologous donation, if a transfusion is "reasonably" anticipated [22]. The US Joint Commission (TJC) requires subject healthcare organizations to establish a process for informed consent prior to transfusion as part of the Patient Blood Management Certification quality program [23]. Furthermore, many hospitals have a requirement in their bylaws for a separate pretransfusion consent.

Several associations have specified the essential elements of a pretransfusion informed consent [1, 18, 21, 23, 24]. The AABB suggests that a transfusion recipient should be informed of the indication for the transfusion as well as its benefits, potential risks, and any alternative therapies [25]. The elements of the consent, including the patient's expressed willingness to proceed with the transfusion, should be clearly documented in the medical record according to institutional guidelines [1]. Studies indicate that the informed consent process is not documented in a substantial percentage of transfusion events and that the patients often do not recall the consent discussion [20, 26, 27]. The ASA, in its *Statement of Documentation of Anesthesia Care* (2018), prioritizes documentation of informed consent as an "essential element of high quality and safe medical care" [28]. In the United Kingdom, national guidelines include informing patients if they have received an emergency or undisclosed blood transfusion prior to hospital discharge, along with the possibility that they may no longer qualify as a blood donor [12, 29, 30].

It may be challenging to properly execute the pretransfusion informed consent process with children who may have limited ability to understand and deliberate about medical decisions. Studies also indicate that the discussion of transfusion risks is often imperfect, with patients having different risk concerns than what is presented to them [20, 26, 31, 32]. One survey found that patients tend to focus on the infectious risks associated with transfusion, whereas physicians emphasized other risks such as allergic and febrile reactions, transfusion-related acute lung injury (TRALI), and transfusion-associated circulatory overload (TACO), although the latter two risks are relatively rare [32]. Reportedly, transfusion specialists have received an increased number of parental requests that their child's transfusion come from a nonvaccinated donor [33]. The AABB has published an online informational document entitled, "Vaccination and Blood Donation", to assist practitioners when obtaining patient informed consent for a blood transfusion.

The pretransfusion consent process may be simplified with the understanding that transfusion-associated risks fall into several general categories: Infectious, non-infectious, and risks amplified by the patient's comorbidities [16]. For example, a neonate is highly susceptible to TACO in part because of its relatively small size as well as the relatively large, recommended transfusion volumes (10–15 mL/kg versus approximately 4 mL/kg in the average adult packed red blood cell (RBC) unit transfusion) [34–36]. In contrast, that same infant may have less risk of a transfusion transmitted infection (TTI) due to the smaller transfusion volume. The patient's developmental level and the parents' assessed ability to understand should guide the discussion, and any risks discussed should reflect what a reasonable person with a particular condition would want to know [10]. Known risks associated with transfusions can be found in *A Compendium of Transfusion Practice Guidelines*, *Appendix II,* published by the AABB and available online or through mobile application [37]. However, this regularly updated report is not specific to the pediatric patient population. Children reportedly have adverse reactions to blood transfusions significantly more often than adults [38, 39]. Currently, the most detailed pediatric-specific hemovigilance data comes from the United Kingdom's annual Serious Hazards of Transfusion (SHOT) hemovigilance report [14, 34].

Healthcare professionals often do not receive formal education in either transfusion therapy or the informed consent process [20, 31, 32]. The difficulty of performing and documenting a transfusion-related informed consent process is underscored by the likelihood that a preoperative interview may last less than 10 min [40]. It is recommended that the informed consent process should be carried out by a licensed physician with sufficient knowledge of bedside transfusions [10, 25]. That physician is unlikely to be a medical student or a relatively inexperienced resident in training. Some institutions credential advanced practice practitioners, such as nurse practitioners (NP's) or certified nurse anesthetists (CRNA's), to obtain consent for transfusion. Institutional policies should also specify the applicable time period for which the consent is valid. Often, transfusion-related consent for hospitalized patients is valid only for a particular admission, but consent for patients requiring chronic transfusions on an outpatient basis may be valid for up to 1 year or more, barring a significant change in medical condition [25].

5.2.2 Refusal of a Blood Transfusion by a Minor Child

As a rule, a patient who is legally competent and has decision-making capacity has a right to refuse a transfusion. However, young children are not considered to be legally competent and are presumed to lack the decision-making capacity necessary to participate in the informed consent process. *Competence* is a legal term determined in a court of law and describes a patient's ability to give informed consent [7]. *Capacity* usually applies to specific situations or events, at a particular place or time, and may be determined through mental status testing. A patient with decision-making capacity has an ability to understand the information relayed and can reason, weigh outcomes, and reach a decision. An example of a patient who is competent to make medical decisions but lacks decision-making capacity is the non-English speaking and reading adult patient who receives the informed consent in English language only; another example is the intermittently psychotic adult patient who is actively hallucinating. In most US states, the age of legal competence is 18 years; the age for consent typically focuses on legally permitted sexual activity and is approximately 16–18 years [10, 41].

Some children are considered to have the decision-making capacity to make certain healthcare decisions, particularly adolescents or chronically ill younger children [42–44]. Initially, a child's chronologic age is used to assess her capacity to consent to a blood transfusion. The American Academy of Pediatrics (AAP) defines a minor as a person less than 18 years; an adolescent is between 13 and 18 years; a child is less than 12 years; an infant is less than 12 months of age [10]. The "Rule of 7" is often used to determine capacity for medical decision-making, which is based on three, age-related categories: For children over 14 years, capacity is *presumed*—but rebuttable—based upon the circumstances of the case; a capacity determination in children 7–14 years must be supported by evidentiary facts; children less than 7 years are not considered to possess decision-making capacity [45].

For children over the age of 7, according to the Rule of 7 paradigm, patients must provide informed *assent* and parents must provide *permission* for transfusion. The dictionary definition of assent is the "expression of approval" [46]. However, children vary significantly in cognitive ability, maturation level, and life experience, so age alone may not determine the capacity to make safe, reasonable medical decisions [9]. Underlying a young patient's ability to provide assent is the ability to understand the information provided, to reason cause-and-effect, and to appreciate the potential outcomes of their decision. The AAP recommends that the physician explain to the child both her condition and the proposed treatment in age-appropriate terms, followed by an evaluation of the child's understanding of the process and any potential factors that may unduly influence the decision [10]. In all cases, except life-sustaining emergency transfusions, feedback should be sought from both the older child and the parent to confirm a voluntary willingness to proceed.

A decision to transfuse a child under the age of 7 should be made according to a "best interest" standard with concomitant *parental permission*. What constitutes a child's best interest should be defined in the context of the individual child while weighing the potential for harm, the effect on the child's lifespan or quality of life, and the likelihood of maintaining the child's physical and psychological well-being. In the past, a "best interest" standard has been used to guide practitioner evaluation of parental decisions for their child; however, other considerations such as the likelihood of harm resulting from the parents' decision may come into play [10].

There are exceptions to general rule that minor patients require parental permission prior to a transfusion. In the US, although each state may have different statutory criteria, the "emancipated minor" may make independent medical decisions for herself. These minors typically include those that are married, pregnant, financially independent, or in military service. Older, more mature minors may obtain "mature minor" independent status through a judicial determination for specific events, including transfusion decisions. In the case of Re E.G. 1989, a 17-year-old adolescent of the Jehovah's Witness faith was allowed to refuse a transfusion for a life-threatening condition, supported by the fact that the parents were in agreement [44]. In the case of 14-year-old Dennis Linberg who was critically ill with leukemia, a Washington court allowed him to refuse a life-saving blood transfusion as the case went through the court system; Daniel died during the legal proceedings [10]. Although these cases illustrate the fact that minors with chronic illness may have advanced maturity and capacity for healthcare decision-making, the acceptance of a transfusion refusal should involve consideration of the likelihood of treatment success, transfusion risks, the patient's prognosis for recovery, and family dynamics or culture. When an older minor refuses a transfusion but has relatively significant life experience (such as a chronic illness requiring regular transfusions) or lives independently, a refusal of transfusion may be considered appropriate as long as it does not create imminent harm, and the consequences of refusal are less burdensome than an involuntary, court-ordered state intervention [10, 47, 48]. In accordance with the duty of beneficence, the practitioner should assist the patient and family in making a decision that is in the best interest for all, which may include consulting extended family or respected community members [7].

Parents are tasked with responsibility for their child's healthcare management as surrogate decision-makers because they are deemed to be knowledgeable about what is best for their child. However, this responsibility has boundaries and is limited when a parental decision has the potential for harm. When assessing the minor patient's capacity for medical decision-making, the practitioner must also examine the appropriateness of the parents as surrogate decision-makers. As early as 1944, the US Supreme Court opined that parents may not freely harm their child, and although "parents may be free to become martyrs themselves, they are not free to make martyrs of their children" [10, 49]. What may be presumed to be in a patient's best interest is a subjective evaluation, and may vary between patients and also surrogate decision-makers. Additionally, the effect that any medical decision may have on the family unit, the child's place within that unit, and the child's future as an autonomous individual is important and should receive strong consideration [7]. Today, parents in the US are not allowed to refuse a life-saving transfusion for their child when the benefit of transfusion outweighs the risk of death or imminent harm [10, 50, 51]. Thus, in some cases of patient or parent refusal, the best interest standard may have to be put aside for a "harm" standard when the risk of refusal is likely to bring about an untoward outcome.

Disagreement over a potential blood transfusion may occur between the minor child, the parents (or surrogate decision-maker), and the physician. Such a conflict should be evaluated in light of potential harm that may arise as a result of refusal [7, 10]. An adverse medical experience (such as an unwanted blood transfusion) may negatively impact family dynamics as well the patient's trust in the medical community. Management dilemmas may present in a variety of ways and are best addressed through multidisciplinary review when circumstances allow [9, 47, 52]:

Transfusions of uncertain benefit:

- A transfusion that is refused but is of unclear benefit should not be performed without further consultation and multidisciplinary review through available hospital legal, ethics, social service, and spiritual services.

Transfusions of clear benefit in a nonemergency situation:

- If the child is refusing a life-saving transfusion, the reasons for refusal and the child's clinical picture should be evaluated in the context of the family dynamic. A state mandated ("court order") transfusion may be required.
- If a blood transfusion is considered lifesaving but is known to be associated with significant side effects (as in the case of a bone marrow transplant), patient or parent refusal should undergo serious consideration through multidisciplinary consultation.
- A most challenging situation is refusal of a nonemergency transfusion that will clearly benefit the child, but the child is hemodynamically stable. An example is the child about to undergo an elective blood loss procedure with a preoperative hemoglobin of 6 g/dL. In this case, a transfusion should not be administered without multidisciplinary case review as well as proactive hemoglobin optimization and assessment of the patient's anemia tolerance.
- If a child is about to undergo an urgent procedure not typically associated with blood loss (such as an appendectomy), the operation may proceed without a consent for blood transfusion. However, the anesthesiologist and surgeon should inform the patient and family that a transfusion may proceed if critically needed.

Transfusions of clear benefit in an emergency:

- In any pediatric surgery where refusal of transfusion is not in the patient's best interest because of imminent threat of severe, life-threatening, or irreversible consequences, the physician may be required to become the decision-maker and proceed with a transfusion while the patient or family refusal is under review.
- A pediatric emergency in which the patient is under imminent threat of harm that can be reversed through a blood transfusion is an exception to the requirement for consent, assent, or parental permission when not feasible. An example is the unconscious child with an intracranial hemorrhage brought into the operating room without parents or guardian present.

In many cases of transfusion refusal, applying the pillars of patient blood management (PBM)—optimization of red cell mass, optimizing the patient's anemia tolerance, and planning to minimize perioperative blood loss—will simultaneously promote patient empowerment, satisfaction, and positive outcomes [53].

5.3 Summary of Key Learning Objectives

5.3.1 Does a Blood Transfusion Require a Separate Informed Consent?

Organizations with oversight of blood transfusion quality and safety—including the AABB, WHO, the JC, and ISBT—recommend that a transfusion-specific consent process should occur prior to any anticipated, nonemergency transfusion event. One basis for this policy is that blood transfusions are not without significant risk, as evidenced by accumulated hemovigilance data over the past several decades. The consent process should include a developmentally appropriate explanation of the indication for transfusion, as well as anticipated benefits, relevant risks, and alternative treatments available. This conversation should be documented in the patient's medical record according to institutional guidelines, along with a statement that the patient and the parents or guardian are willing to proceed.

5.3.2 May a 12-Year-Old Boy Refuse a Blood Transfusion?

A legally competent patient with decision-making capacity has a right to refuse a transfusion. Although this patient is 12 years old and younger than an adolescent, who may be capable of making relatively complex medical decisions, it is likely that this child has significant lifetime and chronic transfusion experience, and his refusal should be given serious consideration. There are no facts presented to suggest that he lacks decision-making capacity. Furthermore, the need for a transfusion is questioned by his parents, who are presumed to be acting in their child's best interest and who have raised him throughout his chronic condition. From a medical standpoint, transfusion refusal is supported by the nonemergency nature of the procedure, a low likelihood of blood loss, and a physiologically compensated chronic anemia. In addition, this child may be at increased risk secondary to a history of iron overload requiring chelation therapy and alloantibody formation. Acceptance of the family's refusal may be appropriate under the biomedical principle of nonmaleficence (avoiding harm to family dynamic by administering a transfusion of unclear benefit). From a legal standpoint, a transfusion at this juncture in care is not lifesaving and thus is not clearly in the patient's best interest to prevent serious or long-lasting harm. Although beyond the scope of this analysis, it is recommended that the RBC transfusion trigger for patients receiving transfusions on a chronic, regular basis should be individualized based on the entire clinical context and not on a single hemoglobin level [54]. If life-threatening bleeding does occur during the surgery, a transfusion may proceed if doing so is in the child's best interest, with appropriate chart documentation of the reason for transfusion. Ideally, the patient and his parents should be informed of any blood transfusion prior to hospital discharge.

Key Points

- Organizations that oversee blood product quality and transfusion safety recommend that a formal consent process occur prior to transfusion.
- When informing a patient and family of the risks, benefits, and alternatives of a proposed blood transfusion, the patient's developmental level and the parents' assessed ability to understand the situation should guide the discussion.
- The "Rule of 7s" is often used to determine capacity for medical decision-making based on the patient's age. However, children vary significantly in cognitive ability, maturation level, and life experience; therefore, age alone may not determine decision-making capacity.
- Some minor patients do not require parental permission prior to a transfusion: those that are married, pregnant, financially independent, in military service, or adjudicated to be emancipated under state law.
- Parental decision-making responsibility has boundaries and is limited when there is a potential for harm. Today, parents in the US are not allowed to refuse a life-saving transfusion for their child when the benefit of transfusion outweighs the risk of death or imminent harm.
- In any pediatric surgery where refusal of transfusion is not in the patient's best interest because of imminent threat of severe, life-threatening, or irreversible consequences, the practitioner may proceed with a transfusion while the patient or family refusal undergoes multidisciplinary review.

References

1. Domen RE, Smith ML. Ethical aspects of informed consent. In: Domen RE, editor. Ethical issues in transfusion and cellular therapies. Bethesda: AABB; 2015. p. 15–26.
2. Slater v Baker and Stapleton (C.B. 1767).
3. Schloendorff v. Society of New York Hospital, 211 NY 125 (1914).
4. Salgo v Leland Stanford Jr University 317 P 2d 170 (Cal App, 1957).
5. Natanson v Klein, 186 Kan. 393; 350 P. 2d 1093 (1960).
6. Mitchell v Robinson, 334 SW 2d 11 (1960).
7. Lo B. Resolving ethical dilemmas: a guide for clinicians. 5th ed. Philadelphia: Lippincott Williams & Wilkins; 2013. p. 79–81, 267–77.
8. Alston C. Institute of Medicine of the National Academies, National Academy of Sciences, Shared Decision-Making Strategies for Best Care. In: Patient Decision Aids. 2014. https://nam.edu/wp-content/uploads/2015/06/SDMforBestCare2.pdf. Accessed 10 Nov 2021.
9. Statement on recommendations for surgeons caring for patients who are Jehovah's witnesses. In: The Bulletin of the American College of Surgeons (ACS). Sept 2018. https://www.facsbulletin.com/acsbulletin/september2018/MobilePagedReplica.action?pm=2&folio=Cover#pg1. Accessed 2 June 2023.
10. Katz AL, Webb SA. Informed consent in decision-making in pediatric practice. Pediatrics. 2016;138(2):e20161485. https://doi.org/10.1542/peds.2016-1485.
11. American Medical Association (AMA). Pediatric decision making. Code of Medical Ethics Opinion 2.2.1. 2021. https://www.ama-assn.org/delivering-care/ethics/pediatric-decision-making. Accessed 10 Nov 2021.

12. NICE National Institute for Health and Care Excellence. Blood transfusion. NICE guideline [NG24]. 2015. https://www.nice.org.uk/guidance/ng24/chapter/Recommendations#patient-information-2. Accessed 22 Mar 2022.
13. Kopko PM. Transfusion reactions. 5th ed. Bethesda: AABB Press; 2021. p. 83, 121, 233–49.
14. Serious Hazards of Transfusion (SHOT). United Kingdom. 2020. https://www.shotuk.org/shot-reports/(2020). Accessed 10 Nov 2021.
15. Serious Hazards of Transfusion (SHOT) Annual Report. 2021. https://www.shotuk.org/wp-content/uploads/myimages/SHOT-REPORT-2021-FINAL-bookmarked-V3-November.pdf. Accessed 2 June 2023.
16. Hart J, Leier B, Nahirniak S. Informed consent for blood transfusion: should the possibility of prion risk be included? Transfus Med Rev. 2004;18(3):177–83.
17. Centers for Disease Control and Prevention (CDC). National Healthcare Safety Network, Blood Safety. https://www.cdc.gov/nhsn/biovigilance/blood-safety/index.html. Accessed 10 Nov 2021.
18. International Society of Blood Transfusion (ISBT). 1999. https://education.isbtweb.org/isbt/document_library?dc_id=829&f=listing%3D0%2Abrowseby%3D8%2Asortby%3D1%2Asearch%3Dinformed+consent. Accessed 10 Nov 2021.
19. Lenet T, Skanes S, Tropiano J, Verret M, McIsaac DI, Tinmouth A, et al. Patient perspectives on intraoperative blood transfusion: a qualitative interview study with perioperative patients. Transfusion. 2023;63(2):305–14.
20. Booth C, Grant-Casey J, Lowe D, Court EL, Allard S, National Comparative Audit of Blood Transfusion Project Group for Patient Information and Consent. National Comparative Audit of blood transfusion: report on the 2014 audit of patient information and consent. Transfus Med. 2018;28(4):271–6.
21. Kaplan A, Arinsburg SA, Puca KE, Coberly E. Informed consent for blood transfusion. The Association for the Advancement of Blood & Biotherapeutics. 2023. https://www.aabb.org/docs/default-source/default-document-library/resources/informed-consent-for-blood-transfusion.pdf?sfvrsn=b2ee9851_2. Accessed 5 June 2023.
22. State of California. Health and safety code. Chapter 4.5. The Paul Gann Blood Safety Act. Section 1645. https://leginfo.legislature.ca.gov/faces/codes_displayText.xhtml?lawCode=HSC&division=2.&title=∂=&chapter=4.5.&article=(2008). Accessed 10 Nov 2021.
23. The Joint Commission, Patient blood management review process guide. 2021. https://www.jointcommission.org/-/media/tjc/documents/accred-and-cert/survey-process-and-survey-activity-guide/2021/2021-patient-blood-mgmt-organization-rpg.pdf. Accessed 11 Nov 2021.
24. Mintz PD. Informed consent for blood transfusion and the joint commission. Am J Clin Pathol. 2013;139(5):693.
25. Fung MK, editor. Technical manual. 19th ed. Bethesda: AABB Press; 2017. p. 489.
26. Cheung D, Lieberman L, Lin Y, Callum J. Consent for blood transfusion: do patients understand the risks and benefits? Transfus Med. 2014;24(5):269–73.
27. Flores CJ, Lakkundi A, McIntosh J, Freeman P, Thomson A, Saxon B, et al. Embedding best transfusion practice and blood management in neonatal intensive care. BMJ Open Qual. 2020;9(1):e000694. https://doi.org/10.1136/bmjoq-2019-000694.
28. American Society of Anesthesiologists (ASA). Statement of documentation of anesthesia care. In: Guidelines, standards, clinical resources. 2018. https://www.asahq.org/standards-and-guidelines/statement-on-documentation-of-anesthesia-care. Accessed 10 Nov 2021.
29. NHS blood and transplant. Blood components mobile application version 2.0.8.: other considerations. https://www.nice.org.uk. Accessed 28 Nov 2021.
30. NICE quality standard QS 138: Blood transfusion. NICE National Institute for Health and Care Excellence. 2016. https://www.nice.org.uk/guidance/qs138/chapter/Quality-statements. Accessed 17 Mar 2022.
31. Vetter TR, Adhami LF, Porterfield JR, Marques MB. Perceptions about blood transfusion: a survey of surgical patients and their anesthesiologists and surgeons. Anesth Analg. 2014;118(6):1301–8.

32. Friedman M, Arja W, Batra R, Daniel S, Hoehn D, Paniz AM, et al. Informed consent for blood transfusion: what do medicine residents tell? What do patients understand? Am J Clin Pathol. 2012;138(4):559–65.
33. Applewhite KY. A look at parental autonomy in pediatric transfusion medicine. AABB News. February 2023. p. 12. https://www.aabb.org/docs/default-source/member-protected-files/news/aabb-news-magazine/news2302.pdf?sfvrsn=1cb84f7c_4.
34. Serious hazards of transfusion and medicines and healthcare products regulatory agency, SHOT Bite No. 4: Lessons in pediatrics. 2018. http://www.isbtweb.org/fileadmin/user_upload/SHOT-Bite-No-4-Lessons-in-Paediatrics-July-2018.pdf. Accessed 11 Nov 2021.
35. Australian government national health and medical research council, patient blood management guidelines: module 6 (neonatal and pediatric). 2016. https://www.blood.gov.au/pbm-module-6. Accessed 11 Nov 2021.
36. Serious hazards of transfusion and medicines and healthcare products regulatory agency (SHOT). United Kingdom. 2020. https://www.shotuk.org/shot-reports/2020. Accessed 25 May 2023.
37. Borge, D (ed). A compendium of transfusion practice guidelines, appendix II. American Red Cross. 2021. https://www.redcrossblood.org/content/dam/redcrossblood/rcb/biomedical-services/components/compendium_v_4.0.pdf. Accessed 10 Nov 2021.
38. Oakley FD, Woods M, Arnold S, Young PP. Transfusion reactions in pediatric compared with adult patients: a look at rate, reaction type, and associated products. Transfusion. 2015;55(3):563–70.
39. Vossoughi S, Perez G, Whitaker BI, Fung MK, Stotler B. Analysis of pediatric adverse reactions to transfusions. Transfusion. 2018;58(1):60–9.
40. Gentry KR, Lepere K, Opel DJ. Informed consent in pediatric anesthesiology. Paediatr Anaesth. 2017;27(12):1253–60.
41. Age of Consent in the United States, Wikipedia. 2020. https://en.wikipedia.org/wiki/Ages_of_consent_in_the_United_States. Accessed 5 Dec 2021.
42. Barbeau JM. The Jehovah's witness patient: ethical and legal issues. In: Domen RE, editor. Ethical issues in transfusion medicine and cellular therapies. Bethesda: AABB Press; 2015. p. 159–70.
43. Cardwell v. Bechtel, 724 S.W.2d 739,750 (Tenn. 1987).
44. In re E.G. 161 Ill. App. 3d 765 (Ill. App. Ct. 1987) N.E.2d 286.
45. Carollo DS, Mann DG. The ethics of pediatric informed consent. American Society of Anesthesiologists. 2018. https://pubs.asahq.org/monitor/article/82/11/10/3403/The-Ethics-of-Pediatric-Informed-Consent. Accessed 28 Nov 2021.
46. "Assent." Merriam-Webster.com Dictionary, Merriam-Webster, https://www.merriam-webster.com/dictionary/assent. Accessed 10 Nov 2021.
47. Waisel DB. Informed consent: the core of pediatric bioethics. 2008. https://www2.pedsanesthesia.org/meetings/2008annual/syllabus/Lecture-Waisel.pdf. Accessed 28 Nov 2021.
48. President's Commission for the Study of Ethical Problems in Medicine and Biomedical and Behavioral Research. Deciding to forego life-sustaining treatment: ethical, medical and legal issues in treatment decisions. Washington, DC: U.S. Government Printing Office; 1983.
49. Prince v. Massachusetts, 321 U.S. 158 (1944).
50. Religious objections to medical care. American Academy of Pediatrics Committee on bioethics. Pediatrics. 1997;99(2):279–81.
51. Clendenin D, Waisel DB. Informed Consent and the pediatric patient. In: Van Norman GA, editor. Clinical ethics in Anesthesiology: a case-based textbook. Cambridge: Cambridge University Press; 2011. p. 33–8.
52. Committee on Pediatric Emergency Medicine and Committee on Bioethics. Consent for emergency medical services for children and adolescents. Pediatrics. 2011;128(2):427–33.
53. Shander A, Hardy JF, Ozawa S, Farmer SL, Hofmann A, Frank SM, et al. A global definition of patient blood management. Anesth Analg. 2022;135(3):476–88.
54. NHS blood and transplant. Blood components mobile application version 2.0.8. 2020. https://www.nice.org.uk. Accessed 28 Nov 2021.

Hospital-Acquired Anemia (HAA) and Blood Conservation

6

Michelle Sheth, Renira Rugnath, John Adams, Forrest Duncan, Patricia Amolenda, and Norma J. Klein

Case Scenario

You are a pediatric intensive care fellow and are moonlighting as a pediatric hospitalist in a large community hospital. When discharging patients, you note that many leave the hospital with a significant decrease in their hemoglobin (Hgb) level. The trend is particularly noteworthy for infants and children who have undergone surgery. You decide to examine the issue more closely as part of a quality project for your fellowship. Your goal is to reduce the number of patients who are anemic upon hospital discharge.

Key Learning Objectives

- What is the burden of anemia in patients presenting for surgery?
- How does one differentiate between physiologic, illness-associated, and HAA?
- Which patients are at greatest risk of HAA?
- What are some of the situational factors that contribute to HAA?
- What specific practice strategies can prevent HAA?

M. Sheth (✉)
Anesthesiology and Pediatrics, Department of Anesthesiology, University of Mississippi Medical Center, Jackson, MS, USA
e-mail: Msheth2@umc.edu

R. Rugnath · J. Adams · F. Duncan · P. Amolenda
Department of Anesthesiology, University of Mississippi Medical Center, Jackson, MS, USA
e-mail: rrugnath@umc.edu; jadams3@umc.edu; fduncan@umc.edu; pamolenda@umc.edu

N. J. Klein
Department of Anesthesiology and Pain Medicine, University of California, Davis, Sacramento, CA, USA
e-mail: nklein@ucdavis.edu

N. J. Klein (ed.), *Perioperative Pediatric Patient Blood Management and Transfusion Safety*, https://doi.org/10.1007/978-3-031-81666-6_6

6.1 Discussion

6.1.1 What Is the Burden of Anemia in Patients Presenting for Surgery?

Anemia is a pathologic condition of global proportions. The World Health Organization (WHO) estimates that more than one-half of pre-school children across the globe are anemic, with the greatest burden in children between 6 and 12 months due to rapid growth and inadequate iron intake [1, 2]. More than two billion persons worldwide are anemic, with the South Asia and Sub-Saharan Africa regions most affected [3, 4]. Before 6 months iron stores and maternal breast milk iron content often forestall the development of iron deficiency anemia, the most common etiology of anemia worldwide [5–8]. Anemia is not a diagnosis per se but a symptom of another untoward process, such as micronutrient deficiency or an underlying disease state [9].

The WHO estimates that one-third of the world's patients who present for surgery are anemic [4]. Large observational studies indicate that up to 40% of patients presenting for surgery are anemic [4, 9–11]. Preoperative anemia is associated with poor surgical outcomes and increased perioperative mortality in both children and adults [4, 12–16]. Hospital-acquired anemia (HAA), a form of iatrogenic anemia developed during any hospital stay, is particularly important because it may exacerbate preoperative anemia [14, 17]. The rate of untoward patient outcomes may be directly proportional to the severity of anemia [12, 16, 18, 19].

Although the definition of anemia is not collectively agreed upon, the WHO defines anemia as hemoglobin (Hgb) <12 g/dL for nonpregnant adult females and <13 g/dL for adult males [1]. Severe anemia is defined as <7 g/dL in children under 5 and pregnant women and <8 g/dL in nonpregnant women [1]. Normal Hgb values in children are often age-based and, despite increased growth and nutritional needs in that population, are lower than corresponding adult norms [20]. Anemia in older infants and children has been defined as Hgb <11 g/dL (6 months to 6 years) and <12–13 g/dL (7–18 years) [20, 21]. Term neonates may have a Hgb mean as high as 16 g/dL with a "physiologic" nadir of approximately 9 g/dL at 3 months of age [20, 22]. Physiologic anemia is a normal adaptation to extrauterine life. At birth, newborns undergo an increase in PaO_2 and O_2 saturation (i.e., 95% versus 50%), followed by a gradual decrease in responsive erythropoietin production. This transition leads to a Hgb nadir of approximately 11 g/dL at 2–3 months that is well tolerated under normal conditions. This physiologic anemia occurs in premature infants sooner (at 3–6 weeks) and with a lower nadir (7–9 g/dL) [7]. As a result, infants hospitalized during their physiologic Hgb nadir are unlikely to compensate for blood loss associated with blood draws and procedures. Low-birth-weight premature infants have an even lower Hgb nadir with a decreased erythropoietin response, placing them at particular risk for iatrogenic anemia.

This discussion will focus on those aspects of patient care that are potentially modifiable but contribute to pediatric HAA, including procedures, blood draws, and well-intended ordering practices.

6.2 How Does One Differentiate Between Physiologic, Illness-Associated, and Hospital-Acquired (HAA) Anemia?

Because anemia in hospitalized patients may be multifactorial, differentiating pure HAA from other causes of anemia may be difficult. Many medical conditions contribute to the development of HAA, including the coagulopathy of sepsis, antibiotic-related hemolysis, massive surgical or traumatic bleeding, and excessive blood draws [23]. In general, red blood cell (RBC) anemia results from decreased production, increased destruction, or increased loss of RBCs. Reduced RBC production is the most common form of anemia, usually seen in inflammatory conditions with associated abnormalities in iron metabolism [8]. However, decreased production may also result from blood loss in the face of low iron and nutritional stores. Blood loss may be acute, such as during procedures, or insidious, as seen with repeated blood draws and bedside interventions. A normal physiologic response to anemia is increased erythropoietin production leading to an increase in reticulocyte levels (>3%) [24]. Reticulocytosis may be seen in both illness- and blood loss-related anemia; however, the mean corpuscular volume (MCV) helps to differentiate the two types of anemia observed in hospitalized patients. In blood loss-associated anemia, the MCV is normal (or "normocytic"), and the reticulocyte count is typically elevated. In contrast, the MCV of chronic disease and inflammation is likely to be microcytic, with a blunted reticulocyte response [20]. However, if a hospitalized child undergoes sequential blood draws or procedures without adequate iron and micronutrient replacement, a low MCV ("microcytic") anemia will eventually develop [7, 25, 26]. Anemia secondary to RBC destruction is likely heralded by external signs of jaundice, dark urine, and scleral icterus, with hyperbilirubinemia and abnormal RBC morphology on blood smear; because reticulocytes are large RBCs, the MCV will reflect the degree of reticulocytosis. Table 6.1 illustrates the MCV and reticulocyte counts in hospitalized patients who have experienced blood loss or sequential blood draws [24]. Note that the MCV is age-based (it is higher in neonates than older children or adults) and that the etiology of anemia can only be ascertained within a clinical context.

Table 6.1 The MCV (mean corpuscular RBC volume) and reticulocyte response in anemic children in the perioperative period. A low MCV is <80–90 fL in neonates and <70 fL in older children

Perioperative anemia	Physiologic (age 2–3 months)	Serial blood draws	Acute blood loss	Chronic illness
MCV	Normal or increased	Low	Normal	Low
Reticulocyte percentage	Normal or decreased	Normal or elevated unless iron deficient	Normal or elevated after 3+ days unless iron deficient	Low or normal with iron and nutrient supplementation

After several months, an infant's reticulocyte count is similar to adult values (<3%). Infants with physiologic anemia will have a low reticulocyte count (<1.5%) due to reduced erythropoietin production in response to extrauterine oxygenation

6.3 Which Patients Are at Greatest Risk of HAA?

Specific patient populations are at particular risk of HAA. These include patients who have preexisting or chronic anemia, intensive care unit (ICU) status, rapid growth, non-White ethnicity, small body size, and prematurity. Awareness of a patient's HAA risk is the first step in mitigating iatrogenic blood loss.

6.3.1 Chronic Anemia

Chronically anemic patients have a relatively lower Hgb level upon hospital admission, increasing the likelihood of a blood transfusion during hospitalization or severe anemia at discharge. In an analysis of over 400 hospitalized adult patients at a Canadian hospital, Thavendiranathan et al. found that over 40% were chronically anemic, with a drop in mean Hgb 0.79 g/dL at hospital discharge. If labs are obtained on a daily basis for 5 days (with a typical daily total volume of 10 mL for blood count, electrolytes, and coagulation studies), a patient's Hgb will decrease by 3.5 g/dL (95% CI; 2.4–4.6) [27]. This margin could conceivably place a patient with an admission Hgb of 8 g/dL close to the RBC transfusion threshold of 7 g/dL often used as a transfusion trigger in stable, hospitalized patients.

6.3.2 Intensive Care Unit Admission

ICU patients are at risk of the severest forms of HAA, particularly during the first day of admission, secondary to patient comorbidities and intense diagnostic blood monitoring [17, 28, 29]. In ICU settings, patients may undergo three to eight blood draws daily at a mean volume of 0.25–5 mL/kg/day, limited only by the nature of the specific tests ordered [21, 29, 30]. A retrospective study by Corwin et al. found that long-term adult ICU patients who received blood transfusions had phlebotomy losses up to 70 mL/day; this daily loss is 1.4% of the average adult's total blood volume of 5 L [31]. If directly extrapolated to the estimated blood volume (EBV) of a 1.5 kg premature neonate (e.g., 90 mL/kg, or 135 mL), 1.4% of 135 mL is 1.9 mL/day of diagnostic blood loss. If sustained, this degree of blood loss is equivalent to 10% of the infant's blood volume per week of hospitalization. Furthermore, a significant percentage of ICU patients are thrombocytopenic or actively bleeding on admission, leading to repeated workups and iatrogenic blood loss [32–35].

6.3.3 Infants

Infants of all ages are particularly susceptible to HAA for several reasons. Diagnostic or procedural blood loss can be relatively significant for small patients. In an observational study of PICU patients, phlebotomy was associated with a daily mean blood loss 7.1 mL (+/– 5.3 mL), with the tiniest patients (e.g., <10 kg) suffering the greatest loss per body weight [36]. A conventional specimen tube for a complete blood count (CBC) requires at least 3–5 mL blood and an electrolyte tube 3–7 mL [37]. Even reduced size specimen tubes (e.g., "pediatric" tubes) may require a significant portion of an infant's EBV. A pediatric-sized tube may need 1–2 mL for a successful specimen but, if obtained daily for 1 week, will remove up to 15% of a 1 kg infant's EBV. In another observational study of 20 premature neonates <28 weeks gestation, Counsilman et al. found the median blood loss associated with phlebotomy and intravenous line starts was 24.2 mL/kg during their first month of life [38]. Figure 6.1 illustrates the daily blood loss attributable to laboratory testing, punctures, and IV placement for these neonates over a 1-month period.

In a premature neonate with an estimated blood volume of 80–90 mL/kg, a 24 mL/kg of blood loss approximates one-quarter of the infant's total blood volume. It is not surprising, then, that the majority of premature infants are transfused during their initial hospital admission (90% in the Counsilman cohort) [39]. Banked umbilical cord blood, characterized as "immunologically naïve" and with a higher concentration of hemoglobin F (HgbF) compared to adult blood, holds promise to reduce iatrogenic blood loss and allogeneic RBC transfusions in both term and preterm neonates [40–42].

An infant requires 8–10 mg/day of iron to support its rapid growth; the USA recommended daily allowance (RDA) is 11 mg [43]. However, both cow's milk and human breast milk from a malnourished mother contain only 1 mg/L iron. Therefore, an infant's daily requirements must be supplemented with iron-fortified milk and foods in order to maintain iron stores [7]. This requirement is complicated by a paucity of nutritional supplementation in low-resource environments and most hospital settings. In high-resource countries, there is a "double burden" of malnutrition (anemia plus obesity) brought about through excessive cow milk ingestion [8].

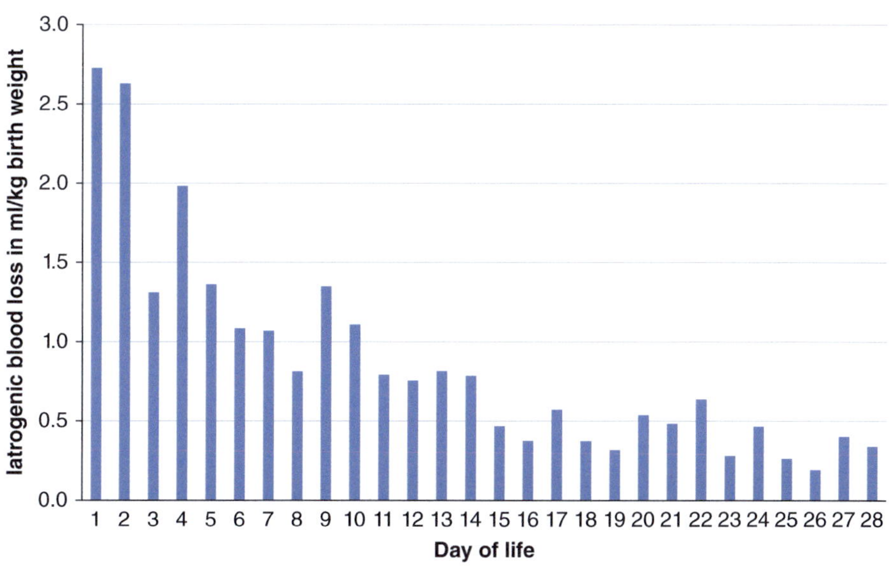

Fig. 6.1 Daily iatrogenic blood loss in 20 premature infants. Reprinted through Creative Commons License: Counsilman et al. [38]

6.3.4 Adolescence

Rapidly growing adolescent males require large iron stores to support an increased RBC volume and muscle mass. In adolescent females, dietary iron replacement is often inadequate to compensate for menstrual losses [44] Observational studies of teenage patients in the ICU have found that they are more likely to be anemic during and following ICU discharge than younger age groups [21, 29]. The Association for the Advancement of Blood and Biotherapies (AABB), recognizing the risk of donation-associated anemia in adolescents as well as a low probability that these donors will quickly recover iron stores, has established increased donation interval requirements for this age group [45].

6.3.5 Extended Hospital Length of Stay (LOS)

A prolonged hospital LOS also increases the risk of HAA. This association partly reflects a sick patient's inability to maintain iron stores while undergoing repeat phlebotomy and other procedures. In a sample of over 600 adult patients hospitalized in the ICU for more than one week, there was a positive correlation between the number of daily RBC transfusions and LOS, mostly attributed to the average daily phlebotomy-related blood loss [31]. In another record review of over 130,000 hospitalized, nonanemic adult patients, 74% developed HAA, with the severity of HAA related to the length of stay (LOS) [13]. An ICU stay longer than 2 days has been found to be associated with an increased rate of transfusion in children with congenital heart disease [46].

6.3.6 Surgery

Surgery is associated with the greatest volumes of blood loss compared to other iatrogenic etiologies, and over one-half of blood transfusions worldwide are given during the perioperative period [17, 23]. In a registry review from the American College of Surgeons National Surgery Improvement Program (ACS NSQIP), over one-third of 2764 neonates (defined as 0–30 days of age) were anemic before noncardiac surgery [12]. In that same study, one-third of the neonates had a gestational age of less than 36 weeks, a population at high risk of severe perioperative anemia and increased mortality. Specific procedures at highest risk for iatrogenic blood loss include, but are not limited to, spine, craniosynostosis, orthopedic, hepatic, and cardiovascular surgery [23].

6.3.7 Race-Based Normative Values

A National Health and Nutrition Examination Survey III (NHANES III) found that African American children had lower mean normal Hgb values compared to non-Hispanic Whites [47]. These discrepant anemia cutoff values are also found in one definition of adult anemia, citing a difference of 0.8 g/dL between White and African American males and 0.7 g/dL for females [23, 24]. In a prospective review of the Hgb and hematocrit (Hct) levels in 1491 African American and 31,005 White adults, the levels were lower in African American men and women even after adjusting for preexisting hemoglobinopathies, suggesting that laboratory reference values vary with ethnicity [48] As a result, African American children and adults are at a disadvantage when facing iatrogenic blood losses. In an ACS NSQIP database study, non-White children were more likely than White children to receive a blood transfusion for femur fracture surgery during the years 2012–2019 [49].

6.4 What Are Some of the Situational Factors That Contribute to HAA?

In addition to patient factors, many situational factors contribute to HAA in hospitalized patients. Table 6.2 lists some of these modifiable, non-patient factors.

6.4.1 Diagnostic Blood Testing

Phlebotomy-related blood losses can be significant, up to several hundred milliliters in adults and up to one-third of a premature newborn's blood volume during a single hospitalization [31, 38, 54]. In a 2008 prospective observational study of over 900

Table 6.2 Situational factors associated with hospital-acquired anemia (HAA)

	Factor	Comment
Factors associated with HAA	Diagnostic phlebotomy	Increased frequency and volumes found in ICU/NICU patients [17, 29]
	Surgery technique, patient selection, patient preparation	High risk iatrogenic blood loss: Spine, cardiovascular, orthopedic, hepatic, craniosynostosis surgery; inadequate preoperative anemia or anticoagulation management [23]
	Indwelling vascular lines	Convenience factor; excessive flushing; absence of line placement criteria [21, 36]
	Bedside procedures	Bleeding is often overlooked or discounted
	Routine orders	Unnecessary testing without individual patient assessment
	Fluid resuscitation	Hemodilution is a diagnosis of exclusion, with a normal RBC count [23]
	Lack of standardization or guidelines	Absence of institutional will and practitioner education [50, 51]
	Diagnostic uncertainty	Levels of training and knowledge often vary [51, 52]
	Non-pediatric specimen tubes	Small-volume tube transition requires institutional costs and commitment.
	Lack of phlebotomy volume documentation	Should be included in I&O tally [32, 50, 53]

critically ill children, three-quarters of daily blood loss was attributed to diagnostic phlebotomy [29]. Francois et al. prospectively studied over 400 children in an ICU and found an association between the volume of blood lost through phlebotomy and anemia at hospital discharge [21]. Children losing more than 5 mL/kg/day from blood tests had a mean drop in Hgb 0.8 g/dL and were at the greatest risk of developing iatrogenic anemia, although the corresponding transfusion rate was not examined in the cohort. The problem is highlighted by the findings of Bateman et al. that age-related blood loss, when adjusted for weight, were inversely related to the number and volume of blood draws in critically ill children. This patient population can least tolerate protracted volume loss. The Prevention and Early Treatment of Acute Lung Injury (PETAL) Network recommends a 120 mL maximum daily withdrawal volume in adult research protocols [32]. However, most institutions do not place a daily cap on the volume of phlebotomy losses.

6.4.2 Blood Wastage

Patient blood waste is a significant contributor to iatrogenic blood loss. A number of studies have examined sources of this waste, including diagnostic sample draws, redundant specimen volumes, line flushing, and bedside procedures. It is estimated that 25–90% of blood samples are discarded [21, 30, 36, 55]. Often, up to twice as much blood is withdrawn than specimen tubes technically require. In 63 PICU patients, Valentine et al. found that patients with central venous lines had specimen volume draws in excess of up to 250%, arterial lines 165%, and peripheral intravenous lines 140%, with a discard volume of 3.8 (±3.6) mL/day [36]. Francois et al. found an average discard volume of 1 (±5.9) mL/kg/hospitalization stay in 423 children in a PICU, with significantly more discard (14 mL for those with central access vs. 2.1 mL) per admission and a greater frequency of blood draws in children with indwelling vascular access [21]. Similarly, in the adult ICU patient population, the presence of an arterial line has been associated with increased frequency and volume of blood tests compared to patients without an arterial line [56]. One explanation for the excess waste associated with central lines is the perceived volumes of flush required to prevent specimen dilution; other authors speculate that indwelling lines may present opportunities of convenience or curiosity [21, 23, 56]. The dead space of most indwelling catheters is rarely greater than 2 mL, and flushing with twice that volume should be adequate [28, 57].

Laboratory analyzers require a minimal blood volume for accurate results. Dale et al. surveyed 140 clinical labs and found that for complete blood counts (CBCs) in adult-sized specimen tubes, collection volumes were 8.5 times what the laboratory analyzers required and 3 times the volume necessary when pediatric-sized specimen tubes were used [37]. Technically, central venous, arterial, and venipuncture sources need only 1 mL, 0.1 mL, and 0 mL of blood discard for accurate lab analysis, respectively [37]. However, a transition away from adult-to pediatric-size specimen tubes and analyzers can be expensive for an institution, particularly when it serves a mixed pediatric and adult patient population.

Significant blood loss may also accompany bedside procedures, including thoracentesis, wound care, and insertion of indwelling vascular access lines. Blood waste in these situations is often overlooked and not included in the patient's intake-and-output (I & O) record, thus concealing its impact on iatrogenic blood loss [23].

6.5 What Specific Practice Strategies Can Prevent HAA?

Varied strategies to reduce iatrogenic blood loss and prevent HAA have been studied. These include small blood tubes, waste reduction techniques, point-of-care-testing (POCT) devices, noninvasive monitors, best practice guidelines, and blood-sparing "bundles."

6.5.1 Small Specimen Tubes

A mainstay solution to the problem of phlebotomy-related blood loss in adults and children has been a recommendation for pediatric-sized specimen tubes. Whereas a standard blood specimen tube is 3–7 mL in capacity, "pediatric" vacuum tubes are 1–2 mL, and "microtainers" hold up to 0.5 mL of blood. Required fill volumes for specific blood tests range from 3 mL (e.g., EDTA tubes for complete blood count) to 4 mL (e.g., citrate tubes for coagulation studies) to 7 mL (e.g., chemistries); a blood gas may require up to 2 mL and a blood culture 10–20 mL [32]. Figure 6.2 illustrates the overall reductions in phlebotomy losses resulting from the substitution of adult tubes for pediatric tubes at an academic center in Germany [32]. Blood sparing may be improved further using microtainer technology.

Other studies have demonstrated a 25–75% reduction in iatrogenic blood losses associated with the introduction of pediatric specimen tubes [21, 37, 50, 54, 58]. An early study examining the substitution of adult- for pediatric-sized specimen tubes in an adult ICU population found a 23 mL/day reduction in diagnostic losses, amounting to a 50% reduction in unnecessary blood loss [54]. In a 2019 systematic review of interventions, Whitehead et al. found that the evidence "generally supported" routine use of pediatric-sized tubes to reduce iatrogenic blood loss, noting

	Normal Sized (mL)	Reduced Size (mL)	Δ (mL)
EDTA	13,317	7891	5425
Citrate tubes	24,871	10,411	14,460
Serum chemistry	39,390	24,684	14,706

Results of a laboratory-chemical extrapolation of the savings achieved by reducing the filling volume of blood tubes per year with about 3700 treatment days on a 12-bed surgical ICU at University Hospital Würzburg. The filling volumes are assumed for EDTA (2.7 mL vs. 1.6 mL), citrate tubes (4.3 mL vs. 1.8 mL), and serum chemistry (7.5 mL vs. 4.7 mL). The last column shows the respective calculated amount of blood saved per year. Δ = delta (normal sized - reduced size).

Fig. 6.2 Patient blood savings through use of reduced size, pediatric specimen tubes. Reprinted from Helmer et al. [32] under the Creative Commons Attribution License 4.0

the number and quality of available studies was limited [59]. A number of the studies included in this systematic review failed to account for the effect of transfusion on Hgb changes, potentially confounding any analysis of the impact of specimen tube size.

The Canadian Choosing Wisely collaboration recommends routine use of pediatric- or smaller- volume blood specimen tubes to prevent HAA [60]. However, not all hospital laboratories have transitioned to small-volume microtechnology [37]. Special analyzers and centrifuges are required, and manual manipulation may be difficult. Unlike regular-sized specimen tubes, microtainers may limit the ability to order add-on labs or dilution studies. Some tests, such as coagulation studies that require specific ratios of blood, typically require the highest volumes and may not be adaptable to microtechnology. A "limited draw" tube with a reduced internal volume but an exterior compatible with standard analyzers has been developed [37]. Ultimately, incorporation of smaller-volume diagnostic tubes requires administrative will and evidence that other measures such as improved ordering practices cannot be achieved.

6.5.2 Waste Reduction

There are currently several strategies used to mitigate unnecessary blood waste. In addition to ordering fewer tests and withdrawing smaller specimen volumes, aspirated "flush" can be returned to the patient. Multiple tests taken from an indwelling catheter should be bundled when possible to avoid repetitive flushing [36]. A venous arterial blood management protection device (VAMP), a closed system designed to return flush and excess blood, has been shown to reduce blood loss by 80% in an adult patient population [28, 32, 61]. Whitehead's systematic review found a 25% reduction in phlebotomy-associated blood loss when these closed systems are used [59]. A readily available solution is the so-called "push-and-pull" technique through a venous line, which has been shown to maintain accuracy for Hgb, blood glucose, and platelet results [51]. Interpretation of test results using the push-and-pull technique must be tempered with the understanding that RBC hemolysis may occur with rapid syringing or if a clave adapter is in the line [62]. A 3-way stopcock located proximal to the patient can also reduce specimen waste by reducing line dead space and facilitating flush return to the patient [57].

Changes in physician practices may help to avoid unnecessary iatrogenic blood loss. All indwelling lines should be placed only for specific, goal-directed purposes, and invasive lines should be removed when no longer necessary [23]. Bedside, procedures by trainees should be supervised to avoid unnecessary bleeding, and all losses should be documented as part of procedural and daily I & O estimated blood loss [21, 32, 50, 53].

6.5.3 Point-of-Care Testing (POCT) Devices

Additional strategies to reduce diagnostic blood loss include the application of point-of-care-testing (POCT) devices and noninvasive physiologic monitors. POCT is currently available for a wide variety of laboratory assays at bedside and in the operating room, including coagulation studies (activated clotting time and viscoelastic testing), complete blood count, Hgb, blood gases, blood dextrose, and chemistries. Commonly encountered POCT devices used in the operating room include the HemoCue (photometry), the iSTAT and EPOC (chemical biosensor cartridges), and the radiometer (spectrophotometric absorbance)[1]. The blood loss-sparing potential of POCT in small patients is evident when one compares the typical sample size for these devices (10–100 μL) to microtube requirements (0.5–1 mL) and to conventional pediatric specimen tubes (2–3 mL) [30, 63]. Use of POCT in one study of extremely low-birth-weight infants was associated with a 43% reduction in transfusion rates when comparing a blood gas analyzer requiring 100 μL samples to the standard spectrophotometric device already in use (e.g., 500 μL) [63]. Widness et al. reported a 30% reduction in transfusion rate and a 25% decrease in diagnostic blood loss using an in-line, umbilical artery radiometer in 225 samples [53]. However, there is a paucity of outcome data on the clinically beneficial use of POCT in children and infants. A recent systematic review on interventions to prevent iatrogenic anemia found insufficient evidence to support routine POCT implementation [59]. POCT does have significant potential to increase efficiency in processing, turnaround times, and provider satisfaction [64]. Reported concordance rates are generally high (e.g., >90%) when comparing POCT results to conventional laboratory analyses [30, 51, 52, 65, 66]. However, practitioners often are unaware of the validity of the machine they are asked to use. Additional caveats of proper POCT management include regulatory requirements that operators (in the US) must be certified under CAP (College of American Pathologists) and Food and Drug Administration (FDA) guidelines [52, 67]. The operator must be a physician or another licensed individual that a physician must supervise. For accurate results, the physician and operator must know the type of blood source required: venous, arterial, or capillary. Finally, validated reference ranges and critical value levels for infants and children are not established for most currently used POCT devices and are usually based on adult values [64]. POCT Hgb values at the extreme of normal values, or in the setting of compromised perfusion, should be confirmed by conventional laboratory testing before making a transfusion decision [52]. The confidence limits for an intraoperative POCT Hgb may vary depending on the device and the specimen source, setting the stage for inaccurate results and unnecessary treatment [68].

6.5.4 Noninvasive Monitors

Several noninvasive devices serve as surrogate markers to indirectly assess oxygenation and perfusion trends. Currently, these monitors include co-oximeters (e.g., Masimo Rainbow® SpHgb), near-infrared spectroscopy (NIRS), CO_2 end-tidal

---

[1] Discussions of infusion devices and equipment are based on information found in current literature and do not reflect the opinions of the authors. Online product information is often distributed throughout multiple URLs and is revised periodically. There was no industry funding contributing to the production of this chapter

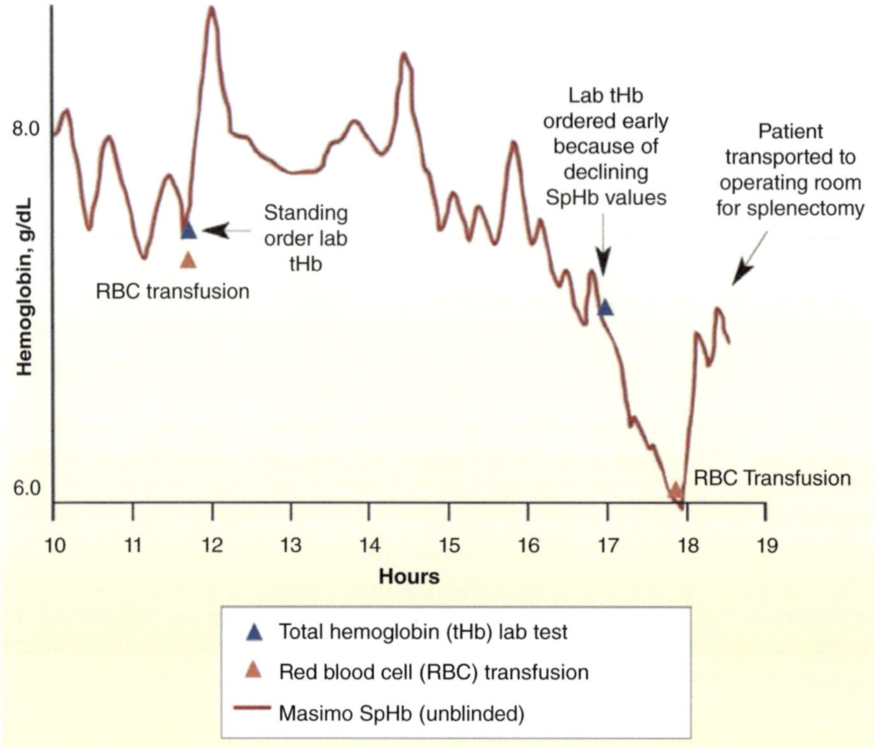

Fig. 6.3 Noninvasive oxygen saturation trend as measured by co-oxymetry in a bleeding patient. Reprinted with permission from McEvoy and Shander [71]. ©2013 by the American Association of Critical-Care Nurses

waveforms ($ETCO_2$), pulse pressure variation (PPV), and stroke volume index (SVI) [21, 23, 69–72]. Although these devices produce informative trends, it is essential to understand the evidence supporting an instrument's validity, age-appropriate reference ranges (if any), and when to back up treatment decisions with conventional technology [52]. For Hgb trend devices, invasive assays may demonstrate high concordance in stable clinical settings but poor correlation in cases of hypoperfusion or at extremes of Hgb values [65, 72–76]. More studies that demonstrate clinically meaningful outcomes are needed as these promising blood-sparing technologies continue to evolve. In the meantime, real-time interpretation and management decisions tend to be a function of the individual practitioner's discretion. Figure 6.3 displays a 9-h Hgb trend measured by co-oximetry in a patient with occult bleeding [71].

6.5.5 Best Practices Guidelines

Unnecessary diagnostic laboratory testing produces unnecessary blood loss. It may also contribute to increased diagnostic sensitivity, leading to further inappropriate testing, increased hospital expense, and patient inconvenience [77, 78]. Recently, the burden of unnecessary blood testing has been quantified in grams of carbon dioxide emission (CO_2e), creating a new outcome measure to address the problem. In a cohort of adult surgery patients, excessive laboratory investigations amounted to 974 g CO_2e per person [79].

Physicians and ordering practitioners may order excessive blood testing for various reasons, including fear of malpractice liability, lack of training, and insufficient knowledge about testing costs (which are often difficult to ascertain in any institution) [78]. However, in a survey of over 40 hospitals in Massachusetts, physicians reported that only 3% of their orders placed the previous day were based entirely on fear of malpractice liability, and only 28% of orders were partly based on litigation concerns [80]. In a record review of 1000 surgical patients, more than one-half had a least one unnecessary test as assessed by the preoperative director [81]. When surveyed, approximately 40% of anesthesiologists responded that how the test might affect perioperative management was extremely important in their decision-making process; another 40% felt that institutional guidelines were not important in the decision to order a perioperative test. The lack of formal blood management education in US anesthesia training is highlighted in a recent study finding that trainees in 37 residency programs scored less than 50% on a validated transfusion medicine exam [82].

Numerous professional societies have recognized the negative impact of excessive blood testing and have promulgated practice guidelines through various Choosing Wisely campaigns [83]. The SABM advises against blood testing that is not necessary for diagnosis and patient management [84]. The American Society of Anesthesiologists (ASA), American Academy of Ophthalmology, and the American Society for Clinical Pathology recommend that preoperative laboratory testing only be performed in patients with clinically relevant diseases undergoing higher-risk procedures [28]. The American Society of Hematology recommends thrombophilia testing only when thrombosis risk is more than "transient" in nature [85]. Unless there is a change in condition, a clinically stable hospitalized patient should not undergo daily, routine laboratory testing. Table 6.3 is an example of the Canadian Choosing Wisely recommendations for placing diagnostic blood orders [60].

6.5.6 Multifaceted Approaches to Reduce Unnecessary Testing

There are several general focus areas in studies that have examined strategies to reduce unnecessary testing: education, performance audits, provider feedback, changes in electronic health record (EHR) functions, or a combination of all four. Laboratory test specifications, including blood volume required, are not readily available to bedside clinicians in many hospitals. The EHR presents tangible blood conservation tools, and various electronic functions may be altered to directly affect practitioner ordering practices. These include replacing order panels with individual options only, eliminating standing orders, hard stops, automatic checks for duplicate orders, and best-practice alerts [28, 86]. When a calculated (weight-based) maximal phlebotomy volume for postoperative patients who weighed less than

Table 6.3 Recommendations for ordering blood tests

Things clinicians and patients should question by the Canadian Society for Medical Laboratory Science	
Recommendation	Caveat
Don't collect more blood than what is needed. Use short draw tubes, consider add-on testing, and reduce or combine duplicate orders	Phlebotomy is not a risk-free event for the patient or the healthcare worker. While rare, injury from needlestick and/or pathogen exposure can occur. Cumulative blood loss due to multiple phlebotomy episodes can result in iatrogenic anemia
Don't proceed with testing or reporting when sample quality or identification is suspect	Any level of error should be avoided to decrease negative impact on clinical decisions and patient care
Don't collect extra blood tubes in anticipation of test orders	This is called a "rainbow draw"; excessive phlebotomy is a recognized contributor to iatrogenic anemia, which is linked to worsened patient outcomes
Don't support repeat test ordering (re-testing) at a frequency that is not backed by evidence	Many analytes have known stability profiles or minimum retesting intervals. Ordering tests more frequently is unlikely to provide clinically meaningful results and may contribute to iatrogenic anemia
Don't routinely repeat critical results for most common analytes before reporting	With modern instrumentation, analytical precision is very high when the result is within the reportable range and no delta checks have failed

Adapted from Choosing Wisely Canada. Fourteen Tests and Treatments to Question in Medical Laboratory Science. 2020. Available online at: Seven Things Clinicians and Patients Should Question. Available online at https://choosingwiselycanada.org/recommendation/medical-laboratory-science/

10 kg was displayed in the EHR, there was a significant reduction in frequency and volume (in mL/kg/hospital stay) accompanied by a high rate of practitioner acceptance [87]. A 2021 quality improvement project focused on unnecessary coagulation test orders (estimated to be almost 90%) during a national shortage of citrate anticoagulant used in blood specimen tubes [88]. A best practice alert (BPA) was embedded into the EHR informing the physician of a "blue top tube" shortage along with evidence-based guidelines for PT, PTT, and INR testing. The result was a 30% sustained reduction in daily tests.

Protocol-driven algorithms embedded in EHR order sets or distributed as pocket cards as decision support tools have succeeded in reducing unnecessary diagnostic blood tests and transfusions [89–91]. Another successful strategy is auditing practitioners' order patterns or costs, followed by peer comparisons and regular feedback. However, interventions that are primarily educational have been reported to have inconsistent success at reducing unnecessary blood testing and are shown to work best when combined with additional interventions such as regular audits, benchmarks, cost reporting, and rounding checklists [78, 92]. Multifaceted approaches to blood conservation tend to have the most success, particularly when education is combined with practitioner feedback and EHR order restrictions [78]. Various interventions that have been used to modify practitioner ordering behavior and reduce inappropriate laboratory testing are listed in Table 6.4 [78].

Table 6.4 Interventions used to change practitioner behavior and reduce unnecessary blood testing

Interventions to reduce unnecessary blood orders	Weight-based maximal phlebotomy volume displayed in EHR order
	Rounding checklists that include the next day's management plan
	Trainees are closely supervised by senior physicians
	Financial incentives are offered to ordering practitioners
	Creation of pocket cards listing guidelines and costs
	Medical teams are rated on basis of ordering patterns and costs
	Educational seminars are held addressing the harm associated with excessive orders
	Hospital administration objectively analyzes clinically useful tests
	Order sets have restrictive ordering functions
	Medicare charges are stated alongside order

Ultimately, sustained improvement entails changing hospital culture, administrative will, and investment, along with practitioner education about the costs, patient inconvenience, and health risks associated with excessive blood testing [78].

6.6 Summary of Key Learning Objectives

6.6.1 What Is the Burden of Anemia for Patients Presenting for Surgery?

The WHO estimates that one-third of the world's patients who present for surgery are anemic. Large observational studies indicate that up to 40% of patients presenting for surgery are anemic.

6.6.2 How Does One Differentiate Between Physiologic, Illness-Associated, and Iatrogenic Anemia?

If the MCV indicates RBC microcytosis, the patient has iron deficiency anemia or another nutritional deficiency unless proven otherwise. If the reticulocyte count is normal, or low in relation to the severity of anemia, the patient may have chronic disease or significant iron deficiency. If the RBC indices are normal, the patient may be hemodiluted or have undergone recent blood loss (e.g., iatrogenic anemia acquired during hospitalization or surgery). Infants age 4–12 weeks may have a physiologic anemia; premature infants will have an earlier onset and more profound physiologic anemia. The record should be reviewed for documentation of blood loss and fluid replacement. Diagnosis of anemia can be complex and further management may require consultation with a hematologist.

6.6.3 Which Patients Are at Greatest Risk of Hospital-Acquired Anemia (HAA)?

The following patient factors are associated the greatest risk of iatrogenic anemia and perioperative blood transfusion:

- Chronic anemia on admission
- Intensive care status
- Prolonged hospital stay
- Infants and small body size
- Adolescents
- Blood loss surgery
- African American ethnicity

Although it is not necessary to perform preoperative diagnostic blood testing in all surgery patients, it is essential to determine which patients are at risk of iatrogenic HAA before surgery.

Preoperative anemia is associated with poor surgical outcomes and increased perioperative mortality in both children and adults.

6.6.4 What Are Some of the Situational factors That Contribute to HAA?

Many practitioner and institutional practices contribute to the development of HAA in at-risk patients. These include but are not limited to adult-sized blood specimen tubes (versus pediatric tubes), indwelling vascular lines, routine orders, an absence of blood loss documentation, and fragmented care between different healthcare teams.

6.6.5 What Specific Practice Strategies Can Prevent HAA?

With a focus on at-risk patients, best practice guidelines can be established at a department or hospital level. Comparison of pre-and post-implementation Hgb values, documentation of blood losses, and transfusion rates may provide the data necessary to achieve crucial buy-in from bedside practitioners and hospital administration. The most successful approach to minimizing anemia at hospital discharge is multipronged, employing a combination of strategies including but not limited to education, monitoring of diagnostic blood orders, focused daily rounding, cost transparency, and EHR optimization.

Key Points

- More than one-third of patients are anemic before surgery.

- Preoperative anemia is exacerbated by HAA and is associated with adverse outcomes including increased perioperative mortality, transfusion rates, and postoperative anemia.
- Specific patient populations are at greatest risk of HAA, including infants, patients in the ICU, and those with indwelling lines.
- The most successful approach to minimize anemia at hospital discharge is multipronged, employing a combination of strategies. These strategies include but are not limited to avoiding waste and unnecessary phlebotomy, use of noninvasive monitors and pediatric-sized specimen tubes, avoiding indwelling lines and routine laboratory orders, and establishing evidence-based practice standards. Blood loss and phlebotomy volumes should be part of the daily I&O documentation. Regular education is essential and requires ongoing monitoring and practitioner feedback.

References

1. World Health Organization. Anaemia in women and children. 2023. https://www.who.int/data/gho/data/themes/topics/anaemia_in_women_and_children#:~:text=Summary%20findings&text=In%202019%2C%20global%20anaemia%20prevalence%20was%2039.8%25%20(95%25,269%20million%20children%20with%20anaemia. Accessed 11 Apr 2022.
2. Dos Santos RF, Gonzalez ES, de Albuquerque EC, de Arruda IK, AaS D, Figueroa JN, et al. Prevalence of anemia in under five-year-old children in a children's hospital in Recife, Brazil. Rev Bras Hematol Hemoter. 2011;33(2):100–4.
3. Pasricha SR. Anemia: a comprehensive global estimate. Blood. 2014;123(5):611–2.
4. World Health Organization (WHO). Policy brief: the urgent need to implement patient blood management. 2021. https://www.who.int/publications/i/item/9789240035744. Accessed 3 Aug 2023.
5. Gallagher PG. The neonatal erythrocyte and its disorders. In: Orkin SH, Fisher DE, Look T, Lux SE, Ginsburg D, Nathan DG, editors. Nathan and Oski's hematology and oncology of infancy and childhood. 8th ed. Philadelphia: WB Saunders; 2015. p. 52.
6. Moraleda C, Rabinovich NR, Menendez C. Are infants less than 6 months of age a neglected group for anemia prevention in low-income countries? Am J Trop Med Hyg. 2018;98(3):647–9.
7. Rothman JA. Iron-deficiency anemia. In: Kliegman RM, St. Geme J, editors. Nelson textbook of pediatrics e-book. 21st ed. Philadelphia: Elsevier; 2020. p. 2522.
8. Moghadam M. Types of anemia and physiological anemia of infancy—a review. Int J Adv Res Biol Sci. 2018;5:26–9.
9. Lin Y. Preoperative anemia-screening clinics. Hematology Am Soc Hematol Educ Program. 2019;2019(1):570–6.
10. Shander A, Corwin HL, Meier J, Auerbach M, Bisbe E, Blitz J, et al. Recommendations from the International Consensus Conference on Anemia Management in Surgical Patients (ICCAMS). Ann Surg. 2023;277(4):581–90.
11. Kloeser R, Buser A, Bolliger D. Treatment strategies in anemic patients before cardiac surgery. J Cardiothorac Vasc Anesth. 2023;37(2):266–75.
12. Goobie SM, Faraoni D, Zurakowski D, DiNardo JA. Association of preoperative anemia with postoperative mortality in neonates. JAMA Pediatr. 2016;170(9):855–62.
13. Koch CG, Li L, Sun Z, Hixson ED, Tang A, Phillips SC, et al. Hospital-acquired anemia: prevalence, outcomes, and healthcare implications. J Hosp Med. 2013;8(9):506–12.

14. Koch CG, Li L, Sun Z, Hixson ED, Tang AS, Phillips SC, et al. From bad to worse: anemia on admission and hospital-acquired anemia. J Patient Saf. 2017;13(4):211–6.
15. Baron DM, Hochrieser H, Posch M, Metnitz B, Rhodes A, Moreno RP, et al. Preoperative anaemia is associated with poor clinical outcome in non-cardiac surgery patients. Br J Anaesth. 2014;113(3):416–23.
16. Musallam KM, Tamim HM, Richards T, Spahn DR, Rosendaal FR, Habbal A, et al. Preoperative anaemia and postoperative outcomes in non-cardiac surgery: a retrospective cohort study. Lancet. 2011;378(9800):1396–407.
17. Makam AN, Nguyen OK, Clark C, Halm EA. Incidence, predictors, and outcomes of hospital-acquired anemia. J Hosp Med. 2017;12(5):317–22.
18. Agathis AZ, Khetan P, Bitner D, Divino CM. Is preoperative anemia a significant risk factor for splenectomy patients? A NSQIP analysis. Surg Open Sci. 2020;2(3):101–6.
19. Faraoni D, DiNardo JA, Goobie SM. Relationship between preoperative anemia and in-hospital mortality in children undergoing noncardiac surgery. Anesth Analg. 2016;123(6):1582–7.
20. Thornburg CD. The Anemias. In: Kliegman RM, Geme JS, editors. Nelson textbook of pediatrics e-book. 21st ed. Elsevier-OHCE; 2019. p. 2505–6.
21. François T, Sauthier M, Charlier J, Dessureault J, Tucci M, Harrington K, et al. Impact of blood sampling on Anemia in the PICU: a prospective cohort study. Pediatr Crit Care Med. 2022;23(6):435–43.
22. Lau W, MD, FRCPC. Clinical guide to transfusion. Chapter 13: neonatal and pediatric transfusions. Canadian Blood Services; 2017. https://professionaleducation.blood.ca/en/transfusion/clinical-guide/neonatal-and-pediatric-transfusion.
23. Martin ND, Scantling D. Hospital-acquired anemia: a contemporary review of etiologies and prevention strategies. J Infus Nurs. 2015;38(5):330–8.
24. Niss O, Quinn CT. Classification and diagnosis of anemia in children and neonates. In: Fish JD, Lipton JM, Lanzkowsky PL, editors. Lanzkowsky's manual of pediatric hematology and oncology. 7th ed. London: Academic Press Elsevier; 2021. p. 37–58.
25. Salami A, Bahmad HF, Ghssein G, Salloum L, Fakih H. Prevalence of anemia among Lebanese hospitalized children: risk and protective factors. PLoS One. 2018;13(8):e0201806.
26. Phiri KS, Calis JC, Siyasiya A, Bates I, Brabin B, van Hensbroek MB. New cut-off values for ferritin and soluble transferrin receptor for the assessment of iron deficiency in children in a high infection pressure area. J Clin Pathol. 2009;62(12):1103–6.
27. Thavendiranathan P, Bagai A, Ebidia A, Detsky AS, Choudhry NK. Do blood tests cause anemia in hospitalized patients? The effect of diagnostic phlebotomy on hemoglobin and hematocrit levels. J Gen Intern Med. 2005;20(6):520–4.
28. Shander A, Corwin HL. A narrative review on hospital-acquired anemia: keeping blood where it belongs. Transfus Med Rev. 2020;34(3):195–9.
29. Bateman ST, Lacroix J, Boven K, Forbes P, Barton R, Thomas NJ, et al. Anemia, blood loss, and blood transfusions in North American children in the intensive care unit. Am J Respir Crit Care Med. 2008;178(1):26–33.
30. Jakacka N, Snarski E, Mekuria S. Prevention of iatrogenic anemia in critical and neonatal care. Adv Clin Exp Med. 2016;25(1):191–7.
31. Corwin HL, Parsonnet KC, Gettinger A. RBC transfusion in the ICU. Is there a reason? Chest. 1995;108(3):767–71.
32. Helmer P, Hottenrott S, Steinisch A, Röder D, Schubert J, Steigerwald U, et al. Avoidable blood loss in critical care and patient blood management: scoping review of diagnostic blood loss. J Clin Med. 2022;11(2):320. https://doi.org/10.3390/jcm11020320.
33. White LJ, Fredericks R, Mannarino CN, Janofsky S, Faustino EVS. Epidemiology of bleeding in critically ill children. J Pediatr. 2017;184:114–9.e6.
34. Aran AA, Karam O, Nellis ME. Bleeding in critically ill children-review of literature, knowledge gaps, and suggestions for future investigation. Front Pediatr. 2021;9:611680.
35. Gunnink SF, Vlug R, Fijnvandraat K, van der Bom JG, Stanworth SJ, Lopriore E. Neonatal thrombocytopenia: etiology, management and outcome. Expert Rev Hematol. 2014;7(3):387–95.

36. Valentine SL, Bateman ST. Identifying factors to minimize phlebotomy-induced blood loss in the pediatric intensive care unit. Pediatr Crit Care Med. 2012;13(1):22–7.
37. Dale JC, Ruby SG. Specimen collection volumes for laboratory tests. Arch Pathol Lab Med. 2003;127(2):162–8.
38. Counsilman CE, Heeger LE, Tan R, Bekker V, Zwaginga JJ, Te Pas AB, et al. Iatrogenic blood loss in extreme preterm infants due to frequent laboratory tests and procedures. J Matern Fetal Neonatal Med. 2021;34(16):2660–5.
39. New HV, Berryman J, Bolton-Maggs PH, Cantwell C, Chalmers EA, Davies T, et al. Guidelines on transfusion for fetuses, neonates and older children. Br J Haematol. 2016;175(5):784–828.
40. Christensen RD, Bahr TM, Christensen TR, Ohls RK, Krong J, Carlton LC, et al. Banked term umbilical cord blood to meet the packed red blood cell transfusion needs of extremely-low-gestational-age neonates: a feasibility analysis. J Perinatol. 2024;44(6):873–9. https://doi.org/10.1038/s41372-023-01833-y.
41. Bahr TM, Carroll PD. Cord blood sampling for neonatal admission laboratory testing—an evidence-based blood conservation strategy. Semin Perinatol. 2023;47(5):151786.
42. Sarin K, Chauhan S, Bisoi AK, Hazarika A, Malhotra N, Manek P. Use of autologous umbilical cord blood transfusion in neonates undergoing surgical correction of congenital cardiac defects: a pilot study. Ann Card Anaesth. 2018;21(3):270–4.
43. NIH Office of Dietary Supplement. Iron: fact sheet for health professionals. National Institutes of Health. 2022. https://ods.od.nih.gov/factsheets/Iron-HealthProfessional/. Accessed 17 Jan 2023.
44. Marx JJ. Iron deficiency in developed countries: prevalence, influence of lifestyle factors and hazards of prevention. Eur J Clin Nutr. 1997;51(8):491–4.
45. Kessler LA, Rossmann SN. Allogeneic and autologous blood donor selection. In: Fung MK, Eder AF, Spitalnik SL, editors. Nineteenth edition technical manual. Bethesda: AABB; 2017. p. 111–122; 175.
46. Zhou D, Luo YL, Luo SH, Feng M, Tang ML. The effect of diagnostic blood loss on anemia and transfusion among postoperative patients with congenital heart disease in a pediatric intensive care unit. J Pediatr Nurs. 2018;38:62–7.
47. Robins EB, Blum S. Hematologic reference values for African American children and adolescents. Am J Hematol. 2007;82(7):611–4.
48. Beutler E, Waalen J. The definition of anemia: what is the lower limit of normal of the blood hemoglobin concentration? Blood. 2006;107(5):1747–50.
49. Malyavko A, Quan T, Kraft D, Mathur A, Ramamurti P, Tabaie S. Racial disparities in outcomes following open treatment of pediatric femoral shaft fractures. Cureus. 2022;14(12):e33149.
50. Wu Y, Spaulding AC, Borkar S, Shoaei MM, Mendoza M, Grant RL, et al. Reducing blood loss by changing to small volume tubes for laboratory testing. Mayo Clin Proc Innov Qual Outcomes. 2021;5(1):72–83.
51. Lokeskrawee T, Muengtaweepongsa S, Patumanond J, Sawaengrat C. Accuracy of laboratory tests drawn by pull-push method from central venous catheterization after routine flushing with 10 ml normal saline in patients with sepsis at the emergency department. Heliyon. 2021;7(6):e07355.
52. Tolich D. Value and accuracy of point-of-care testing. In: AABB patient blood management. 2022. https://www.aabb.org/docs/default-source/default-document-library/resources/value-and-accuracy-of-point-of-care-testing.pdf?sfvrsn=4eb70506_0. Accessed 22 Jun 2022.
53. Widness JA, Madan A, Grindeanu LA, Zimmerman MB, Wong DK, Stevenson DK. Reduction in red blood cell transfusions among preterm infants: results of a randomized trial with an in-line blood gas and chemistry monitor. Pediatrics. 2005;115(5):1299–306.
54. Smoller BR, Kruskall MS, et al. Reducing adult phlebotomy blood loss with the use of pediatric-size blood collection tubes. Am J Clin Pathol. 1989;91(6):701–3.
55. Siegal DM, Belley-Cote EP, Lee SF, Robertson T, Hill S, Benoit P, et al. Small-volume tubes to reduce anemia and transfusion (STRATUS): a pilot study. Can J Anaesth. 2023;70(11):1797–806. https://doi.org/10.1007/s12630-023-02548-6.

56. Low LL, Harrington GR, Stoltzfus DP. The effect of arterial lines on blood-drawing practices and costs in intensive care units. Chest. 1995;108(1):216–9.
57. Rickard CM, Couchman BA, Schmidt SJ, Dank A, Purdie DM. A discard volume of twice the deadspace ensures clinically accurate arterial blood gases and electrolytes and prevents unnecessary blood loss. Crit Care Med. 2003;31(6):1654–8.
58. Sanchez-Giron F, Alvarez-Mora F. Reduction of blood loss from laboratory testing in hospitalized adult patients using small-volume (pediatric) tubes. Arch Pathol Lab Med. 2008;132(12):1916–9.
59. Whitehead NS, Williams LO, Meleth S, Kennedy SM, Ubaka-Blackmoore N, Geaghan SM, et al. Interventions to prevent iatrogenic anemia: a laboratory medicine best practices systematic review. Crit Care. 2019;23(1):278.
60. Choosing Wisely Canada. Seven things clinicians and patients should question. 2020. https://choosingwiselycanada.org/recommendation/medical-laboratory-science/. Accessed 22 Jun 2022.
61. Siegal DM, Manning N, Jackson Chornenki NL, Hillis CM, Heddle NM. Devices to reduce the volume of blood taken for laboratory testing in ICU patients: a systematic review. J Intensive Care Med. 2020;35(10):1074–9.
62. McBride C, Miller-Hoover S, Proudfoot JA. A standard push-pull protocol for waste-free sampling in the pediatric intensive care unit. J Infus Nurs. 2018;41(3):189–97.
63. Madan A, Kumar R, Adams MM, Benitz WE, Geaghan SM, Widness JA. Reduction in red blood cell transfusions using a bedside analyzer in extremely low birth weight infants. J Perinatol. 2005;25(1):21–5.
64. Wilson S, Bohn MK, Adeli K. POCT: an inherently ideal tool in pediatric laboratory medicine. EJIFCC. 2021;32(2):145–57.
65. Young MF, Raines K, Jameel F, Sidi M, Oliveira-Streiff S, Nwajei P, et al. Non-invasive hemoglobin measurement devices require refinement to match diagnostic performance with their high level of usability and acceptability. PLoS One. 2021;16(7):e0254629.
66. Papa F, Rongioletti M, Ventura MD, Di Turi F, Cortesi M, Pasqualetti P, et al. Blood cell counting in neonates: a comparison between a low volume micromethod and the standard laboratory method. Blood Transfus. 2011;9(4):400–6.
67. Schwartz J, Illoh O, Tanhehco YC. Regulatory considerations in transfusion medicine and cellular therapies. In: Cohn C, Delaney M, Johnson ST, Katz LM, editors. Technical manual. 20th ed. Bethesda, MD: AABB; 2020. p. 79.
68. Dietzel F, Dieterich P, Dorries F, Gehring H, Wegerich P. Invasive and non-invasive point-of-care testing and point-of-care monitoring of the hemoglobin concentration in human blood—how accurate are the data? Biomed Tech (Berl). 2019;64(5):495–506.
69. Rabe H, Alvarez RF, Whitfield T, Lawson F, Jungmann H. Spectroscopic noninvasive measurement of hemoglobin compared with capillary and venous values in neonates. Neonatology. 2010;98(1):1–5.
70. Vretzakis G, Georgopoulou S, Stamoulis K, Tassoudis V, Mikroulis D, Giannoukas A, et al. Monitoring of brain oxygen saturation (INVOS) in a protocol to direct blood transfusions during cardiac surgery: a prospective randomized clinical trial. J Cardiothorac Surg. 2013;8:145.
71. McEvoy MT, Shander A. Anemia, bleeding, and blood transfusion in the intensive care unit: causes, risks, costs, and new strategies. Am J Crit Care. 2013;22(6 Suppl):eS1–13; quiz eS4.
72. Kazanasmaz H, Demir M. The comparison of hemoglobin values measured by blood and continuous non-invasive monitoring (SpHb) in newborn infants. J Trop Pediatr. 2021;67(3):fmaa050. https://doi.org/10.1093/tropej/fmaa050.
73. Bhat A, Upadhyay A, Jaiswal V, Chawla D, Singh D, Kumar M, et al. Validity of non-invasive point-of-care hemoglobin estimation in healthy and sick children-a method comparison study. Eur J Pediatr. 2016;175(2):171–9.
74. Kim SH, Lilot M, Murphy LS, Sidhu KS, Yu Z, Rinehart J, et al. Accuracy of continuous noninvasive hemoglobin monitoring: a systematic review and meta-analysis. Anesth Analg. 2014;119(2):332–46.

75. Awada WN, Mohmoued MF, Radwan TM, Hussien GZ, Elkady HW. Continuous and non-invasive hemoglobin monitoring reduces red blood cell transfusion during neurosurgery: a prospective cohort study. J Clin Monit Comput. 2015;29(6):733–40.
76. Mathew SE, Pulido N, Larson AN, Stans AA, Milbrandt TA, Shaughnessy WJ. Noninvasive hemoglobin monitoring for postoperative pediatric orthopaedic patients: a preliminary study. J Pediatr Orthop. 2022;42(8):e897–900.
77. Bodley T, Chan M, Levi O, Clarfield L, Yip D, Smith O, et al. Patient harm associated with serial phlebotomy and blood waste in the intensive care unit: a retrospective cohort study. PLoS One. 2021;16(1):e0243782.
78. Eaton KP, Levy K, Soong C, Pahwa AK, Petrilli C, Ziemba JB, et al. Evidence-based guidelines to eliminate repetitive laboratory testing. JAMA Intern Med. 2017;177(12):1833–9.
79. Spoyalo K, Lalande A, Rizan C, Park S, Simons J, Dawe P, et al. Patient, hospital and environmental costs of unnecessary bloodwork: capturing the triple bottom line of inappropriate care in general surgery patients. BMJ Open Qual. 2023;12(3):e002316. https://doi.org/10.1136/bmjoq-2023-002316.
80. Rothberg MB, Class J, Bishop TF, Friderici J, Kleppel R, Lindenauer PK. The cost of defensive medicine on 3 hospital medicine services. JAMA Intern Med. 2014;174(11):1867–8.
81. Katz RI, Dexter F, Rosenfeld K, Wolfe L, Redmond V, Agarwal D, et al. Survey study of anesthesiologists' and surgeons' ordering of unnecessary preoperative laboratory tests. Anesth Analg. 2011;112(1):207–12.
82. Connelly NR, Adler AC, Vanderberg LE, Conlin F, Mitchell JD, Goldstein S, et al. Anesthesiology resident knowledge of transfusion medicine: results from the anesthesiology transfusion education study. Anesth Analg. 2024;138(3):655–63. https://doi.org/10.1213/ANE.0000000000006327.
83. Five things patients should question. In: Society for the Advancement of Blood Management (SABM). ABIM Foundation. 2022. https://www.choosingwisely.org/clinician-lists/#keyword=transfusion. Accessed 5 June 2022.
84. Burns CD, Brown JP, Corwin HL, Gross I, Ozawa SJ, Shander A. Special report from the Society for the Advancement of Blood Management: the choosing wisely campaign. Anesth Analg. 2019;129(5):1381–6.
85. O'Brien SH, Badawy SM, Rotz SJ, Shah MD, Makarski J, Bercovitz RS, et al. The ASH-ASPHO Choosing Wisely Campaign: 5 hematologic tests and treatments to question. Pediatr Blood Cancer. 2021;68(8):e28967.
86. Rhamy J. Blood belongs in the patient, not in a tube. In: AABB Patient Blood Management. 2021. https://www.aabb.org/docs/default-source/default-document-library/resources/blood-belongs-in-the-patient.pdf?sfvrsn=708bce94_4. Accessed 18 Aug 2023.
87. LaCroix GA, Danford DA, Marshall AM. Impact of phlebotomy volume knowledge on provider laboratory ordering and transfusion practices in the pediatric cardiac ICU. Pediatr Crit Care Med. 2023;24(7):e342–51.
88. Breeden M, Bernstein SJ, Hayward RA, Fendrick AM. Evaluation of a best practice advisory on ordering prothrombin time, international normalized ratio, and partial thromboplastin time tests. JAMA Intern Med. 2022;182(9):999–1000.
89. Haas T, Faraoni D. Viscoelastic testing in pediatric patients. Transfusion. 2020;60(Suppl 6):S75–85.
90. Merlani P, Garnerin P, Diby M, Ferring M, Ricou B. Quality improvement report: linking guideline to regular feedback to increase appropriate requests for clinical tests: blood gas analysis in intensive care. BMJ. 2001;323(7313):620–4.
91. Studnicki J, Bradham DD, Marshburn J, Foulis PR, Straumfjord JV. A feedback system for reducing excessive laboratory tests. Arch Pathol Lab Med. 1993;117(1):35–9.
92. Daichman S, Ostrovsky D, Dreiher J, Pikovsky O. Does training make a difference? Proficiency training in transfusion guidelines and its effect on red blood cell administration. Transfusion. 2022;62(5):1121–7.

Preoperative Autologous and Directed Donation

7

Norma J. Klein

7.1 Case Scenario

A 10-year-old girl presents to the preoperative anesthesia clinic 3 days before a scheduled resection of a newly diagnosed osteosarcoma of the femur. Her parents inform you they want to avoid a blood transfusion and the child concurs. The parents tell you that the surgeon says there is potential for significant blood loss and a transfusion requirement. The child asks if she can donate her own blood. She weighs 40 kg, her hemoglobin (Hgb) is 11 g/dL, her blood type is O positive, and she is in relatively good health as captain of her recreational soccer team. When you respond that you are uncertain if she will quality for a preoperative autologous donation (PAD), the parents respond that they will donate their own blood though a directed donation.

Key Learning Objectives

- May a child donate her own blood prior to surgery for future perioperative use?
- Is it possible for a child with cancer participate in PAD?
- Should parents act as directed blood donors for their child's upcoming cancer surgery?

7.2 Discussion

7.2.1 General

Most blood transfusions in resource rich countries are allogeneic, that is, they come from a person that is different than the transfusion recipient. The blood supply in

N. J. Klein (✉)
Department of Anesthesiology and Pain Medicine, University of California, Davis, Sacramento, CA, USA
e-mail: nklein@ucdavis.edu

N. J. Klein (ed.), *Perioperative Pediatric Patient Blood Management and Transfusion Safety*, https://doi.org/10.1007/978-3-031-81666-6_7

North America is much safer today secondary to rigorous donor screening and advances in infectious disease testing [1–3]. However, much of the public remains fearful of the consequences of allogeneic transfusion, particularly the risk of transfusion transmitted infection (TTI) [4]. Today, many adults recall the early 1980s when the human immunodeficiency virus (HIV) was found to be transmittable through the blood supply; up to 6% of pediatric HIV cases were attributable to transfusions during the peak years 1978 to 1985 [5]. Over a 6-year period at a large hospital in Los Angeles, the risk of a transfusion transmitted HIV infection through 1985 was as high as 1:100 [6]. Modern donor screening in conjunction with nucleic acid testing (NAT) of pools of antibody-negative blood donations in high resource countries has reduced the per unit residual risk of a recipient HIV infection to approximately 1:2.3 million, hepatitis C 1:2.6 million, and hepatitis B 1:1.5 million [1, 3, 7–9]. However, there are TTIs for which there is no available testing (e.g., classic Creutzfeldt-Jakob disease (CJD) and emerging pathogens in the blood supply). This uncertainty has prompted patients to request to donate their own blood for later use (i.e., autologous donation) or to designate a particular person as a donor (i.e., designated donation). Autologous transfusions can occur through self-donation prior to a procedure (PAD), during surgery through hemodilution (acute normovolemic hemodilution; ANH), through cell salvage during or after surgery, or even during the peripartum period (e.g., placental harvest or delayed cord clamping) [10]. Designated donor transfusions typically originate from a family member or an acquaintance of the recipient, often with a misguided belief that the blood of a friend or relative is "safer" than that of a stranger in the general donor pool. However, executing a PAD or directed donation can be difficult, expensive, and not necessarily safer than the voluntary, general pool of banked blood. The following discussion addresses both PAD and directed donations, with emphasis on indications, the procedure, and limitations.

7.3 May a Child Donate Her Own Blood Prior to Surgery for Future Perioperative Use?

PAD rates have declined over the past several decades, most likely because of improved surgical techniques, broader acceptance of restrictive transfusion thresholds, improved safety of the commercial blood supply, and the increased administrative costs associated with PAD [11–15]. In 1990 up to 8% of units transfused in the US were autologous, but by 2019, that percentage dropped to approximately 0.27% [2, 16]. Results from a limited number of studies suggest that pediatric PAD reduces allogeneic (homologous) transfusion rates, and PAD continues to be recommended in specific circumstances despite the existence the few remaining centers that provide the service and an overall decline in the procedure rate [4, 17–19].

Processing a surgical patient's autologous blood unit carries extra administrative costs, special labeling (e.g., "for autologous use only"), and time sensitive donation appointments prior to a planned surgery. As a result, blood centers may view requests for PAD to be burdensome compared to standard, bulk blood inventory management [2, 6, 12, 13, 20–22]. However, given the potential for severe patient anxiety over blood loss surgery requiring a transfusion, it is reasonable to consider PAD as an alternative treatment option. Blood centers have been stressed with a recent trend of parents refusing a blood transfusion for their children if the donor is vaccinated [23, 24]. The Association for the Advancement of Blood and Biotherapies (AABB) has published online position statements to counter the unfounded claim that blood transfusions from vaccinated donors should be avoided [25, 26]. In the State of California, the Paul Gann Act requires that patients are informed of a PAD option if there is a reasonable possibility that a blood transfusion will be required [27, 28]. In Japan, national guidelines have encouraged PAD as a safe alternative to allogeneic blood [29].

7.3.1 PAD Indications

The main indications for PAD include elective surgeries where significant blood loss is anticipated in the following situations [1, 12, 30–32]:

- A rare blood type.
- Patients with multiple alloantibodies (such as the chronically transfused).
- A desire to avoid blood product exposure that may lead to antibody formation against cellular blood products, such as with a potential organ or bone marrow transplant candidate.
- A desire to minimize transfusion-transmitted infection (TTI).
- Severe patient anxiety leading to cancellation of surgery.

In many low-resource countries, the blood supply is critically limited with little regulatory infrastructure, creating another rationale for PAD [33]. PAD may also prevent transfusion reactions in susceptible patients, including allergic and febrile nonhemolytic transfusion reactions (FNHTR), to which children are most susceptible [9, 34, 35]. Some authors claim that use of PAD may preserve the general blood supply [4, 16].

PAD is only suited for planned surgeries with a likelihood of significant blood loss. How much blood loss is appropriate for PAD may be institution dependent, but approximations found in the literature vary from surgeries with a 10–90% likelihood of perioperative transfusion, a perioperative requirement of more than two red blood cell (RBC) units, or, in children, a 20–25% estimated blood volume (EBV) loss [1, 2, 36, 37]. It is important to approximate the potential transfusion requirement because a significant number of autologous units (50–90%) remain unused and may be discarded [1, 38–40]. Many institutions, including the American Blood Cross (ARC), do not move unused autologous blood into the general pool over safety concerns, such as a potential administration error because PAD has comparatively liberal screening criteria [30]. Some blood banks determine the likelihood that certain procedures will require a blood transfusion according to a maximum surgical blood order schedule (MSBOS), specifying which procedures typically require an intraoperative transfusion [12, 41].

7.3.2 PAD Screening and Processing

Donor requirements for PAD may be less than those required of the general, volunteer donor population [40]. Allogeneic blood donors must undergo a lengthy health questionnaire, including sensitive lifestyle information, a focused exam (i.e., blood pressure, body weight, inspection of venipuncture sites for evidence of scarring or infection), and TTI testing [42]. Although there is usually no age limit, blood centers typically set a minimum weight requirement for donation (see below). Regarding donor Hgb level requirements, the minimum value for allogeneic donations is 13 g/dL for males and 12.5 g/dL for females, but the autologous donor threshold is 11 g/dL [1, 36, 39, 40, 42]. If the autologous blood is to be transported to a separate surgical facility or if the institution allows unused units to be crossed over into the general donor pool, the patient's autologous unit must undergo full TTI testing, according to FDA standards [43]. This mandatory TTI testing includes hepatitis B and C, HIV-1, West Nile Virus, and syphilis, with additional testing based on the donor's history or concerns over emerging TTIs [42–44]. The patient must be in good health, without active or unmanaged cardiovascular or pulmonary disease, and have no evidence of systemic infection (including possibly an indwelling urinary catheter) at the time of donation [1]. Blood from donors that test positive for TTI will be discarded for safety reasons [1, 30, 39]. Some blood centers discard all unused units [13]. Each blood center may have additional PAD criteria, and whether or not a donor ultimately qualifies as a suitable PAD donor is at the discretion of the blood center medical director.

There are standard processing requirements that must be followed for a successful PAD [45]. A physician's order is required once the patient and procedure are assessed as appropriate for autologous donation [20, 38, 40, 46]. Informed consent is required from the PAD patient or the parent/guardians of minors as defined by the jurisdiction [47]. Almost all centers require that the blood is donated no less than 72 h prior to the scheduled procedure to allow for processing and appropriate TTI testing. The only exception to these time limitations may be in an emergency situation when a patient with complex blood profile is in critical need of blood [42]. Ideally, donations are performed several weeks prior to the scheduled surgery. The number of blood units and the frequency of donation vary between blood centers, with 1–4 total donations at intervals of every 3–56 days cited in the literature [2, 20, 37, 48, 49]. The maximum storage period is 3–6 weeks, depending on the type of blood component and preservative used: platelets can be stored for only 5–7 days and whole blood for 21–35 days, depending on the preservative used [12, 50, 51]. The most common reason for donor deferral (or rejection) is anemia. A properly managed PAD process entails iron administration, or iron plus an erythropoiesis stimulating agent (ESA) [47, 52–55]. Reportedly, a significant number of blood donors do not take iron therapy between donation events, and depletion of iron stores may prevent serial donations [1, 2, 12, 56]. Donation-associated anemia is of particular concern with female and teen donors [57]. When the inter-donation intervals are short or when iron supplementation is inadequate, there is an increased risk of iatrogenic anemia, with decreases in preoperative hemoglobin 1–3 g/dL [19, 32,

37, 52]. Blood centers may have donor criteria that is different than Association for the Advancement of Blood & Biotherapies (AABB) or US Food and Drug Administration (FDA) standards; however, there is no national registry of deferrals so a rejection at one center may not be known at another [42]. Ultimately, the blood center medical director makes the final decisions about moving forward with a requested PAD.

7.3.3 Pediatric PAD

PAD in children entails special considerations. The advantages are similar to those in the adult patient population, but in children, there is increased concern about potential alloimmunization because it may impact future transfusions, pregnancy, or receipt of organ donation [4, 20, 43, 46]. There are no well-established guidelines addressing pediatric PAD, and standards may vary between institutions and different countries [4, 53]. Surgical case types associated with PAD include spine, cardiac, orthopedic, craniosynostosis, urologic, and even neonatal congenital malformation repairs [4, 53]. Pediatric autologous blood has been harvested from the placenta, umbilical cord, and peripheral and central veins [37, 58]. Commercial donor centers are typically set up to accommodate an older pediatric patient population (e.g., larger body size), and smaller children require specialized equipment and trained personnel to ensure a safe standard of care [52]. Figure 7.1 is an example of a premade pediatric autologous donation bag containing anticoagulant preservative (bags 1 and 2), venipuncture needle [4], and syringe [3, 52].

Although most blood donor centers do not have specific age limits for PAD, a common weight requirement is approximately 50 kg. According to US Centers for Disease Control (CDC) growth charts, 50 kg is an average weight for a 13 y.o. female [59]. PAD has been performed in children as young as 6 months and as small

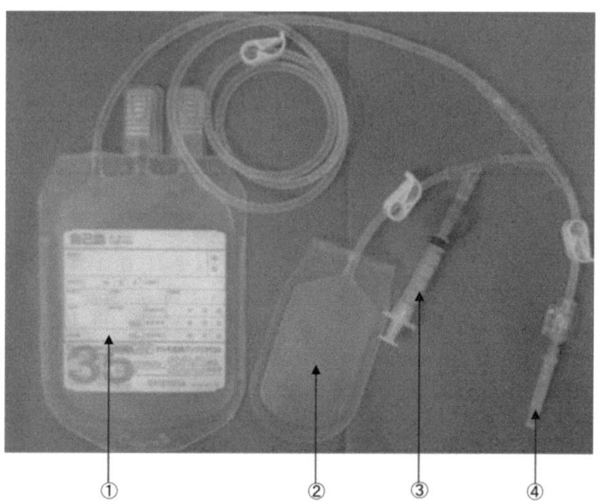

Fig. 7.1 Pediatric autologous donation blood bag containing anticoagulant (1), needle (4), and syringe (3). Bag (2) holds a reduced quantity of anticoagulated blood for aliquot reinfusion. Reprinted with permission from Tasaki T, Ohto H. Nineteen years of experience with autotransfusion for elective surgery in children: more troublesome than we expected. Transfusion. 2007;47 (8):1503–9

as 8 kg, although most reports of smaller children include body weights around 20 kg [49, 52, 53]. Donation volumes documented in the literature range from 6 to 19 mL/kg body weight, most commonly 10 mL/kg per donation event, with frequencies as often as weekly [18, 52]. In a 2007 review of pediatric PAD, four of the 17 studies performed the procedure in a hospital or specialized clinic setting; two reports used intravenous sedation or "light anesthesia" [4, 17, 37, 60, 61]. Most studies in this review were retrospective in nature, with no randomized controlled trials found. It is imperative that PAD be performed in a pediatric-oriented setting and by experts in pediatric critical care (such as pediatric anesthesiologists or intensivists) who are supported by pediatric-trained personnel [4] The risk of human error may be increased for children donating blood in a medical system geared toward adults [62, 63].

7.3.4 PAD Limitations

The literature contains many arguments against routine use of PAD [9, 64]. One meta-analysis found PAD to have a 24% increased the risk of any transfusion (OR 1.24, 95% CI 1.02–1.51) [33]. This same study, however, found that the risk of receiving an allogeneic transfusion was decreased by 68% when PAD was incorporated into a perioperative blood management plan. Results from the limited number of studies suggest that pediatric PAD may lead to a reduced allogeneic (homologous) transfusion rate, and it continues to be recommended in some centers [4, 16–18, 29]. Opponents point out that stored autologous blood does not eliminate the risk of human error and bacterial contamination, and data from the US and Canada indicate that autologous units have been administered to the wrong patient [16]. Although PAD is more costly due to administrative complexities, a well-organized program with institutional support has been shown to reduce costs [18, 29, 65]. Wastage of unused units is significant (up to 50–90% of donated units), although waste may be less severe in a well-structured, standardized system [18, 29]. Acute adverse events associated with PAD have been reported to occur more frequently in children (i.e., > 25% of donation events) compared to adults and include hypotension, dizziness, failure to obtain intravenous access (i.e., size 12 to 19-gauge cannulae), noncooperation, and vasovagal reactions especially in the adolescent population [4, 42, 52, 55, 66].

7.4 Is It Possible for a Child with Cancer to Participate in Preoperative Autologous Donation?

PAD is a controversial alternative in cancer patients [67, 68]. Although transfusion-related immunomodulation (TRIM) is generally accepted as a side effect of blood transfusion, outcome reports are mixed [69]. Graft survival has been shown to improve following allogeneic transfusion in kidney transplants, presumably the result of TRIM [70]. Perioperative allogeneic transfusion has been linked to cancer recurrence in colorectal cancer patients (OR 1.41, 95% CI, 1.2–1.67) and in patients undergoing liver resection, although direct causation is uncertain [71–74]. Early reports also demonstrate an increased risk of postoperative infections and delayed wound healing following allogeneic transfusion [75, 76]. The exact pathophysiology underlying TRIM remains unclear, although leukocyte activity has been described, and leukocyte reduction filters and saline washing of cellular blood components have been proposed as countermeasures [39, 73, 77, 78]. An important blood management alternative, intraoperative cell salvage (ICS), has been used in cancer surgery (e.g., urologic, hepatic, gynecologic) with multiple studies finding that there is not an increased rate of cancer metastasis or recurrence [79, 80]. Blood recovery machine manufacturers may advise against use in cancer surgery, notwithstanding the fact that tumor manipulation during surgery releases cells into the bloodstream. Clinical outcomes have not established that autotransfusion is directly linked to metastatic spread [39, 81]. Another form of autologous transfusion, ANH, did not affect 5-year survival in gynecologic patients undergoing debulking for advanced ovarian cancer [82]. In other cancer patient studies, PAD transfusion has been associated with reduced allogenic blood requirements, enhanced erythropoiesis, and unchanged long-term surgical survival rates [71, 83, 84]. As a result, national organizations with blood donation oversight allow some cancer patients to donate their own blood under certain conditions [42, 85–87]. In general, donation is allowed if the cancer is highly localized (e.g., in situ cervical or skin), solid organ, or nonhematologic, and chemotherapy treatment is complete. A cancer patient who desires PAD is more likely to be disqualified for other reasons, such as anemia, infection, or low body weight. A deferral period of a minimum 1–5 years following curative treatment is likely, and the duration of deferral is at the discretion of the donor center medical director. Adults who have recovered from childhood leukemia are also potential blood donors; however, adulthood hematologic cancers including Hodgkin's lymphoma are likely to result in permanent deferral. Other disqualifying cancer conditions include disease recurrence, active treatment, and a history of Kaposi sarcoma [42].

7.5 Should Parents Act As Directed Blood Donors for Their Child's Upcoming Cancer Surgery?

7.5.1 Directed Donations

A directed donation is made by an individual that a potential blood recipient chooses, and that person is typically an acquaintance or family member. Similar to the rise in popularity of PAD, the peak period of requests for designated donations occurred in the 1980s at the height of the HIV epidemic [20, 43]. However, the percentage of allogeneic donations in the US that are directed has declined appreciably as TTI screening has improved and with increased knowledge about the potential pitfalls of directed donations, discussed below [1, 20, 88]. Some blood centers, including the AABB and the Canadian Blood Services, recommend against directed donations, except in very special circumstances [1, 42]. As with PADs, the ultimate decision to proceed with a directed donations lies with the blood center medical director.

Donor requirements for directed donation are the same as for community, allogeneic blood donors, although the inter-donation interval requirement may be shorter [42]. For this reason, some blood centers allow unused directed donations to be crossed over into the general blood supply. A directed donation cannot proceed without a doctor's order, and the donor must undergo a lengthy and standardized questionnaire that addresses lifestyle behaviors. Directed donations also require heightened informed consent, including the possibility that their blood may be rejected based on a positive infectious disease screen, or that genetic similarity between donor and recipient may set the stage for fatal transfusion-associated graft-vs-host disease (TA-GVHD) [42, 89]. As with PAD blood, 2–5 days processing time is required between donation and blood availability, and the shelf life of the blood is limited (21–35 days). A shorter shelf-life is mandated if the donated blood is irradiated to prevent TA-GVHD when donor and recipient are related [30, 38, 43].

The most common indication for receiving a directed donation is when a patient has multiple alloantibodies to red blood cell (RBC) antigens that exist in high frequency in the population, and the only blood source available is a family member or other specified person [20, 42, 43, 46]. Other indications include platelet refractoriness in the chronically transfused child, IgA-deficiency, and very rare blood types [43, 90, 91]. A rare blood type (e.g., Indian or Bombay) is one that occurs with a frequency of 1:1000–10,000 [43]. A specialized blood bank, the American Rare Donor Program, may meet the needs of chronically transfused patients with sickle cell disease who may have alloimmunization rates up to 47% [43, 92]. Some blood centers deem severe parental psychological distress to be an indication for donating blood to their child [89]. Directed donation from a parent for fetal and neonatal alloimmune thrombocytopenia (FNAIT) is contraindicated because of the possibility that maternal plasma or paternal platelets are incompatible with the fetus [46, 91].

There are risks associated with directed donations, some leading to severe morbidity in the recipient. As with PAD, the directed donations process is viewed by many blood centers as administratively complex and expensive, outweighing any benefits over the safe blood supply in high resource countries [42, 89, 93]. In a retrospective study of over 11 million US blood donors between 2005 and 2010, although the overall viral positivity rates for HIV and hepatitis remained low, the directed donations cohort positivity rate was more than three times that of community volunteers [88]. Adding to this uncertainty is a 2017 donor record review by Jacquot et al. that examined the TTI positivity rate in parents who were screened as directed donors for their children [94]. In a cohort of 1532 parents, the viral positivity rates were 8.66% and 1.25% for first-time and repeat donors, respectively. The same percentages in 4910 nonparent donors were 1.90% for first-time and 0% for repeat donors. As a result of their findings, the Jacquot investigators recommend against the use of parents who are first-time, directed donors [94]. The Jacquot study is crucial because it highlights a concern that designated donors, especially parents, may fail to be fully candid about medical or social history given the sensitive relationship between donor and recipient [20, 30, 46, 95].

A serious consequence of directed donation is transfusion-associated graft-versus-host-disease (TA-GVHD). TA-GVHD may occur when there is genetic similarity of the human lymphocyte antigen (HLA) system between the donor and recipient [96, 97]. TA-GVHD is usually fatal and occurs when donor T-lymphocytes are not recognized by the recipient as "foreign," engraft in the recipient, and produce a massive inflammatory response 4–10 days following transfusion [97]. Certain patients are thought to be susceptible to TA-GVHD, including premature infants, patients with severe congenital immunodeficiency, Hodgkin's disease, and those receiving HLA-matched platelet, intrauterine, or exchange transfusions [46, 91, 98]. In Japan, where there is significant genetic homogeneity, the risk of HLA matching has been estimated to be 1:874 with a random donation, and this risk increases up to 30 times if the donor and recipient are related [97]. In the US, which has a more genetically heterogenous demographic, the risk of HLA similarity has been calculated as 1:7174 for random and 1:475 for related donations [91, 97]. For this reason, designated donation from a related donor is not encouraged, except in cases of a rare blood type in the face of blood scarcity. Irradiation of blood products at a dose of 25 Gy as a preventative measure will inactivate most donor lymphocytes [46]. Most transfusion services provide irradiated cellular blood products for infants under a certain age, whereas others have a blanket policy of universal irradiation with the goal of preventing TA-GVHD in immunocompromised patients who are not yet diagnosed as such. The Pediatric Critical Care Transfusion and Anemia (TAXI) consortium recommends pretransfusion irradiation of all cellular blood components administered to severely immune compromised, critically ill children [98]. Pretransfusion leukoreduction (LR) may be protective against but does not eliminate the risk of TA-GVHD in susceptible individuals because even the highest quality LR process leaves residual leukocytes [99, 100]. In the majority US blood centers, blood products are leukocyte-reduced, either post-donation or, uncommonly, at the bedside [101].

In addition to TA-GVHD, a directed donation may be complicated in other ways due to HLA-system similarity between relatives. If a man donates blood to the mother of his children, their offspring may develop fetal and neonatal autoimmune thrombocytopenia (FNAIT) if their platelets carry the father's HLA genotype. Furthermore, because all transfusions create a risk of alloimmunization or HLA sensitization, if the donor and recipient have HLA relatedness, the recipient may develop HLA antibodies against the donor. In that case, the donor—a family member who may be the only match available—may become unable to serve as a future transplant donor for that recipient [20, 43, 102]. Finally, an additional risk of a mother to child donation is transfusion-associated acute lung injury (TRALI). Women who have been pregnant may develop HLA antibodies against paternally derived white blood cells (WBCs) [68, 103]. As a result, mother to child plasma transfusions may set the stage for TRALI and are likely to be prohibited [38, 46].

7.6 Summary of Key Learning Objectives

7.6.1 May a Child Donate Her Own Blood Prior to Surgery for Future Perioperative Use?

Pediatric patients in relatively good health can donate their own blood for perioperative use if they meet specific criteria. In this case, the 10 y.o., 40 kg child with yet untreated osteosarcoma meets the minimum Hgb requirement (11 g/dL) but weighs less than the usual cutoff of 50 kg. PAD has been performed in children weighing less than 50 kg; thus, an exception may be made if approved by the blood center medical director. Another consideration for PAD is the surgery itself: It must be elective or urgent in nature and must take place at least 2–3 weeks from the date of donation to provide iron therapy and recovery of iron stores. The surgery should also be associated with significant blood loss to substantiate the extra cost and scheduling required. A preoperative donation of 10–20% of the patient's estimated blood volume (2800 mL), or 280 mL–560 mL total, can be donated ideally in two donation events. PAD volumes exceeding perioperative requirements may lead to blood wastage, or unnecessary administration of the patient's PAD blood simply because it is available. The latter situation puts the patient at risk for over transfusion, receipt of a contaminated unit, or receipt of the incorrect unit, the same risks that are associated with blood transfusions in general.

7.7 Is It Possible for a Child with Cancer Participate in Preoperative Autologous Donation?

This patient meets the criteria for PAD under AABB guidelines because she has a newly diagnosed cancer that is untreated, localized, and nonhematologic. Although patients who are undergoing chemotherapy will not be able to donate to the community blood supply, the blood center's policies or medical director may make an exception for an autologous donation in special circumstances. The family's stated desire for autologous blood donation should be discussed with the surgeon and oncologist. An informed consent discussion about the risks of PAD in general in necessary, including but not limited to, anemia, conflicting evidence regarding autologous blood and cancer metastasis, and alternatives such as ICS and intraoperative ANH.

7.8 Should Parents Act As Directed Blood Donors for Their Child's Upcoming Cancer Surgery?

The best options for blood management during this child's elective blood loss surgery include preoperative Hgb optimization, intraoperative ANH or ICS, a restrictive transfusion threshold, coagulation monitoring, the addition of an antifibrinolytic such as tranexamic acid (TXA), and postoperative Hgb surveillance. Because she does not have a rare blood type or other factors supporting a directed donation, the risks of receiving a blood transfusion from one of her parents should receive serious consideration. A 2017 study found that parent blood donors may have a higher likelihood of TTI positivity on initial screening, creating a difficult family dynamic if a parental donation is rejected. Given the donor-recipient genetic similarity in this case, there is also an increased risk of potentially fatal TA-GVHD. Furthermore, if either parent is a blood donor for this patient, recipient HLA sensitization may occur and later disqualify that parent from acting as a future blood, bone marrow, or other transplant donor.

Key Points

- The banked blood supply in high resource countries is as safe as it has ever been and preoperative autologous donation (PAD) rates have declined over the past several decades.
- Donor requirements for PAD may be less than those required of the general, volunteer donor population. For that reason, an unused PAD blood unit is not likely to be used in the general blood supply and will be discarded.
- PAD in children entails special considerations, including a specified weight requirement along with pediatric-oriented equipment and trained staff.
- Cancer patients can participate in PAD if the cancer is highly localized, solid organ, or nonhematologic, and their chemotherapy treatment is complete. A cancer patient who desires PAD is more likely to be disqualified for other reasons such as anemia, infection, or low body weight.
- Many blood centers recommend against directed donations, except in very special circumstances. Risks associated with directed donations include TA-GVHD, TRALI, and TTIs, as well as many of the same risks associated with allogeneic transfusions: misidentification, bacterial contamination, and cytokine release.

References

1. Canadian Blood Services. Chapter 16: Preoperative autologous donation. 2021. https://professionaleducation.blood.ca/en/transfusion/clinical-guide/preoperative-autologous-donation. Accessed 30 Apr 2024.
2. Goodnough LT. Autologous blood donation. Crit Care. 2004;8(Suppl 2):S49–52.
3. Stramer SL, Galel SA. Infection disease testing. In: Fung MK, Eder AF, Spitalnik SL, editors. Technical manual. 19th ed. Bethesda: AABB; 2017. p. 161–4.
4. Lauder GR. Pre-operative predeposit autologous donation in children presenting for elective surgery: a review. Transfus Med. 2007;17(2):75–82.
5. Hayes EV. Human immunodeficiency virus and immunodeficiency syndrome. In: Kliegman RM Blum NJ, Shah SS, editors. Nelson textbook of pediatrics. Philadelphia: Elsevier; 2020. p. 1781.
6. Goldfinger D. Controversies in transfusion medicine. Directed blood donations: pro. Transfusion. 1989;29(1):70–4.
7. Infectious Disease Testing. American Red Cross Blood Services. 2022. https://www.redcrossblood.org/biomedical-services/blood-diagnostic-testing/blood-testing.html#:~:text=The%20

per%2Dunit%20risk%20of%20HIV%2D1%20infection%20through%20blood,HIV%20by%20about%202%20weeks. Accessed 17 Mar 2022.
8. Dodd RY, Crowder LA, Haynes JM, Notari EP, Stramer SL, Steele WR. Screening blood donors for HIV, HCV, and HBV at the American red Cross: 10-year trends in prevalence, incidence, and residual risk, 2007 to 2016. Transfus Med Rev. 2020;34(2):81–93.
9. Sanford KW. Guide to infection Control in the healthcare setting: transfusions. International Society for Infectious Diseases (ISID); 2023. https://isid.org/guide/infectionprevention/transfusions/. Accessed 21 July 2023.
10. Christensen RD, Bahr TM, Christensen TR, Ohls RK, Krong J, Carlton LC, et al. Banked term umbilical cord blood to meet the packed red blood cell transfusion needs of extremely-low-gestational-age neonates: a feasibility analysis. J Perinatol. 2023;44(6):873.
11. Yazer MH, Jackson B, Beckman N, Chesneau S, Bowler P, Delaney M, et al. Changes in blood center red blood cell distributions in the era of patient blood management: the trends for collection (TFC) study. Transfusion. 2016;56(8):1965–73.
12. Fung MK, editor. Technical manual. 19th ed. Bethesda: AABB Press; 2017. p. 115, 120–121, 464–469, 481–489.
13. Etchason J, Petz L, Keeler E, Calhoun L, Kleinman S, Snider C, et al. The cost effectiveness of preoperative autologous blood donations. N Engl J Med. 1995;332(11):719–24.
14. Hamilton CM, Davenport DL, Bernard AC. Demonstration of a U.S. nationwide reduction in transfusion in general surgery and a review of published transfusion reduction methodologies. Transfusion. 2021;61(11):3119–28.
15. HHS.gov. National Blood Collection & Utilization Survey. 15 Sept 2021. https://www.hhs.gov/oidp/topics/blood-tissue-safety/surveys/national-blood-collection-and-utilization-survey/index.html. Accessed 19 Mar 2022.
16. Vassallo R, Goldman M, Germain M, Lozano M, Collaborative B. Preoperative autologous blood donation: waning indications in an era of improved blood safety. Transfus Med Rev. 2015;29(4):268–75.
17. Hibino N, Nagashima M, Sato H, Hori T, Ishitoya H, Tomino T. Preoperative autologous blood donation for cardiac surgery in children. Asian Cardiovasc Thorac Ann. 2008;16(1):21–4.
18. Letts M, Perng R, Luke B, Jarvis J, Lawton L, Hoey S. An analysis of a preoperative pediatric autologous blood donation program. Can J Surg. 2000;43(2):125–9.
19. Forgie MA, Wells PS, Laupacis A, Fergusson D. Preoperative autologous donation decreases allogeneic transfusion but increases exposure to all red blood cell transfusion: results of a meta-analysis. International study of perioperative transfusion (ISPOT) investigators. Arch Intern Med. 1998;158(6):610–6.
20. Joe Chaffin BBGuy Podcast. 062CE: Autologous and Directed Donations with Julie Karp. 2019. https://www.bbguy.org/2019/01/18/062/. Accessed 18 Mar 2022.
21. Foster T, Yan M. Preoperative autologous donation. In: Clinical Guide to Transfusion. Canadian Blood Services; 2021. https://professionaleducation.blood.ca/en/transfusion/clinical-guide-transfusion . Accessed 16 Mar 2022.
22. Patient Blood Management Guidelines. 3.6.1. Preoperative Autologous Donation. National Blood Authority (Australia). https://www.blood.gov.au/system/files/documents/pbm-module-2.pdf . Accessed 16 Mar 2022.
23. Applewhite KY. A look at parental autonomy in pediatric transfusion medicine. In: AABB News. 2023. https://www.aabb.org/docs/default-source/member-protected-files/news/aabb-news-magazine/news2302.pdf?sfvrsn=1cb84f7c_4. 12.
24. Perry N. New Zealand court rules against anti-vax parents of ill baby. AP News. 7 Dec 2022. https://apnews.com/article/health-new-zealand-covid-blood-transfusion-5a2a190d241816a4c26ba2c384ffc012. Accessed 22 July 2023.
25. Association for the Advancement of Blood & Biotherapies (AABB). Policy Statement: Proposals Related to Vaccination and Blood Donation. 2024. https://www.aabb.org/docs/default-source/default-documentlibrary/positions/aabb-position-statement-policy-proposals-related-to-blood-donation-and-vaccines.pdf?sfvrsn=5d533d23_3. Accessed 27 Feb 2025.

26. Association for the Advancement of Blood & Biotherapies (AABB). Policy Statement: Policy Proposals Containing Requirements for Directed and Autologous Blood Donations. 2024. https://www.aabb.org/docs/default-source/default-document-library/positions/aabb-position-statement-policy-proposals-containing-requirements-for-directed-or-autologous-blood-donations.pdf?sfvrsn=400a5a93_5. Accessed 27 Feb 2025.
27. State of California. Health and Safety Code. Chapter 4.5. The Paul Gann Blood Safety Act. Section 1645. 2024. https://www.mbc.ca.gov/Resources/Publications/Mandated-Standardized-Written-Information.aspx. Accessed 30 Mar 2024.
28. Goldfinger D, Pepkowitz SH. Directed blood donations and the concept of individualized care in transfusion medicine. Am J Clin Pathol. 1989;92(4):516–7.
29. Tsuno NH, Nagura Y, Kawabata M, Matsuhashi M, Sone S, Ikeda T, et al. The current status of autologous blood transfusion in Japan—the importance of pre-deposit autologous blood donation program and the needs to achieve patient blood management. Transfus Apher Sci. 2013;49(3):673–80.
30. Autologous and Directed Donations. American Red Cross: Blood Services. 2022. https://www.redcrossblood.org/donate-blood/how-to-donate/types-of-blood-donations/autologous-and-directed-donations.html#:~:text=Autologous%20donations%20are%20donations%20that,for%20example%2C%20before%20a%20surgery.&text=Autologous%20donations%20require%20a%20doctor's,be%20signed%20by%20your%20physician. Accessed 16 Mar 2022.
31. Bandarenko N, editor. Pediatric transfusion: a handbook. 5th ed. American Association of Blood Banks (AABB); 2020. p. 227–30.
32. Frank S, Guinn NR. Patient blood management. In: Cohn C, Delaney M, Johnson ST, Katz LM, editors. Technical manual. 20th ed. Bethesda, MD: AABB; 2020. p. 592–6.
33. Henry DA, Carless PA, Moxey AJ, O'Connell D, Forgie MA, Wells PS, et al. Pre-operative autologous donation for minimising perioperative allogeneic blood transfusion. Cochrane Database Syst Rev. 2002;2001(2):CD003602.
34. Oakley FD, Woods M, Arnold S, Young PP. Transfusion reactions in pediatric compared with adult patients: a look at rate, reaction type, and associated products. Transfusion. 2015;55(3):563–70.
35. Vossoughi S, Perez G, Whitaker BI, Fung MK, Stotler B. Analysis of pediatric adverse reactions to transfusions. Transfusion. 2018;58(1):60–9.
36. Inappropriate Use of Autologous Blood. In: Eichbaum QG, Booth GS, Young PP, editors. Transfusion medicine: quality in laboratory diagnosis. New York: demosMEDICAL; 2013. p. 31–3.
37. Mayer MN, de Montalembert M, Audat F, Brusset MC, Houfani B, Merckx J, et al. Autologous blood donation for elective surgery in children weighing 8-25 kg. Vox Sang. 1996;70(4):224–8.
38. Directed Blood Donation Information. Stanford blood center. 2017–2022. https://stanfordbloodcenter.org/wp-content/uploads/2017/06/03-F09Form_DirectedDonationInfoSheet.pdf. Accessed 17 Mar 2022.
39. Joint United Kingdom (UK) Blood Transfusion and Tissue Transplantation Services Professional Advisory Committee. Autologous blood transfusion (collection and reinfusion of the patient's own red blood cells). In: 6.1.1 Predeposit autologous donation (PAD). Joint United Kingdom (UK) Blood Transfusion and Tissue Transplantation Services Professional Advisory Committee; 2020. https://www.transfusionguidelines.org/transfusion-handbook/6-alternatives-and-adjuncts-to-blood-transfusion/6-1-autologous-blood-transfusion-collection-and-reinfusion-of-the-patient-s-own-red-blood-cells. Accessed 17 Mar 2022.
40. Anon. Process Control. In: Standards for blood banks and transfusion services. 30th ed. Bethesda, MD: AABB; 2016. p. 16–37.
41. Reppucci ML, Meier M, Stevens J, Shirek G, Kulungowski AM, Acker SN. Incidence of and risk factors for perioperative blood transfusion in infants undergoing index pediatric surgery procedures. J Pediatr Surg. 2022;57:1067.

42. Kessler LA, Rossmann SN. Allogeneic and Autologous Blood Donor Selection. In: Fung MK, Eder AF, Spitalnik SL, editors. Technical Manual. 19th ed. Bethesda, MD: AABB; 2017. p. 111–122; 175.
43. Wadge G, Zhang J, Seal J, Cooper ES, Alquist CR. Directed donation: special considerations and review for contemporary clinical practices. Ochsner J. 2021;21(3):281–6.
44. Crowder LA, Steele WR, Stramer SL. Infectious disease screening. In: Cohn C, Delaney M, Johnson ST, Katz LM, editors. Technical manual. 20th ed. Bethesda, MD: AABB; 2020. p. 173, 198, 213.
45. Perioperative Standards Committee. Sections 1, 5, and 7. In: Standards for perioperative autologous blood collection and administration. 10th ed. Bethesda: AABB; 2023.
46. Roseff S, Wong ECC. Donor specific units. In: Pediatric transfusion: a handbook. 5th ed. Bethesda: AABB; 2020. p. 14, 227–230.
47. NICE Quality Standard QS 138: blood transfusion. NICE National Institute for Health and Care Excellence. 2016. https://www.nice.org.uk/guidance/qs138/chapter/Quality-statements. Accessed 17 Mar 2022.
48. Iwase Y, Kohjitani A, Tohya A, Sugiyama K. Preoperative autologous blood donation and acute normovolemic hemodilution affect intraoperative blood loss during sagittal split ramus osteotomy. Transfus Apher Sci. 2012;46(3):245–51.
49. Vanderlinde ES, Heal JM, Blumberg N. Autologous transfusion. BMJ. 2002;324(7340):772–5.
50. Acker J, Razatos A. Whole blood and Aherersis collection of blood components intended for transfusion. In: Cohn C, Delaney M, Johnson ST, Katz LM, editors. Technical manual. 20th ed. Bethesda, MD: AABB; 2020. p. 145–147, 159–161.
51. Alquist C, Harm SK. Transfusion service related activities. In: Cohn C, Delaney M, Johnson ST, Katz LM, editors. Technical manual. 20th ed. Bethesda, MD: AABB; 2020. p. 503–504, 510–517, 522.
52. Tasaki T, Ohto H. Nineteen years of experience with autotransfusion for elective surgery in children: more troublesome than we expected. Transfusion. 2007;47(8):1503–9.
53. Lavoie J. Blood transfusion risks and alternative strategies in pediatric patients. Paediatr Anaesth. 2011;21(1):14–24.
54. Domen RE. Preoperative autologous blood donation: clinical, economic, and ethical issues. Cleve Clin J Med. 1996;63(5):295–300.
55. Sonzogni V, Crupi G, Poma R, Annechino F, Ferri F, Filisetti P, et al. Erythropoietin therapy and preoperative autologous blood donation in children undergoing open heart surgery. Br J Anaesth. 2001;87(3):429–34.
56. Prinsze FJ, de Groot R, Timmer TC, Zalpuri S, van den Hurk K. Donation-induced iron depletion is significantly associated with low hemoglobin at subsequent donations. Transfusion. 2021;61(12):3344–52.
57. Szczepiorkowski Z, Hopkins T. Updated strategies to limit or prevent iron deficiency in blood donors. AABB Bulletin #17–02 2017. https://www.aabb.org/docs/default-source/default-document-library/resources/association-bulletins/ab17-02.pdf . Accessed 21 Mar 2022.
58. Sarin K, Chauhan S, Bisoi AK, Hazarika A, Malhotra N, Manek P. Use of autologous umbilical cord blood transfusion in neonates undergoing surgical correction of congenital cardiac defects: a pilot study. Ann Card Anaesth. 2018;21(3):270–4.
59. Clinical Growth Charts. CDC National Center for Health Statistics. 2017. https://www.cdc.gov/growthcharts/clinical_charts.htm. Accessed 22 Mar 2022.
60. Longatti PL, Paccagnella F, Agostini S, Nieri A, Carteri A. Autologous hemodonation in the corrective surgery of craniostenosis. Childs Nerv Syst. 1991;7(1):40–2.
61. Fukahara K, Murakami A, Ueda T, Doki Y, Tsubata S, Ichida F, et al. Scheduled autologous blood donation at the time of cardiac catheterization in infants and children. J Thorac Cardiovasc Surg. 1997;114(3):504–5.
62. Slusher TM, Kiragu AW, Day LT, Bjorklund AR, Shirk A, Johannsen C, et al. Pediatric critical Care in Resource-Limited Settings-Overview and Lessons Learned. Front Pediatr. 2018;6:49.

63. Newton MW, Hurt SE, McEvoy MD, Shi Y, Shotwell MS, Kamau J, et al. Pediatric perioperative mortality in Kenya: a prospective cohort study from 24 hospitals. Anesthesiology. 2020;132(3):452–60.
64. Schved JF. Preoperative autologous blood donation: a therapy that needs to be scientifically evaluated. Transfus Clin Biol. 2005;12(5):365–9.
65. Frank SM, Waters JH, editors. Patient blood management: multidisciplinary approaches to optimizing care. Bethesda: AABB Press; 2016. p. 6, 29–47, 180–186, 241.
66. Murto KT, Splinter WM. Perioperative autologous blood donation in children. Transfus Sci. 1999;21(1):41–62.
67. Morris-Stiff G, Steel A, Savage P, Devlin J, Griffiths D, Portman B, et al. Transmission of donor melanoma to multiple organ transplant recipients. Am J Transplant. 2004;4(3):444–6.
68. Yang H, Lee J, Seed CR, Keller AJ. Can blood transfusion transmit cancer? A literature review. Transfus Med Rev. 2010;24(3):235–43.
69. Blajchman MA. Immunomodulation and blood transfusion. Am J Ther. 2002;9(5):389–95.
70. Opelz G, Graver B, Terasaki PI. Induction of high kidney graft survival rate by multiple transfusion. Lancet. 1981;1(8232):1223–5.
71. Heiss MM, Mempel W, Delanoff C, Jauch KW, Gabka C, Mempel M, et al. Blood transfusion-modulated tumor recurrence: first results of a randomized study of autologous versus allogeneic blood transfusion in colorectal cancer surgery. J Clin Oncol. 1994;12(9):1859–67.
72. Bennett S, Baker LK, Martel G, Shorr R, Pawlik TM, Tinmouth A, et al. The impact of perioperative red blood cell transfusions in patients undergoing liver resection: a systematic review. HPB (Oxford). 2017;19(4):321–30.
73. Amato A, Pescatori M. Perioperative blood transfusions for the recurrence of colorectal cancer. Cochrane Database Syst Rev. 2006;2011(1):CD005033.
74. Heiss MM, Fraunberger P, Delanoff C, Stets R, Allgayer H, Ströhlein MA, et al. Modulation of immune response by blood transfusion: evidence for a differential effect of allogeneic and autologous blood in colorectal cancer surgery. Shock. 1997;8(6):402–8.
75. Jensen LS, Andersen AJ, Christiansen PM, Hokland P, Juhl CO, Madsen G, et al. Postoperative infection and natural killer cell function following blood transfusion in patients undergoing elective colorectal surgery. Br J Surg. 1992;79(6):513–6.
76. Tartter PI. Transfusion-induced immunosuppression and perioperative infections. Beitr Infusionsther. 1993;31:52–63.
77. Refaai MA, Blumberg N. Transfusion immunomodulation from a clinical perspective: an update. Expert Rev Hematol. 2013;6(6):653–63.
78. Cata JP, Owusu-Agyemang P, Kapoor R, Lonnqvist PA. Impact of anesthetics, analgesics, and perioperative blood transfusion in pediatric cancer patients: a comprehensive review of the literature. Anesth Analg. 2019;129(6):1653–65.
79. Waters JH, Yazer M, Chen YF, Kloke J. Blood salvage and cancer surgery: a meta-analysis of available studies. Transfusion. 2012;52(10):2167–73.
80. Trudeau JD, Waters T, Chipperfield K. Should intraoperative cell-salvaged blood be used in patients with suspected or known malignancy? Can J Anaesth. 2012;59(11):1058–70.
81. Waters JH. Intraoperative blood recovery and reinfusion. In: Frank SM, Waters JH, editors. Patient blood management: multidisciplinary approaches to optimizing care. Bethesda: AABB Press; 2016. p. 186.
82. Boerner T, Tanner E, Filippova O, Zhou QC, Iasonos A, Tew WP, et al. Survival outcomes of acute normovolemic hemodilution in patients undergoing primary debulking surgery for advanced ovarian cancer: a memorial Sloan Kettering cancer center team ovary study. Gynecol Oncol. 2021;160(1):51–5.
83. Kang R, Seath BE, Huang V, Barth RJ. Impact of autologous blood transfusion on survival and recurrence among patients undergoing partial hepatectomy for colorectal cancer liver metastases. J Am Coll Surg. 2019;228(6):902–8.
84. Hoynck van Papendrecht MA, Hop W, Langenhorst BL, Kothe FC, Marquet RL, Jeekel J. Feasibility of a predeposit autologous blood donation program in colorectal cancer patients: results from a randomized clinical study. Vox Sang. 1992;62(2):102–7.

85. Can I Donate Blood If I'm a Cancer Survivor? American Cancer Society 2022. https://www.cancer.org/treatment/treatments-and-side-effects/treatment-types/blood-transfusion-and-donation/blood-donation-by-cancer-survivors.html . Accessed 16 Mar 2022.
86. I have had cancer. Can I donate? Australian Red Cross Lifeblood. 2021–2022. https://www.lifeblood.com.au/faq/eligibility/medical-conditions-and-procedures/cancer . Accessed 16 Mar 2022.
87. Eligibility Criteria. American Red Cross Blood Services. https://www.redcrossblood.org/donate-blood/how-to-donate/eligibility-requirements/eligibility-criteria-alphabetical.html. Accessed 22 Mar 2022.
88. Dorsey KA, Moritz ED, Steele WR, Eder AF, Stramer SL. A comparison of human immunodeficiency virus, hepatitis C virus, hepatitis B virus, and human T-lymphotropic virus marker rates for directed versus volunteer blood donations to the American red Cross during 2005 to 2010. Transfusion. 2013;53(6):1250–6.
89. Canadian Blood Services, Lau W. Chapter 13: neonatal and pediatric transfusions. 2017. https://professionaleducation.blood.ca/en/transfusion/clinical-guide/neonatal-and-pediatric-transfusion . Accessed 23 February 2025..
90. Ballas SK, Draper EK, Harris M, MacCarthy V. Designated blood donations. N Engl J Med. 1984;310(2):124–5.
91. Klein HG, Anstee DJ, editors. Mollison's blood transfusion in clinical medicine. New Jersey: Wiley Blackwell; 2014. p. 14, 188, 194, 335, 500, 667–668.
92. Flickinger C. REGGI and the American rare donor program. Transfus Med Hemother. 2014;41(5):342–5.
93. Cordell RR, Yalon VA, Cigahn-Haskell C, McDonough BP, Perkins HA. Experience with 11,916 designated donors. Transfusion. 1986;26(5):484–6.
94. Jacquot C, Seo A, Miller PM, Lezama N, Criss VR, Colvin C, et al. Parental versus non-parental-directed donation: an 11-year experience of infectious disease testing at a pediatric tertiary care blood donor center. Transfusion. 2017;57(11):2799–803.
95. Kruskall MS, Umlas J. Acquired immunodeficiency syndrome and directed blood donations. A dilemma for American medicine. Arch Surg. 1988;123(1):23–5.
96. Ohto H, Yasuda H, Noguchi M, Abe R. Risk of transfusion-associated graft-versus-host disease as a result of directed donations from relatives. Transfusion. 1992;32(7):691–3.
97. Schroeder ML. Transfusion-associated graft-versus-host disease. Br J Haematol. 2002;117(2):275–87.
98. Zantek ND, Parker RI, van de Watering LM, Josephson CD, Bateman ST, Valentine SL, et al. Recommendations on selection and processing of RBC components for pediatric patients from the pediatric critical care transfusion and anemia expertise initiative. Pediatr Crit Care Med. 2018;19(9S Suppl 1):S163–S9.
99. Klein HG, Anstee DJ. Mollison's blood transfusion in clinical medicine. 12th ed. New York: Wiley-Blackwell; 2014.
100. Elliot J, Narayan S, Poles D, Tuckley V, Bolton-Maggs PHB. Missed irradiation of cellular blood components for vulnerable patients: insights from 10 years of SHOT data. Transfusion. 2021;61(2):385–92.
101. Spinella PC, Tucci M, Fergusson DA, Lacroix J, Hébert PC, Leteurtre S, et al. Effect of fresh vs Standard-issue red blood cell transfusions on multiple organ dysfunction syndrome in critically ill pediatric patients: a randomized clinical trial. JAMA. 2019;322(22):2179–90.
102. Lau W. Clinical guide to transfusion: chapter 13: neonatal and pediatric transfusions: Canadian Blood Services. 2017. https://professionaleducation.blood.ca/en/transfusion/clinical-guide/neonatal-and-pediatric-transfusion. Accessed 30 Mar 2024.
103. Dunbar N, Cooke M, Diab M, Toy P. Transfusion-related acute lung injury after transfusion of maternal blood: a case-control study. Spine (Phila Pa 1976). 2010;35(23):E1322–7.

Pediatric Perioperative Transfusion-Related Equipment

8

Amy Graham-Carlson and Norma J. Klein

8.1 Case Scenario

A 6 kg, 8-month-old male is scheduled for an emergency craniotomy to evacuate bilateral subdural hematomas secondary to non-accidental trauma. When he arrives to the operating room (OR), he is intubated and has bilateral antecubital fossae peripheral intravenous catheters (PIVCs) in place: a 22 gauge in the right arm and a 24 gauge in the left. His blood pressure (BP) is 50/25 and heart rate (HR) 162, and his initial hemoglobin is 7 g/dL. The anesthesia technician places a rapid infusion device (RID) in your OR setup. The surgeon has not yet opened the dura mater. You consider the options available to transfuse large volumes of blood rapidly and safely in this infant. His baseline estimated blood volume (EBV) is 480 mL (e.g., 80 mL/kg body weight).

The equipment-related data in this chapter are based on published information and do not necessarily reflect the opinion or advice of the authors. Manufacturer-related data may be updated at times and may differ or be incomplete in online sources. There was no industry funding contributing to the production of this chapter.

A. Graham-Carlson (✉)
Department of Anesthesiology, Critical Care, McGovern Medical School Children's Memorial Hermann Hospital, Houston, TX, USA
e-mail: Amy.d.grahamcarlson@uth.tmc.edu

N. J. Klein
Department of Anesthesiology and Pain Medicine, University of California, Davis, Sacramento, CA, USA
e-mail: nklein@ucdavis.edu

N. J. Klein (ed.), *Perioperative Pediatric Patient Blood Management and Transfusion Safety*, https://doi.org/10.1007/978-3-031-81666-6_8

Key Learning Objectives

Discuss available options to support blood volume replacement in children including:

- Rapid infusion devices.
- Vascular access.
- Vascular access insertion sites.
- Fluid warmers.
- Blood filters.

What adverse events are associated with rapid blood transfusions in pediatric patients?

8.2 Discussion

8.2.1 General

There are many challenges during management of pediatric hemorrhagic shock, particularly with respect to neonates and infants. As healthcare practitioners we are often confronted with difficult vascular access that is compounded by an inconsistent availability of warming devices and the adverse consequences of rapid blood replacement. There are many efficacy and safety issues surrounding perioperative transfusions in children because large volumes given at rapid infusion rates are often necessary. Most studies on pediatric fluid administration rates are done with crystalloid solutions, and little is known about optimal blood administration rates. Most studies on pediatric infusion rates are small with numerous confounding variables, and study results often conflict. Recommended packed red blood cell (RBC) transfusion volumes in infants and children are relatively large compared to adult patients (e.g., 10–15 mL/kg versus 3.6 mL/kg for a 250 mL bag of RBCs in a 70 kg adult.)

8.2.2 Rapid Transfusion Techniques and Devices[1]

8.2.2.1 Infant Resuscitation

RIDs have no place in neonatal resuscitation, although the acceptable weight cutoff for using these devices in older children is unclear [1, 2]. Rapid transfusion options for neonates and infants therefore include gravity flow, syringe pumps, manual "syringing," and pressure bags. In a 2013 survey of staff at a large tertiary children's hospital, 43% responded that they had infrequent experience with RIDs (e.g., once or twice yearly), with the majority limiting RID use to patients weighing more than 20 kg [3].

[1] Discussions of infusion devices and equipment are based on information found in current literature and do not necessarily reflect the authors' opinions. Online product information is often distributed throughout multiple URLs and is revised periodically.

8.2.2.2 Gravity Flow

Table 8.1 illustrates single manufacturer-supplied data on hourly volumes of crystalloid that may be infused under gravity through size 24 gauge to 18 gauge peripheral intravenous catheters (PIVCs), with a delivery rate range of 20–295 mL/min: (Table 8.1) [4].

Table 8.1 IV catheter flow rates for crystalloid solutions under gravity. Reprinted with permission from A Practice of Anesthesia for Infants and Children. sixth ed. Ross PA, Lerman J, Cote CJ. Chapter 52: Pediatric Equipment, Patient Warming, Fluid & Blood Warmers. p. 1176–1177. Copyright Elsevier. 2019

IV Catheter flow rate by gauge and length[a]		
Gauge	Length (inches)	Flow Rate (mL/minute)
Peripheral IV		
24	0.75	20
22	1.0	37
20	1.0	63
20	1.16	61
20	1.88	54
18	1.16	95
18	1.88	87
16	1.16	193
16	1.77	185
14	2.0	295
Central Venous Line		
4F Double-Lumen		
20		23
22		12
5F Double-Lumen		
20		15
20		20
5F Triple-Lumen		
18		20
23		2
23		2
7F Triple-Lumen		
16		49
18		20
18		20
8F Cordis (4-inch)[b]		133
Percutaneous Intravenous Central Catheters (PICO)		
4F Single-lumen		21.2
5F Single-lumen		20
5F Dual (each lumen)		9.6
6F Dual (each lumen)		12.5

[a]The standard by which flow rate is measured (by gravity) is that the intravenous bag of crystalloid is suspended 1 m above the height of measurement

[b]Cordis (Milpitas, CA)

Information regarding central venous catheters was abstracted from Cook Medical "Quick Reference Guide for Spectrum" catheters (https://www.cookmedical.com/data/resources/4%20CC-BM-ABRMQR-EN-201111.pdf). PICC line information is for the PowerPICC Catheter from Bard Access Systems (Salt Lake City, UT)

Table 8.2 illustrates gravity flow rate data supplied by a variety of manufacturers for 20-gauge (1 inch) to 26-gauge (3/4 inch) PIVCs

Flow rate by gravity (mL/min)	20 gauge (1″)	22 gauge (1″)	24 gauge (3/4″)	26 gauge (3/4″)	Manufacturer
	63	37	20		Cook Medical [4]
	51	37	17		BD [5]
	59	31	24	15	ICU Medical [6]
	60–70	30–40	20	10–15	CIA [7]
	65	35	22		Braun [8]
	65	35	15		Terumo [9]

Table 8.2: PIVC flow rates of crystalloid solutions under gravity according to available manufacturer information fact sheets

In a study applying the American College of Critical Care Medicine (ACCM) guidelines for resuscitation of children in septic shock, Stoner et al. found that fluid administration by gravity provided only one-third of the recommended initial requirements (i.e., 20 mL/kg of fluid in the first 5 min) [10]. This administration rate is reduced by approximately 30–70% for blood because it has a much higher viscosity than crystalloid [11, 12]. From these flow rate estimations, blood replacement by gravity alone is unlikely to achieve the updated 2014 ACCM recommended 20–60 mL/kg fluid volume over an initial 5 min through PIVC sizes typically placed in the infants. RBC hemolysis secondary to pressurized administration of RBCs, an important consideration with rapid infusions, is of limited concern with gravity administration.

8.2.3 Syringe Pumps

Syringe or volumetric infusion pumps are often used for routine blood transfusion in infants at rates between 2 and 5 mL/kg/h [13–15]. Modern syringe pumps cannot administer fluids at a rate greater than 999 mL/hr. (16.7 mL/min); however, they are capable of downstream occlusion, high pressure, and air emboli detection. Syringe pumps cannot warm fluids, an important function in all large volume, rapid transfusions [1, 11, 14]. Volumetric and syringe pumps have pressure limits close to 500 mmHg (10 psi) to prevent injury, namely, infiltration. The older "peristalic" pumps had pressure limits as high as 3000 mmHg [16]. However, infiltration or extravasation can occur at pressures as low as 100 mmHg. To put the risk of infiltration into perspective, peripheral venous pressure is only 10–30 mmHg (0.2–0.6 psi), and interstitial pressure is 2–5 mmHg [17]. Newer volumetric or syringe pumps may have customizable, user-set pressure limits. However, end users are often uninformed of pump pressure limits, capacity for air detection, or alarm delay periods. Safety standards include regular monitoring of pump settings and maintaining PIV site visibility for regular inspection, the latter standard of particular importance for nonverbal patients [18, 19].

8.2.4 Manual Syringe Administration

Intraoperative administration of blood via a handheld syringe generates transfusion rates that are not only highly variable between practitioners, but that may be significantly faster per child body weight than pressurized adult transfusions [20]. The manual syringe or "push-pull" methods are often employed to rapidly transfuse neonates and infants due to the small volumes needed for infusion [3]. However, manual "syringing" may generate very high intraluminal pressures, leading to RBC disruption and hemolysis. This hemolysis has been attributed partly to the irregular force created during episodic, pulsatile hand movements. Syringing-related hemolysis (and resultant hyperkalemia) may be exacerbated through a number of factors, including small intravenous catheter sizes (23 gauge and smaller), rapid infusion rates, pretransfusion cell washing, and the presence of a one-way valve (e.g., needleless IV connectors) [20–22]. In addition, a hemolysis effect is directly proportional to the size of syringe used: a 1 mL capacity syringe may produce significantly greater driving pressure (363 psi) compared to a 3 mL syringe (177 psi) or a 10 mL syringe (53 psi) [23]. Under simulated conditions, Miller et al. found increased hemolysis when blood was manually administered through a 23-gauge or smaller needle, as well as a notable increase in needle-associated hemolysis when the smallest (24—and 25-gauge) needles were used [22]. However, the Miller study found no increased hemolysis or increased effluent potassium when syringing RBCs through using 18-and 20-gauge needles. In another in vitro study prompted by the presence of discolored urine in four, 10 kg surgery patients, investigators examined the hemolysis effect of RBC syringing on free Hb, visual hemolysis index, and hematocrit (Hct) [20]. All RBC samples in the study were irradiated, less than 10 days old, and washed in a cell salvage machine. They were then administered with and without a "clave" adapter through 24-gauge and 16-gauge PIVCs (Fig. 8.1). Significant hemolysis was found in post-syringing samples administered by hand through the clave adapter. In addition, investigators found significant hemolysis related to rapid, manual syringing through the 24 gauge but not the 16-gauge catheters. Component

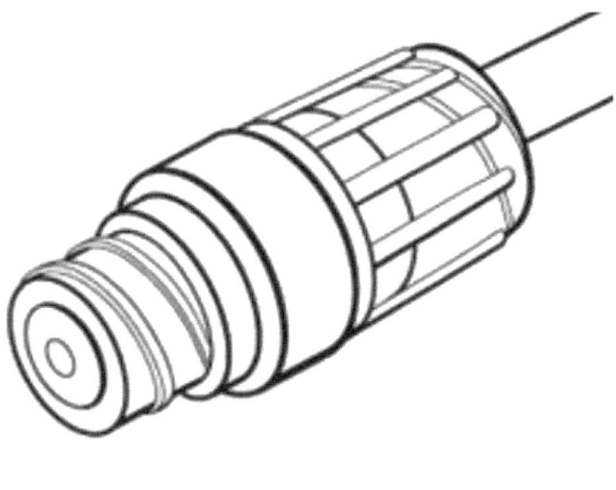

Fig. 8.1 A clave, one-way, needleless adapter

RBCs administered via a syringe pump at 2 mL/min (120 mL/h) with and without the clave adapter did not show signs of hemolysis. These findings suggest that manual syringing through PIVC catheters less than 22 gauge in size should be performed slowly when possible and without using an inline clave adapter. In the alternative, rapid blood administration in small patients may be given through a fluid pump that generates a nonpulsatile flow pattern, which may minimize hemolysis.

RBC hemolysis can also occur with forceful aspiration from an RBC blood bag.

8.2.5 Pressurized Infusion Bags

Another option for rapid fluid administration in neonates and infants is the pressure bag. In a study following up on the ACCM recommendation that children in septic shock receive a minimum of 20 mL/kg of fluid in the first 5 min of resuscitation, Stoner et al. found that fluid administration requirements were met 68% of the time using the syringe method but 58% of the time using a pressured bag [10]. Both the pressurized bag (at 300 mmHg) and the "push-and-pull" administration through a three-way stopcock provided delivery of 20 mL/kg within the first 5 min of resuscitation in children weighing less than 40 kg. The ACCM standard was not achieved using either technique in children >40 kg; however, the PIVC sizes used in this study were not mentioned. A pressurized bag infusion was compared to manual syringing in a 2017 in vitro study, finding that the pneumatic pressure bag held to 300 mmHg through a 22G PIVC resulted in tenfold less hemolysis than the manual syringe method [21]. It is important to keep in mind that the in vivo administration of blood to small patients under pressure—despite a steady 300 mmHg pressure head—may produce fluid overload and air entrainment leading to air embolism [24]. The default pressure limit of 300 mmHg is an industry standard for pressurized infusion devices that has an unclear scientific basis.

8.2.6 Rapid Fluid Administration in the Older Child

8.2.6.1 Rapid Infusion Devices (RIDs)

Currently, there are no standardized guidelines addressing RID use in children [11]. The default pressure set on automated power infusers, or RIDs such as the Level 1 (now discontinued at many institutions secondary to concerns over aluminum leaching) and the "Belmont" (Belmont® Rapid Infuser), is 300 mmHg. The final infusion rate is mitigated by the gauge of the PIVC, the IV tubing, and the type of fluid administered. Healthcare providers often lack knowledge of the preset pressures, flow rates through different devices, or whether the pressure transmitter at hand has crucial safety features (e.g., air entrapment capability or a high pressure alarm) [3]. Power infusers—lacking pediatric-based modes but with the ability to infuse up to 1 L of fluid per minute—require specific training to avoid air embolism, circulatory overload, and hyperkalemia that can be seen in children who undergo rapid blood transfusion [11, 25–27]. Belmont® advises against its RID use as a massive transfusion device in neonates, as well as for required flow rates <2.5 mL/min (150 mL/h) [28]. In clinical practice, the minimum body weight limit for RID fluid administration is often cited as 20–40 kg [29, 30].

In the older pediatric population, several options exist for the rapid transfusion of blood products. The new LifeFlow Plus ®Plus (LifeFlow) is a handheld gun-shaped infuser that is reported to have the capacity to infuse an adult-sized unit of RBCs in approximately 2 min in PIVCs as small as 22G; data is currently lacking for use of smaller gauge PIVCs (Fig. 8.2) [31]. In one prospective study, the LifeFlow significantly increased fluid administration rates and time to bladder filling in females requiring pelvic ultrasound for abdominal pain [32]. The LifeFlow device is now commonly used by EMS agencies for the rapid delivery of blood for patients with hemorrhagic shock [33]. The LifeFlow infuser can be hooked up to the QinFlow Warrior fluid warmer [34].

Two other rapid infusion devices commercially available in the United States for use in larger patients include the Belmont® Rapid Infusion System RI-2 and the 3 M™Ranger™ Pressure Infuser system [28, 35]. Belmont reports that the RI-2 can be user-adjusted to flow rates as low as 2.5 mL/min using a 20 gauge PIVC [36]. It is also important to note that the RI-2 has an integral pressure limit of 300 mmHg but the ability to produce infusion rates as high as 1000 mL/min on demand. As an

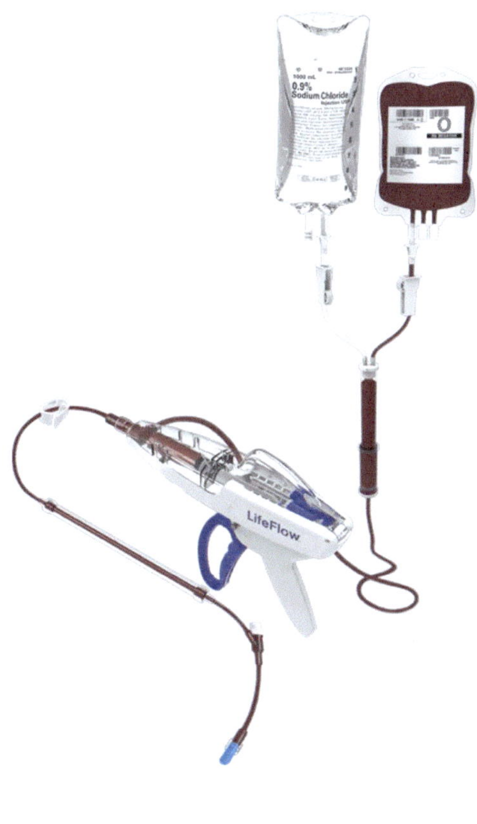

Fig. 8.2 LifeFlow Rapid Infuser. Reprinted with permission from Mark Peihl. Image found online at https://410medical.com/about/how-it-works/

example, the "bolus" function of the Belmont RI-2 is defaulted at 200 mL, to be delivered at 200 mL/min [28]. Currently, there are no standardized pediatric guidelines for age or weight applicable to the Belmont Rapid Infusion System RI-2™. Because of its automated touchscreen functions, the absence of pediatric-specific programming, and the ability to infuse at rates up to 1000 mL/min, the Belmont rapid infuser system should never be used in children without expert management and close supervision.

The 3 M™Ranger Pressure Infuser has a maximum pressure of 300 mmHg applied by two bladders, and pressure adjustment is not possible [35]. It provides low-and high-pressure alerts but not real time infusion rates. The smallest fluid bag size possible with the 3 M™Ranger Pressure Infuser is 250 mL, thus making apparatus dead space an obstacle in small patients who may be receiving divided RBC bags (e.g., pediatric units). At the time of this writing, the Level 1® Rapid Infuser has been discontinued in many institutions due to concerns for aluminum leaching [37].

8.2.7 Intravascular Devices for Pediatric Resuscitation

8.2.7.1 General

Multiple factors must be considered when determining vascular access for resuscitation in children, including patient size, available insertion sites, and the desired infusion rate. In an effort to fill in the evidence-based gap in guidance on PIVC selection and management in children, a consortium of hospitals has developed standards through the Michigan Appropriateness Guide for Intravenous Catheters (MAGIC) in Pediatrics [38]. Figure 8.3 illustrates the consortium recommendations for intravenous device selection in neonates; this group has also put forth guidance for infants and older children [38].

Additional sources of standardized guidance addressing PIVC selection, maintenance, and training requirements include the European Recommendations for Proper Indication and Use of Peripheral venous access (ERPIUP) consensus and the UK Vessel Health and Preservation (VHP) Framework [39, 40].

8.2.7.2 Catheter Sizing

Under the Hagen-Poiseuille's equation for linear flow, intra-catheter flow rates decrease exponentially as the radius of the catheter lumen decreases and the length increases (Fig. 8.4):

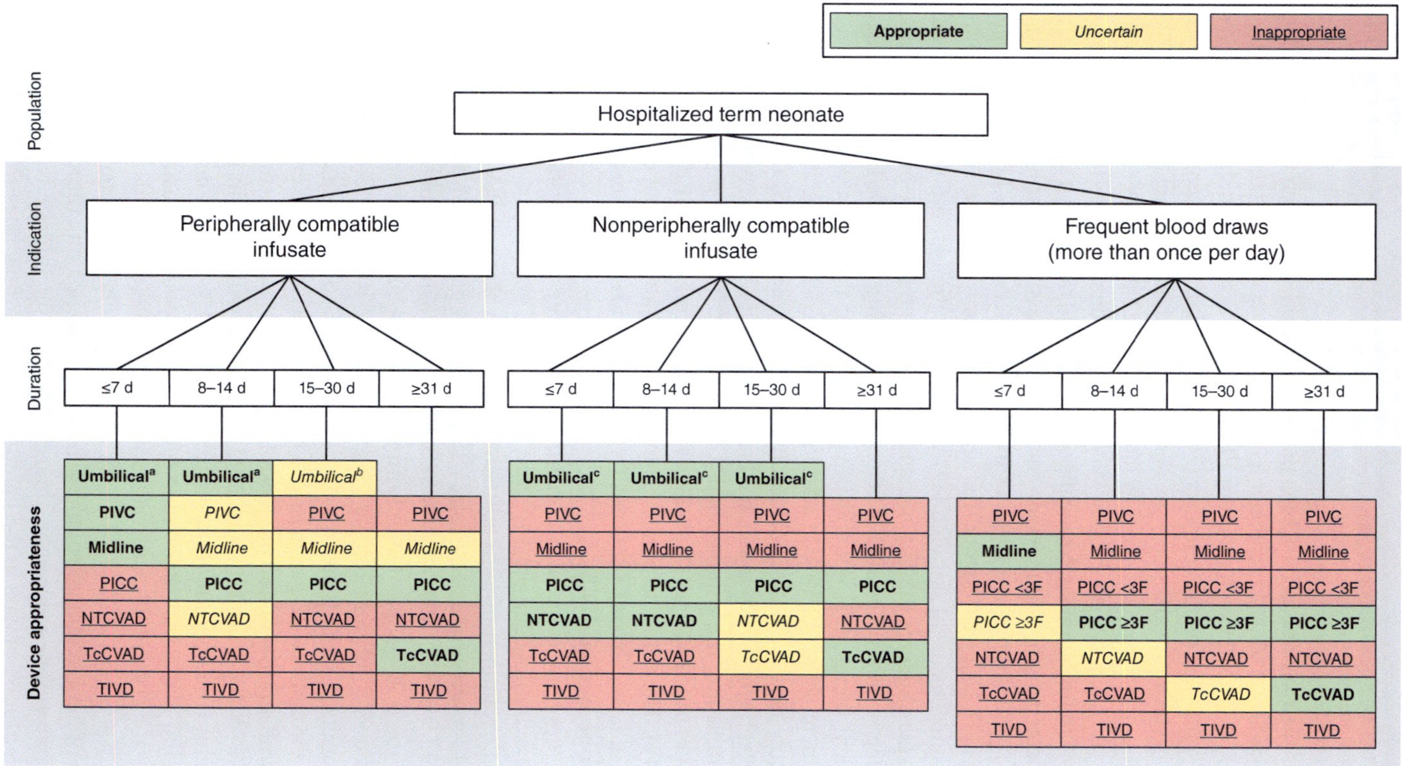

Fig. 8.3 miniMagic recommendations for appropriate device selection for hospitalized, term neonates. (**a**) Less than or equal to 2 days after birth. (**b**) All neonatal ages. (**c**) Less than or equal to 5 days after birth. NTCVAD, nontunneled central venous access device; TcCVAD, tunneled, cuffed central venous access device; TIVD, totally implanted venous device. (Reprinted with permission from Ullman AJ, Bernstein SJ, Brown E, Aiyagari R, Doellman D, Faustino EVS, et al. The Michigan Appropriateness Guide for Intravenous Catheters in Pediatrics: miniMAGIC. Pediatrics. 2020;145(Suppl 3):S269-S84)

Fig. 8.4 Poiseuille's Equation

$$Q = \frac{(P_2 - P_1)\pi r^4}{8\eta \ell}$$

whereby Q is the flow rate, P2—P1 the pressure difference between two points, π is 3.14, r is the catheter radius, l is catheter length, and η is viscosity of the fluid. In order to calculate flow rates through different PIVC gauges, assume that the driving force generated by a pressure or power infuser (300 mmHg), the catheter length, and viscosity of RBCs (which is 4–10 times greater than crystalloid) are held constant [12]. Applying Poiseuille's equation, the flow rate through a 22-gauge PIVC (0.4 mm internal diameter (ID)) is less than the flow rate of an 18-gauge catheter (ID 0.84 mm) by a factor of 19. Optimal laminar flow in the setting of rapid transfusion also requires the shortest catheter length. Milne et al. conducted a massive transfusion simulation (RBC:FFP 1:1 ratio) through a series of infusion catheters, size 7–9 French (Fr) and 14–18 gauge [41]. Using a Belmont RID set to a maximum flow rate of 1000 mL/min, the mean conductance (mL/min/mmHg) was greatest through the 9 Fr-sheath and least through the 18-gauge PIVC. Conductance was also found to be indirectly related to catheter length: conductance fell when extension tubing was added to the system.

The medical literature is not consistent about what flow rates can be achieved through different sizes of PIVs. In addition to the viscosity of the infusate, factors that have been shown to affect achievable flow rates under pressure include the length of the catheter, as discussed, the brand of catheter, the presence of a clave or needleless connector, the volume status of the patient, the PIVC insertion site, the infusate temperature (warmer fluids flow faster), and the blood vessel size or capacity [29, 42–47]. The ability to predict actual infusion rates is further complicated by the fact that at lower driving pressures (e.g., < 450 mmHg), the pressure-flow relationship may be nonlinear [48].

Table 8.3 contains manufacturer-published flow rates for crystalloid solutions under both gravity flow and pressure for various PIVC sizes [5].

Lehn et al. examined in vitro crystalloid flow rates through PIVCs under pressures 370–417 mmHg for catheter sizes 22 gauge to 14 gauge [46]. Using a Level 1 fast flow fluid warmer, flow rates were similar to previously published findings: 88 mL/min for a 22-gauge, 134 mL/min for the 20-gauge, 235 mL/min for the 18-gauge, and 438 mL/min for the 16-gauge PIVCs. Rates for 24-gauge PIVCs were not examined. Lehn found the flow rate for RBCs fell by almost one half, to 47 mL/min, through the 22-gauge PIVC. If these observations are extrapolated to a 6 kg infant with an EBV of 480 mL (80 mL/kg), 18% of her circulating volume may be replaced with crystalloid through a 22-gauge PIV within 1 min if administered under pressure; if the crystalloid is replaced with RBCs, 10% of her EBV may be replaced during that same time frame. Manufacturer-published data indicates that the flow rate for crystalloid under gravity through different brands of a 22-gauge, 1-inch PIVCs is 30–37 mL/min [4–7, 9]. If crystalloid is administered under gravity, only 7% of her circulating volume can be replaced in 1 min through a 22-gauge PIVC. This rate will be reduced by almost one-half if the infusate is blood.

There is a paucity of data in the literature regarding flow rates for 24 PIVCs. In infants and toddlers, it is often possible to achieve PIVC access with catheters as large as 22 gauge or even 20 gauge. The Association for the Advancement of Blood

Table 8.3 Flow rates for crystalloid solutions under gravity and pressure. Reprinted from Greene N et al. Vascular access, fluid resuscitation, and blood transfusion in pediatric trauma. Int J Crit Illn and Inj Sci. 2012;2:135–42 under Creative Common License 4.0

Gauge	Published flow rate (mL/min)[a]	Flow rate gravity (mL/min) [2]	Flow rate level 1 (mL/min) [3]	Flow rate RIS (mL/min) [3]	10 cc syringe pum (mL/min) [4]
4 Fr	Not published	286	450	516	Not published
5 Fr	Not published	380	533	667	Not published
6 Fr	Not published	480	548	702	Not published
7 Fr	Not published	Not published	564	772	Not published
8.5 Fr	Not published	674	596	857	Not published
14	330	Not published	488	584	Not published
16	220	Not published	368	412	Not published
18	105	92	209	205	Not published
20	60	51	140	144	Not published
22	35	37	Not published	Not published	106
24	17	Not published	Not published	Not published	78

[a]All values are for crystalloid solutions, published flow rate from BD packaged IV catheters

& Biotherapies (AABB) advises that 24-gauge catheters and 25-gauge needles are the smallest that can be safely used for blood transfusion under conditions of constant flow or pressure [1]. PIVC development continues, however, in search of safe alternatives for contrast injection under high pressures in children with small PIVCs in place. An "integrated port" system has been developed that is claimed to contain a main line that withstands high pressures, with additional ports for medication or other fluid administration [6].

Newly developed "integrated" PIVCs may allow longer indwelling periods in hospitalized patients if properly maintained [49]. Infusion rates for contrast media using a power infusing device are reported to be greater than 300 mL/min through both the 24 gauge and the 22 gauge integrated catheter [47].

An early resuscitation goal in a hemodynamically unstable child is to achieve vascular access as fast as possible with a device appropriate for the type of fluid and flow rate necessary (see *Initial Vascular Access Anatomic Locations for Volume Resuscitation*, below) [38]. It is difficult to achieve venous access in neonates with a PIVC external diameter greater than 0.7 mm (25 gauge). A 2017 systematic review of pediatric massive transfusion recommends that 18 gauge or larger PIVCs be used with RIDs during for pediatric resuscitation [11]. In a prospective in vitro study, examining flow and warming capabilities of two different RIDs, other investigators recommend against using PIVCs less than 16 gauge in pediatric resuscitation based on efficiency consideration [29]. Another author recommends a 20-gauge or larger PIVC for rapid volume resuscitation in children [50]. In a review on pediatric trauma resuscitation, Greene et al. suggest that one circulating blood volume can be replaced in a 20 kg child in less than 6 min using a RID with two, 20-gauge PIVCs; in a 5 kg infant, one blood volume may be better replaced using a 10 mL syringe [5]. However, excessive pressure and flows can have side effects, including catheter disruption, migration, fluid extravasation, hemolysis, hyperkalemia, and transfusion-associated circulatory overload (TACO) [51, 52]. The maximum flow rate associated with clinically significant adverse transfusion events in children is unknown, but the highest incidence is seen in patients with multiple comorbidities, a positive fluid balance, high transfusion volumes, old age, and small body weight [52–56]. A large volume, weight-based RBC transfusion in children has been defined as 25 mL/kg and a "massive" transfusion 40 mL/kg [13, 57]. The transfusion rate associated with acute reactions is unclear but has been reported to be greater than 19 mL/kg/hour and as high as 120 mL/kg/h [14, 58–60]. Extrapolating these rates to a 70 kg adult patient produces transfusion rates of 1.3 L/h–8.4 L/h, respectively. RBC infusion rate limits in the literature that are focused on preventing transfusion-associated hyperkalemia (TAH) vary widely, from 0.17 mL/kg/min to 2 mL/kg/min, but these estimates tend to be based on small retrospective analyses [52, 60–62]. These infusion rates are equivalent to 1.8 mL/min and 12 mL/min in a 6 kg infant, rates that are notably less than the flow rates achievable through a pressurized 22-gauge PIVC: 88 mL/min for crystalloid and 47 mL/min for RBCs [46].

8.2.8 Central Venous Catheters (CVCs)

Multilumen central venous catheters (CVCs) are not recommended as the primary vascular access for trauma resuscitation of adults and children when a suitable PIVC is available [63]. This is because multilumen CVCs are often less than 20–21 gauge in diameter and are longer than their PIVC counterparts, leading to a significant reduction in flow rate capacity. However, if already in place, a CVC may be used for initial resuscitation until PIVC or IO access can be obtained [64]. Under simulated conditions, Milne et al. found that shorter 14-gauge and 16-gauge PIVCs (32–50 mm length) outperformed CVCs (300 mm length) of the same caliber [41]. Interposition of clave (needleless) connectors attached to a 7–9-Fr-size introducer sheath produces flow rates similar to that of a 20-gauge PIVC [63]. In another in vitro simulation using 16 different catheter sizes to determine flow rates for fluid administered by an RID, a 2.5 cm-long, 20-gauge PIVC produced faster flow rates than a 16 cm-long, 16-gauge-single CVC (65 mL/min versus 59.2 mL/min, respectively) [12]. In addition to flow rate limitations through central lines, rapid administration of unwarmed RBCs through a CVC has been associated with hypothermia and hyperkalemic arrest in small patients [52].

8.2.9 Peripherally Inserted Central Catheters (PICCs)

Neonates often present to the OR with PICC lines. Like CVCs, PICC lines are not recommended for rapid volume replacement when a suitable PIVC is available. These intravenous lines may be as small as 1 Fr (28 gauge) and 2 cm in length [65, 66]. Shorter indwelling IV catheters are more likely to infiltrate than their longer counterparts. Size 4 Fr and 5 Fr PICCs allow slow flow rates (2–3 mL/min) under gravity and 10–13 mL/min through a pump [67]. Wong et al. found that when blood was administered at pump rates as high as 20 mL/hr., intraluminal PICC pressures exceeded 300 mmHg, but without evidence of clinically significant hemolysis [68]. In recent in vitro study, there was no evidence of hemolysis or occlusion when 15 mL of irradiated RBCs was infused at a rate of 4 mL/h using either a 24-gauge short PIVC, a 24-gauge (30 cm) silicone PICC catheter, or a 28-gauge (20 cm) polyurethane PICC catheter [65]. However, the internal pressure in the 28-gauge PICC line reached 183 mmHg (± 12 mmHg) during transfusion, as opposed to 55 mmHg in the 24-gauge, 30 cm PICC and 7.6 mmHg in the 24-gauge short PIVC. This driving pressure of 183 mmHg is considered to fall within the "safe" infusion driving pressure of less than 300 mmHg (the default pressure set in power infusers). The authors of this study concluded that blood can be safely transfused through either 24-gauge or 28-gauge PICC line at 4 mL/h.

At driving pressures and flow rates required for rapid volume resuscitation, PICC lines may migrate, malposition, or fracture [69]. Power injections of radiographic contrast or other RIDs may generate intraluminal pressures as high as 15,000 mmHg (300 psi) [67]. Silicone PICCS are more likely to break or dislodge, with a maximum safe limit of 60 psi, compared to polyurethane catheters that reportedly can tolerate pressures up to 100 psi [51, 67]. In 2004, following reports of mechanical damage to venous lines exposed to high driving pressures, the US FDA issued an advisory that when power injectors are used with PICC lines, they must be specifically designated as "power PICCs" [67]. The maximum driving pressure allowable in a PICC may be embedded on the external part of the catheter itself. Another management caveat is that strict adherence to a post-use flushing protocol is required to prevent thrombosis formation; their small caliber and long length lend to a high rate of clotting, occurring in up to one-third of PICC lines [70].

8.2.10 Long Peripheral Intravenous Catheters (LPCs)

LPCs (6–15 cm in length) offer an alternative to PIVCs when a longer dwell time is desired and to CVCs when central venous access is not necessary, or there is a desire to preserve central veins such as in patients who may require hemodialysis. LPCs can be inserted using sedation although many are inserted under general anesthesia. The most common insertion sites are the basilic and saphenous veins [71]. An X-ray is not required to confirm tip placement. In a randomized prospective trial of 72 children (age 1–17 years) requiring ≥ 2 days intravenous therapy, LPCs had improved life span (4.7 versus 3.5 days; $p = 0.01$) and significantly fewer children required catheter replacement during therapy [72]. Adverse side effects associated with LPCs are similar to PIVCs and CVCs: phlebitis, infiltration, occlusion, and venous thromboembolism (up to 30%) [71, 72].

8.2.11 Portacaths

A portacath is a tunneled, indwelling, central venous catheter often placed in patients needing long-term therapies. Access to all "ports" should be made using a specialized needle (e.g., the "Huber" needle) [73]. These special needles, with a 90-degree turn and inserted into a reservoir port, can be used to infuse blood products but should not be subjected to high infusion pressures or flow rates for extended periods; a portacath is not suitable for sustained, rapid volume replacement. If high infusion pressure is required such as with IV contrast injection, the needle should be fastened in place with a specialized "power lock" device. According to one manufacturer, a 20-gauge port needle can withstand non-sustained flow rates up to 5 mL/s (300 mL/min) and a 22-gauge port needle can withstand 2 mL/sec (120 mL/min) when used for contrast injection [74].

8.2.12 Anatomic Sites for Vascular Access in Pediatric Resuscitation

Another important consideration in pediatric fluid resuscitation is the vascular access site. Successful cannulation with a 20-gauze catheter in an emergency can be difficult at best. Knowledge of the relative calibers and anatomic peculiarities of the small patient's vascular system can be critical. In a 2004 literature review, Haas et al. categorized various PIVC sites according to the difficulty of approach and likelihood of complications [75] (Table 8.4).

8.2.13 Catheter-to-Vein Ratio

Commonly used PIVC sites for pediatric fluid resuscitation include the veins of the antecubital fossa, the saphenous vein, and the external jugular vein. Rapid fluid resuscitation requires judgment about the necessary balance between the anatomic site(s) available, the flow capabilities of the catheter, and the reality that a PIVC acts as its own form of intravascular obstruction [50, 66]. Barone et al. examined the various access options in 100 neonates and found the brachiocephalic vein to be favorable because it is relatively large (e.g., ≥ 3 mm in diameter) in infants weighing as little as 500 g (Table 8.5) [105].

Table 8.4 PIVC sites in children listed according to the difficulty of approach. Reprinted with permission from Haas NA. Clinical review: vascular access for fluid infusion in children. Crit Care. 2004;8 (6):478–84

Features of the different sites for intravenous access for fluid infusion in children							
	IO access	Subclavian vein	Femoral vein	Internal jugular vein	External jugular vein	Axillary vein	Venous cutdown
Emergency access	++++	++	+++	++	+++	+	++
Ease of access for unexperienced clinician	++++	++	+++	++	+++	+	+
Infection	+	++	++	++	+	+	++
Thrombosis	0	+	++	+	+	+	++++
Other complications	+	++	+	+	0	+	0
Long-term use	0	+++	++	++	+	+	0
Short-term use	++++	++	+++	+++	++	+++	++

IO intraosseous, *0* no effect/not suitable/no risk, ++++ excellent effect/very suitable/high risk

Table 8.5 Deep vein diameters as measured by ultrasound in newborns, weights 500–3000 g. Reprinted with permission from Barone G, D'Andrea V, Vento G, Pittiruti M. A Systematic Ultrasound Evaluation of the Diameter of Deep Veins in the Newborn: Results and Implications for Clinical Practice. Neonatology. 2019;115 (4):335–40

Vein	Whole cohort (*n* = 100)	500–1.000 g (*n* = 20)	1.001–1.500 g (*n* = 20)	1.501–2.000 g (*n* = 20)	2.001–2.500 g (*n* = 20)	2.501–3.000 g (*n* = 20)	ICC
R IJV	3.1±0.8 (1.8–6.0)	2.4±0.5 (1.8–3.1)	2.8±0.5 (2.0–3.3)	3.0±0.6 (2.1–4.2)	3.2±0.3 (2.8–3.6)	4.2±0.7 (3.2–6.0)	0.85
L IJV	3.2±0.8 (1.9–7.0)	2.5±0.4 (1.9–3.1)	2.7±0.5 (2.0–3.4)	3.2±0.6 (2.2–4.4)	3.2±0.2 (2.8–3.6)	4.4±0.9 (3.3–7.0)	0.87
R BCV	3.6±0.6 (2.6–5.7)	3.0±0.3 (2.6–3.6)	3.3±0.3 (2.7–3.7)	3.4±0.3 (2.7–3.6)	3.8±0.4 (3.1–4.2)	4.5±0.6 (3.7–5.7)	0.96
L BCV	3.5±0.8 (2.0–7.5)	3.0±0.3 (2.2–3.3)	2.9±0.4 (2.0–3.6)	3.4±0.5 (2.4–4.2)	3.5±0.3 (2.9–4.1)	4.6±0.9 (3.5–6.5)	0.97
R SBV	1.8±0.6 (0.8–3.0)	1.1±0.3 (0.8–1.7)	1.5±0.3 (1.2–2.2)	1.8±0.3 (1.3–2.3)	2.0±0.3 (1.5–2.4)	2.5±0.4 (2.0–3.0)	0.91
L SBV	1.8±0.6 (0.8–3.2)	1.1±0.3 (0.8–1.6)	1.4±0.3 (0.8–1.7)	1.8±0.3 (1.3–2.2)	2.0±0.3 (1.5–2.3)	2.5±0.3 (1.9–3.2)	0.92
R EJV	1.3±0.3 (0.8–2.2)	1.0±0.2 (0.8–1.3)	1.3±0.2 (0.9–1.5)	1.2±0.2 (0.9–1.5)	1.3±0.2 (1.0–1.5)	1.7±0.3 (1.1–2.2)	0.89
L EJV	1.4±0.4 (0.6–2.4)	0.9±0.2 (0.6–1.2)	1.2±0.3 (0.8–1.5)	1.4±0.2 (1.1–1.7)	1.5±0.2 (1.2–1.7)	1.8±0.2 (1.5–2.4)	0.90
R AxVc	1.9±0.5 (1.2–3.5)	1.5±0.1 (1.2–2.0)	1.7±0.4 (1.3–2.3)	1.8±0.3 (1.3–2.2)	2.0±0.3 (1.5–2.3)	2.5±0.5 (1.9–3.5)	0.91
L AxVc	2.0±0.4 (1.3–3.2)	1.6±0.2 (1.3–1.9)	1.9±0.5 (1.3–2.8)	2.0±0.3 (1.4–2.2)	2.2±0.2 (1.9–2.5)	2.5±0.4 (2.0–3.2)	0.93
R AxVa	1.6±0.4 (0.8–2.4)	1.2±0.3 (0.8–1.5)	1.5±0.3 (1.0–1.9)	1.5±0.3 (1.1–2.1)	1.8±0.3 (1.3–2.2)	2.1±0.2 (1.5–2.4)	0.92
L AxVa	1.6±0.4 (0.8–2.6)	1.2±0.2 (0.8–1.7)	1.5±0.4 (1.0–2.1)	1.7±0.3 (1.0–2.1)	1.8±0.2 (1.4–2.1)	2.0±0.3 (1.6–2.6)	0.91
R BrV	1.0±0.3 (0.5–2.1)	0.9±0.2 (0.7–1.2)	0.8±0.2 (0.5–1.0)	0.8±0.2 (0.6–1.1)	1.1±0.1 (0.9–1.3)	1.5±0.2 (1.2–2.1)	0.89
L BrV	1.1±0.4 (0.6–1.9)	0.9±0.2 (0.7–1.3)	0.8±0.2 (0.6–1.0)	1.0±0.2 (0.7–1.3)	1.2±0.1 (1.0–1.4)	1.6±0.2 (1.3–1.9)	0.90
R BaV	1.0±0.3 (0.5–1.5)	0.7±0.2 (0.5–1.1)	1.0±0.2 (0.7–1.2)	0.9±0.2 (0.6–1.2)	1.2±0.2 (0.7–1.4)	1.3±0.1 (1.1–1.5)	0.91
L BaV	1.0±0.3 (0.5–1.5)	0.7±0.1 (0.5–1.0)	0.9±0.1 (0.7–1.1)	0.9±0.1 (0.6–1.1)	1.3±0.2 (0.8–1.5)	1.3±0.1 (1.1–1.5)	0.92
R FeV	2.3±0.7 (1.1–3.5)	1.4±0.2 (1.1–1.8)	2.1±0.4 (1.3–2.7)	2.2±0.3 (1.8–2.6)	2.8±0.4 (2.1–3.4)	3.2±0.2 (2.9–3.5)	0.89
L FeV	2.3±0.7 (1.1–3.5)	1.4±0.3 (1.1–1.9)	2.1±0.5 (1.6–2.9)	2.0±0.4 (1.4–2.6)	2.9±0.2 (2.5–3.3)	3.1±0.2 (2–9–3.5)	0.91
R SaV	1.3±0.5 (0.5–2.3)	0.8±0.2 (0.5–1.2)	1.0±0.3 (0.7–1.8)	1.3±0.2 (0.9–1.5)	1.7±0.4 (1.2–2.3)	1.8±0.3 (1.3–2.3)	0.88
L SaV	1.3±0.5 (0.4–2.3)	0.8±0.2 (0.4–1.1)	1.1±0.2 (0.7–1.5)	1.2±0.2 (0.8–1.4)	1.8±0.3 (1.4–2.3)	1.8±0.3 (1.4–2.3)	0.89

Values are expressed in millimeters as mean ± standard deviation (range). *ICC* intraclass correlation, *R* right, *L* left, *IJV* internal jugular vein, *BCV* brachiocephalic vein, *SBV* subclavian vein, *EJV* external jugular vein, *AxVc* axillary vein at the chest, *AxVa* axillary vein at the axilla, *BrV* brachial vein, *BaV* basilic vein, *FeV* femoral vein, *SaV* saphenous vein

Table 8.6 IV catheter sizes and approximations of external diameters under the Birmingham and French gauge systems

IV catheter gauge	External diameter (mm)	French (Fr) size	External diameter (mm)
24	0.7	**1**	0.33
22	0.9	**2**	0.66
20	1.1	**3**	1.0
18	1.3	**4**	1.34
17	1.5	**5**	1.67
16	1.7	**6**	2.0
14	2.1	**7**	2.3

A recent systematic review by the American Academy of Pediatrics (AAP) noted that a "catheter-to-vein" ratio of <33% in neonates and a catheter-to-vein ratio of <50% in older children may be necessary to minimize line occlusion and thrombosis [106]. Modern ultrasound machines contain software that suggest PIVC sizing based on this criteria. One recommendation is that a catheter will meet the desired 33% catheter-to-vein ratio if the French size of the catheter is less than or equal to the patient's vessel size in millimeters [99]. Approximations of the external diameter of IV cannulae, which vary with the material used, are listed below (Table 8.6) [66, 100, 101]. If a catheter is to be used for blood sampling, a size 3 Fr (20 gauge) or larger is recommended, with the clave adapter removed to avoid specimen hemolysis [66].

There are two main catheter diameter systems: the Birmingham gauge system and the French system. In the Birmingham system, a smaller gauge number reflects a larger catheter size; in the French system, a low Fr number reflects a smaller catheter diameter. The outer diameter of a catheter, in millimeters, can be estimated by dividing the French size number by 3 [100].

8.2.14 Initial Vascular Access Anatomic Locations for Volume Resuscitation

8.2.14.1 Newborns

8.2.14.2 Umbilical Vein Cannulation

The American Heart Association Pediatric Advanced Life Support (AHA PALS) 2020 guideline recommends an umbilical vein catheter (UVC) for initial resuscitation in newborns, followed by intraosseous (IO) cannulation if concomitant PIVC attempts fail [102]. The UV approach should be limited to neonates less than 5–7 days old, whose cord has no signs of infection [103]. A "high" UVC is recommended to prevent gastrointestinal ischemia or thrombosis. Depth can be calculated using a variety of formulae; however, the Shukla formula has been shown to be the most reliable (Table 8.7) [103, 104].

Table 8.7 Technical considerations when selecting a UVC in newborns. (Adapted from D'Andrea et al. Umbilical Venous Catheter Update: A Narrative Review Including Ultrasound and Training. Front Pediatr. 2021; Nakamura H, Nakamura R, Paran TS. Chapter 16. Vascular Access in Infants and Children. In: Puri P, editor. Pediatric Surgery. Germany: Springer-Verlag GmbH. 2020. P. 263–272)

Patient weight (kg)	Less than 1500 grams	Equal to or > 1500 grams	Considerations
UVC catheter size	2.5–3.5 French	5–8 French	Average size 5 Fr
"High" tip position (cm)	$\frac{[(3 \times \text{birthweight in kg}) + 9]}{2+1}$		Preferred tip location; multiple formulae available, but there is a high malposition rate (~50%)
"Low" tip position (cm)	Insert 2–4 cm maximum for short-term, rapid fluid resuscitation only		Avoid hyperosmolar substances (25% dextrose)

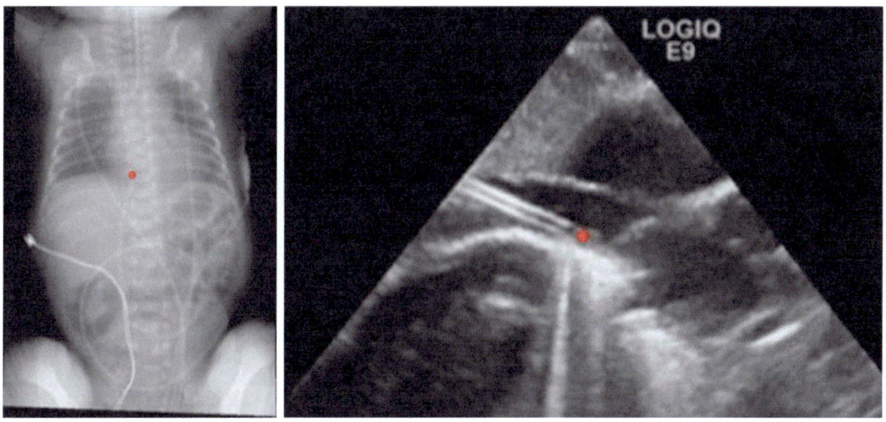

Fig. 8.5 Correct level for umbilical catheter placement in a neonate as determined by plain X-ray (left) and ultrasound (right). Reprinted from D'Andrea V, Prontera G, Rubortone SA, Pezza L, Pinna G, Barone G, et al. Umbilical Venous Catheter Update: A Narrative Review Including Ultrasound and Training. Front Pediatr. 2021;9:774705 under Creative Commons Attributions License

Figure 8.5 illustrates a plain abdominal chest X-ray as well as ultrasound image indicating correct UVC tip placement at the level of the diaphragm (i.e., at the level of the IVC and right atrial junction, or thoracic vertebrae levels 6–9, which places it outside the hepatic circulation) [103]. A UVC tip lying below the diaphragm (e.g., below thoracic vertebra 11) is considered to be a peripherally placed line that may be in the portal vein and should be used only for rapid volume resuscitation of non-hypertonic solutions. When feasible, the UVC location should be confirmed by X-ray or, preferably, ultrasonography; the latter technique may hasten diagnosis and reduce neonatal radiation exposure [103, 110].

8.2.15 Infants and Older Children

The American Academy of Pediatrics recommends transition to IO access after ≥ 2 PIVC attempts or 60 seconds in older children requiring emergency fluid resuscitation [106]. Attempting immediate central venous access through the internal jugular vein (IJV) or the subclavian vein (SCV) is not recommended in pediatric resuscitation before peripheral access has been attempted.

8.2.15.1 Peripheral Venous Sites

The largest caliber PIVC access points in infants are the upper arm venous system and the saphenous vein of the lower extremity [50]. The right basilic and both median cubital veins are relatively superficial and offer a direct course to the superior vena cava (SVC) (Fig. 8.6).

Another rapid access and easily accessible option is the saphenous vein, located immediately anterior to the medial malleolus (Fig. 8.7) [111]. The external jugular vein (EJ), which is sharply angulated and close to the major vessels and apex of the lung, should be accessed only if PIVC attempts fail.

The tip of any venous catheter should not lie beyond the right atrium-superior vena cava (RA-SVC) junction. The RA-SVC junction can be identified by plain chest X-ray at approximately two vertebral bodies below the carina [99]. If a femoral vein is used to achieve central access, the catheter tip should lie below the diaphragm (e.g., below the RA—inferior vena cava (IVC) junction). Improperly positioned CVCs that are utilized prior to placement confirmation may lead to cardiac perforation and thrombosis, phlebitis, extravasation, and irreversible extremity tissue damage.

All techniques used to guide vascular access in children—whether it be transillumination, electrocardiogram, or fluoroscopy—have been shown to provide higher success rates and fewer complications than the "landmark" technique [106]. In particular, ultrasound-guided (US) vascular access is recommended for placement of both central and peripheral lines in children when available [75, 106].

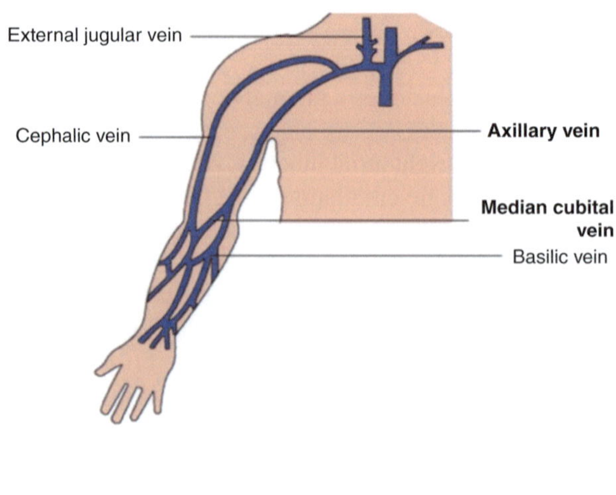

Fig. 8.6 The basilic and median cubital veins with direct route to the SVC (from [Moreau NL, editor. Vessel Health and Preservation: The Right Approach for Vascular Access. Springer Open; 2019.], licensed under CC-BY 4.0)

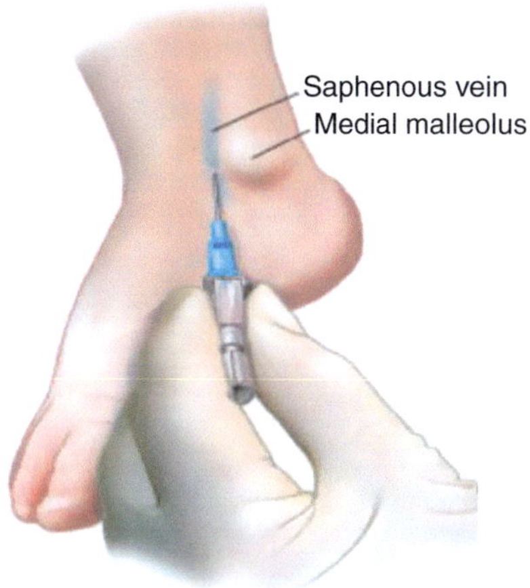

Fig. 8.7 Saphenous vein cannulation. Reprinted with permission from A Practice of Anesthesia for Infants and Children. sixth ed. New York: Elsevier. 2019. Wald SH, Mendoza J, Mihm FG, Cote CJ. Chapter 49: Procedures for Vascular Access. p. 1131

8.2.15.2 Interosseus (IO) Access

In an emergency situation when rapid vascular access is critical but cannot be obtained or is not feasible, the IO approach should be considered [102]. The 2014 ACCM resuscitation guidelines recommend achieving definitive IV or IO access in children in septic shock within 5 min [27]. The 2015 European Resuscitation Council Guidelines recommend establishing IO access in cardiac arrest if PIVC attempts are unsuccessful after 1 min [64]. Recommended IO insertion sites in the small child include the upper medial tibia (one patient fingerbreadth medial and two fingerbreadths caudal to the tibial tuberosity), the lower medial tibia (above the medial malleolus), the distal femur, the proximal humerus, and the anterior iliac crest [111, 112]. The needle should be inserted in a direction opposite to the epiphyseal plate. Figure 8.8 illustrates a basic IO insertion technique [111].

Proper IO placement is confirmed by observing free flow of fluid under gravity or by flushing with normal saline and observing an absence of extravasation. Any needle with a stylet can be used, including IV catheters and spinal needles [113]. A variety of premade IO devices are commercially available that contain stylets and fastening systems to prevent dislodgement, with age-based lengths to prevent piercing the entire bone. Acute complications include excessive insertion depth, needle kinking, growth plate disruption, and dislodgement. Once appropriate peripheral or central vascular access is achieved, the IO needle should be removed.

In a 2010 review by Tobias and Kinder Ross, blood as well as a number of medications were found to have been safely administered through an IO needle, including epinephrine, sodium bicarbonate, dopamine, propofol, succinylcholine, and even ampicillin [113]. Hypertonic medications, such as 25% dextrose, should not be administered through an IO unless highly diluted.

Medications and fluid administered into the tibial medullary cavity flow into the popliteal then femoral venous systems at rates similar to IV administration; blood is likely to flow more slowly than crystalloid secondary to its greater viscosity. The onset times for medications administered through the IO route are similar to PIVC

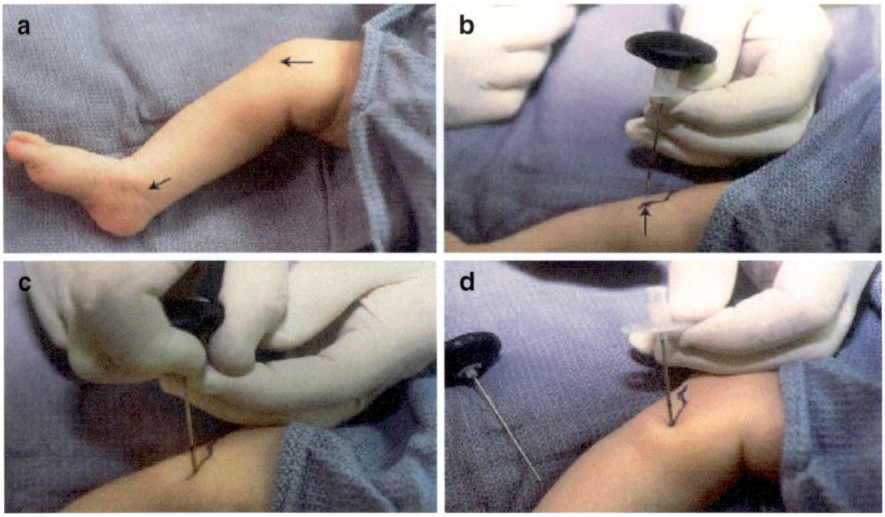

Fig. 8.8 Basic IO needle insertion technique: (**a**) The IO needle can be inserted 1 to 2 cm below and medial to the tibial tuberosity, or at the medial malleolus. (**b–d**) After sterile preparation of the insertion site(s), the needle is inserted with a twisting motion in a direction away from the growth plate(s). Reprinted with permission from A Practice of Anesthesia for Infants and Children. sixth ed. 2019. Wald SH, Mendoza J, Mihm FG, Cote CJ. Chapter 49: Procedures for Vascular Access. New York: Elsevier. p. 1139

or central routes [64]. Depending on the size of the medullary cavity, the substance infused, and size of the IO needle, flow rates of 0.5–41 mL/min have been achieved under gravity in an animal model [113]. Various studies have examined flow rates associated with pressurized and power drill devices. Using a 15-gauze, drill-powered IO needle intended for patients >3 kg body weight, Ong et al. achieved rates of 73 mL/min under gravity and up to 165 mL/min with a pressure bag in 24 adult patients [114]. There was no difference in flow rates between the tibial and humeral sites tested.

In a swine model study in which the animals were bled 30% of blood volume, the flow rates of autologous whole blood via a 15-gauge, 45 mm IO needle were compared with a 20G PIVC using three different techniques: a pressure bag (300 mmHg), the push-pull technique, and the LifeFlow Rapid Infuser device. The LifeFlow device delivered average IO and IV flow rates of 172 mL/min, or fourfold higher than the pressure bag (average 44 mL/min) and 80% higher than the push-pull method (91 mL/min) [76]. However, there was significant hemolysis in the PIVC arm as evidenced by free hemoglobin levels. This study informed device modifications that ultimately led to development and FDA-approval of LifeFlow Plus for the delivery of blood products for 22G PIVCs and larger. This study highlights the need for future investigation of what flow rates are obtainable and safe for IO blood administration in pediatric resuscitation.

8.2.15.3 Cut Downs, Femoral and Internal Jugular Vein

The venous cutdown has been replaced by other preferred sites secondary to infection risk and the significant time required to achieve cutdown access in children (e.g., > 6 min) [75]. In addition, the femoral vein was once considered optimal for resuscitation in small patients due to ease of access and its direct route to the central circulation. However, recent data indicates that femoral cannulation is associated with an increased rate of thromboembolism, particularly in neonates. The risk is increased following multiple attempts or if a femoral line is in place for prolonged periods [50, 75, 77]. The internal jugular (IJ) vein is relatively large in infants; however, it may lie directly in front of the carotid artery in one-half of patients, and access attempts may be complicated by pneumothorax, hematoma formation, and carotid artery puncture. SCV cannulation is likewise associated with similar risks in children, particularly when placed under duress.

8.2.16 Blood Filters and Fluid Warming Devices[2]

Currently, warming is not strictly advised for standard transfusion volumes when administered over the recommended 4-hour interval, even in the smallest ex-premature patients. However, rapidly administered, large volumes of cold-stored blood should be given through a warming device to prevent the multitude of associated side effects, including hypothermia, coagulopathy, acidosis, and apnea in neonates [1]. The AABB recommends all devices be validated and approved by the US FDA [78]. The National Institute for Health and Care Excellence (NICE; United Kingdom) has set a standard that all intravenous infusions over 500 mL should be warmed during the intraoperative phase of surgery [79]. The AABB cautions against warming blood with a radiant warmer due to a risk of RBC hemolysis [1].

When choosing fluid and blood warmers for pediatric patients, it is important to consider priming volumes, warming efficiency, and portability for bedside use. Technical information about the actual warming abilities of fluid warmers varies significantly between manufacturer and independent research results [80–82]. Examples of commercially available hospital fluid warming devices for perioperative use include the Belmont Buddy Lite™, the Warrior (QinFlow), the HOTLINE® (Smiths-Medical, Dublin, OH), the Pediatric 3 M™Ranger™ (3 M Health Care, St. Paul, MN), the Belmont® Rapid Infusion System RI-2, and the Fluido. There are additional warming devices for combat and prehospital settings [83]. Fluid warmers operate through a variety of techniques, including heating plates ("dry heat"; the Buddy Lite and 3 M Ranger), electromagnetic infrared induction (the RI-2 and the Fluido), water bath or coaxial heat exchange (the Hotline), and even forced hot air surrounding a coil (the Baire Hugger) [80, 82]. The maximum temperature suggested to avoid RBC hemolysis is 42 °C blood at the device outlet. The ability of

[2] Discussions of infusion devices and equipment are based on information found in current literature and do not reflect the opinions of the authors. Online product information is often distributed throughout multiple URLs and is modified periodically by the manufacturers

fluid warmers to meet this requirement varies with the device technology, the rate of blood flow, the time in contact with the warming element, and the length of the IV tubing. There are significant differences in output temperatures between the different devices and also between gravity and pressurized flow, as illustrated in Table 8.8 [78, 80, 84, 85].

The temperature of the fluid entering the patient's IV device varies indirectly with the length of the extension tubing leaving the warmer (due to ambient heat loss); thus, small devices that can be positioned with minimal extension tubing are more efficient. The heating efficiency of a fluid warmers takes on greater importance as they are designed to be smaller and more portable [85]. Examples of small size fluid warmers with the ability to operate near the patient include the Fluido and the Buddy Lite [87]. Of the warming devices mentioned, the priming volume is smallest with Buddy Lite (7.5 mL), intermediate for the Pediatric Ranger, the HOTLINE, and QinFlow (20 mL), and largest with Ranger® High Flow (150 mL) [86].

There are concerns over aluminum leaching from the heating elements of certain fluid warmers, and several have been recalled by the US FDA, including the enFlow IV fluid warmer (Vyaire Medical, Mittawa, IL), the ThermaCor 1200® disposable

Table 8.8 Warming capabilities of various fluid warmers found in the literature. [a]All fluids were infused at room temperature unless otherwise stated

Fluid warmer	[a]Output temp°C	Study mean infusion rate (mL/min)	Residual volume (mL)	Comments
Buddy lite (Belmont) [28, 58, 81, 86, 87]	30.5 °C	50	7.5	Stopped working at 200 mL/min; maximum recommended rate 50 mL/min
Warrior QinFlow [34]	38 °C	200	20	
3 M ranger pediatric [80, 88]	33 °C–41 °C	100	20	High temp alarm at 43 °C; no DEHP
3 M ranger high flow [35, 80]	35.2 °C	Gravity	40	Rated up to 150 mL/min
	31.2 °C	407 (300 mmHg pressure)		
Belmont RI-2 (28)	38 °C	100 mL/min	100	No warming 2.5–5 mL/min; unclear warming at max 1000 mL/min
Fluido [80, 85]	35.3 °C	Gravity	90	Output T ° 24.1 °C infusing cold saline <6 °C; designed for 15–800 mL/min
	35.5 °C	446 (300 mmHg pressure)		
	37 °C	800		
Hotline [82, 89]	31.1 °C	Gravity	20	Gravity flow recommended
	26.3 °C	375 (300 mmHg pressure)		
	37 °C	83 mL/min		
Bair Hugger [80]	26.3 °C	Gravity	34	Recommended 50 mL/min
	23.9 °C	225 (300 mmHg pressure)		
	28.5 °C at patient	0.38 mL/min		

sets (Smisson-Cartledge, Macon, GA), and the Level 1®H-1200 fast flow fluid warmer (Smiths Medical ASD Inc., Minneapolis, MN) [37]. Both the Belmont RI-2, HOTLINE, and Fluido warmers contain air detectors (as well as the majority of modern warmers); however, these functionalities are imperfect and blood tubing should always be monitored for entrained air to prevent air embolism. Additional safety concerns surrounding fluid heating devices include bacterial infection (inside the fluid warming jackets), plasticizer exposure, hypothermia secondary to inadequate fluid warming capability at high flow rates (e.g., using a forced air mattress devices), and hyperthermia from devices with manually set output temperatures; once the patient's core temperature exceeds 37–41° C, the warming unit temperature should be reduced and monitored regularly [90, 91].

Several fluid warmers—the Belmont Rapid Infusion System RI-2™ and the 3 M™Ranger Pediatric/Neonatal warmer (3 M Health Care, St. Paul, MN)—double as RIDs. The pediatric ranger advertises a needless port for calibrated fluid aspiration and administration (syringe "bolus" capability), latex-and Di-(2-ethylhexl) phthalate (DEHP; a plasticizer)-free material, an air bubble trap, tolerance of infusion pressure up to 300 mmHg, and a high temperature alarm [88]. The FDA has published a warning against the use of plasticizer materials (particularly DEHP) in male fetuses, neonates, and prepubertal children [92, 93]. Blood transfusion tubing and containment devices often contain plasticizers to improve container performance; however, manufacturer product labeling is often absent or incomplete [94]. Lastly, platelet function is affected when infused through a warming device [95]. Both platelets and cryoprecipitate are released from the blood bank at room temperature and do not need to be transfused through a warmer during resuscitation unless administered as part of a cold-stored whole blood transfusion. In vitro studies suggest that running either room temperature or cold stored apheresis platelets through a warming device may affect platelet aggregometry and viscoelastic results (i.e., MA or maximum amplitude and alpha angle), but the clinical significance of these findings is unclear [96, 97].

8.2.16.1 Blood Filters

A blood filter that can remove blood clots and macroparticles is required for all blood transfusions [19]. Standard "blood tubing" contains an in-line "macroaggregate" filter usually in the range of 170–260 microns, intended to filter out most cellular debris and clots accumulated during blood storage. The size of the filter signifies the size of the substance filtered and not the pores in the filter itself. Specialized add-on filters include the 20–40 micron "microaggregate" filter once used as a "leukocyte reduction" filter (LRF), which is now recommended to filter blood collected through an autologous transfusion device (e.g., a "cell saver") or for intraoperative whole blood autologous administration (e.g., autologous normovolemic hemodilution; ANH) [19]. An example of a commonly encountered microaggregate (e.g., 40 micron) filter can be found online at https://www.medline.com/media/catalog/Docs/MKT/SQ40%20FILTER.PDF.

Microaggregate filters are thought to remove fibrin strands, leukocytes, fat globules, and cytokines associated with transfusion reactions. They are not for routine use and should never be used to transfuse platelets, as they tend to stick to the filter elements. Microaggregate filters also should not be used with pressure devices or power infusers because they will shear RBCs and activate platelets.

Blood filters as small as 5 microns (reportedly capable of filtering shards of glass ampules) and 1.2 microns (reportedly capable of reducing bacteria and endotoxin content) are commercially available. Neonatal in-line filter sets are routinely used for calibrated syringe administration of small volume aliquots (Figs. 8.9 and 8.10) [107, 108].

Although manufacturers may supply a recommendation for how often a blood filter should be replaced, they should be changed once there is a noticeable decrease in the gravity flow rate or, in the case of automated infusing devices, as indicated by the high pressure alarm. Coadministration of blood products (particularly

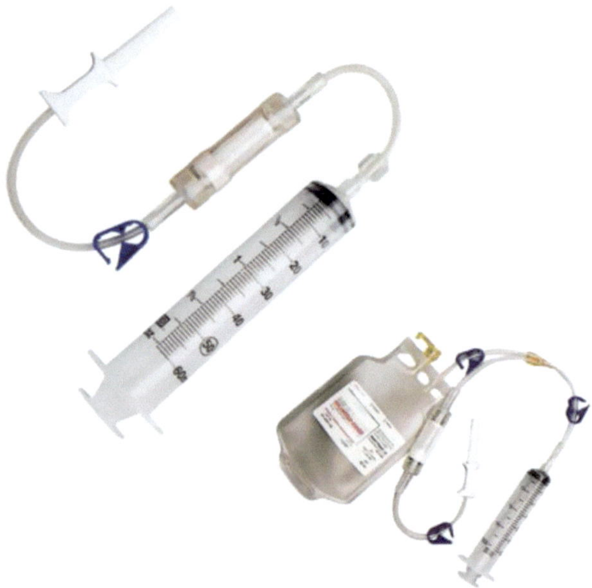

Fig. 8.9 A neonatal blood administration set with an inline 150-micron filter for removing small aliquots of blood. Reprinted with permission from Charter Medical. (Image found online at https://chartermedical.com/syringe-sets/)

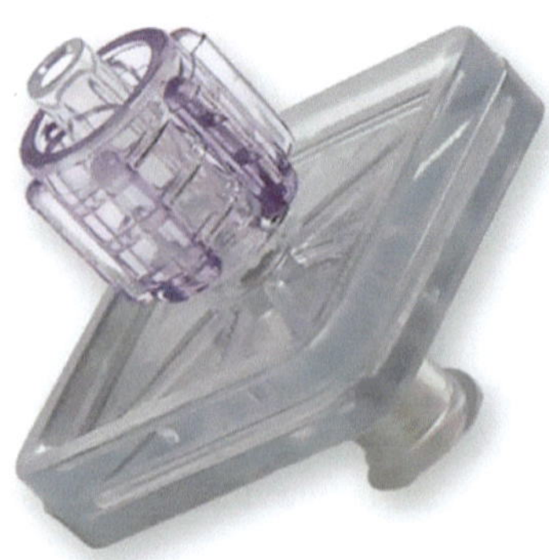

Fig. 8.10 The 18-micron Hemo-Nate® neonatal filter, with a prime volume 0.7 mL, can be attached to any syringe. Image reprinted with permission from Utah Medical Products, Inc. and found online at http://www.utahmed.com/hemo-nate.html

cryoprecipitate and platelets) in an administration set that is not designed for blood administration, or admixture with a calcium-containing carrier fluid (such as Lactated Ringer's), may lead to line clotting and product wastage [109, 115].

Leukocyte reduction (LR) is usually performed today on cellular blood products (e.g., RBCs and platelets) just after donation and before storage in the hospital blood bank. LR has been associated with fewer nonhemolytic febrile transfusion reactions (seen more frequently in children compared to adults), HLA alloimmunization, and CMV transmission. The objective of leukocyte reduction is to remove 99% of white blood cells from the RBC or platelet unit [19]. Bedside LR filters (LRFs), which operate through electrostatic adhesion of particles to the filter material (rather than simple pore filtration) are used to filter particles smaller than the sieve pore size (Fig. 8.11) [116]. Bedside LRFs are commercially available but are not present in many hospitals. Individual LRFs may be specific for platelets or RBCs only and should never be used to transfuse leukocytes or stem cells [19]. Furthermore, they are not as efficient at removing leukocytes as the filtration process employed in large-scale donor centers before storage [98]. Low volume RBC unit, platelet, and plasma LRF sets have also been developed.

Bedside LRFs have been associated with hypotensive reactions, particularly when transfusing platelets through negatively charged LRFs (versus positively charged) in patients taking angiotensin-coenzyme (ACE) inhibitors [19, 117]. The observed hypotension is thought to be secondary to bradykinin release [117–119]. Some experts recommend using LRFs when administering blood obtained through cell salvage [120].

Other specialty filters may be required in certain clinical situations such as inside cell salvage machines, cardiac bypass, and ECMO circuits. These filters are upstream of the macro-and macroaggregates filters discussed in the preceding section and are included within the device tubing sets.

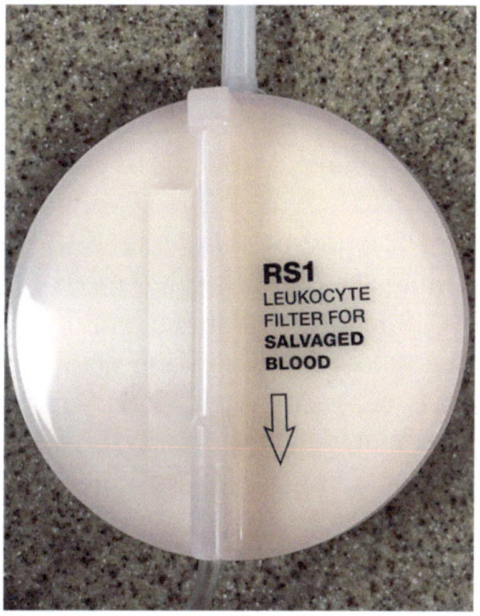

Fig. 8.11 A bedside, single-use leukocyte reduction filter for intraoperatively salvaged blood. It can reduce levels of white blood cells, fat globules, and microaggregates in up to 450 mL of concentrated and washed "cell saver" blood. Reprinted with permission from Jonathan Waters, MD (personal collection)

8.3 The Double Effect of Rapid Transfusions in Small Children

Many noninfectious adverse events are associated with the rapid transfusion of blood products to pediatric patients [4, 25, 52, 91, 121–123]. They include, but are not limited to:

- Hyperkalemia
- Administration error
- Transfusion-associated circulatory overload (TACO)
- Transfusion-related dyspnea (TAD)
- Hypothermia
- Hypocalcemia (citrate toxicity)
- Dilutional coagulopathy
- Hypoglycemia
- Lactic acidosis
- Thromboembolism
- Hemolysis
- Hypotension
- Infiltration and extravasation

Transfusion reactions associated with transfusion equipment include transfusion-associated hyperkalemia (TAH), transfusion-associated hemolysis, venous thromboembolism (VTE), transfusion-associated circulatory overload (TACO), hypothermia, and venous air embolism (VAE). Detailed discussion of these side effects can be found in Chap. 14. At times, these events are the result of life-saving blood resuscitation and, at best, can only be managed but not prevented.

8.4 Summary of Recommendations

It is likely that this 6 kg patient is in hypovolemic shock and must be treated aggressively prior to surgical incision and further volume loss. The patient's estimated blood volume is 480 mL. A starting hematocrit of 22% suggests that the patient has lost up to half of his blood volume. This means one must rapidly transfuse a significant fraction of this volume to restore hemodynamic stability. If the goal is to administer 20 mL/kg (120 mL) of RBCs during the first 5 min per ACCM and AHA PALS recommendations, gravity flow through existing PIVCs may be inadequate. The use of a pressurizing device may not accommodate the small, aliquoted volumes necessary, and a RID will produce excessive volumes. Appropriate alternatives include a volumetric infusion pump at a rate of 999 mL/hr (16.7 mL/min) or manual administration using a 10 mL syringe through a three-way stopcock for a push-pull technique. This will allow careful volume titration and, if syringe pressure is firm but nonpulsatile, RBC hemolysis will be minimized.

The preexisting 22-gauge PIVC is the preferable access alternative because it will allow a faster transfusing rate with less RBC hemolysis compared to the 24-gauge PIVC. The 24-gauge PIVC can be utilized for medications, other fluids, or, if essential, further blood administration. When possible, a 20-gauge or larger PIVC should be inserted into the saphenous vein if surgical blood loss is persistent. The saphenous vein diameter in an 8-month-old that will meet the recommended catheter-to-vein ratio (< 50%) to avoid vein occlusion or thrombosis formation is ≥2 ms. According to the table below, a 22-gauge and a 20-gauge PIVC will provide a total crystalloid infusion volume of 95 mL/min under gravity or 228 mL/min under pressure; the potential blood administration rate is approximately 50% of those rates, or 48 mL/min to 114 mL/min within the first minute of resuscitation.

	24-gauge PIVC		22-gauge PIVC		20-gauge PIVC	
Achievable flow rate (mL/minute)	Gravity	Pressure	Gravity	Pressure	Gravity	Pressure
Crystalloid solution	20	Unknown	35	88	60	140
Blood	Reduce rate by 30–70% (average 50%)					

The latter blood volume administration rate (114 mL/min) is one-quarter of the patient's 480 mL total blood volume. All PIVCs are at risk of infiltration and clotting; therefore, the option to insert an IO line into the proximal tibia or humerus should be present if the existing PIVCs are unable to meet fluid demands in a timely manner.

Because relatively large volumes must be administered to this small patient at relatively rapid rates, RBCs and plasma should be warmed prior to administration. If a validated fluid warmer is available, it should have minimal dead space, be placed close to the patient (avoiding direct skin contact), and should be connected to relatively short IV tubing to prevent ambient heat loss. If a dedicated IV fluid warmer with the ability to monitor output temperature is not available, the patient's IV tubing can be surrounded by a forced air body warmer or a bath of warm water, keeping in mind that overheating of IV fluid can occur using any external warming technique. The patient's body temperature must be monitored, and all fluid warming devices should be turned off if the blood loss has ceased and the patient's core temperature has normalized. Platelets and cryoprecipitate should not be run through a warming device unless administered as part of a cold-stored whole blood transfusion.

If this patient's IV set up contains "blood tubing," the required "macroaggregate" blood filter (170–260 microns) used to remove storage-related clots will be self-contained in the tubing. Other blood filters, specifically the "microaggregate" filters used to remove cytokines, fat globules, or glass shards, should not be used under pressure because they will traumatize the blood cells. If blood loss has ceased and it is feasible to administer blood at a slow rate (e.g., 2–4 mL/kg/h), a variety of neonatal blood filters can be safely utilized.

As a small patient, this 6 kg child is particularly susceptible to adverse, device-related transfusion events. The challenge of estimating ongoing blood loss in a bleeding infant can lead to over transfusion and TACO during rapid blood replacement. This is a dilemma because diagnosing TACO during the intraoperative period can be difficult if not impossible. Forceful blood administration may produce RBC hemolysis and high supernatant potassium concentrations, with resultant hyperkalemia that overwhelms the infant's ability to excrete excess potassium. Citrate toxicity, leading to hypocalcemia, will ensue if the infant's electrolyte values are not closely followed or if calcium is not administered proactively during periods of massive blood replacement (e.g., 25–40 mL/kg body weight). All infusion devices, including pressure bags and RIDs with "air traps," place patients at risk of air embolism and must be scrupulously inspected before and during all rapid transfusions. RBCs and plasma released from the blood bank are stored at temperatures less than 10 °C and, if not warmed through a validated fluid warmer, will produce hypothermia and eventually a lethal coagulopathy if administered rapidly in large doses.

Key Points

Rapid infusion devices (RIDs): Currently, there are no standardized pediatric guidelines for RIDs. The classic RIDs have no place in neonatal resuscitation, and the acceptable weight cutoff for using these devices in older children is unclear; a body weight between 20 and 40 kg is cited in the literature. Some of the newer volumetric or syringe pumps have customizable, user-set pressure limits.

Vascular access devices: Patient body size, available insertion sites, and the desired infusion rate must be considered when selecting vascular access for resuscitation. The Association for the Advancement of Blood & Biotherapies (AABB) advises that 24-gauge catheters and 25-gauge needles are the smallest that can be safely used for blood transfusion under conditions of constant flow or pressure. Multilumen CVCs and PICC lines are not recommended for primary vascular access in rapid volume replacement when a suitable PIVC is available. A portacath may be used to infuse blood products but is not suitable for rapid volume replacement.

Vascular access sites: A "catheter-to-vein" ratio < 33% in a 24-gauge PIVC and < 50% in a 22-gauge PIVC may be necessary to minimize line occlusion and thrombosis. The largest caliber PIVC access point in infants are the upper arm venous system and the saphenous vein of the lower extremity. When rapid vascular access is critical but cannot be obtained, the intraosseous approach should be considered.

Fluid warmers: Rapidly administered, large volumes of cold-stored blood should be administered through a warming device.

Blood filters: A blood filter that can remove blood clots and macroparticles is required for all blood transfusions. Standard "blood tubing" contains an in-line filter usually in the range of 170–260 microns, intended to filter out most cellular debris and clots accumulated during blood storage.

Equipment-related adverse transfusion events: There are many adverse events associated with the rapid transfusion of blood products to small patients. These include, but are not limited to, hyperkalemia, over-transfusion, hypocalcemia, and venous air embolism.

References

1. Wong ECC, Punzalan RC. Neonatal and pediatric transfusion practice. In: Cohn C, Delaney M, Johnson ST, Katz LM, editors. Technical manual. 20th ed. Bethesda: AABB; 2020. p. 676, 685, 689–692.
2. Canadian Blood Services. Chapter 13: Neonatal and Pediatric Transfusion. In: Clinical Guide to Transfusion. 2017. https://professionaleducation.blood.ca/en/transfusion/clinical-guide/neonatal-and-pediatric-transfusion. Accessed 31 July 2023.
3. Parker MJ, Manan A. Translating resuscitation guidelines into practice: health care provider attitudes, preferences and beliefs regarding pediatric fluid resuscitation performance. PLoS One. 2013;8(3):e58282.
4. Ross PA, Lerman J, Cote CJ. Chapter 52: Pediatric equipment, patient warming, fluid & blood warmers. In: Cote CJ, Lerman J, Anderson B, editors. A practice of anesthesia for infants and children. 6th ed. Philadelphia: Elsevier; 2019. p. 1176–90.
5. Greene N, Bhananker S, Ramaiah R. Vascular access, fluid resuscitation, and blood transfusion in pediatric trauma. Int J Crit Illn Inj Sci. 2012;2(3):135–42.
6. ICUMedical. DeltaVen® Fast Flash™. https://www.icumed.com/products/infusion-therapy/vascular-access/peripheral-iv-catheters/deltaven-fast-flash. Accessed 3 Aug 2023.
7. Clinical Infusion Alliance (CIA). Guide to IV Catheter Sizes: Gauge, Diameter, Length, Flow Rate. 2023. https://www.ciamedical.com/insights/iv-catheter-sizes/#:~:text=24%20gauge%20catheters%20have%20yellow,and%20other%20kinds%20of%20infusions. Accessed 3 Aug 2023.
8. B. Braun Medical Inc. (2019). Introcan Safety IV Catheter with Automatic Passive Safety. Bethlehem, PA: B. Braun Medical Inc. Retrieved from https://www.bbraunusa.com/en/products/b/introcan-safety-ivcatheterstraight.html. Accessed on February 23, 2025.
9. Terumo Europe. Surflash I.V. Catheter. 2023. https://www.terumo-europe.com/en-emea/products/surflash%E2%84%A2-i-v-catheter?TermStoreId=70aa3b4e-82ed-47d3-b1dc-9d7951d9228f&TermSetId=2fa1bbfb-d558-4262-9605-3c31f742e996&TermId=55bd1bb5-5905-4733-a1d0-4ffcac69b092. Accessed 3 Aug 2023.
10. Stoner MJ, Goodman DG, Cohen DM, Fernandez SA, Hall MW. Rapid fluid resuscitation in pediatrics: testing the American College of Critical Care Medicine guideline. Ann Emerg Med. 2007;50(5):601–7.
11. Skelton T, Beno S. Massive transfusion in pediatric trauma: we need to focus more on "how". J Trauma Acute Care Surg. 2017;82(1):211–5.
12. Berman DJ, Schiavi A, Frank SM, Duarte S, Schwengel DA, Miller CR. Factors that influence flow through intravascular catheters: the clinical relevance of Poiseuille's law. Transfusion. 2020;60(7):1410–7.
13. Strauss RG. Data-driven blood banking practices for neonatal RBC transfusions. Transfusion. 2000;40(12):1528–40.
14. Whyte RK, Jefferies AL. Canadian Paediatric society FtaNC. Red blood cell transfusion in newborn infants. Paediatr Child Health. 2014;19(4):213–22.
15. Tyler DC. Wake up safe®: the pediatric anesthesia quality improvement initiative. 2015. https://wakeupsafe.org/wp-content/uploads/2018/10/Hyperkalemia_statement.pdf . Accessed 31 July 2023.
16. Davis WOM. Infusion devices training tutorial. In: EBME & Clinical Engineering Articles. https://www.ebme.co.uk/articles/clinical-engineering/infusion-devices-training-tutorial. Accessed 31 July 2023.
17. Tobias MD, Hanson CW 3rd, Heppenstall RB, Aukburg SJ. Compartment syndrome after pressurized infusion. Br J Anaesth. 1991;67(3):332–4.
18. Kim JT, Park JY, Lee HJ, Cheon YJ. Guidelines for the management of extravasation. J Educ Eval Health Prof. 2020;17:21.

19. Jorgenson M. Administration of blood components. In: Cohn CS, Delaney M, Johnson ST, Katz LM, editors. Technical manual. 20th ed. Bethesda: AABB; 2020. p. 537, 541–546.
20. Gniadek TJ, Richtsfeld M, Pulkrabek S, Hansen KR, Barnett SL, Joyner N, et al. Mechanical hemolysis in pediatric patients associated with rapid transfusion and one-way valve. Transfusion. 2018;58(5):1228–33.
21. De Villiers WL, Murray AA, Levin AI. Expediting red blood cell transfusions by syringing causes significant hemolysis. Transfusion. 2017;57(11):2747–51.
22. Miller MA, Schlueter AJ. Transfusions via hand-held syringes and small-gauge needles as risk factors for hyperkalemia. Transfusion. 2004;44(3):373–81.
23. Hayward WA, Haseler LJ, Kettwich LG, Michael AA, Sibbitt W, Bankhurst AD. Pressure generated by syringes: implications for hydrodissection and injection of dense connective tissue lesions. Scand J Rheumatol. 2011;40(5):379–82.
24. Shamim F, Abbasi S. Fatal vascular air embolism during fluid resuscitation as a complication of pressure infuser bag. J Emerg Trauma Shock. 2016;9(1):46–7.
25. Serious Hazards of Transfusion (SHOT). SHOT Annual Reports and Summaries. 2023. https://www.shotuk.org/shot-reports/. Accessed 16 June 2023.
26. Bhananker SM, Ramamoorthy C, Geiduschek JM, Posner KL, Domino KB, Haberkern CM, et al. Anesthesia-related cardiac arrest in children: update from the pediatric perioperative cardiac arrest registry. Anesth Analg. 2007;105(2):344–50.
27. Davis AL, Carcillo JA, Aneja RK, Deymann AJ, Lin JC, Nguyen TC, et al. American College of Critical Care Medicine Clinical Practice Parameters for hemodynamic support of pediatric and neonatal septic shock. Crit Care Med. 2017;45(6):1061–93.
28. 3M. The Belmont® Rapid Infuser RI-2 Operators Manual (English). In: Belmont Medical Technologies. Resources. https://belmontmedtech.com/resources. Accessed 31 July 2023 https://belmontmedtech.com/resources?field_related_product_target_id_verf=All&type_1=brochure&resource_language=140&sort_by=created&sort_order=DESC and https://www.bhs.org.au/bhsapps/govdoc/gdhtml/gdcpp0440%2D%2D25610-the%20belmont%20rapid%20infuser%20ri-2%20operators%20manual.pdf. Accessed 2 Aug 2024.
29. Barcelona SL, Vilich F, Coté CJ. A comparison of flow rates and warming capabilities of the level 1 and rapid infusion system with various-size intravenous catheters. Anesth Analg. 2003;97(2):358–63. table of contents
30. Parker RI. Transfusion in critically ill children: indications, risks, and challenges. Crit Care Med. 2014;42(3):675–90.
31. 401 Medical: LifeFlowPlus Blood & Fluid Infuser. 2020. https://410medical.com/wp-content/uploads/2021/01/LifeFlow-PLUS-In-Service-Training-Guide.pdf. Accessed 2 Aug 2024.
32. Chang TP, Ringold SM, Lichtenfeld N, Nguyen P, Paz D, Festekjian A. The effect of rapid fluid infusions on transabdominal pelvic ultrasound timing among female pediatric patients: a randomized controlled pilot trial. Acad Emerg Med. 2020;27(11):1191–3.
33. Coyle C, Zitek T, Pepe PE, Stotsenburg M, Scheppke KA, Antevy P, et al. The implementation of a prehospital whole blood transfusion program and early results. Prehosp Disaster Med. 2023;38(4):513–7.
34. QinFlow. Warrior Extreme. 2022. https://www.qinflow.com/product/warrior-warrior-extreme/. Accessed 1 Aug 2023.
35. 3M™Ranger™Pressure Infuser. 2022. https://www.3m.com/3M/en_US/p/?Ntt=3m+ranger. Accessed 1 Aug 2024.
36. McGonigal M. Rapid Infusers: How Fast Can They Go? In: The Trauma Pro. 2021. https://thetraumapro.com/2021/07/28/rapid-infusers-how-fast-can-they-go/. Accessed 2 Aug 2024.
37. US FDA. Urgent voluntary recall: level 1 fast flow fluid warming systems, NORMOFLO fluid warmer and level 1 Normothermic IV fluid administration set. 2021. https://www.fda.gov/medical-devices/letters-health-care-providers/potential-risk-aluminum-leaching-use-certain-fluid-warmer-devices-letter-health-care-providers. Accessed 31 July 2023.
38. Ullman AJ, Bernstein SJ, Brown E, Aiyagari R, Doellman D, Faustino EVS, et al. The Michigan appropriateness guide for intravenous catheters in pediatrics: miniMAGIC. Pediatrics. 2020;145(Suppl 3):S269–S84.

39. Pittiruti M, Van Boxtel T, Scoppettuolo G, Carr P, Konstantinou E, Ortiz Miluy G, et al. European recommendations on the proper indication and use of peripheral venous access devices (the ERPIUP consensus): a WoCoVA project. J Vasc Access. 2023;24(1):165–82.
40. Hallam C, Denton A, Weston V, Dunn H, Jackson T, Keeling S, et al. UK vessel health and preservation (VHP) framework: a commentary on the updated VHP 2020. J Infect Prev. 2021;22(4):147–55.
41. Milne A, Teng JJ, Vargas A, Markley JC, Collins A. Performance assessment of intravenous catheters for massive transfusion: a pragmatic in vitro study. Transfusion. 2021;61(6):1721–8.
42. Rosen KR, Rosen DA. Comparative flow rates for small bore peripheral intravenous catheters. Pediatr Emerg Care. 1986;2(3):153–6.
43. Warren DW, Kissoon N, Sommerauer JF, Rieder MJ. Comparison of fluid infusion rates among peripheral intravenous and humerus, femur, malleolus, and tibial intraosseous sites in normovolemic and hypovolemic piglets. Ann Emerg Med. 1993;22(2):183–6.
44. Iserson KV, Reeter AK, Criss E. Comparison of flow rates for standard and large-bore blood tubing. West J Med. 1985;143(2):183–5.
45. Tan BK, Chong S, Koh ZX, Ong ME. EZ-IO in the ED: an observational, prospective study comparing flow rates with proximal and distal tibia intraosseous access in adults. Am J Emerg Med. 2012;30(8):1602–6.
46. Lehn RA, Gross JB, McIsaac JH, Gipson KE. Needleless connectors substantially reduce flow of crystalloid and red blood cells during rapid infusion. Anesth Analg. 2015;120(4):801–4.
47. Barton A. Clinical use of closed-system safety peripheral intravenous cannulas. Br J Nurs. 2018;27(8):S22–S7.
48. Miyoshi H, Nakamura R, Noda Y, Kimura H, Kamiya S, Morio A, et al. Relationship between the loaded pressure and flow rate of packed red blood cells and various infusion solutions in Normal infusion lines and catheters. Anesth Analg. 2021;133(5):1107–15.
49. Pinelli F, Pittiruti M. The integrated short peripheral cannula: a new peripheral venous access device? J Vasc Access. 2023;24(3):353–7.
50. Kleidon T, Ullman A. Right pediatric site selection and technology. In: Moreau NL, editor. Vessel health and preservation: the right approach for vascular access. New York: Springer Open; 2019. p. 192–208.
51. Seckold T, Walker S, Dwyer T. A comparison of silicone and polyurethane PICC lines and postinsertion complication rates: a systematic review. J Vasc Access. 2015;16(3):167–77.
52. Lee AC, Reduque LL, Luban NL, Ness PM, Anton B, Heitmiller ES. Transfusion-associated hyperkalemic cardiac arrest in pediatric patients receiving massive transfusion. Transfusion. 2014;54(1):244–54.
53. Wiersum-Osselton JC, Whitaker B, Grey S, Land K, Perez G, Rajbhandary S, et al. Revised international surveillance case definition of transfusion-associated circulatory overload: a classification agreement validation study. Lancet Haematol. 2019;6(7):e350–e8.
54. Bulle EB, Klanderman RB, Pendergrast J, Cserti-Gazdewich C, Callum J, Vlaar APJ. The recipe for TACO: a narrative review on the pathophysiology and potential mitigation strategies of transfusion-associated circulatory overload. Blood Rev. 2022;52:100891.
55. Delaney M, Wendel S, Bercovitz RS, Cid J, Cohn C, Dunbar NM, et al. Transfusion reactions: prevention, diagnosis, and treatment. Lancet. 2016;388(10061):2825–36.
56. Cote CJ, Grabowski EF, Stowell CP. Chapter 12: strategies for blood product management, reducing transfusions, and massive blood transfusion. In: Cote CJ, Lehman J, Anderson BJ, editors. Cote and Lerman's A practice of anesthesia for infants and children. 5th ed. Amsterdam: Elsevier; 2019. p. 208–210, 257–280, 307, 317.
57. Neff LP, Cannon JW, Morrison JJ, Edwards MJ, Spinella PC, Borgman MA. Clearly defining pediatric massive transfusion: cutting through the fog and friction with combat data. J Trauma Acute Care Surg. 2015;78(1):22–8; discussion 8–9.
58. Barcelona SL, Thompson AA, Coté CJ. Intraoperative pediatric blood transfusion therapy: a review of common issues. Part II: transfusion therapy, special considerations, and reduction of allogenic blood transfusions. Paediatr Anaesth. 2005;15(10):814–30.

59. Yamada C, Edelson M, Lee A, Saifee NH, Bahar B, Delaney M. Transfusion-associated hyperkalemia in pediatric population: prevalence, risk factors, survival, infusion rate, and RBC unit features. Transfusion. 2021;61(4):1093–101.
60. Cote C, Lerman J, Todres DI. A practice of anesthesia for infants and children. 4th ed. Philadelphia: Saunders; 2008. p. 207–9.
61. Strauss RG. RBC storage and avoiding hyperkalemia from transfusions to neonates & infants. Transfusion. 2010;50(9):1862–5.
62. Vraets A, Lin Y, Callum JL. Transfusion-associated hyperkalemia. Transfus Med Rev. 2011;25(3):184–96.
63. Williams JH. Goodbye, Large-Bore IV Access. In: Anesthesia Experts. 2016. https://anesthesiaexperts.com/uncategorized/goodbye-large-bore-iv-access/#:~:text=Needleless%20connectors%20have%20distinct%20advantages,needleless%20connectors%20should%20be%20removed. Accessed 27 July 2023.
64. Maconochie IK, de Caen AR, Aickin R, Atkins DL, Biarent D, Guerguerian AM, et al. Part 6: pediatric basic life support and pediatric advanced life support: 2015 international consensus on cardiopulmonary resuscitation and emergency cardiovascular care science with treatment recommendations. Resuscitation. 2015;95:e147–68.
65. Rosa-Mangeret F, Waldvogel-Abramowski S, Pfister RE, Baud O, Fau S. Safety of red blood cell transfusion using small central lines in neonates: an. Front Pediatr. 2021;9:606611.
66. Scott-Warren VL, Morley RB. Paediatric vascular access. BJA Education. 2015;15:199–206.
67. Pittiruti M, Brutti A, Celentano D, Pomponi M, Biasucci DG, Annetta MG, et al. Clinical experience with power-injectable PICCs in intensive care patients. Crit Care. 2012;16(1):R21.
68. Wong EC, Schreiber S, Criss VR, LaFleur B, Rais-Bahrami K, Short B, et al. Feasibility of red blood cell transfusion through small bore central venous catheters used in neonates. Pediatr Crit Care Med. 2004;5(1):69–74.
69. Gonzalez R, Cassaro S. Percutaneous central catheter. In: StatPearls. Treasure Island, FL: StatPearls Publishing; 2021. https://www.ncbi.nlm.nih.gov/books/NBK459338/. Accessed 22 Aug 2022.
70. Wall C, Moore J, Thachil J. Catheter-related thrombosis: a practical approach. J Intensive Care Soc. 2016;17(2):160–7.
71. Ostlund A, Flaring U, Norberg A, Kaiser S, Frisk T, Larsson P, et al. Complications of pediatric midline catheters: a prospective observational pilot study. Anesth Analg. 2024;138(3):572–8.
72. Qin KR, Ensor N, Barnes R, Englin A, Nataraja RM, Pacilli M. Standard versus long peripheral catheters for multiday IV therapy: a randomized controlled trial. Pediatrics. 2021;147(2):e2020000877.
73. Eldridge L. Get to know your Huber needle for chemo port access. In: Verywellhealth. 2022. https://www.verywellhealth.com/get-to-know-your-huber-needle-for-chemo-port-access-430073. Accessed 31 July 2023.
74. BD. PowerLoc Safety Infusion Set. 2024. https://www.bd.com/en-uk/products-and-solutions/products/product-families/powerloc-safety-infusion-set. Accessed 31 Oct 2024.
75. Haas NA. Clinical review: vascular access for fluid infusion in children. Crit Care. 2004;8(6):478–84.
76. Bianchi W, George T, McEvoy C, Piehl M, Manzano A, Boboc M, et al. Intravenous and intraosseous blood transfusion with three different pediatric pressure transfusion strategies in an immature swine (Sus scrofa) model of hemorrhagic shock: a pilot study. Mil Med. 2020;185(Suppl 1):121–9.
77. Bhatt MD, Chan AK. Venous thrombosis in neonates. Fac Rev. 2021;10:20.
78. Fung MK. Technical manual. 19th ed. Bethesda: AABB Press; 2017. p. 115, 120–121, 127, 265–291, 464–469, 481–489, 492–493, 632.
79. NICE. National Institute for Health and Care Excellence. https://www.nice.org.uk/guidance/cg65/chapter/Recommendations#intraoperative-phase. 2016. Accessed 6 Sept. 2022.
80. Turner M, Hodzovic I, Mapleson WW. Simulated clinical evaluation of four fluid warming devices*. Anaesthesia. 2006;61(6):571–5.

81. Weatherall A, Gill M, Milligan J, Tetlow C, Harris C, Garner A, et al. Comparison of portable blood-warming devices under simulated pre-hospital conditions: a randomised in-vitro blood circuit study. Anaesthesia. 2019;74(8):1026–32.
82. Hooper CM. Warming devices. In: Davey A, Diba A, editors. Ward's anaesthetic equipment. 6th ed. Philadelphia: Saunders Elsevier; 2011. p. 514.
83. Martin SM, Fisher AD, Meledeo MA, Wampler D, Nicholson SE, Raczek K, et al. More sophisticated than a drink cooler or an old sphygmomanometer but still not adequate for pre-hospital blood: a market review of commercially available equipment for prehospital blood transport and administration. Transfusion. 2021;61(Suppl 1):S286–S93.
84. Horowitz PE, Delagarza MA, Pulaski JJ, Smith RA. Flow rates and warming efficacy with hotline and ranger blood/fluid warmers. Anesth Analg. 2004;99(3):788–92.
85. Zoremba N, Bruells C, Rossaint R, Breuer T. Heating capabilities of small fluid warming systems. BMC Anesthesiol. 2018;18(1):98.
86. QinFlow. What is the Priming Volume of Each Hospital Warmer (ml)? 2022. https://www.qinflow.com/compare-blood-fluid-warmers/compare-hospital-blood-fluid-warmers/what-is-the-priming-volume-of-each-hospital-warmer-ml/. Accessed 29 July 2023. .
87. Belmont Medical. Emergency transport. buddy lite. https://belmontmedtech.com/ems-hypothermia-devices?utm_source=google&utm_medium=cpc&utm_campaign=buddylite_competitor&gclid=EAIaIQobChMIwpjz7dvZhwMVmyZ7Bx0DRDXTEAAYASAAEgLYe_D_BwE. Accessed 2 Aug 2024.
88. 3M. 3M™ Ranger™ Pediatric/Neonate Disposable Set. 2023. https://www.3m.com/3M/en_LB/p/d/v000525507/. Accessed 1 Aug 2023.
89. ICU Medical. Hotline Blood and Fluid Warmer. https://www.icumed.com/products/critical-care/temperature-management/hotline#:~:text=The%20HOTLINE%20Blood%20and%20Fluid,temperatures%20under%20gravity%20flow%20conditions. Accessed 31 July 2023.
90. Nemeth M, Miller C, Brauer A. Perioperative hypothermia in children. Int J Environ Res Public Health. 2021;18:7541. https://pubmed.ncbi.nlm.nih.gov/34299991/. Accessed 22 Aug 2022
91. Chiravuri SD. Chapter 135. Rapid fluid and blood delivery systems. In: Fleisher LA, Rosenbaum SH, editors. Complications in anesthesia. 3rd ed. Philadelphia: Elsevier; 2018. p. 119, 553–5.
92. Health Care Without Harm. Summary of the FDA safety assessment of DEHP. 2022. https://noharm-uscanada.org/documents/summary-fda-safety-assessment-dehp-released-pvc-medical-devices-what-it-says-what%E2%80%99s-next. Accessed 1 Aug 2023.
93. Sampson J, de Korte D. DEHP-plasticised PVC: relevance to blood services. Transfus Med. 2011;21(2):73–83.
94. Panneel L, Malarvannan G, Jorens PG. Plasticizers in the neonatal intensive care unit: a review on exposure sources and health hazards. Crit Rev Environ Sci Technol. 2022;52:3947–72.
95. Hoyos Gomez T, El Haddi SJ, Grimstead-Arnold SL, Schreiber MA. The effect of the Belmont rapid infuser on cold stored whole blood coagulability. Injury. 2023;54(1):29–31.
96. Mattson MK, Groves C, Smith MM, Christensen JM, Chen D, Stubbs JR, et al. Platelet transfusion: the effects of a fluid warmer on platelet function. Transfusion. 2021;61(1):52–6.
97. Valencia Morales DJ, Klompas AM, Torbenson JM, Finney RE, Chen D, Stubbs JR, et al. Cold platelet transfusion: the effects of a fluid warmer on platelet function. Transfusion. 2024;64(1):47–52.
98. Mishima Y, Tsuno NH, Matsuhashi M, Yoshizato T, Sato T, Ikeda T, et al. Effects of universal vs bedside leukoreductions on the alloimmunization to platelets and the platelet transfusion refractoriness. Transfus Apher Sci. 2015;52(1):112–21.
99. Georgeades C, Rothstein AE, Plunk MR, Arendonk KV. Iatrogenic vascular trauma and complications of vascular access in children. Semin Pediatr Surg. 2021;30(6):151122.
100. Gibson CM. French catheter scale. In: WikiDoc. 2014. WikiDoc https://www.wikidoc.org/index.php/French_catheter_scale. Accessed 31 July 2023.
101. Gibson MC. Needle gauge comparison chart. WikiDoc. 2012. WikiDoc. https://www.wikidoc.org/index.php/French_catheter_scale. Accessed 31 July 2023.

102. Aziz K, Lee HC, Escobedo MB, Hoover AV, Kamath-Rayne BD, Kapadia VS, et al. Part 5: neonatal resuscitation: 2020 American Heart Association guidelines for cardiopulmonary resuscitation and emergency cardiovascular care. Circulation. 2020;142(16_suppl_2):S524–S50.
103. D'Andrea V, Prontera G, Rubortone SA, Pezza L, Pinna G, Barone G, et al. Umbilical venous catheter update: a narrative review including ultrasound and training. Front Pediatr. 2021;9:774705.
104. Nakamura H, Nakamura R, Paran TS. Vascular access in infants and children. In: Puri P, editor. Pediatric surgery. Cham: Springer; 2020. p. 263–72.
105. Barone G, D'Andrea V, Vento G, Pittiruti M. A systematic ultrasound evaluation of the diameter of deep veins in the newborn: results and implications for clinical practice. Neonatology. 2019;115(4):335–40.
106. Paterson RS, Chopra V, Brown E, Kleidon TM, Cooke M, Rickard CM, et al. Selection and insertion of vascular access devices in pediatrics: a systematic review. Pediatrics. 2020;145(Suppl 3):S243–S68.
107. Charter Medical. Neonatal syringe set. 2023. https://chartermedical.com/syringe-sets/. Accessed 18 July 2024.
108. Utah Medial Products Inc. Hemo-Nate blood filtration system. 2023. http://www.utahmed.com/hemo-nate.html. Accessed 29 July 2023.
109. Shulman AB, Kase YH, Arrigo RT, Hess AS. Coagulated cryoprecipitate in an intravenous line. Anesthesiology. 2022;137(5):602–3.
110. Harabor A, Soraisham A. Rates of intracardiac umbilical venous catheter placement in neonates. J Ultrasound Med. 2014;33(9):1557–61.
111. Wald SH, Mendoza J, Mihm FG, Cote CJ. Procedures for vascular access. In: Cote CJ, Lerman J, Anderson B, editors. A practice of anesthesia for infants and children. 6th ed. New York: Elsevier; 2019. p. 1129–45.
112. Neuhaus D. Intraosseous infusion in elective and emergency pediatric anesthesia: when should we use it? Curr Opin Anaesthesiol. 2014;27(3):282–7.
113. Tobias JD, Ross AK. Intraosseous infusions: a review for the anesthesiologist with a focus on pediatric use. Anesth Analg. 2010;110(2):391–401.
114. Ong MEH, Chan YH, Oh JJ, Ngo AS. An observational, prospective study comparing tibial and humeral intraosseous access using the EZ-IO. Am J Emerg Med. 2009;27(1):8–15.
115. Eyzaguirre Pellon MT, Walsh AM, Willis J, Forbes J, Cone SJ. Inappropriate intravenous infusion set occluded by cryoprecipitate. Transfusion. 2022;62(9):1697–8.
116. Blue Everest Medical. Red Cell Filter. https://bemedical.co.za/store/blood-bank-laboratory-red-cell-filter/. Accessed 31 July 2023.
117. Shiba M, Tadokoro K, Sawanobori M, Nakajima K, Suzuki K, Juji T. Activation of the contact system by filtration of platelet concentrates with a negatively charged white cell-removal filter and measurement of venous blood bradykinin level in patients who received filtered platelets. Transfusion. 1997;37(5):457–62.
118. Gauvin F, Lacroix J, Robillard P, Lapointe H, Hume H. Acute transfusion reactions in the pediatric intensive care unit. Transfusion. 2006;46(11):1899–908.
119. Abe H. Hypotension reactions with a white cell-reduction filter: activation of kallikrein-kinin cascade in a patient. Transfusion. 1998;38:411–2.
120. Waters JH. Intraoperative blood recovery and reinfusion. In: Frank SM, Waters JH, editors. Patient blood management: multidisciplinary approaches to optimizing care. Bethesda: AABB Press; 2016. p. 186.
121. Mohamed A, Shah PS. Transfusion associated necrotizing enterocolitis: a meta-analysis of observational data. Pediatrics. 2012;129(3):529–40.
122. Kopko PM. Transfusion reactions. 5th ed. Bethesda: AABB Press; 2021. p. 41, 83, 90–92, 98, 102–103, 121, 182, 233–249, 380, 408, 428, 457–453, 478, 2512–2513.
123. De Cloedt L, Savy N, Gauvin F, Taylor S, Lacroix J, Emeriaud G. Transfusion-associated circulatory overload in ICUs: a scoping review of incidence, risk factors, and outcomes. Crit Care Med. 2019;47(6):849–56.

Patient Blood Management Through Electronic Health Record [EHR] Optimization

9

Norma J. Klein

You work as your anesthesia department's quality assurance (QA) representative in a busy children's hospital and are assigned to oversee blood ordering workflows in the EHR. The hospital blood bank is asking for your assistance in dealing with numerous improperly made red blood cell (RBC) orders. The hospital has a busy stem cell transplant service that requires special blood treatments, such as RBC irradiation and CMV-negative antibody product. In addition, the administration has become concerned over recent adverse transfusion events, including incorrect patient identification, overtransfusion, and noncompliance with the new transfusion guidelines. Unfortunately, certain members of your department dislike using the EHR because they find it difficult to navigate and irrelevant to their busy workflows. You decide to investigate potential solutions through EHR optimization and PBM principles.

Key Learning Objectives

- What is EHR "optimization"?
- Can the EHR facilitate patient-centered, evidence-based, safe blood management practices for perioperative pediatric patients?
- Does the EHR improve patient outcomes?
- What are limitations of the EHR in advancing perioperative pediatric blood management?

N. J. Klein (✉)
Department of Anesthesiology and Pain Medicine, University of California, Davis, Sacramento, CA, USA
e-mail: nklein@ucdavis.edu

N. J. Klein (ed.), *Perioperative Pediatric Patient Blood Management and Transfusion Safety*, https://doi.org/10.1007/978-3-031-81666-6_9

9.1 Discussion

9.1.1 What Is EHR "Optimization"?

EHR optimization has been defined as, "post-EHR implementation efforts to improve organization performance" [1]. The vast majority of US hospitals have implemented an EHR, including over one-half of pediatric hospitals [2]. In 2009, the United States (US) Congress established the Health Information Technology for Economic and Clinical Health (HITECH) Act, which incentivizes physicians and healthcare institutions that transition to EHRs (and reduces Medicare reimbursement for those who do not) at a cost of approximately 27 billion dollars [3, 4]. There are many potential advantages to implementing an EHR: rapid notification and communication, minimized testing redundancy, clinical guidance for practitioners, reduced resource expenditure, standardization of care, and, as illustrated in some specialties, EHR-related improvements in medication-related patient safety events [2, 5, 6]. When and how these purported advantages translate into reality is a source of continued investigation.

The EHR sets the stage for "big data" mining because it is an electronic database of healthcare data on millions of patients. An audit of the American College of Surgeons National Surgical Quality Improvement Program (ACS NSQIP) public files revealed a 28% decrease in transfusion rates between 2012 and 2018 [7]. From this (big) data, the authors identified successful PBM strategies potentially contributing to this trend: restrictive transfusion thresholds, use of antifibrinolytics, waste reduction, and clinical decision support (CDS). Frank et al. retrospectively examined anesthesia information systems (AIMS) in two separate studies, noting significant variation among physicians in hemoglobin transfusion triggers and a modifiable excess in pretransfusion testing in over 100,000 perioperative patients [8, 9]. Suggested future uses of EHR-derived data to advance PBM include preoperative anemia management, cell salvage use, efficient blood delivery during massive bleeding, quality control, and identification of patient populations at risk for transfusion-associated circulatory overload (TACO) [10–13]. However, unlike traditional scientific inquiry, where a hypothesis is created in advance and patient information is collected in a prospective manner, bag data analysis generates hypotheses from data already in existence [14]. Nevertheless, the sheer volume of data in the EHR—whether collected retrospectively or prospectively—can uncover trends in blood management that serve as benchmarks, inform policy development, and eventually produce enough data necessary to implement artificial intelligence (AI) and machine learning (ML) analytics.

PBM has been defined as a, "patient-centered, systemic, evidence-based approach to improve patient outcomes by managing and preserving a patient's own blood, while promoting patient safety and empowerment" [15]. The following discussion will address the role of EHR-optimization in advancing the various elements of PBM as covered in the pediatric and adult literature.

9.2 Can the EHR Facilitate Patient-Centered, Evidence-Based, Safe Blood Management Practices for Perioperative Pediatric Patients?

9.2.1 Patient-Centered Transfusion Practice

Studies on the outcome effects of patient-centered EHRs have shown conflicting results [16]. The EHR has the potential to support patient-centered blood management through greater transparency in the informed consent process and laboratory results. It also assists blood banks in guiding practitioners to order specialized blood treatments for patients with specific comorbidities.

9.2.2 The Electronic Informed Consent

All blood transfusions should involve a shared decision between the patient and ordering practitioner and should be accompanied by an informed consent process [15, 17, 18]. Paper-based consent forms are fraught with errors, including misplacement and loss, missing signatures, incorrect procedure, and incorrect surgical site [19]. Some patients may refuse a blood transfusion or request modifications based on religious orientation. An EHR-based informed consent for transfusion is being increasingly implemented in US hospitals and has been shown to reduce errors by over 40% [19]. Furthermore, an electronic consent form is immediately available for patient review of the surgery site, provider, and stated exceptions, thus providing improved transparency and a patient-centered focus.

A special challenge for the anesthesiologist is the patient who refuses all transfusions or who accepts some but not all products and procedures. The ASA has created a patient-oriented consent template that can be adapted to the EHR (Fig. 9.1) [20].

An electronically based (versus paper) consent is available to the patient and all practitioners involved in advance of surgery and throughout the perioperative period and is likely to minimize perioperative communication gaps that can occur with complex transfusions requests.

9.2.3 Patient-Specific Order Modifications

At times, a patient's vital signs, baseline laboratory values, or comorbid conditions have direct bearing on the correct type and volume of blood to order. Initial computerized physician order entry (CPOE) development attempts often did not provide enough flexibility in physician orders to properly address a varied patient population, creating an inability to provide relevant guidance for specific patient conditions [21]. CPOE can be optimized, however, to direct special blood treatments for a specific patient's condition. Many physicians are unaware of specialized blood product treatments required in pediatric patients, including the need for weight-based dosing, age-related immunodeficiency cutoffs (i.e., approximately 6 months),

GENERAL CONSENT FOR BLOOD PRODUCTS – Page 1 of 2

PATIENT NAME: ______________________ DATE OF BIRTH: ____/____/_____ MRN: ____________

Please mark whether you Accept or Decline each of the following:

WHOLE BLOOD COMPONENTS (*some people call these Major Fractions*) Blood carries oxygen and nutrients through the body. The 4 main parts (or components) can be separated and used for treatment.	
RED BLOOD CELLS (Other Names: Erythrocytes, RBCs) take oxygen from your lungs to your organs and tissues. They also take carbon dioxide back to your lungs to breathe out. We give RBCs if your blood count is too low.	☐ Accept ☐ Decline
WHITE BLOOD CELLS (Other Names: Leukocytes, WBCs) are one of your body's defenses against bacteria, viruses, and diseases the body produces. We give WBCs to help you fight certain diseases.	☐ Accept ☐ Decline
PLATELETS (Other Name: Thrombocytes) are small pieces of cells. They help your blood make clots that prevent or stop bleeding. We give Platelets if your bleeding is hard to stop or if your Platelet count is very low.	☐ Accept ☐ Decline
PLASMA is the liquid part of blood. It is made of water, albumin, clotting factors, salts, sugars, fats, vitamins, and hormones. We give this if you need more Plasma or Clotting Factors.	☐ Accept ☐ Decline
TYPES OF PLASMA ▸ **Frozen (or thawed) plasma (FFP)** is Plasma removed from whole blood. It is frozen so it can be used later. ▸ **Solvent detergent-treated plasma** is Plasma that is cleaned to reduce the chance of infection or allergic reaction.	
FRACTIONATED BLOOD COMPONENTS are separated from whole blood components (*some people call these Minor Fractions*).	
*–– **Clotting Factors** are proteins in Plasma. They help your blood make clots that stop bleeding. ––*	
CRYOSUPERNATANT is plasma that has most of the solid parts taken out. The leftover liquid is called Cryosupernatant. We give Cryosupernatant to replace plasma.	☐ Accept ☐ Decline
CRYOPRECIPITATE is plasma that has the liquid part taken out. The leftover clotting factors are called Cryoprecipitate. We give Cryoprecipitate to help stop bleeding.	☐ Accept ☐ Decline
PROTHROMBIN COMPLEX CONCENTRATE is a mix of many clotting factors. We give this mix to help stop bleeding or to reverse the effects of blood thinning medicine.	☐ Accept ☐ Decline
CONCENTRATED CLOTTING FACTORS are single clotting factors. We give them to help stop bleeding.	☐ Accept ☐ Decline
ALBUMIN is the main protein in plasma. We give Albumin to increase blood volume.	☐ Accept ☐ Decline
ANTIBODIES (Other Name: Immune Globulins) are proteins your body makes to fight disease. We can also give you Antibodies to help your body fight some types of infections.	☐ Accept ☐ Decline
YOUR OWN BLOOD can be used in the procedures below in a closed system. Your blood is not mixed with any other blood.	
APHERESIS (Other Names: Plasma exchange, Plasmapheresis) is when a closed-system machine replaces bad plasma with a good plasma substitute. It is used if your plasma has antibodies that are attacking your body.	☐ Accept ☐ Decline
AUTO-TRANSFUSION (Other Names: Cell Saver, Cell Salvage, Salvaged Autologous Blood) is when your blood is collected during surgery, washed and filtered, and then given back to you in a closed system.	☐ Accept ☐ Decline
HEMODILUTION is when your blood is replaced with IV fluids during surgery. After surgery, we give your blood back to you in a closed system.	☐ Accept ☐ Decline
HEART AND LUNG MACHINE is when your blood flows into a machine that adds oxygen to it. Your blood then flows back into your body in a closed system primed with non-blood fluid. It is used during some surgeries.	☐ Accept ☐ Decline
DIALYSIS (Other Names: Renal Dialysis, Hemodialysis) is when your blood flows into a machine that filters and cleans it, then flows back into your body in a closed system. It is used if your kidneys are not working well or harmful substances need to be taken out of your blood.	☐ Accept ☐ Decline
EPIDURAL BLOOD PATCH is when your blood is injected around your spinal cord to stop a spinal fluid leak.	☐ Accept ☐ Decline
PLATELET GEL is made of your platelets and white blood cells. We use it to cover wounds and help stop bleeding.	☐ Accept ☐ Decline
RECOMBINANT PRODUCTS are like Whole Blood Components, but they are made with protein technology and do not come from blood.	
RECOMBINANT CLOTTING FACTORS are like the clotting factors that come from Whole Blood Components that are listed above. We give them to help stop bleeding.	☐ Accept ☐ Decline
RECOMBINANT ERYTHROPOIETIN (Other Names: EPO, ESA, Hematopoietin) is like your body's Erythropoietin. It is a hormone that tells bone marrow to make more red blood cells. We give it if your blood count is too low.	☐ Accept ☐ Decline
OTHER TREATMENT (Please Specify):	☐ Accept ☐ Decline

Fig. 9.1 ASA blood transfusion consent and refusal form for patient-specific preferences. Reprinted with permission of the American Society of Anesthesiologists, 1061 American Lane, Schaumburg, Il 60,173–4973

institutional rhesus (Rh) antigen guidelines, or blood bank leukoreduction practices [22–24]. At NYU Langone Health, an order to prepare RBCs explicitly provides tick boxes guiding special blood treatment requirements for certain neonatal conditions (Fig. 9.2) [25]. These conditions may include an immunocompromised state, a hemoglobinopathy, or a very low birthweight, which can predispose to

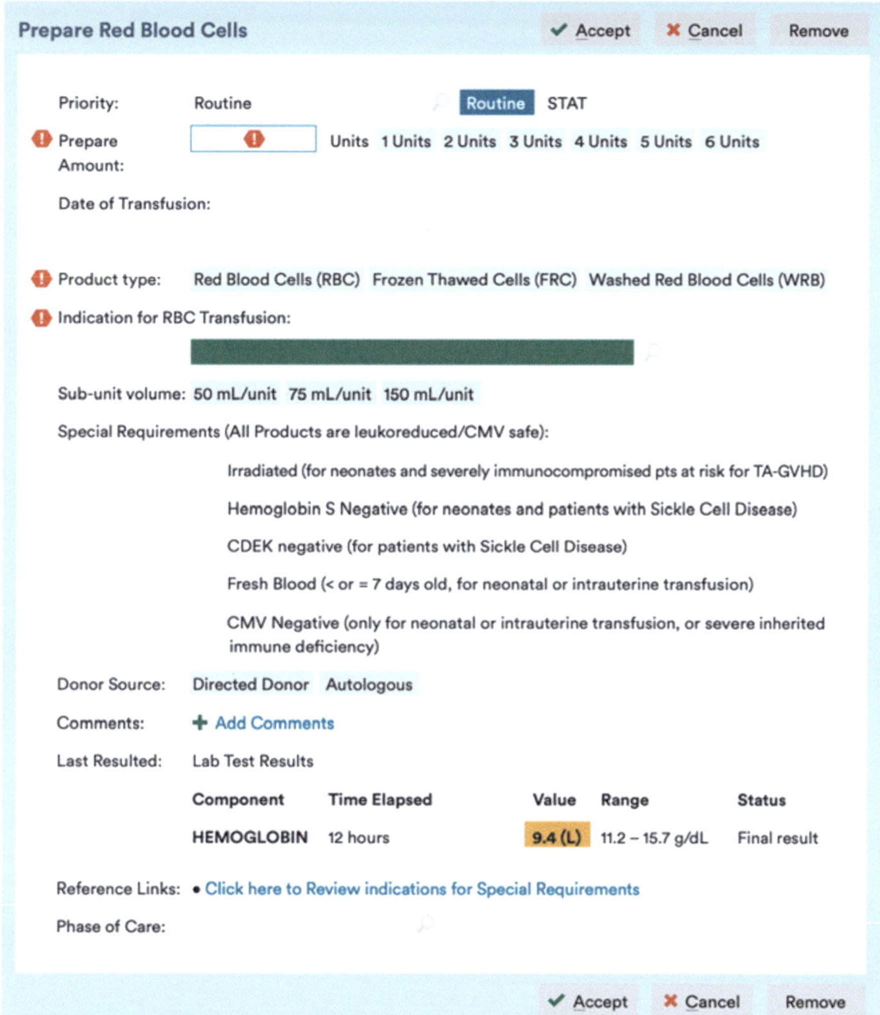

Fig. 9.2 EHR RBC order screen. Reprinted with permission from the Association for the Advancement of Blood Biotherapies (AABB) found in Friedman M. How Do I Use Clinical Decision Support for Patient Blood Management? Oct 2022

transfusion-associated hyperkalemia (TAH) or transfusion-associated circulatory overload (TACO).

Figure 9.3 is another example of an order set with decision support in which the ordering provider is asked whether the patient has a specific condition, thus allowing the blood bank to determine the appropriate special blood treatment [26].

Pediatric CPOE orders sets that explicitly state the patient's weight (with the specific unit of measurement: kilogram versus pounds) and require a weight-based

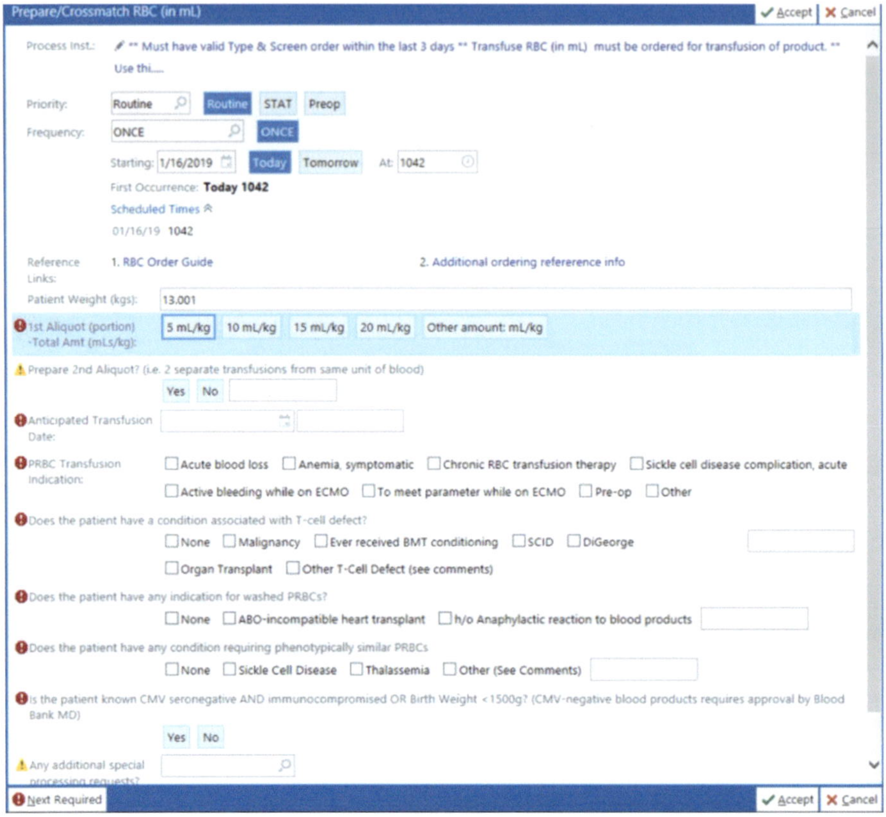
Prepare/Crossmatch RBC (in mL) ✔ Accept ✖ Cancel

Process Inst.: ** Must have valid Type & Screen order within the last 3 days ** Transfuse RBC (in mL) must be ordered for transfusion of product. ** Use thi....

Priority: Routine | Routine | STAT | Preop

Frequency: ONCE | ONCE

Starting: 1/16/2019 | Today | Tomorrow | At: 1042

First Occurrence: Today 1042

Scheduled Times

01/16/19 1042

Reference Links: 1. RBC Order Guide 2. Additional ordering refererence info

Patient Weight (kgs): 13.001

1st Aliquot (portion) -Total Amt (mLs/kg): 5 mL/kg | 10 mL/kg | 15 mL/kg | 20 mL/kg | Other amount: mL/kg

Prepare 2nd Aliquot? (i.e. 2 separate transfusions from same unit of blood) Yes | No

Anticipated Transfusion Date:

PRBC Transfusion Indication: Acute blood loss | Anemia, symptomatic | Chronic RBC transfusion therapy | Sickle cell disease complication, acute | Active bleeding while on ECMO | To meet parameter while on ECMO | Pre-op | Other

Does the patient have a condition associated with T-cell defect? None | Malignancy | Ever received BMT conditioning | SCID | DiGeorge | Organ Transplant | Other T-Cell Defect (see comments)

Does the patient have any indication for washed PRBCs? None | ABO-incompatible heart transplant | h/o Anaphylactic reaction to blood products

Does the patient have any condition requiring phenotypically similar PRBCs None | Sickle Cell Disease | Thalassemia | Other (See Comments)

Is the patient known CMV seronegative AND immunocompromised OR Birth Weight < 1500g? (CMV-negative blood products requires approval by Blood Bank MD) Yes | No

Any additional special processing requests?

Next Required ✔ Accept ✖ Cancel

Fig. 9.3 EHR order with decision support requesting the blood bank to prepare blood for patients with specific transfusion requirements. Reprinted with permission from the AABB as found in Orenstein EW, Rollins M, Jones J, Kandaswamy S, Boudreaux J, Carter AB, et al. Influence of user-centered clinical decision support on pediatric blood product ordering errors. 2022. Blood Transfus

volume order (e.g., mL/kg) add further personalization and a significant measure of safety for small patients at risk of volume overload [22].

Following enactment of the 21st Century Cures Act in the US, patients now have electronic access to personal health information that was inaccessible to them in the past [27]. Less than 60% of US residents are aware of their own blood type [28]. Knowing one's blood type may have positive impact on several patient choices, including a decision to donate in the case of a rare blood antigen or emergency blood requirements. It may also guide pregnancy decisions in the case of rhesus D-antigen status and the need for rhesus immunoglobulin (RhIG) therapy to prevent hemolytic disease of the fetus and newborn (HDFN). Self-knowledge of a history of an adverse transfusion reaction (ATR) may also empower a patient about future transfusion decisions since ATRs may recur in individuals.

9.2.4 Evidence-Based Transfusion Practice as Supported Through the EHR

Blood transfusions are one of the most common and overly prescribed procedures in the USA [29, 30]. As a result, the American Board of Internal Medicine (ABIM) and the Association for the Advancement of Blood and Biotherapies (AABB) have identified transfusion as a target for utilization reduction using a variety of patient blood management strategies, including modification of practitioner behavior through computerized order sets. There is now ample evidence based on randomized controlled trials of RBC transfusion triggers in the adult patient literature that "less is more": hemodynamically stable patients may fare better or no worse when managed with restricted RBC transfusion protocols [29]. However, because of the complexities encountered in clinical practice and the dynamic nature of medical judgment, practitioners may be slow or even resistant to incorporate practice guidelines into the multitude of decisions required on a daily basis. Over 15 professional societies have established guidelines for adult RBC transfusions [25]. There are fewer recommendations for transfusion triggers in the pediatric literature, partly due to less available data [31]. Furthermore, local institutional guidelines may vary depending on the patient population served, whether it be trauma patients, a general hospital, or a center serving patients with chronic anemia.

Clinical decision support functions embedded into the EHR are now widely adopted under the belief that CDS is an effective and efficient tool to improve compliance with evidence-based guidelines. CDS is defined as, "any software designed to directly aid in clinical decision-making in which characteristics of individual patients are matched to a computerized knowledge base for the purpose of generating patient-specific assessments or recommendations that are then presented to clinicians for consideration" [32]. CDS has been formatted into physician orders as order "sets," laboratory results, guideline links, evidence-based literature links, and descriptions of noncompliant orders. Unfortunately, existing CDS studies tend to exclude intraoperative and emergency blood orders that are most relevant to anesthesiologists and other intensive care practitioners [7]. A recent simulation trial comparing an electronic, user-oriented CDS tool for massive transfusion protocol (MTP) implementation to a paper-based MTP found a significantly higher rate of correct decisions per hour (8.5 versus 6.9; 95% CI 0.6–2.6) in the electronic CDS group [33]. The simulation analyzed the decisions of 35 acute care specialists over 20 minutes, including patient assessment, MTP activation, RBC administration, and calcium administration. Participants rated the CDS tool's usability as excellent.

In a systematic review, Hibbs et al. identified 20 studies published between 2000 and 2014 that examined the impact of CDS on transfusion ordering practices. Although decision support systems had an overall positive effect on RBC ordering practices, the impact of guideline-compliant plasma, platelet, and cryoprecipitate orders was weak, most likely related to an insufficient number of studies [34]. Hibbs found three pediatric studies addressing CPOE-embedded CDS tools for RBC transfusions in the newborn intensive care unit (NICU) and pediatric ICU and one addressing an exchange transfusion protocol in sickle cell patients. Guideline compliance for RBC orders increased from 65% to 90% in a multicenter NICU study after embedding a CDS tool that required an explanation for ordering blood products outside of guidelines [35]. In another study, there was a decrease in the RBC transfusion rate in a single center PICU following implementation of an interruptive alert (when an order was outside guidelines), which was interpreted as evidence that the CDS was effective in increasing guideline adherence [36]. In another single center NICU study, orders for plasma and platelets were accompanied by the patient's most recent prothrombin time (PT) and partial thromboplastin time (PTT) and then audited when outside guidelines; whereas inappropriate plasma orders decreased, inappropriate platelet orders continued [37]. Although real-time CDS alerts have been shown to reduce inappropriate plasma and cryoprecipitate orders in adult patients, there are no studies examining a CDS effect on cryoprecipitate orders in pediatrics at this point in time [38].

It is unclear what types of CDS are most successful in modifying practitioner blood ordering practices and whether observed improvements in ordering practices are the result of CDS, educational efforts, or something else [39]. Existing studies addressing the issue are usually surveys or single center reports about what has worked. Ideally, the CDS is supported by the most recent and highest level of evidence. However, some CPOEs include order sets that are based on bundles or enhanced recovery after surgery (ERAS) protocols that may reflect local practices or expert consensus at best. Although CPOE-based CDS has been shown to improve guideline adherence in a number of specialties, including cardiovascular surgery, intensive care, and pediatrics, the effectiveness of CDS to guide evidence-based transfusion ordering practices remains unclear [39, 40]. Table 9.1 lists various CDS approaches that have been reported to be successful in advancing evidence-based blood ordering practices.

9.2.5 Promoting Transfusion Patient Safety through the EHR

The EHR is thought to facilitate continuity of patient care, improved access to medical history, and increase the speed of information access. However, there is little to no structural oversight of potential risks to patient safety once the EHR is integrated into the clinical environment [48]. As the EHR has taken over prescribing and other practices, current information about patient safety events comes largely from retrospective or observational data analysis. Because severe adverse outcomes associated with blood transfusions are rare, even AI that is grounded in big data has yet to inform actionable best transfusion safety practices. Specific blood management safety topics that have been addressed through EHR optimization studies include patient verification, patient handovers, and the diagnosis and management of adverse transfusion reactions. The following sections address patient handovers and the management of adverse transfusion reactions using the EHR; patient verification and the EHR is discussed in more detail in the chapter entitled "Patient Verification."

Table 9.1 EHR optimization through various CDS tools for blood transfusions found in the adult and pediatric literature. Most data are based on before-and-after observations

Investigator/year	EHR intervention	Reported results
Petaja/2004 [37]	Most recent coagulation laboratory value accompanying plasma orders, with required explanation of basis for order	Significant improvement (7.8% to 0.9%) in plasma orders outside guidelines but not seen with platelet orders.
Adams/2011 [36]	Hemodynamic parameters plus recent hemoglobin (Hgb) value creates a best practice alert (BPA) and a link to current literature; no hard stop	Decrease in RBC units transfused per PICU patient-day and the Hgb transfusion trigger
Baer/2011 [35]	NICU orders that are noncompliant with suggested guidelines for all blood products requires an explanation	Guideline compliance increased 65–90% for all blood products and decrease in RBC transfusions per patient
Cohn/2014 [41]	Blood bank audit of orders outside recommended guidelines; medical director report to noncompliant clinicians and positive feedback to compliant clinicians	Appropriate RBC orders increased 70–95%
McCrory/2014 [42]	CPOE based on established protocol for infrequently performed manual exchange transfusion in sickle cell patients; education	Protocol violations decreased from $n = 20$ to $n = 3$
Goodnough/2015 [39]	Order outside suggested RBC trigger threshold creates BPA and link to supporting literature; no hard stop	Overall RBC transfusions reduced 24%
Harb/2019 [43]	BPA triggered by phlebotomy orders that are duplicate or irrelevant; clinician required to contact blood bank; hard stop; education; dashboard	"Modest" decrease in patient phlebotomy rate
Goodnough/2019 [29]	BPA and audit if Hgb transfusion trigger is outside guideline threshold or for multiunit RBC orders; link to guidelines; no hard stop	42% decrease in RBC units per number of patient-days (follow up on 2015 study)
Ikoma/2021 [44]	"Dynamic" vs "interruptive" BPA; pre-implementation education; explicit guidelines	RBC guideline compliance increased 43.6–54.2%; multiunit orders decreased 8.6%
Metcalf/2021 [45]	CPOE appearance: Default option for multiunit RBC order changed from "keep" to "remove"	35% improvement in acceptance of single RBC unit order option
Friedman/2022 [25]	CPOE with patient's most recent Hgb and coagulation studies, along with dropdown indicating special treatment needed; audit letters sent to clinician if order outside guidelines	25% decrease in RBC transfusion rate
Murphy/2022 [46]	BPA for platelet orders outside guidelines; randomized alert with controls; clinician interviews post-BPA	Reduction in total platelets transfused but not per patient-day; 92% of alerts overridden
Adkins/2023 [47]	Interruptive BPA if RBC transfusion outside guidelines, with reference link and most recent Hgb; required acknowledgement and explanation if BPA bypassed	14.5% reduction in RBC transfusion within 24 h; $51,000 cost savings annually

9.2.6 Computerized Patient Handovers

A handover has been defined as "the transfer of information and professional responsibility and accountability between individuals and teams" [49]. In the perioperative setting, the handover is often a casual, verbal relay of information [50]. Closed loop communication is a hallmark of safe patient handoffs but is not always possible when there are multiple personnel changes. Anesthesiologists perform numerous handovers throughout a workday, at shift change, during a break, or when transferring a patient from the intraoperative phase of care to a postoperative location. However, there is recent evidence that although a second-look or a "copilot" may facilitate care, handovers are associated with worse patient outcomes [51–57]. Failure in communication was determined to be the root cause of one-quarter of the most frequently identified healthcare-related sentinel events reported to The Joint Commission (TJC) in 2015 [58]. The Joint Commission estimates that only 2% of sentinel events are reported annually. A 2018 handover "toolkit" from the Royal College of Physicians and Surgeons of Canada estimated that of 7.5% adverse events in hospitalized patients, 37% were preventable [59]. The Joint Commission made communication a national patient safety goal (NPSG) in its 2009 objectives; the 2022 NPSG's include two additional categories that are analogous to the safe handover of transfusion-related patient care: NPSG.02.03.01 (timely relay of correct test information to the correct provider) and NPSG.03.06.01 (correct relay and documentation of patient's medication information) [60].

From sample collection to bedside administration, the blood transfusion process presents many openings for failed handover communication. Blood ordered inside the operating room may involve more than 20 steps between the blood bank and the intraoperative transfusionist [61]. Oftentimes, there is no handover report about an ongoing or pending transfusion [50, 51, 62]. In an early landmark report of critical events related to failed intraoperative handovers, Cooper et al. reported eight cases of hypovolemia and one case of wrong component transfused (WCT) due to not checking the patient's name [52]. In the SHOT (Serious Hazards of Transfusion) 2021 annual report, there were 13 errors associated with verbal handovers (versus written or electronic handover reports), including four unnecessary transfusions, five transfusions based on incorrect laboratory results, and four based on an outdated treatment plan [63]. In the case of pediatric patients, an incomplete handover report in the laboratory or at bedside can lead to overtransfusion, hypervolemia, or dyspnea. The most recent SHOT report described a death due to a failure to call for a life-saving transfusion in a premature infant with a hemoglobin of 5 g/dL, and three cases of pediatric TACO [64].

An electronic handover report is a centralized and readily accessible source of documentation that is increasingly favored as a technology that can improve communication safety [65–68]. The ideal handover process is to be determined. However, experts generally agree that it should be structured (or standardized), tailored to accommodate the particular workflow, developed with direct provider input and feedback, and performed in a face-to-face manner [49, 53, 65, 69]. Most sources of miscommunication (or no communication) in the perioperative environment—such as distraction, lack of documentation, knowledge deficits, patient comorbidities, and lack of contingency planning—may be obviated with an electronic, structured format that can serve as a resource for relieving anesthesiologists and practitioners in other departments. Despite the complexity of patient information that may be included in a perioperative handover, a few transfusion-related details may be key to preventing a single sentinel event. Based on a 2012 systematic review of postoperative handovers, Segall et al. pinpointed fluid volumes and blood products administered, estimated blood loss, and bleeding issues as important handover subject matter [49]. These transfusion specifics are particularly relevant in blood loss cases. As part of a quality improvement project, a retrospective review of intraoperative anesthesia handovers lasting more than one-half hour (n = 48,986) found improved mortality and major morbidity rates when a structured handoff, embedded in the EHR, was utilized (6.2% versus 7.2%; OR 1.08, 95% CI, 1.04–1.12) [70]. Among other details, the handover function in this study contained blood related information including patient ABO type, product availability, estimated blood loss, and blood administered. Relaying such information may not only prevent avoidable exsanguination but a fatal hemolytic transfusion event.

9.2.7 Adverse Transfusion Reactions (ATRs) Diagnosis and Reporting

Adverse transfusion reactions are relatively rare but occur more frequently in children compared to adults [71–73]. Reaction rates reported in the literature vary significantly but range from 0.34% to 1.3%, with serious and life-threatening events occurring in 16 per 100,000 transfusions [74, 75]. The precise rate is unclear due to a number of factors, including passive versus active reporting, practitioner knowledge, and the degree of bedside monitoring. In the US, only fatal transfusion reactions must be reported, whereas the United Kingdom (UK) has a robust hemovigilance database partly attributable to a mandatory reporting requirements [76]. SHOT reports a transfusion-related fatality rate of 0.92 per 100,000 transfusions; the US FDA in contrast advises that the absolute number of reported fatalities (29 in year 2020) be interpreted with caution due to the inherent bias in voluntary reporting systems [77]. Transfusion reactions are significantly underreported in most hemovigilance registries [48, 74, 75, 78]. Thus, the stage is set for underdiagnosis, delayed or inappropriate management, and a failure to identify patients at high risk for an ATR or a transfusion-related untoward event.

The EHR, when properly integrated with blood bank software, the anesthesia information system (AIMS), and real-time remote patient monitoring, offers an algorithmic solution to improved diagnosis, management, and reporting of transfusion reactions [79, 80]. Successful event surveillance using the EHR has been achieved in other specialties, including early detection of hypotension during surgery, ventilator-induced lung injury, anticoagulation medication warning prior to neuraxial analgesia, and pediatric sepsis [81–86]. Villamin et al. reported a 524%

increase in transfusion reaction reporting and diagnosis following implementation of a structured, digitally-based system that monitors patient vital signs in real time from multiple medical campuses [75]. A centralized dashboard is monitored around-the-clock by trained nurses who can review a patient's medical records and risk factors and then directly contact the transfusionist. In addition, an event can be reviewed by a trained practitioner who determines further action to be taken. Another electronic notification system that relays vital signs changes before, during, and following transfusion was associated a significant increase in both detection and reporting, although vital signs alone made detection possible in only one-half cases [79]. Transfusion reactions may involve not only vital sign changes but subjective symptoms (e.g., itching and dyspnea) and objective signs (e.g., rash, flushing) that cannot be detected through remote wireless monitors. However, unstructured data associated with an ATR may be incorporated into algorithms followed by ongoing optimization through machine learning [21, 74, 87, 88]. Examples include plain language (e.g., nurse documentation of flushing or back pain), pharmacy records indicating antihistamine or diuretic administration, or laboratory orders (e.g., chest x-rays or blood gas results) made at the time of transfusion. Diagnosis codes have been used to identify transfusion reactions but often do not match the diagnosis made by the transfusion specialist in the blood bank and typically come too late to prevent or manage an acute reaction [89, 90]. Furthermore, there is not an ICD (International Classification of Diseases) code 9 or 10 for several types of transfusion reactions, including hypotensive and mild allergic reactions [89]. Often, clinicians do not report transfusion reactions to the blood bank. This may be due to limited knowledge about transfusion reactions, improper classification, or lack of understanding that reporting transfusion reactions to the blood bank is crucial to possible blood sequestration and process improvement [79].

As EHR and hemovigilance technology improves, practitioner education at all levels should include the basics of transfusion therapy. In a recent survey of 423 anesthesiology residents in 37 US training programs, less than one-quarter correctly answered a keyword-based question on the diagnosis and management of ATRs [91]. The ability to recognize, manage, and report transfusion reactions is critical to patient safety. The EHR can compensate for educational gaps because it is suited to data mining, algorithms, and CPOE development. Optimal impact requires education efforts focused on bedside nurses and anesthesiology practitioners who are at the front lines of perioperative blood administration.

9.3 Does the EHR Improve Patient Outcomes?

9.3.1 EHR-Related Patient Outcomes, Costs, and IT-Related Errors

Despite the perceived or documented advantages of an EHR, there is little validation about how best to optimize EHR functionalities to improve patient outcomes [29, 48]. Single studies have found EHR-related improvements in blood waste, utilization, laboratory testing and orders, compliance with evidence-based guidelines, and patient identification [92]. However, meta-analyses and systematic reviews over the past decade (since HITECH incentivization) have not established a definite association between EHR implementations and improved patient morbidity and mortality rates [16, 25, 29, 74]. Most studies examining the effect of the EHR on patient outcomes are underpowered, of short duration, lack controls, or vary in the functionality studied [34]. Although the US Food and Drug Administration (FDA) provides regulatory oversight of blood bank IT systems, the agency does not oversee EHR implementation [48]. Many hospital administrations, in response to HITECH regulation, have implemented EHRs in a "big bang" approach with limited practitioner input or outcome data [1, 93]. It is estimated that one-half of EHR projects fail at implementation [94]. The failure is often blamed on the bedside practitioner, with mandatory further education programs and design changes mounting into a pyre of dissatisfaction. Recognizing the inherent weakness created by a lack of structural guidance, the Australian and New Zealand Society of Blood Transfusion (ANZSBT) has proposed a detailed draft outlining guidelines for EHR implementation [48]. Many of the most common EHR functions employed to improve healthcare outcomes are aimed at modifying practitioner behavior. These functions include CPOE, CDS, guideline suggestions, and decision-making audits [6]. Practitioner acceptance has been slow and inconsistent, attributed to a variety of limitations including poor workflow integration, mistrust in guideline quality, loss of practice autonomy, lack of patient-specific relevance, intrusiveness, alert fatigue, and inadequate IT support [2, 25, 95].

Moja et al. performed a meta-analysis on 28 randomized controlled trials examining evidence-based CDS tools and found little effect on cost, morbidity, or mortality [3]. Later reviews suggest that little progress has been made in definitively clarifying the power of CDS tools [16, 96]. With a recognition that successful EHR optimization may be complicated by the dynamic behavior of both patients and practitioners who are required to make complex decisions, a 2018 systematic review factored in the role of specific disease entities and, again, found that although most studies (70%) reported a positive effect, there was no apparent improvement in clinical impact [97]. The authors of this review identified blood management as one of six disease categories "promising" for effective CDS implementation because it has potential to decrease the rate of serious adverse events.

An important goal of every hospital administration is reduction of costs through increased efficiency. However, there is limited transparency about what hospitals pay for initial EHR adoption and maintenance. The costs of optimization may be significant when one considers the expense of new software and upgrades, personnel training, and technological back-peddling when systems fail [1, 98–100]. One investigation into a popular EHR described it as lacking "straightforward pricing plans" [99]. Software charges for this EHR included an average of $500,000 USD for clinic and hospital startup, $2000 USD for training, and monthly maintenance fees as high as $35,000 USD, and these costs may be unaffordable to small practices. Cost savings reported in the literature range from $36,000 to over $1 million USD secondary to EHR data mining or successful optimization [35, 36, 43, 44, 46,

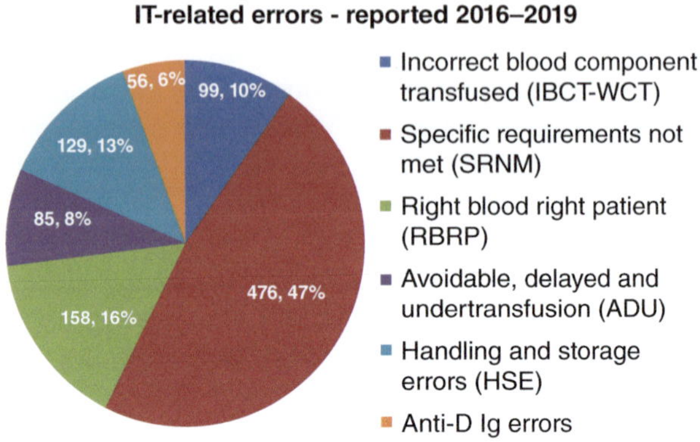

Fig. 9.4 A breakdown of 1003 IT-related errors reported between 2016–2019 as reported to the SHOT registry. Reprinted with permission from SHOT, found online at https://www.shotuk.org/resources/current-resources/shot-bites/. (SHOT data is updated regularly; refer to https://www.shotuk.org/ for up-to-date content)

101–103]. A 2006 literature review examining the relative benefits and costs of health information technology (IT) estimated that the institutional benefits should eventually compensate for EHR investment costs over a 3 to 13 year period [98].

Between 2016 and 2019, the SHOT registry received 1003 IT-related error reports [104]. Thirty-six errors involved incorrect sample request forms, leading to blood issued with an incorrect patient identification in those cases [104]. In a 2021 SHOT report, there were 399 IT-related error reports, including wrong-component-transfused ($n = 41$), administration delays, overtransfusion, and unmet special treatment requirements ($n = 116$) [105]. This report emphasized an urgent need for improved staff and IT expert training (with a focus on transfusion-related knowledge), as well as collaboration between interfacing departments. Fig. 9.4 illustrates a general breakdown of IT-related errors as reported to SHOT [104].

9.4 What are the Limitations of the EHR in Advancing Perioperative Pediatric Blood Management?

Improper integration of an intraoperative blood transfusion system with an EHR can reflect a variety of operational weaknesses, including the following [6, 48, 74, 104]:

- Functions that are irrelevant or do not follow transfusionist workflow.
- Absence of a direct or real-time link between the blood bank and the anesthesia information system.
- Functions that produce extra work (including extra "clicks") for the end-user.
- Implementation of EHR functions before end-user education.
- Failure to regularly update guidelines that direct clinical decision support.
- Different software vendors in different departments with different workflow priorities.
- Hospital consolidations creating the potential for decreased interoperability and increased system complexity.
- Absence of a universal healthcare system resulting in delayed development of standardized guidelines for alerts and interoperability.

Successful EHR optimization includes proactive end-user education and what is called "usability testing," or real-time observation of how end-users interact with a system. When comparing a computerized order entry system based on real-time provider feedback to an original order set initiated by committee, Orenstein et al. found that the user-centered order set was associated with a 30% increase in error-free task completion [26]. Another important safety concern in the physical appearance of an order set, which can impact the ability of providers to order the correct blood product. As an example, 30% (116/399) of IT-related errors reported to SHOT in 2021 included "special requirements not met" [76]. Unfortunately, few physicians, particularly trainees, understand which patients should receive irradiated, CMV-antibody negative, or fresh RBCs, particularly in the context of a harried OR environment [91, 106]. Figures 9.2 and 9.3 illustrate computerized orders to prepare RBCs that reduce the likelihood of special-requirement-related errors because they provide explicit, real-time decision support about the patient's condition [25, 26].

There remains much room for EHR-related outcomes research [107]. As the EHR is not going away anytime soon—considering current financial incentives and regulatory constraints—data collection regarding hospital and practitioner EHR experience, along with newly identified associations uncovered through AI networks, will be fundamental to answering the question of EHR effectiveness [21].

9.5 Summary of Key Learning Objectives

9.5.1 What Is EHR "Optimization"?

EHR optimization has been defined as "post-EHR implementation efforts to improve organization performance." The EHR startup is process is expensive and often fraught with operational inexperience leading to user dissatisfaction and unintended consequences. EHR optimization is necessary for electronic medical record sustainability, regulatory compliance, and practitioner buy-in.

9.5.2 Can the EHR Facilitate Patient-Centered, Evidence-Based, and Safe Blood Management Practices for Pediatric Patients in the Perioperative Period?

The EHR has significant potential to facilitate PBM metrics for both adult and pediatric patients. Because medical record transparency is a priority of the US 21st Century Cures Act, personalized and electronically based consents for blood transfusion are accessible to patients and practitioners alike when faced with complex blood management plans. Orders for RBC preparation may be designed so that patients with specialized blood requirements receive the correct blood product. Women may find out for the first time that they are rhesus (Rh) antigen negative, thereby informing future childbearing decisions.

The EHR can facilitate evidence-based PBM practices through CPOE and CDS that are based on regularly updated best practice guidelines, are in sync with practitioners' real workflows, and are optimized through regular end-user usability testing. Although a number of CDS "tools" have been integrated into CPOEs, it remains to be seen what are the best patient-centered CDS interventions to promote evidence-based PBM practices.

There is a paucity of literature addressing how to preserve patients' blood supply through EHR optimization. Using big data in the ACS NSQIP registry, a 28% decrease in transfusion rates between 2012 and 2018 was attributed to PBM strategies, including restrictive transfusion thresholds, use of antifibrinolytics, waste reduction, and CDS. Through AI, future big data mining from the EHR may yield information on successful practices likely to minimize blood loss and preserve pediatric patients' circulating blood volume.

The EHR has shown potential to advance safe transfusion practices through electronic patient identification, wristband and specimen bar code labeling, and computer-based, standardized handover reports. When properly integrated with blood bank software, AIMS, and real-time remote patient monitoring, the EHR can support algorithmic solutions to improved diagnosis, management, and reporting of transfusion reactions. Active surveillance programs using the EHR have been associated with improved patient safety in several specialties.

9.5.3 Does the EHR Improve Patient Outcomes?

Meta-analyses and systematic reviews over the past decade have failed to establish a direct association between EHR implementations and improved patient morbidity and mortality rates. Most studies examining the effect of the EHR on patient outcomes are underpowered, of short duration, lack controls, or vary in the functionality studied. There is a significant need for EHR- and IT-related outcomes research in blood management, particularly perioperative PBM.

9.5.4 What Are Limitations of the EHR in Advancing Perioperative Pediatric Blood Management?

There are few studies examining the relationship between perioperative pediatric PBM and the EHR. A 2015 review found three pediatric studies addressing blood utilization and guideline compliance, each one retrospective in design. At the current time, there are no studies examining the role of EHR in blood management for children undergoing surgery. Limitations in an institution's approach to both the EHR and adult perioperative PBM affect children as well. These limitations include implementation of an EHR function prior to end-user education, electronic processes that are viewed by practitioners as irrelevant or burdensome, and multiple types of software programs within and across hospital systems. At the present time, absent further prospective research, hemovigilance IT-related events as reported to the hospital blood bank or large registries (such as SHOT), are the best available tools to advance safe perioperative pediatric PBM.

Key Points

- EHR optimization is the process of improving EHR's contribution to organizational performance after initial implementation.
- The EHR may provide patient-centered care through electronic blood consents by specifying alternatives to blood management and CPOE that directs specific blood product requirements.
- The EHR can prevent pediatric transfusion associated circulatory overload (TACO) through standardized electronic orders sets that state the patient's weight in explicit units of measurement (e.g., kilogram versus pounds) and orders that require a weight-based volume order (e.g., mL/kg). The EHR can also support patient safety through electronic patient verification, patient handovers, and the diagnosis and management of adverse transfusion reactions.
- The EHR may improve compliance with evidence-based guidelines through CDS functions, but guidelines must be regularly updated.
- Successful EHR optimization includes proactive end-user education and "usability testing" or real-time observation of how end-users interact with a system.

References

1. Hagland M. What does EMR optimization actually mean? So much more than just working out the kinks. Healthcare Innovation. 2016. https://www.hcinnovationgroup.com/policy-value-based-care/blog/13025919/what-does-emr-optimization-actually-mean-so-much-more-than-just-working-out-the-kinks. Accessed 4 Dec 2022.
2. Wang E, Brenn BR, Matava CT. State of the art in clinical decision support applications in pediatric perioperative medicine. Curr Opin Anaesthesiol. 2020;33(3):388–94.
3. Moja L, Kwag KH, Lytras T, Bertizzolo L, Brandt L, Pecoraro V, et al. Effectiveness of computerized decision support systems linked to electronic health records: a systematic review and meta-analysis. Am J Public Health. 2014;104(12):e12–22.
4. Lite S, Gordon WJ, Stern AD. Association of the Meaningful use Electronic Health Record Incentive Program with Health Information Technology Venture Capital Funding. JAMA Netw Open. 2020;3(3):e201402.
5. Callum J, Etchells E, Shojania K. Addressing the identity crisis in healthcare: positive patient identification technology reduces wrong patient events. Transfusion. 2019;59(3):899–902.
6. Williams CN, Bratton SL, Hirshberg EL. Computerized decision support in adult and pediatric critical care. World J Crit Care Med. 2013;2(4):21–8.
7. Hamilton CM, Davenport DL, Bernard AC. Demonstration of a U.S. nationwide reduction in transfusion in general surgery and a review of published transfusion reduction methodologies. Transfusion. 2021;61(11):3119–28.
8. Frank SM, Savage WJ, Rothschild JA, Rivers RJ, Ness PM, Paul SL, et al. Variability in blood and blood component utilization as assessed by an anesthesia information management system. Anesthesiology. 2012;117(1):99–106.
9. Frank SM, Rothschild JA, Masear CG, Rivers RJ, Merritt WT, Savage WJ, et al. Optimizing preoperative blood ordering with data acquired from an anesthesia information management system. Anesthesiology. 2013;118(6):1286–97.
10. Pendry K. The use of big data in transfusion medicine. Transfus Med. 2015;25(3):129–37.
11. Bright RA, Bright-Ponte SJ, Palmer LAM, Rankin SK, Blok SV. Use of diagnosis codes to find blood transfusion adverse events in electronic health records. J Patient Saf. 2022;18(5):e823–e66.

12. Song WJ, Kim HJ, Kang SG, Seo BF, Choi NK, Lee JH. Big data analysis of the risk factors and rates of perioperative transfusion in immediate autologous breast reconstruction. Sci Rep. 2022;12(1):5314.
13. Lopes MGM, Recktenwald SM, Simionato G, Eichler H, Wagner C, Quint S, et al. Big data in transfusion medicine and artificial intelligence analysis for red blood cell quality control. Transfus Med Hemother. 2023;50(3):163–73.
14. Ning S, Li N, Barty R, Arnold D, Heddle NM. Database-driven research and big data analytic approaches in transfusion medicine. Transfusion. 2022;62(7):1427–34.
15. Shander A, Hardy JF, Ozawa S, Farmer SL, Hofmann A, Frank SM, et al. A global definition of patient blood management. Anesth Analg. 2022;135(3):476–88.
16. Brands MR, Gouw SC, Beestrum M, Cronin RM, Fijnvandraat K, Badawy SM. Patient-centered digital health records and their effects on health outcomes: systematic Review. J Med Internet Res. 2022;24(12):e43086.
17. Domen RE, Smith ML. Ethical aspects of informed consent. In: Domen RE, editor. Ethical issues in transfusion and cellular therapies. Bethesda, MD: AABB; 2015. p. 15–26.
18. The Joint Commission (TJC). Certification Through the Joint Commission and AABB. 2023. https://www.amsect.org/Certification/PBMT-Exam. Accessed 4 June 2023.
19. Chan LJ. Electronic consent forms on ancillary applications with electronic medical record integration: reducing consent error rates. Digital UCD 2022. https://doi.org/10.22371/07.2022.003. Accessed 4 Dec 2022.
20. Jorgensen TD, Golbaba B, Guinn N, Smith CE. When blood is not an option: the case for a standardized blood transfusion consent form. ASA Monitor. 2017;81:48. https://pubs.asahq.org/monitor/issue/81/6. Accessed 4 Dec 2022.
21. Meier JM, Tschoellitsch T. Artificial intelligence and machine learning in patient blood management: a scoping Review. Anesth Analg. 2022;135(3):524–31.
22. SHOT Bite No. 4: Lessons in Paediatrics (including neonates). Serious Hazards of Transfusion (SHOT). 2018. https://www.shotuk.org/resources/current-resources/shot-bites/. Accessed 4 Dec 2022.
23. Halford B, Pinheiro A, Haspel RL. Hospital medicine Providers' transfusion knowledge: a survey study. Transfus Med Rev. 2021;35(2):140–5.
24. Elliot J, Narayan S, Poles D, Tuckley V, Bolton-Maggs PHB. Missed irradiation of cellular blood components for vulnerable patients: insights from 10 years of SHOT data. Transfusion. 2021;61(2):385–92.
25. Friedman M. How do i Use clinical decision support for patient blood management? Association for the Advancement of Blood & Biotherapies (AABB); 2022. https://www.aabb.org/docs/default-source/default-document-library/resources/how-do-i-use-clinical-decision-support.pdf?sfvrsn=a9315ba1_0. Accessed 4 Dec 2022.
26. Orenstein EW, Rollins M, Jones J, Kandaswamy S, Boudreaux J, Carter AB, et al. Influence of user-centered clinical decision support on pediatric blood product ordering errors. Blood Transfus. 2022;21:1.
27. 21st Century Cures Act. FDA US Food & Drug Administration. Congressgov 2020. https://www.fda.gov/regulatory-information/selected-amendments-fdc-act/21st-century-cures-act. Accessed 4 Dec 2022.
28. Marples M. Many people don't know their blood type. Here's how to find out yours. CNN Health. 2023. Cable News Network. https://www.cnn.com/2020/07/18/health/how-to-find-blood-type-wellness/index.html. Accessed 7 Sept 2023.
29. Goodnough LT, Hollenhorst MA. Clinical decision support and improved blood use in patient blood management. Hematology Am Soc Hematol Educ Program. 2019;2019(1):577–82.
30. Society for the Advancement of blood management (SABM). Transfusion Overuse. 2019. https://www.sabm.org/wp-content/uploads/SABM-Transfusion-Overuse-2019.pdf. Accessed 28 Aug 2023.
31. Downey LA, Goobie SM. Perioperative pediatric erythrocyte transfusions: incorporating hemoglobin thresholds and physiologic parameters in decision-making. Anesthesiology. 2022;137(5):604–19.

32. Fisher SA, Docherty AB, Doree C, Hibbs SP, Murphy MF, Estcourt LJ. Computerised decision support systems to promote appropriate use of blood products. Cochrane Database Syst Rev. 2017;2017(2):CD012545.
33. Sanderson BJ, Field JD, Kocaballi AB, Estcourt LJ, Magrabi F, Wood EM, et al. Clinical decision support versus a paper-based protocol for massive transfusion: impact on decision outcomes in a simulation study. Transfusion. 2023;63(12):2225–33.
34. Hibbs SP, Nielsen ND, Brunskill S, Doree C, Yazer MH, Kaufman RM, et al. The impact of electronic decision support on transfusion practice: a systematic review. Transfus Med Rev. 2015;29(1):14–23.
35. Baer VL, Henry E, Lambert DK, Stoddard RA, Wiedmeier SE, Eggert LD, et al. Implementing a program to improve compliance with neonatal intensive care unit transfusion guidelines was accompanied by a reduction in transfusion rate: a pre-post analysis within a multihospital health care system. Transfusion. 2011;51(2):264–9.
36. Adams ES, Longhurst CA, Pageler N, Widen E, Franzon D, Cornfield DN. Computerized physician order entry with decision support decreases blood transfusions in children. Pediatrics. 2011;127(5):e1112–9.
37. Petäjä J, Andersson S, Syrjälä M. A simple automatized audit system for following and managing practices of platelet and plasma transfusions in a neonatal intensive care unit. Transfus Med. 2004;14(4):281–8.
38. Collins RA, Triulzi DJ, Waters JH, Reddy V, Yazer MH. Evaluation of real-time clinical decision support systems for platelet and cryoprecipitate orders. Am J Clin Pathol. 2014;141(1):78–84.
39. Goodnough LT, Shah N. Is there a "magic" hemoglobin number? Clinical decision support promoting restrictive blood transfusion practices. Am J Hematol. 2015;90(10):927–33.
40. Adams ES, Longhurst CA. Clinical decision support for pediatric blood product prescriptions. J Pediatr Intensive Care. 2016;5(3):108–12.
41. Cohn CS, Welbig J, Bowman R, Kammann S, Frey K, Zantek N. A data-driven approach to patient blood management. Transfusion. 2014;54(2):316–22.
42. McCrory MC, Strouse JJ, Takemoto CM, Easley RB. Computerized physician order entry improves compliance with a manual exchange transfusion protocol in the pediatric intensive care unit. J Pediatr Hematol Oncol. 2014;36(2):143–7.
43. Harb R, Hajdasz D, Landry ML, Sussman LS. Improving laboratory test utilisation at the multihospital Yale New Haven health system. BMJ Open Qual. 2019;8(3):e000689.
44. Ikoma S, Furukawa M, Busuttil A, Ward D, Baldwin K, Mayne J, et al. Optimizing inpatient blood utilization using real-time clinical decision support. Appl Clin Inform. 2021;12(1):49–56.
45. Metcalf RA, Goodfellow J, Cail K, Blaylock R, Kawamoto K, Enniss T, et al. Electronic clinical decision support: evidence that default settings influence end-user behavior. Transfusion. 2021;61(3):669–70.
46. Murphy C, Mou E, Pang E, Shieh L, Hom J, Shah N. A randomized study of a best practice alert for platelet transfusions. Vox Sang. 2022;117(1):87–93.
47. Adkins BD, Murfin R, Luu HS, Noland DK. Paediatric clinical decision support: evaluation of a best practice alert for red blood cell transfusion. Vox Sang. 2023;118(9):746–52.
48. Crispin P, Akers C, Brown K, Delaforce A, Keegan A, King F, et al. A review of electronic medical records and safe transfusion practice for guideline development. Vox Sang. 2022;117(6):761–8.
49. Segall N, Bonifacio AS, Schroeder RA, Barbeito A, Rogers D, Thornlow DK, et al. Can we make postoperative patient handovers safer? A systematic review of the literature. Anesth Analg. 2012;115(1):102–15.
50. Nagpal K, Abboudi M, Manchanda C, Vats A, Sevdalis N, Bicknell C, et al. Improving postoperative handover: a prospective observational study. Am J Surg. 2013;206(4):494–501.
51. Joseph MM, Mahajan P, Snow SK, Ku BC, Saidinejad M. Optimizing pediatric patient safety in the emergency care setting. J Emerg Nurs. 2022;48(6):652–65.

52. Cooper JB, Long CD, Newbower RS, Philip JH. Critical incidents associated with intraoperative exchanges of anesthesia personnel. Anesthesiology. 1982;56(6):456–61.
53. Agarwala A. The evidence base for optimal conduct of handoffs. Anesthesia Patient Safety Foundation (APSF); 2017. https://www.apsf.org/wp-content/uploads/newsletters/2017/Oct/pdf/APSF201710.pdf. Accessed 4 Dec 2022.
54. Saager L, Hesler BD, You J, Turan A, Mascha EJ, Sessler DI, et al. Intraoperative transitions of anesthesia care and postoperative adverse outcomes. Anesthesiology. 2014;121(4):695–706.
55. Hudson CC, McDonald B, Hudson JK, Tran D, Boodhwani M. Impact of anesthetic handover on mortality and morbidity in cardiac surgery: a cohort study. J Cardiothorac Vasc Anesth. 2015;29(1):11–6.
56. Boet S, Djokhdem H, Leir SA, Theberge I, Mansour F, Etherington C. Association of intraoperative anaesthesia handovers with patient morbidity and mortality: a systematic review and meta-analysis. Br J Anaesth. 2020;125(4):605–13.
57. Jones PM, Cherry RA, Allen BN, Jenkyn KMB, Shariff SZ, Flier S, et al. Association between handover of anesthesia care and adverse postoperative outcomes among patients undergoing major surgery. JAMA. 2018;319(2):143–53.
58. TJC. Sentinel event statistics released for 2015. Jt Comm Perspect. 2016;36:10. https://info.jcrinc.com/rs/494-MTZ-066/images/Sentinel39.pdf. Accessed 11 Sept 2023.
59. Bismilla Z, Wong B. Handover Toolkit. Royal College of Physicians and Surgeons of Canada. 2018. \Users\normaklein\Downloads\canmeds-handover-toolkit-e.pdf. Accessed 4 Dec 2022.
60. TJC. Hospital National Patient Safety Goals. 2022. https://www.jointcommission.org/-/media/tjc/documents/standards/national-patient-safety-goals/2022/simple_2022-hap-npsg-goals-101921.pdf. Accessed 14 Sept 2023.
61. Wyne L, Sayyad T, Hairston R. Making Blood Available "Just-in-Time"—Eliminating Supply Chain Complexities and Improving Efficiencies. Haemonetics Healthcare IT News 13 Sept 2018, 6 Jan 2020. https://www.healthcareitnews.com/news/why-it-matters-advancing-your-clinical-blood-transfusion-workflows. Accessed 12 Sept 2023.
62. Tuckley V, Davies J, Poles D, Robbie C, Narayan S. Safe handovers: safe patients-why good quality structured handovers in the transfusion laboratory are important. Transfus Med. 2022;32(2):135–40.
63. Serious Hazards of Transfusion and Medicines and Healthcare Products Regulatory Agency (SHOT) Annual SHOT Report 2021. https://www.shotuk.org/shot-reports/report-summary-and-supplement-2021/. Accessed 12 Sept 2023. 110, 218, 225–226.
64. Kelly A, New H. Paediatric Cases n=137. Serious Hazards of Transfusion (SHOT). 2021. https://www.shotuk.org/shot-reports/. Accessed 13 Sept 2023.
65. Coughlan JJ, Mross T, Gul F, Abbott A, Say R, Nawaz A, et al. Implementing an electronic clinical handover system in a university teaching hospital. Ir J Med Sci. 2018;187(2):309–12.
66. Tan XL, Park H, Patel J, Murden M. Improving clinical handover on an electronic communication platform: a quality improvement project. Cureus. 2021;13(10):e19156.
67. Skelton L, Rogers J, Kalafatis C. Development and implementation of electronic medical handovers across psychiatric hospitals: quality improvement initiative. BMJ Open Qual. 2019;8(4):e000630.
68. Aronson T, Oertle S, Piscotty R. Key characteristics of a successful EHR-supported e-handoff tool: a systematic review. Online J Nurs Inform (OJNI). 2021;25:1. https://www.himss.org/resources/key-characteristics-successful-ehr-supported-e-handoff-tool-systematic-review. Accessed 12 Sept 2023.
69. Burgess A, van Diggele C, Roberts C, Mellis C. Teaching clinical handover with ISBAR. BMC Med Educ. 2020;20(Suppl 2):459.
70. Saha AK, Segal S. A quality improvement initiative to reduce adverse effects of transitions of anesthesia care on postoperative outcomes: a retrospective cohort study. Anesthesiology. 2024;140(3):387–98.
71. Vossoughi S, Perez G, Whitaker BI, Fung MK, Stotler B. Analysis of pediatric adverse reactions to transfusions. Transfusion. 2018;58(1):60–9.

72. Oakley FD, Woods M, Arnold S, Young PP. Transfusion reactions in pediatric compared with adult patients: a look at rate, reaction type, and associated products. Transfusion. 2015;55(3):563–70.
73. Kopko PM. Transfusion reactions. 5th ed. Bethesda: AABB Press; 2021. p. 659.
74. Poisson JL, O'Leary MF. Improving our reaction time—using technology to identify transfusion reactions sooner. Transfusion. 2022;62:923–7.
75. Villamin C, Bates T, Mescher B, Benitez S, Martinez F, Knopfelmacher A, et al. Digitally enabled hemovigilance allows real time response to transfusion reactions. Transfusion. 2022;62(5):1010–8.
76. Serious Hazards of Transfusion and Medicines and Healthcare Products Regulatory Agency (SHOT) Annual SHOT Report. 2021. https://www.shotuk.org/shot-reports/report-summary-and-supplement-2021/. Accessed 12 Sept 2023.
77. US Food & Drug Administration. Transfusion/donation fatalities. 2020. https://www.fda.gov/media/160859/download#:~:text=During%20FY%202016%20there%20were,2019%2C%20and%2029%20in%202020. Accessed 15 June 2023.
78. Kopko PM. Transfusion reactions. 5th ed. Bethesda: AABB Press; 2021. p. 41, 83, 90–92, 98, 102–103, 121, 182, 233–249, 380, 408, 457–453, 2512–2513.
79. Lim YA, Kim J, Park C. Early recognition of possible transfusion reactions using an electronic automatic notification system for changes in vital signs in patients undergoing blood transfusions. Transfusion. 2020;60(9):1950–9.
80. White SK, Walker BS, Schmidt RL, Metcalf RA. The incidence of transfusion-related acute lung injury using active surveillance: a systematic review and meta-analysis. Transfusion. 2024;64(2):289–300.
81. Herasevich V, Tsapenko M, Kojicic M, Ahmed A, Kashyap R, Venkata C, et al. Limiting ventilator-induced lung injury through individual electronic medical record surveillance. Crit Care Med. 2011;39(1):34–9.
82. Gupta RK. Using an electronic clinical decision support system to reduce the risk of epidural hematoma. Am J Ther. 2014;21(5):327–30.
83. Wijnberge M, Geerts BF, Hol L, Lemmers N, Mulder MP, Berge P, et al. Effect of a machine learning-derived early warning system for intraoperative hypotension vs standard care on depth and duration of intraoperative hypotension during elective noncardiac surgery: the HYPE randomized clinical trial. JAMA. 2020;323(11):1052–60.
84. Harinstein LM, Kane-Gill SL, Smithburger PL, Culley CM, Reddy VK, Seybert AL. Use of an abnormal laboratory value-drug combination alert to detect drug-induced thrombocytopenia in critically ill patients. J Crit Care. 2012;27(3):242–9.
85. Weiss SL, Balamuth F, Chilutti M, Ramos MJ, McBride P, Kelly NA, et al. Identification of pediatric sepsis for epidemiologic surveillance using electronic clinical data. Pediatr Crit Care Med. 2020;21(2):113–21.
86. Benson M, Junger A, Fuchs C, Quinzio L, Bottger S, Hempelmann G. Use of an anesthesia information management system (AIMS) to evaluate the physiologic effects of hypnotic agents used to induce anesthesia. J Clin Monit Comput. 2000;16(3):183–90.
87. Whitaker B, Pizarro J, Deady M, Williams A, Ezzeldin H, Belov A, et al. Detection of allergic transfusion-related adverse events from electronic medical records. Transfusion. 2022;62(10):2029–38.
88. Murff HJ, Patel VL, Hripcsak G, Bates DW. Detecting adverse events for patient safety research: a review of current methodologies. J Biomed Inform. 2003;36(1–2):131–43.
89. Jhaveri P, Bozkurt S, Moyal A, Belov A, Anderson S, Shan H, et al. Analyzing real world data of blood transfusion adverse events: opportunities and challenges. Transfusion. 2022;62(5):1019–26.
90. Fung MK, AuBuchon JP, Stephens LD. Classification of posttransfusion adverse events using a publicly available artificial intelligence system. Transfusion. 2024;64:590.
91. Connelly NR, Adler AC, Vanderberg LE, Conlin F, Mitchell JD, Goldstein S, et al. Anesthesiology resident knowledge of transfusion medicine: results from the anesthesiology transfusion education study. Anesth Analg. 2024;138(3):655–63.

92. Shulman I, Hudgins J, Maramica I. Approaches to blood utilization. In: Cohn CS, Delaney M, Johnson ST, Katz LM, editors. Technical manual. 20th ed; 2020. p. 620–47.
93. Blumenthal D, Tavenner M. The "meaningful use" regulation for electronic health records. N Engl J Med. 2010;363(6):501–4.
94. Jimenez A. E-learning supports EHR implementations. In addition to meaningful use, we need to define meaningful training. Health Manag Technol. 2010;31(11):22–3.
95. Roshanov PS, Fernandes N, Wilczynski JM, Hemens BJ, You JJ, Handler SM, et al. Features of effective computerised clinical decision support systems: meta-regression of 162 randomised trials. BMJ. 2013;346:f657.
96. Chen W, O'Bryan CM, Gorham G, Howard K, Balasubramanya B, Coffey P, et al. Barriers and enablers to implementing and using clinical decision support systems for chronic diseases: a qualitative systematic review and meta-aggregation. Implement Sci Commun. 2022;3(1):81.
97. Varghese J, Kleine M, Gessner SI, Sandmann S, Dugas M. Effects of computerized decision support system implementations on patient outcomes in inpatient care: a systematic review. J Am Med Inform Assoc. 2018;25(5):593–602.
98. Shekelle PG, Morton SC, Keeler EB. Costs and benefits of health information technology. Evid Rep Technol Assess (Full Rep). 2006;132:1–71.
99. Danao M, Main K. Epic EMR Review. 2022 Features, pricing & more forbes advisor. 2022. https://www.forbes.com/advisor/business/software/epic-emr-review/. Accessed 12 Sept 2023.
100. Tan BT, Fralick J, Flores W, Schrandt C, Davis V, Bruynell T, et al. Implementation of epic beaker clinical pathology at Stanford University medical center. Am J Clin Pathol. 2017;147(3):261–72.
101. Rinehart JB, Lee TC, Kaneshiro K, Tran MH, Sun C, Kain ZN. Perioperative blood ordering optimization process using information from an anesthesia information management system. Transfusion. 2016;56(4):938–45.
102. Frank SM, Oleyar MJ, Ness PM, Tobian AA. Reducing unnecessary preoperative blood orders and costs by implementing an updated institution-specific maximum surgical blood order schedule and a remote electronic blood release system. Anesthesiology. 2014;121(3):501–9.
103. Jenkins I, Doucet JJ, Clay B, Kopko P, Fipps D, Hemmen E, et al. Transfusing wisely: clinical decision support improves blood transfusion practices. Jt Comm J Qual Patient Saf. 2017;43(8):389–95.
104. SHOT Bite No. 13: Information Technology in Transfusion—Highlights and Lessons. Serious Hazards of Transfusions (SHOT). 2020. https://www.shotuk.org/resources/current-resources/shot-bites/. Accessed 12 July 2024.
105. Davies J, McGrann A, Rowley M. 15: errors related to information technology. In: Serious hazards of transfusion annual report; 2021. https://www.shotuk.org/shot-reports/report-summary-and-supplement-2021/. Accessed 12 Sept 2023.
106. Lin Y, Tinmouth A, Mallick R, Haspel RL, Investigators B-T. BEST-TEST2: assessment of hematology trainee knowledge of transfusion medicine. Transfusion. 2016;56(2):304–10.
107. Mueller MM, Van Remoortel H, Meybohm P, Aranko K, Aubron C, Burger R, et al. Patient blood management: recommendations from the 2018 Frankfurt consensus conference. JAMA. 2019;321(10):983–97.

Part II

Intraoperative Phase of Care

Whole Blood Administration for Pediatric Patients

10

Meera Gangadharan, Alfredo Burgos, Deirdre L. Wyrick, and Destiny F. Chau

10.1 Case Scenario

A 3-year-old, 16 kg female child was involved in a motor vehicle accident and arrives emergently in the operating room. She has multiple scalp lacerations and a deformity in her right lower extremity, and the focused assessment with sonography for trauma (FAST) is positive for fluid in the peritoneal cavity. The child has received 40 mL/kg of crystalloid during resuscitation in the emergency room. As she enters the operating room, her blood pressure is 60/40 mmHg, heart rate 170 bpm, Hgb 7 g/dL, base deficit (−) 8 mmol/L, and lactate 4 mmol/L. Her core body temperature is 35 °C. She is intubated and unresponsive to physical stimulation. Whole blood is available from your blood bank, and you consider using it for this patient.

Key Learning Objectives

- What are the advantages of whole blood over component therapy?
- What is the current availability of whole blood for administration?
- What are the current criteria for whole blood for administration in children?

M. Gangadharan (✉)
Department of Anesthesiology, Critical Care and Pain Medicine University of Texas Health Science Center at Houston, McGovern Medical School, Houston, TX, USA
e-mail: meera.gangadharan@uth.tmc.edu

A. Burgos · D. F. Chau
Department of Anesthesiology and Pain Medicine, University of Arkansas for Medical Sciences, Arkansas Children's Hospital, Little Rock, AK, USA
e-mail: aburgosbriceno@uams.edu; dchau@uams.edu

D. L. Wyrick
Division of Pediatric Surgery and Section of Pediatric Critical Care Medicine, University of Arkansas for Medical Sciences Trauma Medical Director Arkansas Children's Hospital, Little Rock, AK, USA
e-mail: DLWyrick2@uams.edu

N. J. Klein (ed.), *Perioperative Pediatric Patient Blood Management and Transfusion Safety*, https://doi.org/10.1007/978-3-031-81666-6_10

- In what pediatric patient populations is whole blood currently used?
- Does the use of whole blood improve patient outcomes in the pediatric patient population?
- What is the risk of hemolysis from whole blood administration?
- Are there special considerations when administering whole blood to female patients?
- What are the components of whole blood, including preservatives?
- What is the known coagulation profile and efficacy of platelets in cold-stored whole blood?
- Does whole blood undergo leukocyte reduction (LR)?
- How might whole blood administration to trauma patients fit into a patient blood management (PBM) program?

10.2 Discussion

For centuries, whole blood was the only form of blood product available for transfusion. While whole blood continued to be used in combat settings ("walking blood bank"), its use was abandoned in civilian healthcare facilities after the development of separated blood components in the 1970s [1]. Component therapy allowed the therapeutic targeting of different deficits such as isolated anemia or thrombocytopenia, and it maximized the utility of a whole blood unit as its components could serve several patients. Additionally, component separation increased the overall shelf life of the blood unit. Blood components have different storage requirements, and some may be stored for longer period than others. For example, the shelf-life of component red blood cells (RBCs) is 21–42 days, fresh frozen plasma (FFP) 12 months, cryoprecipitate 12 months, and platelets 5–7 days [2]. Consequently, separation into components reduced blood product wastage.

The decades that followed the change to component therapy witnessed an era of crystalloid-heavy trauma resuscitation which was associated with adult respiratory distress syndrome (ARDS), abdominal compartment syndrome, coagulopathy, and acidosis. During the conflicts in Afghanistan and Iraq in early 2000, there was high mortality associated with severe injuries, prompting a reconsideration of early crystalloid resuscitation. Hemostatic resuscitation thus developed as a component of damage control resuscitation. It emphasized the importance of early administration of packed red cells, plasma, and platelets (in approximately equal ratios) during trauma resuscitation to restore oxygen delivery and to mimic the coagulation profile of whole blood. The provision of platelets in combat zones is challenging because platelets are conventionally stored at room temperature, with a recommended shelf life of 5–7 days in continuous physical agitation [2]. Additionally, storage and transport of RBC, FFP, and cryoprecipitate components to an austere environment also require refrigeration. The use of fresh whole blood made it possible to administer all three components to exsanguinating soldiers without the above logistic challenges associated with component therapy. Additionally, using fresh whole blood for resuscitation in the combat zone has been associated with equivalent or improved outcomes compared to component resuscitation [3, 4]. The renewed interest in whole blood transfusion in the military then expanded to the civilian arena [5, 6]. Figure 10.1 shows the timeline and evolution of whole blood products for pediatric transfusion which did not become popular until the 1990s.

Several whole blood classifications are found in the medical literature which will be clarified later in this chapter:

- Cold-stored low titer type O whole blood (LTOWB).

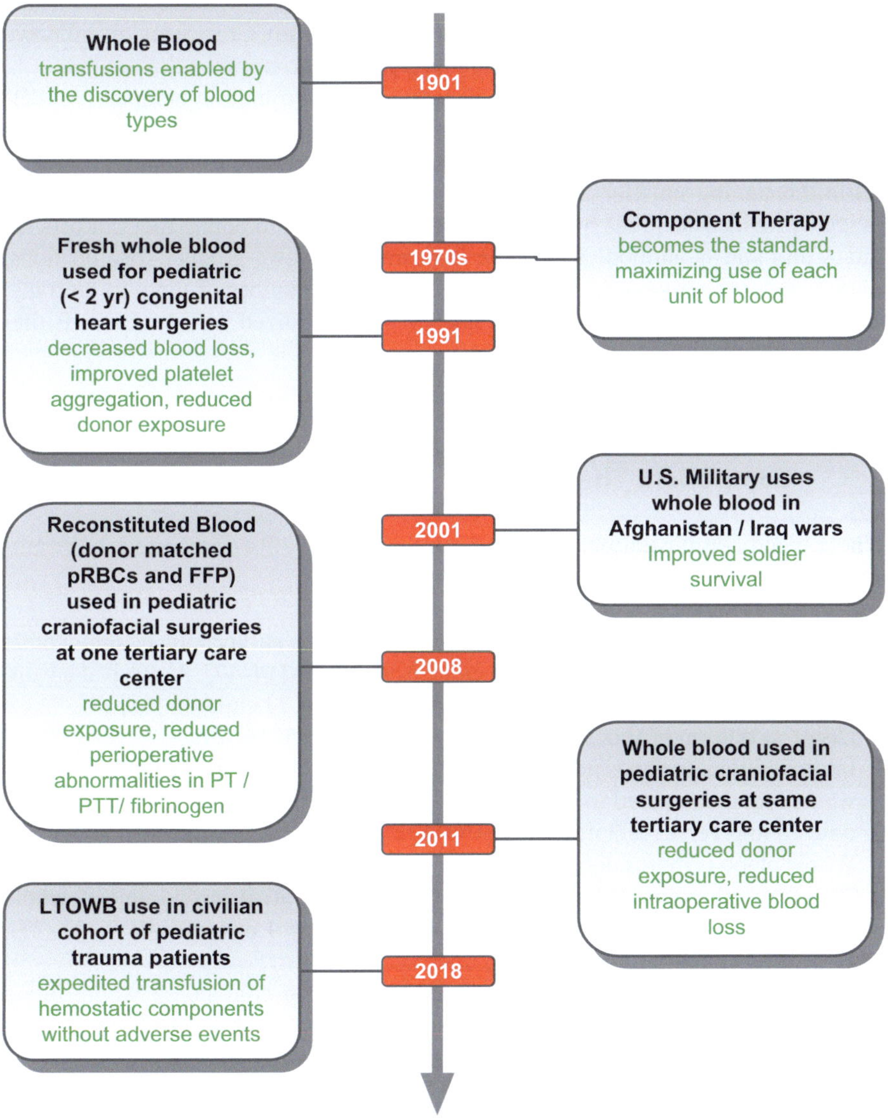

Fig. 10.1 Timeline and evolution of whole blood products used for pediatric transfusion

- Cold-stored fresh whole blood (administered within 48 h of collection).
- Cold-stored type-specific whole blood.
- Warm fresh whole blood (procured through a "walking blood bank") [3, 7].

Some institutions report the use of whole blood in pediatric congenital heart, craniofacial, and spine surgery [8–12]. These surgeries are elective and done in situations in which type-specific, cross-matched whole blood is available, in contrast to the exsanguinating trauma patient who typically receives type O whole blood because their blood type is unknown. There is no whole blood universal donor that guarantees both antigen and antibody compatibility with a recipient of unknown blood type; only group-identical whole blood fits that criterion.

In 2018, the Association for the Advancement of Blood and Biotherapies (AABB) approved conditional use of type-specific whole blood and LTOWB. The AABB recommends that whole blood be ABO group-specific with the recipient; however, in life-threatening situations, "group O whole blood may be administered to non-O patients provided facilities have policies and procedures to define titer cut-offs for anti-A and anti-B antibodies, specific indications for use, product specifications, administration instructions, and a defined maximum number of units to be transfused to each patient" [13]. There is not yet a standardized anti-A or anti-B titer required for whole blood processing.

10.3 What Are the Advantages of Whole Blood over Component Therapy?

Whole blood administration includes the following benefits as reported in the current literature:

- Adult studies indicate improved early and 30-day survival in coagulopathic trauma patients and an overall reduced mortality rate [14–17]. A survival advantage was found in at least one observational study of 27 children [18, 19].
- Faster resolution of shock in traumatized children [15, 16, 20].
- Improved transfusion efficiency, including reduced time to transfuse one unit of whole blood compared to one unit each of RBCs, plasma, and platelets (median time 15 min versus 303 mins; $p < 0.001$) [21].
- Whole blood is more concentrated, with less diluents and anticoagulants: there is 70 mL of citrate-phosphate-dextrose (CPD) preservative in one unit of whole blood versus 180 mL in the equivalent volume of 1:1: 1 components [5, 22, 23].
- Platelet advantages.
  - Increased shelf life of platelets contained within cold-stored whole blood (21–35 days) compared to component platelets stored at room temperature (5 days) or platelets cold stored at 1–6 °C under strict criteria (7 days) [2].
  - Cold-stored platelets have improved hemostatic function in vitro [9, 24–28].

  - Cold-stored whole blood platelets show a decline of platelet numbers and function over time; however, hemostatic properties are preserved for longer than room temperature platelets at end of a 5-day shelf life [29, 30].
  - Decreased bacterial contamination in cold platelet products compared to room temperature platelets [31].
- LTOWB is transported under the same conditions as RBCs, so no further practice alteration is required [32].
- Reduced donor exposure [9, 11, 15, 33].
- Theoretically reduced risk of clerical error in busy settings when group O whole blood is dispensed, with reduced "balanced ratio confusion" [23].
- More convenient for prehospital care by emergency medical teams when transporting blood in the field [1].

10.4 What Is the Current Availability of Whole Blood for Resuscitation?

Several recent surveys examining hospitals that provide whole blood for trauma resuscitation suggest that LTOWB is becoming more available in prehospital and hospital settings as clinical experience broadens and safety studies continue to support its use [34]. Currently, the major role for LTOWB is in trauma resuscitation, although its use has now expanded to nontraumatic and obstetric hemorrhage as well as prehospital first response vehicle transport, intraoperative hemorrhage, and severe anemia [4, 12, 35–38]. A 2020 survey found 37 hospitals supply LTOWB (US 35, Norway 1, Israel 1), a 130% increase from a prior study in 2018 [39]. In a 2021 survey of US Children's Hospitals (response rate greater than 80%), 18.8% ($n = 6/32$) of pediatric trauma directors used LTOWB in traumatized children [40]. The median number of times these centers activated their massive transfusion protocol (MTP) was 12 per year (5.8–20 IQR), suggesting a low rate of experience in managing massive hemorrhage and therefore a reduced impetus to provide this administratively complex blood product. In a more recent study of 72 level I pediatric trauma centers in the USA, 16% stocked LTOWB, and one-half of respondents felt that a controlled study on the matter is warranted [41].

10.5 What Are the Current Criteria for Whole Blood for Administration in Children?

Whole blood administration in children is currently limited to LTOWB. The criteria for LTOWB in children are primarily trauma-related with limitations for patient age and weight, as well as cutoffs for the maximum quantity allowed per resuscitation. The results from the first civilian cohort of pediatric patients to receive LTOWB for trauma resuscitation were published in 2018 from the Children's Hospital of Pittsburgh [21]. In 2016, the original criteria for administering LTOWB included male or female children $\geq$3 years old, weight $\geq$ 15 kg, and maximum allowed

Table 10.1 Criteria for administration of LTOWB to children during prehospital hemorrhagic resuscitation. Any one criterion qualifies for LTOWB administration in hemorrhagic shock. Adapted from Weymouth W, Long B, Koyfman A, Winckler C. Whole Blood in Trauma: A Review for Emergency Clinicians. J Emerg Med. 2019;56 (5):491–8

Systolic blood pressure (SB)	< 70 mmHg
SBP	< 90 mmHg with heart rate > 110 beats per minute
End-tidal CO_2	< 25 mmHg
Cardiac arrest	If witnessed and < 5 min with uninterrupted cardiopulmonary resuscitation since arrest

volume of 20 mL/kg LTOWB [18]. Following this original research experience, the same center liberalized the age limit to ≥2 years and weight ≥ 10 kg, which was again modified in 2019 to age ≥ 1 year without a minimum weight requirement [20]. The liberalization of criteria was primarily based on research indicating that LTOWB was not associated with hemolysis or increased adverse events in the short term. The current Pittsburgh guidelines now allow up to 40 mL/kg of LTOWB in children age ≥ 1 year with signs of hemorrhagic shock due to either trauma or non-traumatic hemorrhage, without a minimum weight criterion [42]. Following the transfusion of 40 mL/kg of LTOWB, conventional blood components are provided based on the patient's clinical and laboratory findings. The dose of 40 mL/kg was based on the maximum dose of LTOWB that is used at adult trauma hospitals in the same geographic location (i.e., 6 units or 3 L volume); in a 70 kg individual, the dose is approximately 40 mL/kg. Another pediatric trauma center administers 10 mL/kg of LTOWB initially followed by a maximum of 40 mL/kg for children >1 year [38].

LTOWB is now available as part of the massive transfusion protocol (MTP) in some pediatric centers [40–42]. An example of one medical center's guideline for pediatric LTOWB resuscitation focuses on patients with current or anticipated critical blood loss and is illustrated in Tables 10.1 and 10.2 [43].

Recent prospective observational and retrospective studies of children who have received LTOWB continue to report relatively successful outcomes, adequate hemostatic resuscitation, and safety in younger age groups [18, 44, 45]. Administration of low antibody titer (e.g., < 200) whole blood has even been used in nontraumatic bleeding in a neonatal ICU MTP, where Carr et al. reported resuscitation of a severely anemic, 25-week preterm neonate with 20 mL/kg of whole blood processed by the American Red Cross through a platelet-sparing leukoreduction filter [37].

10.6 In What Pediatric Patient Populations Is Whole Blood Currently Used?

At the time of this writing, whole blood transfusion for pediatric patients has been described in the following populations:

Table 10.2 LTOWB overall volume limits for children during hemorrhagic resuscitation. Adapted from Weymouth W, Long B, Koyfman A, Winckler C. Whole Blood in Trauma: A Review for Emergency Clinicians. J Emerg Med. 2019;56 (5):491–8

Age (years)	Maximum volume LTOWB recommended
< 6	Permission must be obtained from medical director
6–10	500 mL
11–13	1 liter (L)
>13	> 1 L

- Trauma patients who present in hemorrhagic shock [18, 20, 21, 38, 42, 44, 45].
- Craniofacial surgery [11].
- Congenital cardiac surgery [8–10, 46].
- Complex spine surgery [12].
- Hemorrhage secondary to medical hemorrhage, gastrointestinal bleeding, surgical bleeding, menorrhagia, and severe anemia [37, 41, 42].

10.7 Does the Use of Whole Blood Improve Patient Outcomes in the Pediatric Patient Population?

Available LTOWB studies in children are relatively small with the result that a mortality benefit has not yet been conclusively demonstrated. In general, current data suggests that LTOWB use in pediatric trauma does not lead to increased adverse events compared to resuscitation with component therapy [21, 42, 44]. More recent studies indicate improved survival or other outcomes when administered early in trauma resuscitation [18, 20, 45, 47]. The current published studies on LTOWB report modest doses (median 15 to 20 mL/kg) and a conservative titer threshold (< 1:50–1:200), which appear to be serologically safe among non-group O pediatric trauma recipients in the short term. Reassuring results in initial studies has led to the expansion of the conservative selection criteria for pediatric LTOWB use; large, controlled trials are needed to validate LTOWB efficacy under liberalized protocol parameters.

The following discussion addresses currently published research on the use of whole blood in children:

10.7.1 Pediatric Trauma

Research continues to evolve on clinical outcomes in traumatized children who receive LTOWB for resuscitation, compared to conventional blood components. Early studies found no difference in mortality between LTOWB and conventional blood therapy groups [20, 21, 45]. A database analysis of the American College of Surgeons (ACS) 2017 Trauma Quality Improvement Program (TQIP) examined 135 injured patients between 1 and 17 years who received any volume of LTOWB (with or without conventional components) and propensity score matched with 270 patients receiving component therapy only for resuscitation [45]. In-hospital and 24-h mortality were similar between groups. No differences were found in other endpoints (i.e., ARDS, acute kidney injury, sepsis, and venous thromboembolism). However, the LTOWB group had fewer ventilator days and reduced volumes of transfused products compared to the conventional component group. A single-center study propensity score matched 36 LTOWB pediatric trauma patients with 36 trauma patients who received only conventional blood components for resuscitation [47]. Again, there was no difference between groups for in-hospital mortality as well as other outcome parameters (i.e., organ failure, acute kidney injury, transfusion reaction, sepsis, venous thromboembolism, ventilator days, and functional disability at discharge). However, ICU length of stay (LOS) was shorter in the LTOWB group (median 3 days versus 6 days; $p = 0.03$). A third study, also with propensity score matching, found lower plasma and platelet volumes as well as faster resolution of base deficit i.e., shock; (2 versus 6 h, $p < 0.001$) in 28 children who received LTOWB compared to 28 conventional component recipients; there was no difference in secondary outcomes including in-hospital deaths, hospital LOS, ICU LOS, and ventilator days [20].

In contrast, a 2021 prospective observational study found a survival benefit of LTOWB in pediatric trauma resuscitation [18]. The study compared 80 children between the ages of 1 and 17 years who received a massive transfusion with LTOWB as the first resuscitative fluid (up to the protocol limit 40 mL/kg), followed by component blood (WB + CB group), with patients who received component blood (CB) alone. The primary outcome was survival at 28 days. The LTOWB group were older with higher body weight. Thirty three percent of patients in the LTOWB group received 20 mL/kg (median IQR, 15–33). Total blood product volumes were as follows: WB + CB group ($n = 27$) 50 mL/kg versus CB group ($n = 53$) 61 mL/kg ($p = 0.06$). After age adjustment, the WB + CB group had decreased mortality at 72 h (odds ratio (OR) 0.23; $p = 0.009$) and at 28 days (OR 0.41; $p = 0.02$), but not at 6 h. Investigators also found fewer hospital and ventilator days in the WB + CB group.

In a secondary analysis of data from the US Department of Defense Trauma Registry, a survival benefit for fresh whole blood was sought in pediatric casualties that received at least one unit of blood [48]. In the military, two types of whole blood are available: "fresh" whole blood refers to whole blood that is collected in the field, stored at room temperature, and used within 24 h of collection. The second type (since 2016) is cold-stored LTOWB, the preferred resuscitation blood. There were 1244 survivors meeting inclusion criteria, of which 23 received fresh whole blood (in addition to component blood), at a mean total volume 55.4 mL/kg. The odds ratio for survival in this group was 2.86 (95% CI, 0.4–20.45) compared to those who received component blood alone. After adjustment for confounders and removal of head injury victims, the survival odds were 58.63 (95% CI, 2.7–1272.67) in the fresh whole blood group.

Total transfused blood product volumes between whole blood and component recipients have been examined in several studies, with varied results. Due to protocol limits in the initial amount of LTOWB administered, these studies are usually based on comparison between those patients receiving any LTOWB (WB + CB) to component blood therapy alone (CB). Anand et al. conducted a database study and found a lower 24-h total blood product volume administration in those that received any whole blood: WB + CB group (n = 135) 39 mL/kg versus CB group (n = 270) 53 mL/kg CB ($p < 0.001$) [45]. Other studies have not found a statistically significant difference in the WB + CB group (maximum WB 15 mL/kg) versus CB group in 24-h total blood product volume transfused [20, 47]. In a 2023 multicenter prospective observational study of pediatric level 1 trauma centers including 90 children who received at least one unit of whole blood during early trauma resuscitation, there was also no statistically significant difference in volumes of whole blood (n = 62) versus component therapy (n = 28) administered within the first 24 h of admission (median 8.5 units vs 5.5 units, respectively; $p = 0.825$) [44].

10.7.2 Pediatric Craniofacial Surgery

Type-specific whole blood was compared to reconstituted whole blood in a single-center retrospective review of the Pediatric Craniofacial Surgery Perioperative Registry [11]. The primary outcomes sought were donor exposure and postoperative coagulation status. Type-specific whole blood is blood of the same ABO- and Rhesus (Rh) group as the intended recipient. In that study, reconstituted whole blood was made of separate components (FFP and RBCs mixed in a 1:1 ratio) and, in this case, from the same donor. There were 111 patients with a mean age of approximately 1 year. The type-specific whole blood group (n = 52) had significantly less donor exposure (1 versus 2 units; $p = 0.02$) and less calculated intraoperative blood loss (61.1+/− 30.7 mL/kg versus 86 +/− 43.3 mL/kg; p value not mentioned) compared to the reconstituted whole blood group (n = 59). Postoperative drain output and coagulation profile studies were similar between groups. The type-specific whole blood in this case was administered within 3 days of donation. Investigators postulate the results may be related to the fact that the type-specific, non-reconstituted whole blood contains platelets and possibly "superior hemostatic activity." Although logistically difficult to obtain, type-specific whole blood was used because it does not present a mismatch between recipient anti-A or anti-B RBC antigens and donor plasma antibodies that may occur when type O whole blood is administered to a non-type O recipient.

10.7.3 Pediatric Spine Surgery

A prospective randomized controlled trial examined the potential effects of fresh whole blood (administered within 24 h of collection) versus component therapy on postoperative outcomes in children undergoing spine correction surgery ≥ 6 levels [12]. Approximately one-half of patients in each group had idiopathic scoliosis, and approximately one-quarter had neuromuscular scoliosis. The blood in both groups underwent leukoreduction. Component therapy was administered in a 1:1:1: ratio of RBC/plasma/platelets to simulate balanced resuscitation. The whole blood group ($n = 30$) demonstrated a shorter ICU LOS (40.6 h versus 46.51 h, $p = 0.02$) and a reduced inflammatory response as assessed through interleukin-6 levels ($p = 0.019$), compared to the component blood group ($n = 35$). Intraoperative blood loss and total blood volumes transfused were similar between groups.

10.7.4 Pediatric Congenital Cardiac Surgery

Manno et al. prospectively studied postoperative hemostasis associated with 3 blood preparations in 161 randomized children undergoing complex congenital heart surgery [8]. The blood types were very fresh whole blood (VFWB, administered within 6 h of donation), whole blood administered within 24–48 h of donation, and reconstituted blood (e.g., RBC, FFP, and platelets combined). In children less than 2 years ($n = 93$), the 24-h blood loss in the reconstituted blood group was 85% more than either whole blood group. In children older than 2 years, no difference in blood loss was seen among the three groups. The highest volume blood loss was in the reconstituted blood group for children <2 years undergoing complex procedures ($p = 0.002$). Although laboratory coagulation parameters were altered in all blood groups, platelet aggregation was most affected in the reconstituted group. Differences in total volumes of blood products transfused were not reported.

A single-center, randomized, double-blind, controlled trial examined survival and ICU LOS in patients younger than 1 year undergoing congenital cardiac surgery with cardiopulmonary bypass [46]. Pump prime using fresh whole blood (within 48 h of donation) was compared to reconstituted blood made at bedside (i.e., RBCs plus FFP). Power analysis resulted in a sample size of 100 for each blood group; there were 96 patients in the fresh whole blood prime group and 104 in the reconstituted blood prime group. A composite score was created for analysis: 1 point for each day in the ICU, up to 7 days maximum, and a score of 8 for death within 28 days of surgery. The patient characteristics, demographics, and illness severity were similar between groups. Investigators found no difference in the composite score between the blood prime groups; however, the fresh whole blood group had a longer ICU LOS as an individual data point and significantly more fluid overload. There was no difference in the overall volume of blood products transfused between groups. Based on this study, some transfusion medicine experts have concluded that fresh whole blood offers no clinical benefit when used in cardiopulmonary bypass prime but, if locally available, may have a role in postoperative transfusion therapy following congenital cardiac surgery [33].

Even though infants less than 4–6 months old are unlikely to mount an immunologic response to foreign blood cell antigens, it is common practice to set a goal of reducing the number of different donors a child is exposed to through blood transfusions. There are several reasons for this, including prevention of excessive alloimmunization, avoiding sensitization to HLA (human lymphocyte antigen) antigens in white blood cells, and minimizing the rate of transfusion reactions including transfusion-transmitted infections. Jobes et al. examined a retrospective cohort of 4111 patients younger than 2 years of age who received whole blood transfusion for congenital cardiac surgery [9]. The hospital registry was retrospectively reviewed for the number of donor exposures per patient, and the results were then compared to donor exposure reports published in the literature for children <2 years undergoing congenital cardiac surgery. The institution had a fresh whole blood donor program for cardiac surgery during the study period (1995–2010) whereby children received two units of fresh whole blood (administered within 48 h of donation) for the first blood required and component therapy thereafter. The fresh whole blood recipients had a median of 2 (range 0–28) donor exposures, whereas studies in similar patients over a similar period found more than twice as many exposures. In an earlier retrospective study, Valleley et al. reported reduced blood donor exposure in patients < 5 kg body weight who received whole blood in the bypass prime as opposed to RBC prime [10]. Sixty four percent of the children in the fresh whole blood group had only one donor exposure ($n = 61$; $p < 0.0001$), but more than three-quarters of the RBC group had ≥3 donor exposures ($n = 39$; $p < 0.0003$). Postoperative blood loss and other outcomes were similar among the two groups.

10.8 What Is the Risk of Hemolysis from Whole Blood Administration?

A safety consideration when transfusing type O whole blood to patients of unknown or non-type O blood type is a risk of immune-related hemolysis. Type O whole blood contains anti-A and -B antibodies in plasma which may lead to clinical incompatibility with A and B antigens on type A, B, or AB recipient RBCs (Table 10.3).

ABO antigens are present on RBCs (and in platelets suspended in plasma) as well as many other tissues including the heart, lungs, kidneys, bowel, pancreas, and endothelium [51]. Naturally occurring antibodies ("autoantibodies") against type A and B blood group antigens are of two types: IgM and IgG. IgM antibodies are largest in size, do not cross the placenta, and can be produced in response to multiple stimuli including gut flora, vaccines, and probiotics. The IgM isotype is predominant in blood groups A and B, while the IgG isotype is most predominant in type O blood group. A hemolytic transfusion reaction can occur from either of these antibodies when encountering the corresponding antigen [52, 53].

The risk of hemolysis from a non-identical whole blood transfusion can be mitigated by selecting units with low titers of anti-A and anti-B antibodies. While older studies from a major institution report usage of LTOWB with titers less than 50, this same institution has increased the threshold to <100 as the safety profile of more liberal titers has been demonstrated and the demand for LTOWB has increased [21, 42]. A 2022 survey of US level 1 pediatric trauma center guidelines found titers ranging from <50 to <256 [41, 54].

Thus far, hemolysis marker studies following LTOWB transfusions have not found evidence of hemolysis in short-term follow-up. Concerning short-term

Table 10.3 ABO and Rh antigens in RBCs and corresponding plasma antibodies. Also shown is the distribution of blood group types in the US. *W* White, *AA* African American, *Latin-Am* Latino-American [49, 50]

Blood type	Distribution in the US (per Red Cross)	Antigens expressed on RBCs	Antibodies expressed in plasma
O	O+ (37% W, 47% AA, 39% Asian, 53% Latin-am) O− (12% W, 4% AA,1% Asian, 4% Latin-am)	None	Anti-A Anti-B Anti-AB
A	A+ (33% W, 24% AA, 27% Asian, 29% Latin-am) A− (7% W, 2% AA, 0.5% Asian, 2% Latin-am)	A	Anti-B
B	B+ (9% W, 18% AA, 25% Asian, 9% Latin-am) B− (2% W, 1% AA, 0.4% Asian, 1% Latin-am)	B	Anti-A
AB	AB+ (3% W, 4% AA, 7% Asian, 2% Latin-am) AB− (1% W, 0.3% AA, 0.1% Asian, 0.2% Latin-am)	AB	None
Rhesus D positive	Overall 85%	Rh	None
Rhesus D negative	Overall 15%	None	[a]None

[a]An RhD negative patient may develop anti-RhD antibodies if past exposure to RhD positive RBCs or platelets, in certain circumstances. Similarly, any patient may have antibodies other than the ones described in the table if exposed to foreign non-ABO antigens undetected on routine pretransfusion screening

results, Leeper et al. found no difference in biochemical hemolytic markers in 18 traumatized children older than 3 years who were treated with a maximum volume 20 mL/kg of LTOWB with anti-A and anti-B titers <50 [21]. Another study sought laboratory evidence of hemolysis on post-transfusion days 0–3 in 47 traumatically injured children who received a median 16 mL/kg (IQR 10–25) cold-stored, Rh-negative, titer <50, LTOWB obtained from male donors [42]. The laboratory markers included lactate dehydrogenase (LDH), haptoglobin, total bilirubin, reticulocyte count, potassium, and creatinine. There were not statistically or clinically significant differences in the median values of the biochemical markers of hemolysis between type O and non-type O recipients at any of the time points measured. There were also no adverse events reported or direct antiglobulin test (DAT) tests performed in blood type O patients within 48 h of whole blood transfusion [42]. The lack of positive hemolysis markers in these studies is consistent with results reported in the adult trauma populations resuscitated with LTOWB [16, 22, 55]. Although these preliminary results are promising, some authors caution that the ability to mount an immunologic response may be impaired in previously healthy but traumatized patients as opposed to those who have comorbidities such as cancer or severe trauma [53].

10.9 Are there Special Considerations When Administering Whole Blood to Female Patients?

Women of childbearing age and younger face additional risks of transfusion with incompatible blood types. While the type O RhD negative RBCs are the universal donor, the transfusion of RhD positive RBCs to an RhD negative female may result in the production of anti-RhD antibodies in the recipient. If an RhD negative sensitized female becomes pregnant with a RhD positive fetus, antibodies from the mother may cross the placenta and cause hemolysis of fetal RBCs or hemolytic disease of the fetus and newborn (HDFN). For this reason, some centers will not administer RhD positive blood to females of childbearing age or younger whose RhD antigen status is unknown. However, a recent survey of US level 1 adult trauma centers found that up to one half ($n = 22/43$) report resuscitation with RhD positive blood to females of childbearing age who are RhD negative or those whose blood type is unknown, often because of the increasing shortage of available type O RhD negative blood [56]. In another survey of 117 US level 1 and 2 pediatric trauma centers, 92.7% provided only RhD negative product for girls ≤ 18 years, and 54.5% did so for boys in that age range [57]. Three years later, a more recent survey of US transfusion service directors found that approximately one half of centers that use LTOWB dispense only RhD negative product for massive bleeding in females of childbearing potential (adult and pediatric) with an unknown blood type, and one quarter do so for boys [58]. A 2019 AABB bulletin calling for a reduction in misuse of RhD negative type O blood notes that 6.9% of the US blood donors are blood type O and RhD negative; however, the amount of RhD negative blood that is administered continues to increase beyond that percentage [59]. The AABB recommends reserving RhD negative type O blood for females of childbearing potential; when not available, lifesaving RhD positive O blood may be administered, since a patient's likelihood of dying from hemorrhagic shock is estimated to be more than four times the risk of inducing HDFN if she is pregnant at the time of resuscitation [14, 54, 59, 60]. Although the American College of Gynecologists (ACOG) recommends administration of anti-D immune globulin (e.g., Rhogam) to RhD negative women who have experienced abdominal trauma, a policy of routine surveillance for RhD antigen and antibody status in women resuscitated with RhD positive blood has not been universally implemented [61–63]. According to a recent survey, one quarter of centers have no policy for mitigating RhD alloimmunization in RhD negative females resuscitated for massive bleeding, such as RhD immunoglobulin administration or patient counseling [58]. Furthermore, anti-D immune globulin has inherent side effects and must be administered in a timely fashion, usually within several days of the transfusion event.

10.10 What Are the Components of Whole Blood, Including Preservatives?

Whole blood has a higher hematocrit, platelet count, percentage of coagulation factors, and less anticoagulant volumes than the equivalent components administered together in a 1:1:1 ratio (RBC/plasma/platelets) (Table 10.4) [2, 13].

10.11 What Is the Known Coagulation Profile and Efficacy of Platelets in Cold-Stored Whole Blood?

Conventional platelets are stored at room temperature with a limited shelf life of 5–7 days. This storage temperature promotes bacterial growth, setting the stage for wastage and critical supply chain shortages [29]. These concerns have led to a renewed interest in cold-stored platelets. In February 2023 the US Food and Drug Administration (FDA) approved the use of cold-stored platelets for actively bleeding patients when conventional platelets are unavailable [64]. The platelets must be obtained by apheresis technique, leukoreduced, and stored at 1–6 °C for not more than 14 days; agitation is not required under this exception.

Cold-stored platelets (1–6 °C) demonstrate improved hemostatic function compared to conventional room temperature platelets in in vitro studies [65]. Specifically, cold-stored platelets have been shown to have superior contractile function, thromboelastographic (TEG) parameters, reduced inflammatory markers, and enhanced convenience with an extended shelf life [9, 24–26, 28, 66]. However, translating in vitro results into improved clinical outcomes is difficult because of the paucity of data on cold-stored platelets in the pediatric patient population. Platelet counts and viscoelastic parameters were examined in 8 children >2 years of age who received

Table 10.4 Composition of whole blood versus 1:1:1 ratio combination of packed red cells, plasma, and platelets

Features of whole blood versus fractionated components	Fresh whole blood (one unit)	Blood components (1:1:1 administration)
Hematocrit % (median IQR)	39 (33–41)	31 (29–32)
Platelet count K/mm^3 (median IQR)	195 (190–220)	150 (110–180)
Coagulation factors (%)	92–100	68–93
Volume (mL)	450–500	650–675
Shelf life	21–35 days	*RBC*: 21–42 days *Plasma:* FFP frozen 12 months; thawed 24 h to 5 days *Platelets*: Room temperature: 5–7 days under continuous gentle agitation; cold-stored, per manufacturer *Cryoprecipitate*: Frozen 12 months; thawed 4–6 h
Anticoagulant CPD (mL)	70	180

up to 30 mL/kg of cold-stored LTOWB for trauma resuscitation and compared to 14 children who received component therapy (including room temperature platelets) for resuscitation [67]. Post-transfusion maximum amplitude (MA) on TEG was similar between groups (59.5 mm versus 60.2 mm), as were the platelet counts (median 129/L versus 135/L). In another retrospective record review, 48 children <24 months undergoing cranial vault reconstruction received whole blood when available [27]. All patients were treated with an antifibrinolytic. The patients who received conventional room temperature platelets (n = 18) demonstrated a greater post-transfusion decrease in MA on TEG (7.7 mm versus 2.1 mm; $p < 0.001$). Investigators attributed this finding to decreased fibrinogen levels found in the component group. In a prospective randomized controlled study designed to assess post-operative hemostasis in 161 children undergoing cardiopulmonary bypass, Manno et al. found an 18 mL/kg increase in blood loss in children <2 years who received reconstituted whole blood (1:1:1 RBC/plasma/platelets) compared to fresh whole blood [8]. This difference in blood loss was attributed to reduced ADP-induced platelet aggregation, although there were differences in additional coagulation parameters between groups.

In vitro studies have found decreased platelet counts in leukoreduced, cold-stored whole blood with increasing storage time [68–70]. This may occur as early as 5 days of cold storage [69]. Huish et al. compared platelet counts and activity in cold-stored and leukoreduced whole blood to room temperature component platelets and found a 50% decrease in count and decrease in platelet aggregation by day 21 in the cooled whole blood [70]. The type of filter used (or, not) can also affect the coagulation profile of whole blood. In the past, whole blood did not undergo leukoreduction (LR), but, today, application of an LR filter before release from the blood center or at the bedside is standard. "Platelet-sparing" filters are also becoming the norm in processing whole blood. The coagulation profile in five units of cold-stored leukoreduced whole blood was assessed after processing through a platelet-sparing LR filter and compared to five units processed through a LR filter that was not platelet-sparing [71]. The maximum amplitude as measured by TEG was 54.9 mm in the platelet-spared units compared to 13.9 mm in the units run through a LR filter that was not platelet-sparing ($p < 0.001$). Furthermore, the whole blood platelet hemostatic function as measured by a PFA-100 analyzer as well as the whole blood platelet counts was also decreased in the LR-filtered units without platelet-sparing. However, these changes were not apparent until after 2 weeks of storage. Pathogen reduction treatment (PRT) is also commonplace today to prevent transfusion transmitted infections. Jobes et al. compared the coagulation profiles of cold-stored whole blood from 32 volunteers that was treated with riboflavin and ultraviolet light [26]. Although platelet aggregation was reduced, TEG parameters were preserved, and fibrinolysis was reduced in all units during 3 weeks of storage. In another study of whole blood run through a rapid infusion device up to 100 mL/min and also a pneumatic pressure bag, the platelet counts of five units tested decreased, but the overall hemostatic function including viscoelastic parameters remained stable [72].

An additional concern in the safe administration of cold-stored LTOWB is the use of fluid warmers. Platelet function and aggregation studies performed in vitro suggest that fluid warmer-induced alterations in platelet function may vary depending on whether the transfused platelets are administered at room temperature or after cold storage. In a 2024 prospective observational study of 23 cold-stored, pathogen reduced platelets units, the ADP-induced aggregation but not the platelet count was reduced after running through a warming device (set point 41 °C) over 1 min [73]. An earlier in vitro study of 31 room temperature apheresis platelet units run through the same brand warmer found no change in aggregometry and only small changes in TEG MA and alpha angle readings remained within normal parameters [74]. The clinical significance of these warming effects is unclear.

In conclusion, while in vitro studies focusing on cold-stored platelets indicate abnormalities in quantity and function related to storage time, there is a lack of clinical data establishing that cold platelets—alone or within whole blood—lead to excessive bleeding or a coagulopathic state. Given the complexity of the coagulation properties of whole blood and the special pretransfusion treatments used in the interest of patient safety (e.g., LR and platelet filtration, preservatives, additive solutions, and pathogen reduction), more studies exploring this precious resource are necessary [29, 30]. At this point in time, there is no evidence that the hemostatic function of platelets or any other coagulation factor contributes to a clinical coagulopathy in traumatized children resuscitated with cold-stored LTOWB.

10.12 Does Whole Blood Undergo Leukocyte Reduction (LR)?

Leukocyte reduction (LR) filters reduce the risk of transmission of intra-leukocyte pathogens such as HTLV, CMV, and EBV, reduce the rate of febrile nonhemolytic transfusion reactions (FNHR), mitigate transfusion-related host versus graft disease, and decrease the risk of HLA alloimmunization [52, 75]. LR does not consistently eliminate the risk of transfusion-transmitted prion disease, notwithstanding the fact that the incidence is very rare (there has not been a reported case of sporadic prion disease in the USA and the UK for decades) [76]. There are now "prion reduction" filters available; however, it is unclear if these newer generation filters can consistently prevent the Creutzfeldt-Jakob disease variant (vCJD) [75].

Blood component LR is now the standard of care in the majority of US blood centers. In most cases, LR is performed before release from the blood center, after whole blood donation and before splitting the whole unit into components, but bedside filters are also available for individual patient use [31]. No filtration process removes 100% of leukocytes. Commercial-level LR is highly regulated; in the USA, 95% of units filtered must have residual leukocytes less than 5×10^6 per unit, and, in Europe, restrictions are even greater [31]. Most filters that remove leukocytes also remove platelets. The US FDA has approved a whole blood LR filter that is platelet-sparing, improving the ability to optimally process whole blood as the demand for it continues to increase [77]. Platelet- sparing filters, with or without LR capability, still remove up to one-quarter of platelets [78, 79]. An additional limitation of any bedside, in-line blood filter less than 150 microns is that rapid transfusions under pressure will produce cell lysis and a shortened filter life.

TA-GVHD, a potentially fatal response to the transfusion of cellular blood products, is best prevented in susceptible patient populations through irradiation of whole blood and cellular blood components [80].[1] These include fetuses undergoing intrauterine transfusion, neonates undergoing exchange transfusion, congenital T lymphocyte immunodeficiency, and HLA-matched or related donor cellular products.[2] Frozen plasma (but, not fresh plasma), cryoprecipitate, as well as RBCs cold stored for more than 14 days do not require irradiation to prevent TA-GVHD. Importantly, although large volume transfusions prepared for susceptible neonates should be administered within 24 h of irradiation, emergency transfusions and those administered under a massive transfusion protocol (MTP) are exempt from irradiation requirements for practical reasons [80].

10.13 How Might Whole Blood Administration to Trauma Patients Fit Into a Patient Blood Management (PBM) Program?

Whole blood fits into a PBM program in several ways. Although existing studies are relatively small, the current use of whole blood in civilian children is supported by evidence-based research using gradually increasing volumes, older patients, and relatively low plasma anti-A and -B antibody titers [20, 21, 42, 47]. The AABB, which credentials US hospital blood banks and centers, requires institutional protocols specifying indications, blood characteristics, and volume limits before any institution may administer whole blood [43, 81]. Its use in children who require larger volume transfusions is patient-centered because LTOWB reduces donor exposure [9, 11, 15]. Early studies indicate that it reduces blood loss and therefore preserves the patient's RBC mass [20, 44, 45, 47]. This latter advantage may be secondary to the fact that it contains less anticoagulant preservative and platelets, and coagulation proteins are present in natural ratios. Some studies have established that cold-stored platelets may have superior hemostatic function [24–28, 82]. Finally, although there are no large prospective trials of outcomes in children receiving whole blood, early studies suggest no difference in adverse events and at least one recent observational study of 80 traumatized children found a survival benefit of LTOWB compared to MTP component therapy [18].

---

[1] A more detailed discussion of the pathophysiology of TA-GVHD may be found in the chapter entitled, "Preoperative Autologous and Designated Donations."

[2] For a more complete list of patients susceptible to TA-GVHD, refer to the Australian and New Zealand Society of Blood Transfusion Guidelines for the Prevention of Transfusion-Associated Graft-Versus-Host-Disease, second ed.

10.14 Summary of Key Learning Objectives

10.14.1 What Are the Advantages of Whole Blood Over Component Therapy?

Under current guidelines as required by the AABB and adopted by various pediatric hospitals, this 3 y.o.,16 kg, acutely traumatized and anemic child is a candidate for whole blood resuscitation. Ideally, the whole blood is type specific, although in a trauma setting. LTOWB becomes the option when the patient's blood type is unknown and there is no time for blood typing. Improved efficiency of product delivery and administration, superior hemostatic function in vitro, reduced donor exposure, less confusion when delivering balanced ratios, and, in one pediatric observational study and in numerous adult studies, improved survival in trauma patients who are coagulopathic are some of the advantages of whole blood for this patient.

10.14.2 What Is the Current Availability of Whole Blood for Administration?

According to a recent survey, up to 18% of pediatric trauma centers provide whole blood, but that percentage is increasing along with the types of cases and patient conditions treated with whole blood.

10.14.3 What Is the Current Criteria for Whole Blood for Administration in Children?

The current criteria for whole blood administration in children are usually limited by patient age and transfusion volume. Permitted only under institutional protocol that addresses indications, blood characteristics, and maximum volumes, whole blood up to 40 mL/kg is now administered to children as young as newborn age in the US.

10.14.4 In What Pediatric Patient Populations Is Whole Blood Currently Used?

Trauma is the major indication for whole blood (LTOWB) in children, but its use is expanding to surgeries with large blood loss and severely anemic patients.

10.14.5 Does the Use of Whole Blood Improve Patient Outcomes in the Pediatric Patient Population?

Recent prospective observational and retrospective studies of children who have received LTOWB continue to report relatively successful outcomes, adequate hemostatic resuscitation, and safety in younger age groups.

10.14.6 What Is the Risk of Hemolysis from Whole Blood Administration?

ABO blood type incompatibility between the donor(s) and recipient is a concern with the use of type O whole blood in random patients with unknown blood type. Recent clinical studies in both children and adults suggest that LTOWB does not produce laboratory evidence of hemolysis from the anti-A and anti-B antibodies in the plasma of LTOWB (with titers <256) when administered to trauma patients of unknown blood type. Recent small studies have not found differences in the clinical safety profiles between LTOWB and component therapy resuscitation in this patient population.

10.14.7 Are There Special Considerations When Administering Whole Blood to Female Patients?

Female patients who are RhD negative blood type and are transfused with RhD positive blood cells may become "sensitized" and develop antibodies against the RBC RhD positive antigen. If they become pregnant with an RhD positive fetus, HDFN may result. The practice of administering RhD positive type O whole blood to females of childbearing age and unknown blood type remains controversial; however, it's use may be lifesaving in certain situations and should not be withheld because RhD negative blood is unavailable.

10.14.8 What Are the Components of Whole Blood, Including Preservatives?

Whole blood has a higher hematocrit, platelet count, percentage of coagulation factors, and less anticoagulant volumes than the equivalent components administered together in a 1:1:1 ratio (RBC/plasma/platelets).

10.14.9 What Is the Known Coagulation Profile and Efficacy of Platelets in Cold-Stored Whole Blood?

At this point in time, there is no evidence that the hemostatic function of platelets or any other coagulation factor in cold-stored LTOWB contributes to a clinical coagulopathy when used for the resuscitation of traumatized children.

10.14.10 Can Whole Blood Undergo Leukocyte Reduction (LR)?

Yes, and if the whole blood is distributed by a donor center, the leukocyte reduction is probably performed before distribution to the hospital. If not, the whole blood can be infused through a bedside LR filter; however, this will significantly reduce the potential flow rate. Furthermore, LR filters are not always available in many hospitals for bedside use.

10.14.11 How Might Whole Blood Administration to Trauma Patients Fit Into a Patient Blood Management (PBM) Program?

- Decreased blood loss during resuscitation, thus preserving the patient's RBC mass.
- Individualizing the patient's care through reduced donor exposure.
- Possible improved outcomes including likelihood of survival and total volumes of transfused blood product.

Key Points

- Many pediatric hospitals are expanding the use of whole blood to include patients with massive hemorrhage from any cause, thus adding to the research on the potential benefits of whole blood use in children.
- Concerns about hemolysis from administering type O whole blood to patients of unknown blood type are currently mitigated by screening for low titer anti-A and anti-B antibodies in plasma of donor whole blood.
- Many hospital centers administer RhD positive blood products to women of childbearing age and young children who are exsanguinating to preserve the patient's life and also the scarce type O (universal donor) blood supply.
- When type-specific blood is not available, administration of type ABO-compatible blood components or LTOWB may be lifesaving.

References

1. Zielinski MD, Stubbs JR, Berns KS, Glassberg E, Murdock AD, Shinar E, et al. Prehospital blood transfusion programs: capabilities and lessons learned. J Trauma Acute Care Surg. 2017;82(6S Suppl 1):S70–S8.
2. Alquist C, Harm SK. Transfusion service related activities. In: Cohn C, Delaney M, Johnson ST, Katz LM, editors. Technical manual. 20th ed. Bethesda, MD: AABB; 2020. p. 503–504, 510–517, 522–523, 525, 528–530.
3. Shackelford SA, Gurney JM, Taylor AL, Keenan S, Corley JB, Cunningham CW, et al. Joint trauma system, defense committee on trauma, and armed services blood program consensus statement on whole blood. Transfusion. 2021;61(Suppl 1):S333–S5.
4. Braverman MA, Smith A, Pokorny D, Axtman B, Shahan CP, Barry L, et al. Prehospital whole blood reduces early mortality in patients with hemorrhagic shock. Transfusion. 2021;61(Suppl 1):S15–21.
5. McCoy CC, Brenner M, Duchesne J, Roberts D, Ferrada P, Horer T, et al. Back to the future: whole blood resuscitation of the severely injured trauma patient. Shock. 2021;56(1S):9–15.
6. Spinella PC, Cap AP. Whole blood: back to the future. Curr Opin Hematol. 2016;23(6):536–42.
7. Mendoza AB, Ngamsuntikul S, Quesada JF. Integrated programs for trauma and disaster response: a regional blood center perspective. AABB NEWS; 2023. p. 16–7.
8. Manno CS, Hedberg KW, Kim HC, Bunin GR, Nicolson S, Jobes D, et al. Comparison of the hemostatic effects of fresh whole blood, stored whole blood, and components after open heart surgery in children. Blood. 1991;77(5):930–6.
9. Jobes DR, Sesok-Pizzini D, Friedman D. Reduced transfusion requirement with use of fresh whole blood in pediatric cardiac surgical procedures. Ann Thorac Surg. 2015;99(5):1706–11.
10. Valleley MS, Buckley KW, Hayes KM, Fortuna RR, Geiss DM, Holt DW. Are there benefits to a fresh whole blood vs. packed red blood cell cardiopulmonary bypass prime on outcomes in neonatal and pediatric cardiac surgery? J Extra Corpor Technol. 2007;39(3):168–76.
11. Thottathil P, Sesok-Pizzini D, Taylor JA, Fiadjoe JE, Vincent A, Stricker PA. Whole blood in pediatric craniofacial reconstruction surgery. J Craniofac Surg. 2017;28(5):1175–8.
12. Vasan PK, Rajasekaran S, Viswanathan VK, Shetty AP, Kanna RM. Is fresh, leucodepleted, whole blood transfusion superior to blood component transfusion in pediatric patients undergoing spinal deformity surgeries? A prospective, randomized study analyzing postoperative serological parameters and clinical recovery. Eur Spine J. 2021;30(7):1943–9.
13. AABB. Circular of Information For the Use of Human Blood and Blood Components. 2021. https://www.aabb.org/docs/default-source/default-document-library/resources/circular-of-information-watermark.pdf. Accessed 6 July 2023.
14. Hanna M, Knittel J, Gillihan J. The use of whole blood transfusion in trauma. Curr Anesthesiol Rep. 2022;12(2):234–9.
15. Shea SM, Staudt AM, Thomas KA, Schuerer D, Mielke JE, Folkerts D, et al. The use of low-titer group O whole blood is independently associated with improved survival compared to component therapy in adults with severe traumatic hemorrhage. Transfusion. 2020;60(Suppl 3):S2–9.
16. Williams J, Merutka N, Meyer D, Bai Y, Prater S, Cabrera R, et al. Safety profile and impact of low-titer group O whole blood for emergency use in trauma. J Trauma Acute Care Surg. 2020;88(1):87–93.
17. Torres CM, Kent A, Scantling D, Joseph B, Haut ER, Sakran JV. Association of Whole Blood with Survival among Patients Presenting with Severe Hemorrhage in US and Canadian adult civilian trauma centers. JAMA Surg. 2023;158:532.
18. Gaines BA, Yazer MH, Triulzi DJ, Sperry JL, Neal MD, Billiar TR, Leeper CM. Low titer group O whole blood in injured children requiring massive transfusion. Ann Surg. 2023;277(4):e919–e24.
19. Abou Khalil E, Morgan KM, Gaines BA, Spinella PC, Leeper CM. Use of whole blood in pediatric trauma: a narrative review. Trauma Surg Acute Care Open. 2024;9(Suppl 1):e001127.

20. Leeper CM, Yazer MH, Triulzi DJ, Neal MD, Gaines BA. Whole blood is superior to component transfusion for injured children: a propensity matched analysis. Ann Surg. 2020;272(4):590–4.
21. Leeper CM, Yazer MH, Cladis FP, Saladino R, Triulzi DJ, Gaines BA. Use of Uncrossmatched cold-stored whole blood in injured children with hemorrhagic shock. JAMA Pediatr. 2018;172(5):491–2.
22. Seheult JN, Bahr M, Anto V, Alarcon LH, Corcos A, Sperry JL, et al. Safety profile of uncrossmatched, cold-stored, low-titer, group O+ whole blood in civilian trauma patients. Transfusion. 2018;58(10):2280–8.
23. Dishong D, Cap AP, Holcomb JB, Triulzi DJ, Yazer MH. The rebirth of the cool: a narrative review of the clinical outcomes of cold stored low titer group O whole blood recipients compared to conventional component recipients in trauma. Hematology. 2021;26(1):601–11.
24. Nair PM, Pandya SG, Dallo SF, Reddoch KM, Montgomery RK, Pidcoke HF, et al. Platelets stored at 4 degrees C contribute to superior clot properties compared to current standard-of-care through fibrin-crosslinking. Br J Haematol. 2017;178(1):119–29.
25. Nair PM, Meledeo MA, Wells AR, Wu X, Bynum JA, Leung KP, et al. Cold-stored platelets have better preserved contractile function in comparison with room temperature-stored platelets over 21 days. Transfusion. 2021;61(Suppl 1):S68–79.
26. Pidcoke HF, Cap AP. Refrigerated platelets for the treatment of acute bleeding: a review of the literature and reexamination of current standards: reply. Shock. 2015;44(6):616–7.
27. Nelson O, Wu L, Swanson JW, Hsu G, Lambert MP, Obstfeld A, et al. Thromboelastography changes of whole blood compared to blood component transfusion in infant Craniosynostosis surgery. J Craniofac Surg. 2022;33(1):129–33.
28. Strandenes G, Austlid I, Apelseth TO, Hervig TA, Sommerfelt-Pettersen J, Herzig MC, et al. Coagulation function of stored whole blood is preserved for 14 days in austere conditions: a ROTEM feasibility study during a Norwegian antipiracy mission and comparison to equal ratio reconstituted blood. J Trauma Acute Care Surg. 2015;78(6 Suppl 1):S31–8.
29. van der Meer PF, Klei TR, de Korte D. Quality of platelets in stored whole blood. Transfus Med Rev. 2020;34(4):234–41.
30. Kristoffersen EK, Apelseth TO. Platelet functionality in cold-stored whole blood. VOXS. 2019;14:308–14. https://doi.org/10.1111/voxs.12501.
31. Acker J, Razatos A. Whole blood and apheresis collection of blood components intended for transfusion. In: Cohn C, Delaney M, Johnson ST, Katz LM, editors. Technical manual. 20th ed. Bethesda, MD: AABB; 2020. p. 145–147, 159–161.
32. Yazer MH, Woolley T. Introduction to THOR supplement. Transfusion. 2020;60(Suppl 3):S1.
33. Wong ECC, Punzalan RC. Neonatal and pediatric transfusion practice. In: Cohn C, Delaney M, Johnson ST, Katz LM, editors. Technical manual. 20th ed. Bethesda, MD: AABB; 2020. p. 676, 685, 689–692.
34. McCartney J. Whole blood in resuscitating trauma patients is making a comeback. ACS/American College of Surgeons Bulletin; 2023. https://www.facs.org/for-medical-professionals/news-publications/news-and-articles/bulletin/2023/april-2023-volume-108-issue-4/whole-blood-in-resuscitating-trauma-patients-is-making-a-comeback/. Accessed 7 July 2023.
35. Nowadly CD, Fisher AD, Borgman MA, Mdaki KS, Hill RL, Nicholson SE, et al. The use of whole blood transfusion during non-traumatic resuscitation. Mil Med. 2022;187(7–8):e821–e5.
36. Morris DS, Braverman MA, Corean J, Myers JC, Xenakis E, Ireland K, et al. Whole blood for postpartum hemorrhage: early experience at two institutions. Transfusion. 2020;60(Suppl 3):S31–S5.
37. Carr NR, Hulse WL, Bahr TM, Davidson JM, Ilstrup SJ, Christensen RD. First report of transfusing low-titer cold-stored type O whole blood to an extremely-low-birth-weight neonate after acute blood loss. Transfusion. 2022;62(9):1923–6.
38. Lucisano AC, Leeper CM, Gaines BA. Trauma-induced coagulopathy in children. Semin Thromb Hemost. 2020;46(2):147–54.
39. Yazer MH, Spinella PC. An international survey on the use of low titer group O whole blood for the resuscitation of civilian trauma patients in 2020. Transfusion. 2020;60(Suppl 3):S176–S9.

40. Kolodziej JH, Leonard JC, Josephson CD, Gaines BA, Wisniewski SR, Yazer MH, Spinella PC. Survey to inform trial of low-titer group O whole-blood compared to conventional blood components for children with severe traumatic bleeding. Transfusion. 2021;61(Suppl 1):S43–S8.
41. Meshkin D, Yazer MH, Dunbar NM, Spinella PC, Leeper CM. Low titer group O whole blood utilization in pediatric trauma resuscitation: a National Survey. Transfusion. 2022;62(Suppl 1):S63–71.
42. Morgan KM, Yazer MH, Triulzi DJ, Strotmeyer S, Gaines BA, Leeper CM. Safety profile of low-titer group O whole blood in pediatric patients with massive hemorrhage. Transfusion. 2021;61(Suppl 1):S8–S14.
43. Weymouth W, Long B, Koyfman A, Winckler C. Whole blood in trauma: a review for emergency clinicians. J Emerg Med. 2019;56(5):491–8.
44. Perea LL, Moore K, Docherty C, Nguyen U, Seamon MJ, Byrne JP, et al. Whole blood resuscitation is safe in pediatric trauma patients: a multicenter study. Am Surg. 2023;89(7):3058.
45. Anand T, Obaid O, Nelson A, Chehab M, Ditillo M, Hammad A, et al. Whole blood hemostatic resuscitation in pediatric trauma: a nationwide propensity-matched analysis. J Trauma Acute Care Surg. 2021;91(4):573–8.
46. Mou SS, Giroir BP, Molitor-Kirsch EA, Leonard SR, Nikaidoh H, Nizzi F, et al. Fresh whole blood versus reconstituted blood for pump priming in heart surgery in infants. N Engl J Med. 2004;351(16):1635–44.
47. Leeper CM, Yazer MH, Morgan KM, Triulzi DJ, Gaines BA. Adverse events after low titer group O whole blood versus component product transfusion in pediatric trauma patients: a propensity-matched cohort study. Transfusion. 2021;61(9):2621–8.
48. Lauby RS, Cuenca CM, Borgman MA, Fisher AD, Bebarta VS, Moore EE, et al. An analysis of outcomes for pediatric trauma warm fresh whole blood recipients in Iraq and Afghanistan. Transfusion. 2021;61(Suppl 1):S2–7.
49. American Red Cross. Facts About Blood and Blood Types (2022). https://www.redcrossblood.org/donate-blood/blood-types.html . Accessed 9 July 2023.
50. Kelley JM, Cushing MM. Transfusion support for hematopoietic stem cell transplant recipients. In: Cohn C, Delaney M, Johnson ST, Katz LM, editors. Technical manual. 20th ed. Bethesda, MD: AABB; 2020. p. 771.
51. Cavagnetto C, Alejo Blanco R, McKenna H, Willmott L, Aydogdu E, Akinyemi N, et al. Residual red cells in blood components: a multisite study of fully automated enumeration using a hematology analyzer. Transfusion. 2021;61(2):568–78.
52. Fung MK. Technical manual. 19th ed. Bethesda: AABB Press; 2017. p. 115, 120–121, 127, 265–291, 464–469, 481–489, 492–493, 632.
53. Berséus O, Boman K, Nessen SC, Westerberg LA. Risks of hemolysis due to anti-a and anti-B caused by the transfusion of blood or blood components containing ABO-incompatible plasma. Transfusion. 2013;53(Suppl 1):114S–23S.
54. Braverman MA, Smith AA, Ciaraglia AV, Radowsky JS, Schauer SG, Sams VG, et al. The regional whole blood program in San Antonio, TX: a 3-year update on prehospital and in-hospital transfusion practices for traumatic and non-traumatic hemorrhage. Transfusion. 2022;62(Suppl 1):S80–S9.
55. Harrold IM, Seheult JN, Alarcon LH, Corcos A, Sperry JL, Triulzi DJ, Yazer MH. Hemolytic markers following the transfusion of uncrossmatched, cold-stored, low-titer, group O+ whole blood in civilian trauma patients. Transfusion. 2020;60(Suppl 3):S24–30.
56. Yazer MH, Spinella PC, Anto V, Dunbar NM. Survey of group a plasma and low-titer group O whole blood use in trauma resuscitation at adult civilian level 1 trauma centers in the US. Transfusion. 2021;61(6):1757–63.
57. Yazer MH, Dunbar NM, Delaney M, Collaborative BEfST. Survey of the RhD selection and issuing practices for uncrossmatched blood products at pediatric trauma hospitals in the United States: the BEST collaborative study. Transfusion. 2021;61(12):3328–34.

58. Clayton S, Leeper CM, Yazer MH, Spinella PC. Survey of policies at US hospitals on the selection of RhD type of low-titer O whole blood for use in trauma resuscitation. Transfusion. 2024;64:S111.
59. Murphy M, BenAvram D. Recommendations on the Use of Group O Red Blood Cells. AABB. 2019 (update 2022). https://www.aabb.org/docs/default-source/default-document-library/resources/association-bulletins/ab19-02.pdf. Accessed 21 July 2023.
60. Yazer MH, Panko G, Holcomb JB, Kaplan A, Leeper C, Seheult JN, et al. Not as "D"eadly as once thought - the risk of D-alloimmunization and hemolytic disease of the fetus and newborn following RhD-positive transfusion in trauma. Hematology. 2023;28(1):2161215.
61. Practice Bulletin No. 181 summary: prevention of Rh D Alloimmunization. Obstet Gynecol. 2017;130(2):481–3.
62. Jain V, Chari R, Maslovitz S, Farine D, Maternal Fetal Medicine C, Bujold E, et al. Guidelines for the management of a pregnant trauma patient. J Obstet Gynaecol Can. 2015;37(6):553–74.
63. Munisteri M, Wong R, Brown VG. Preventing Alloimmunization in the trauma setting: a case report and development of a multidisciplinary protocol. J Womens Health Reproduct Med. 2021;5(6):23.
64. US Food and Drug Administration (FDA). Exceptions and Alternative Procedures Approved Under 21 CFR 640.120(a). 2023. https://www.fda.gov/media/124235/download. Accessed 10 July 2023.
65. Shea SM, Reisz JA, Mihalko EP, Rahn KC, Rassam RMG, Chitrakar A, et al. Cold-stored platelet hemostatic capacity is maintained for three weeks of storage and associated with taurine metabolism. J Thromb Haemost. 2023;22:1154.
66. McRae HL, Kara F, Milito C, Cahill C, Blumberg N, Refaai MA. Whole blood haemostatic function throughout a 28-day cold storage period: an in vitro study. Vox Sang. 2021;116(2):190–6.
67. Leeper CM, Yazer MH, Cladis FP, Saladino R, Triulzi DJ, Gaines BA. Cold-stored whole blood platelet function is preserved in injured children with hemorrhagic shock. J Trauma Acute Care Surg. 2019;87(1):49–53.
68. Thomas KA, Shea SM, Yazer MH, Spinella PC. Effect of leukoreduction and pathogen reduction on the hemostatic function of whole blood. Transfusion. 2019;59(S2):1539–48.
69. Keneally RJ, Gonzalez-Almada A, Wargowsky R, Fernandez X, Kochar O, Cresswell G, et al. In vitro analysis of platelet adhesion, aggregation, and surface GP1balpha expression in stored refrigerated whole blood: a pilot study. Anesth Analg. 2023;136(5):920–6.
70. Huish S, Green L, Kempster C, Smethurst P, Wiltshire M, Prajapati C, et al. A comparison of platelet function in cold-stored whole blood and platelet concentrates. Transfusion. 2021;61(11):3224–35.
71. Haddaway K, Bloch EM, Tobian AAR, Frank SM, Sikorski R, Cho BC, et al. Hemostatic properties of cold-stored whole blood leukoreduced using a platelet-sparing versus a non-platelet-sparing filter. Transfusion. 2019;59(5):1809–17.
72. Zaza M, Meyer DE, Wang YW, George M, Daniels K, Cardenas JC, Cotton BA. The impact of rapid infuser use on the platelet count, platelet function, and hemostatic potential of whole blood. J Surg Res. 2021;260:76–81.
73. Valencia Morales DJ, Klompas AM, Torbenson JM, Finney RE, Chen D, Stubbs JR, Nuttall GA. Cold platelet transfusion: the effects of a fluid warmer on platelet function. Transfusion. 2024;64(1):47–52.
74. Mattson MK, Groves C, Smith MM, Christensen JM, Chen D, Stubbs JR, et al. Platelet transfusion: the effects of a fluid warmer on platelet function. Transfusion. 2021;61(1):52–6.
75. Bianchi M, Vaglio S, Pupella S, Marano G, Facco G, Liumbruno GM, Grazzini G. Leucoreduction of blood components: an effective way to increase blood safety? Blood Transfus. 2016;14(2):214–27.
76. Crowder LA, Steele WR, Stramer SL. Infectious disease screening. In: Cohn C, Delaney M, Johnson ST, Katz LM, editors. Technical manual. 20th ed. Bethesda, MD: AABB; 2020. p. 173, 198, 213.

77. Rice J, Bill JR, Razatos A, Marschner S. Platelet aggregation in whole blood is not impaired by a platelet-sparing leukoreduction filter and instead depends upon the presence of leukocytes. Transfusion. 2021;61(Suppl 1):S90–S100.
78. Snyder EL, Whitley P, Kingsbury T, Miripol J, Tormey CA. In vitro and in vivo evaluation of a whole blood platelet-sparing leukoreduction filtration system. Transfusion. 2010;50(10):2145–51.
79. Turner CP, Sutherland J, Wadhwa M, Dilger P, Cardigan R. In vitro function of platelet concentrates prepared after filtration of whole blood or buffy coat pools. Vox Sang. 2005;88(3):164–71.
80. Australian and New Zealand Society of Blood Transfusion, Guidelines for the Prevention of Transfusion-Associated Graft-Versus-Host Disease (TA-GVHD), 2nd ed., 2024. https://anzsbt.org.au/wp-content/uploads/2024/02/TAGVHD-Guideines-2024.pdf. Accessed 7 Mar 2024.
81. Association for the Advancement of Blood & Biotherapies (AABB). Regulatory & Advocacy. Whole Blood and Red Blood Cell Components. 2023. https://www.aabb.org/regulatory-and-advocacy/regulatory-affairs/regulatory-for-blood/whole-blood-and-red-blood-cell-components. Accessed 13 July 2023.
82. Jobes D, Wolfe Y, O'Neill D, Calder J, Jones L, Sesok-Pizzini D, Zheng XL. Toward a definition of "fresh" whole blood: an in vitro characterization of coagulation properties in refrigerated whole blood for transfusion. Transfusion. 2011;51(1):43–51.

11 Intraoperative Cell Salvage (ICS)

Destiny F. Chau, Timothy Hunsinger, and Jonathan H. Waters

11.1 Case Scenario

A 5-year-old, 20 kg child with hepatoblastoma is scheduled for a liver tumor resection. He has undergone preoperative anemia treatment. His hemoglobin (Hgb) is 13 g/dL and coagulation studies are normal. The surgeon warns you that a large blood loss is expected. There is a national shortage of blood donations, and the blood bank has asked for judicious use of this resource. You are planning intraoperative cell salvage (ICS) as part of perioperative patient blood management (PBM) to minimize the need for an allogeneic transfusion. The parents have given informed consent to the use of ICS.

Key Learning Objectives

- What are the advantages of ICS?
- What are the indications for ICS?
- What are absolute and relative contraindications to ICS?
- Does ICS reduce allogeneic transfusions?
- Is ICS cost-effective?
- How does the ICS process work?
- What is the quantity and quality of red blood cells (RBCs) in a unit of ICS-recovered blood?
- What adverse effects are associated with ICS-recovered blood administration?
- Is ICS recommended by professional organizations?

D. F. Chau (✉) · T. Hunsinger · J. H. Waters
Department of Anesthesiology and Pain Medicine, University of Arkansas for Medical Sciences, Arkansas Children's Hospital, Little Rock, AR, USA

University of Pittsburgh Medical Center, Magee-Womens Hospital, Pittsburgh, PA, USA
e-mail: dchau@uams.edu; HunsingerTS@archildrens.org; watejh@upmc.edu

N. J. Klein (ed.), *Perioperative Pediatric Patient Blood Management and Transfusion Safety*, https://doi.org/10.1007/978-3-031-81666-6_11

11.2 Discussion

11.2.1 General

Patient blood management (PBM) planning in blood loss cases is a multidisciplinary task and includes the preoperative optimization of hemoglobin levels along with intra-and postoperative strategies for blood conservation. Autologous blood salvage for reinfusion conserves the patient's own red blood cells (RBCs) and reduces allogeneic blood requirements. Several professional organizations support ICS as part of a perioperative pediatric PBM program such as the Network for the Advancement of PBM (NATA), the National Blood Authority (Australia), and the Association of Anaesthetists (United Kingdom, UK) [1–3]. This chapter will discuss the clinical considerations in the decision to utilize ICS, its effectiveness in minimizing allogeneic blood transfusion, and the technical implications for patient safety.

11.2.2 What Are the Advantages of ICS?

Intraoperative cell salvage (ICS)—also commonly referred to as cell saver, autologous blood recovery, or autotransfusion—is a blood conservation technique in which the patient's operative blood loss is collected and processed so that RBCs can be reinfused as needed. Intraoperative autologous blood recovery is recommended in invasive procedures where substantial blood loss is anticipated. ICS offers several advantages, including the following:

- No preoperative screening or testing is necessary.
- Provides prompt availability of red cells and in amounts proportional to blood loss.
- Reduces exposure to allogeneic red cells and associated complications.
- Preserves the community blood supply.
- Serves as a blood supply for patients who are a difficult crossmatch because they possess multiple alloantibodies.
- A staged or "collect only" mode can be set up in cases where major blood loss is possible but difficult to predict.
- Supports donor exposure reduction for children undergoing heart surgery with cardiopulmonary bypass.
- Setup is relatively easy for unexpected major bleeding, such as is seen in trauma and obstetrics.

ICS had its beginnings in the1970s, with its popularity increasing into the 1980s, due to concerns over transfusion transmitted infections (TTIs), particularly the emergence of HIV. Over the next few decades, improvement in blood screening significantly decreased the risk of TTIs with a return to allogeneic blood use and a decline in ICS. At present, there is an increased awareness of the non-infectious hazards associated with allogeneic blood transfusions along with a critical global shortage of blood that is expected to continue [4, 5]. Adverse transfusion-related events are reported to occur more frequently in children compared to adults [6, 7]. There is also evidence in the literature that implementation of patient blood management (PBM) bundles, including ICS, may improve patient outcomes [8–14]. As a result, there is increased interest in cell salvage use during the perioperative period. This renewed interest has been bolstered by modern advances in ICS technology permitting more efficient use in children [3, 15].

11.2.3 What Are the Indications for ICS?

11.2.3.1 The Patient

In adults, ICS has been traditionally recommended when a surgical procedure is expected to be associated with the following degrees of blood loss [2, 3, 14, 16, 17]:

- A surgical procedure where the maximum surgical blood ordering schedule (MSBOS) predicts that one unit of allogeneic blood may need to be transfused, on average.
- Greater than 10% of patients undergoing a particular procedure are historically transfused.
- An anticipated blood loss greater than 500 mL or 1000 mL.
- An anticipated blood loss greater than 10% or 20% of the patient's estimated blood volume (EBV).

ICS should also be considered when a patient has a rare RBC antigen and procuring compatible blood is difficult. Furthermore, many patients who refuse allogeneic blood transfusions are willing to undergo ICS.

While ICS use is widely accepted and commonplace in adult surgeries, its use in children can be somewhat limited. The primary constraint is reconciling cost expenditure against the ability to procure adequate amounts of blood to process (which is relatively small due to children's small total blood volumes). The indication for pediatric cell salvage as determined by anticipated blood loss varies in the literature: greater than 10–40% of the patient's EBV, the latter volume of blood loss being most commonly used to trigger a pediatric massive transfusion protocol (MTP) [3, 18–22]. In all cases of unpredictable blood loss, a cell salvage machine can be set up in "collect" mode for salvage of lost blood that can be processed on an as-needed basis (see below). The Association of Anaesthetists (in the United Kingdom; UK) recommends that at a minimum, the "collect only" or "reserve" mode be considered when anticipated blood loss is greater than 8 mL/kg or 10% of EBV and the child's weight is at least 10 kg [3]. ICS is routinely used today in pediatric cardiac surgery under cardiopulmonary bypass; in these cases children less than 2 kg have undergone autotransfusion via ICS [19].

11.2.4 The Procedure

Preoperative hematocrit (Hct), gender, age, and body weight influence the risks associated with receiving allogeneic blood components versus ICS. Blood recovery may be indicated in different surgery types, and these cases should be individualized based on the judgment of the anesthesiologist and the surgeon. Common indications for ICS in pediatric and adult patient populations include craniofacial, spinal, liver transplant, major orthopedic, vascular, general, and cardiothoracic surgery [18, 23]. In addition, the American College of Obstetricians and Gynecologists (ACOG) approves the use of cell salvage during cesarean section (C-section) when properly conducted post-delivery [24–26]. This includes copious irrigation of the surgical field, use of two separate suction setups, and a greater volume of saline bowl wash. Select indications for use during C-section include severe anemia, thrombocytopenia, placental abruption, and abnormal placentation.

11.2.5 What Are Absolute and Relative Contraindications to ICS?

Although the science of cell salvage is still evolving, the literature and various machine manufacturers list contraindications based on either known or theoretical adverse effects. There are few *absolute* contraindications to ICS, including:

- Aspiration of substances from the surgical field that could destroy red cells in the collection reservoir or are toxic (e.g., sterile water, alcohol, hydrogen peroxide, hypotonic solutions, iodine)
- Microfibrillar collagen hemostatic agents and tissue adhesives such as topical thrombin and fibrin glue in the surgical field
- Vasoactive drugs in the surgical field (e.g., oxymetazoline (Afrin), epinephrine)
- Frank stool in the surgical field
- Patient or guardian refusal

Table 11.1 illustrates common *relative* contraindications to ICS [3, 18]. In cancer cases and others in which bacteremia may be an issue, the use of leukocyte reduction filters (LRFs) may reduce the infection or systemic cancer risk. Studies are ongoing and inconclusive. During tumor surgery, hematogenous spread of cancer cells is common at baseline [23, 27, 28]. Also, bacteria, cancer cells, and amniotic fluid will be removed with proper washing and filtration. As aptly stated by the National Blood Authority (Australia), "All staff operating cell salvage devices should receive appropriate training, to ensure knowledge of the technique and proficiency in using it" [2]

Table 11.1 Relative contraindications to intraoperative cell salvage (ICS)

Relative contraindication	Rationale	Alternative
Immune-mediated, heparin-induced thrombocytopenia (HIT)	Residual heparin solution (used for ICS) in salvaged red cells could cause destruction of circulating platelets	Use acid-citrate-dextrose (ACD) solution for anticoagulation
Red cell disorders (sickle cell trait, thalassemia)	Salvaged red cells could hemolyze or sickle	Consult with hematology before utilizing ICS; check for lysis or sickling of salvaged red cells prior to transfusion. Obtain patient consent for ICS. Proceed with caution Reports describe the successful use of ICS in patients with sickle cell trait and thalassemia. However, increased sickling has been reported with up to 50% of RBCs after processing [29–31] Increased hemolysis in patients with spherocytosis has also been reported
Contamination or infection at surgical site	Residual bacteria in salvaged red cells may cause bacteremia	Utilize ICS on a case-by-case basis for surgery involving open bowel or an infected wound There are multiple reports of successful use of ICS (washing) and specific use of leukocyte reduction filter (LRF) in cases with potential or unobserved contamination/infection (vs. gross/observed); no bacteremia or sepsis in outcomes reported [32]
Cancer at surgical site	Residual tumor cells in salvaged red cells could disseminate cancer	Utilize ICS on a case-by-case basis for surgery involving resection of a malignant tumor There are multiple reports of successful use of ICS and additional specific use of LRF in cases of cancer resection [33–35]
Obstetrics	Aspiration of amniotic fluid along with the aspirated blood. Residual amniotic fluid in ICS blood can lead to poor outcomes	Many centers routinely use ICS successfully in cesarean deliveries, now approved by ACOG [25] Use separate suctions and copious irrigation after uterine closure If mother is RhD antigen negative, monitor for antibody formation and also cord blood for fetal RhD status; consider anti-D immunoglobulin administration if mother not already RhD-sensitized [36]

(continued)

Table 11.1 (continued)

Relative contraindication	Rationale	Alternative
Orthopedics	Contamination of salvaged red cells with bone cement (methyl methacrylate), bone graft, bone substitutes or titanium fragments (with revision surgery) could cause aggregation of circulating platelets or embolus with ensuing sequela	Do not utilize ICS until bone cement (methyl methacrylate) is fully set Utilize standard (waste) suction, with generous irrigation for removal of other contaminants Transfusion should include use of LRF Exercise caution with revision cases; a 40-micron microaggregate filter will not eliminate the smallest of titanium fragments
Biologics/hemostatic agents	Clotting of equipment by hemostatic agents used for processing during ICS Contamination of salvaged red cells from biologics or hemostatic agents could cause aggregation of circulating platelets or embolus	Utilize standard (waste) suction, with generous irrigation for removal of contaminants Processing should include washing of red cells; transfusion should include use of LRF
Electrocautery (carbon monoxide in plume)	Hemoglobin has a higher affinity for carbon monoxide (CO); salvaged red cells with COHb could significantly reduce total oxygen-carrying capacity.	ICS (aspiration line) should not be used for electrocautery plume reduction

LRF leukocyte reduction filter

11.3 Does ICS Reduce Allogeneic Transfusions?

A primary goal of ICS is to reduce a patient's likelihood of receiving an allogeneic transfusion. Current evidence supports a role for ICS in decreasing allogeneic blood transfusions in blood loss surgeries. The literature for ICS comes primarily from the adult patient population, demonstrating no increased risk of adverse events when properly managed. A 2016 database review of a nine-hospital system providing quality oversight of ICS examined 43,198 patients who were managed with perioperative ICS over an 11-year period [37]. Potential adverse events were observed in two patients: dyspnea with rigors after a cesarean delivery and dyspnea plus hypotension following postpartum hemorrhage. It was unclear if the symptoms were related to ICS; both patients recovered without sequelae.

A Cochrane systematic review analyzed 67 prospective randomized ICS trials and found a 38% decrease in the rate of exposure to allogeneic transfusions (odds ratio, OR 0.62; 95% confidence interval, CI 0.55–0.70; NNT 4.8) [38] The largest relative risk reduction (RRR) occurred among orthopedic surgery patients (RRR 54%; 95% CI 43%–63%). Secondary outcomes such as thrombotic events, wound complications, infections, length of stay, and mortality were not impacted by cell salvage usage. A subgroup analysis of eight trials using ICS alone showed that the relative risk of exposure to allogeneic blood transfusion was 0.59 (95% CI 0.46 to 0.76). Heterogeneity was high among all trials. A meta-analysis of 31 randomized controlled trials including over 2000 cardiac surgery patients found that ICS reduced the rate of exposure to allogeneic blood products by 37% (OR 0.63, 95% CI: 0.43–0.94) or RBC transfusion by 40% (OR 0.60, 95% CI: 0.39–0.92) [39]. ICS also reduced the total volume of transfused allogeneic blood products per patient by a weighted mean difference of 256 mL. All other outcomes—stroke, renal dysfunction, atrial fibrillation, infection, and in-hospital mortality—were similar between groups. A more recent meta-analysis of 15 controlled trials found that ICS during cardiac surgery did not lead to a reduction on the transfusion rates of RBC, platelets, or FFP [40]. These authors noted the high heterogeneity of available studies.

A limitation of the meta-analysis design is that the included studies often cover a period of many years during which practices and techniques undergo significant modification. A meta-analysis of clinical trials that examined cell salvage use in total hip and knee arthroplasty found that cell salvage reduced the rate and the volume of allogeneic RBCs transfused during both procedures in studies published before 2010 [41]. However, in later trials, ICS was found to not impact exposure rate or volume of allogeneic RBCs. Investigators in the meta-analysis speculated that this apparent change in ICS efficacy may be attributed to a wider acceptance of PBM's multimodal perioperative strategies such as preoperative anemia treatment, antifibrinolytic use, and restrictive transfusion thresholds. In any event, restrictive transfusion thresholds and a general awareness of the potential hazards of blood transfusion have led to lower overall use of transfusions in general [42]. Over the past two decades, minimally invasive surgical methods and advances in surgical techniques have also been associated with decreased blood loss and transfusion requirements [43]. In summary, the general consensus is that ICS remains as a valuable adjunct to perioperative PBM in blood loss surgeries and, when used in selected patients in conjunction with other blood conservation strategies, leads to a reduction in the need for allogeneic blood transfusion, less donor exposure, and improved outcomes without an increase in complication rates [3, 44–46].

11.3.1 ICS in Pediatric Surgery

As with adult surgeries, ICS is most successful in the pediatric surgical population when used as part of a comprehensive PBM program. As an example, spinal correction surgery is associated with significant blood loss. A retrospective review studied the effects of a quality improvement (QI) program for children undergoing scoliosis correction surgeries (n = 1039). The program included preoperative hemoglobin optimization, ICS, tranexamic acid use, and transfusion criteria awareness education. This practice bundle was associated with large and sustained reductions in allogeneic blood transfusions. Another retrospective study found that ICS decreased allogeneic transfusion rates and volume in surgeries longer than 6 h and EBL greater than 30% EBV [47]. Two other relatively small studies randomized consecutive scoliosis patients into ICS and non-ICS groups [48, 49]. Both studies found that lower intra-and perioperative allogeneic blood rates were associated with ICS.

Studies in craniosynostosis surgery have also found a reduction in allogeneic blood transfusion rates with ICS implementation [50–52]. Similar to scoliosis surgery, ICS is more likely to be effective when used as part of a bundle with other blood conservation modalities such as preoperative anemia treatment [53, 54]. Beethe et al. tested initiatives as part of a QI program including the use of ICS [54]. The result was an increase in the number (0–87%) of perioperative transfusion-free patients despite yields as small as 25 mL recovered from the surgical field.

ICS has also been shown to benefit pediatric cardiac surgery. Cholette et al. randomized 106 pediatric patients scheduled for cardiac surgery under cardiopulmonary bypass (CPB) to ICS and no-ICS groups [19]. The ICS group had a reduced mean number of RBC transfusions within 24 and 48 h postoperatively, although there was no difference between groups at day 7. In this study, the ICS blood was stored and administered 24 h following collection in the postoperative period. A 2018 retrospective review of children undergoing cardiac surgery with ICS implemented as a standard (which also included using residual circuit volume) found ICS decreased intraoperative RBC transfusions by a median difference of 138 mL/m^2 [55]. A trend toward reduced blood bank cost expenditure was also found. There was a decrease in adverse events in the ICS cohort, although the study was not powered to detect statistically significant differences in adverse events which are rare at baseline. Similarly, a study of 309 consecutive patients undergoing cardiac surgery where ICS was performed using residual pump prime showed decreased perioperative allogeneic RBC transfusion rates, without an increase in adverse events [56]. This study was also not powered to detect real differences in ICS-associated adverse events.

11.4 Is ICS Cost-Effective?

Case selection is important when considering the monetary costs of ICS. The benefit of avoiding allogeneic blood transfusion is an intangible source of potential "cost-savings." Waters et al. reported that cell salvage is cost-effective in adult surgical patients when at least one unit of RBCs is returned to the patient [57]. The cost of consumable equipment for one case is estimated to be one-half the cost of a unit of allogeneic RBCs, with the consideration that blood and other indirect costs such as labor vary between locations [14, 57]. Cost-effectiveness is improved when multiple units of blood are recovered and processed. In a "collect-only" mode, such as when the collection reservoir is set up for lower blood loss cases, the centrifuge bowl and processing tubing are opened only if the shed blood is sufficient to process (usually over 500 mL in adults and a function of the processing bowl size in children). Furthermore, if managed through a standardized and quality controlled program, an ICS device can be used to "wash" allogeneic blood (as in the case of pediatric cardiac surgery or massive transfusion when low-potassium units are sought) more rapidly and conveniently than washed blood from the blood bank (e.g., > 1 h) [58–60].

11.5 How Does the ICS Process Work?

RBC salvage, or ICS, refers to the collection, filtration, washing, and administration of blood lost into the surgical field. It can be done intra-and postoperatively. The following discussion addresses what is currently known about the RBC salvage process including some basic technical details of the cell-saver machine.

11.5.1 The Machine

The cell-saver is a free-standing machine that collects and processes blood suctioned from the surgical field, drapes, and drains. Blood can also be collected when saturated field gauze is allowed to soak in compatible crystalloid solution; large gauze are capable of holding up to approximately 100 mL of blood [14]. Figure 11.1 is a schematic illustration of a generic cell salvage machine containing collection reservoir, processing chamber, and irrigation solutions.

There are now several cell salvage devices available, classified as intermittent or continuous systems. An intermittent system fills the bowl and washes the collected blood in batches. A continuous system uses ongoing processing which enables the treatment of smaller amounts of shed blood that become available in a timely fashion [15, 61].

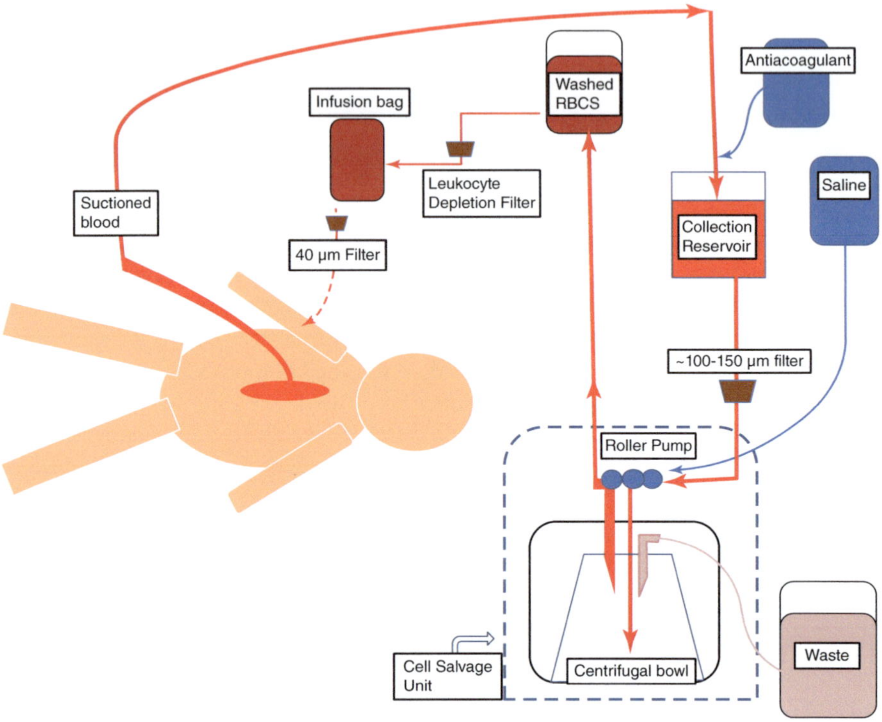

Fig. 11.1 Schematic diagram of the path of surgical site blood to the cell salvage unit and returned to the patient. The patient's untreated salvaged blood is mixed with anticoagulant-treated normal saline or Plasma-Lyte as it is suctioned from the surgical field. It is then filtered, centrifuged, washed, and ultimately returned to the patient from an infusion bag that is "burped" to eliminate air

11.5.2 The Process

The cell salvage process involves two major steps: collection and processing [23].

Collection phase*:* Blood in the surgical field is suctioned into a collection reservoir. The blood is suctioned through a coaxial tube arrangement that mixes suctioned blood with heparinized saline (30 units/mL; citrate is the anticoagulant of choice in patients who have a heparin allergy). This saline is set to run at 2–3 drops per second (or, 100 mL heparinized saline for every 500 mL blood collected). The flow of heparinized saline must be increased during periods of rapid bleeding to ensure anticoagulation. Only *trained* OR personnel are qualified to adjust the flow of the anticoagulant solution. To prevent undue RBC trauma, the tip of the suction catheter is best kept within the blood pool to avoid excessive atmospheric air bubbling. Baseline suction pressure must be fairly low (80–120 mmHg) to prevent shear-induced hemolysis, but the suction pressure should be increased during rapid bleeding [62]. Furthermore, shed blood must be quickly suctioned into the collection reservoir because static RBCs release cytokines and other inflammatory substances that may produce hemodynamic consequences when transfused.

Blood suctioned from the field is stored in the collection reservoir after passing through a system filter (100–150 micron) and is then stored until the proper ratio of blood to processing bowl size is collected. The bowl size chosen at the outset must be proportional to the anticipated blood loss for maximum efficiency. For example, a 250 mL processing bowl requires approximately 750 mL of blood in the collection reservoir; a 125 mL processing bowl requires approximately 375–500 mL of collected blood; a 70 mL bowl requires 200–300 mL collected blood. Once the proper ratio is achieved, your collection reservoir is ready to process (or, "spin"). It is important to note whether the spin cycle is set to automatic mode or if the spin must be manually triggered. If in the manual spin mode, you may need the assistance of the perfusionist or trained anesthesia technician to begin the processing phase.

The 40-to 150-micron filter in the collection reservoir is effective in sifting out macroaggregates such as fat, bone fragments, tissue, and gauze fibers. Other soluble substances, such as heparin, free hemoglobin, and potassium, are removed in the "wash out" phase (see below). If a lot of blood appears to be trapped in the collection reservoir filter, suctioning up more saline along with a shake of the reservoir can free up much of the trapped RBCs.

Processing phase: Often called the "spin" phase, once the proper amount of field blood is in the collection reservoir, the blood is then pumped via a roller pump into the processing bowl that spins to generate a centrifugal force. Relatively heavier cells (e.g., RBCs) are forced toward the sides of the bowl, whereas lighter cells or products (e.g., platelets and plasma) collect in the center of the processing bowl. As the bowl spins, the lighter products such as plasma and platelets exit the bowl into the waste bag along with the saline suction fluid. This pumping of surgical field blood from the collection reservoir into the processing bowl continues until RBCs reach the *upper shoulder* of the processing bowl. At that point, the bowl contains predominantly RBCs that are now ready for "wash out": the fluid pumped into the processing bowl is now transitioned from blood to saline and allowed to saturate the mass of RBCs. A typical baseline saline wash volume should be three (3) times the processing bowl volume. Furthermore, *this wash volume must be doubled for cesarean sections* or any other case where gross field contamination is suspected.

Note that if during the initial pumping-in phase the field blood is suctioned into the bowl too quickly (as in the case of massive exsanguination), RBCs will not have enough time to settle along the sides of the bowl and will be dispensed into the waste container. Once the wash out is complete (4–5 min are required for complete spin plus wash cycle), the roller pump direction is reversed, and the washed RBCs are sent into an infusion bag. While this processing phase is taking place, another collection phase can begin.

Infusion: Cell salvaged blood is sometimes infused at the patient's bedside using a 40-micron "microaggregate" filter or a bedside LRF [14, 63]. The 40-micron filter is considered by some to be a final safety net to filter out macro-and microaggregates; a LRF will remove most bacteria, fat, and leukocytes [14, 64]. In general, cell salvage machine processing and washing alone can remove significant amounts of these contaminants, but one can increase the safety margin of the system's capabilities by adding filters. Note that pressure devices applied to the cell-saver bag may clog a microaggregate or leukoreduction filters. Pressure devices also produce excessive hemolysis as the blood is forced through a 40-micron or smaller pore size filter; bedside LRFs have a pore size as small as 4 micron (RBCs are reported to be approximately 8 micron in diameter) [65]. The standard "blood transfusion tubing" available in many operating rooms contains a 150-micron filter (on average) that can withstand external pressure without producing undue hemolysis. As with any transfusion filter, it must be replenished when the transfusion rate has notably decreased or the when the infuser high-pressure alarm sounds.

11.5.3 Special Considerations for Safe ICS Blood Collection and Administration

- The patient should be informed of planned cell salvage use, with a documented discussion of risks, benefits, and alternatives [3, 18].
- Blood collection needs to include the blood shed into various objects and compartments including surgical sponges. Seventy five percent of collected blood is retrievable by rinsing the sponge in a basin of isotonic solution. The rinse solution can be added to the cell salvage reservoir when it is grossly bloody. This practice can increase red cell retrieval rates by more than 25% [66, 67].
- Adequate anticoagulant must be used while suctioning the blood to prevent blood clotting in the collection system. Use normal saline or Plasma-Lyte for suction fluid; do *not* use Lactated Ringers.
- Low suction pressures minimize cell shear stress damage to the RBCs. Normal wall suction of (−) 300 mmHg needs downregulation to a level of (−) 80 mmHg to (−) 120 mmHg through a suction regulator. Some blood salvage devices incorporate their own suction source, allowing various suction pressures to be applied. Adding two suction ports allows the surgeon to have a clear operative field.
- Separating safer blood from potentially contaminated blood that is suctioned off the surgical field can be achieved using two suction setups. One suction line is connected to the cell salvage reservoir for re-infusion purposes, and the other is used to aspirate the contaminated blood for disposal.
- Each collected bag of blood should be properly labeled per Association for the Advancement of Blood & Biotherapies (AABB) standards. All cell-saver units must be labeled with the at least two patient identifiers (e.g., patient name and medical record number or date of birth) if the unit is not immediately attached to the patient's IV tubing, as well as a date and time of expiration.
- The blood bag may be maintained at room temperature for 8 h or at 1–6 °C in a blood bank-controlled refrigerator or blood cooler for 24 h. These time intervals begin at the start of collection. However, cold storage must be started within 4 h of processing completion [68].
- It is important to consult the hospital blood bank because each institution's requirements for room storage duration may vary.

- For RhD-antigen negative pregnant women, the British Society of Haematology recommends evaluating the fetal cord blood for RhD-antigen status at delivery. If the neonate is RhD-antigen positive, maternal anti-RhD immunoprophylaxis should be considered if she is not already sensitized [36].

11.6 What Is the Quantity and Quality of Red Blood Cells (RBCs) in a Unit of ICS-Recovered Blood?

A bag of cell salvaged blood is strictly erythrocytes suspended in wash solution (normal saline or Plasma-Lyte solution). The bag typically contains RBCs at a Hct of 55–70% in saline (similar to a banked RBC unit) and is devoid of platelets, plasma, and coagulation factors. The goal of each processing phase is to produce a bag with a final Hgb value of 15–25 g/dL; thus the saline-heparin-blood solution collected must contain an appropriate red cell mass. If the patient's blood loss is replaced with large quantities of ICS blood, coagulation parameters must be closely monitored [23]. Currently, there are newer ICS system setups that will also recover platelets [69].

It is nearly impossible to recover 100% of surgical blood loss. A significant portion goes into the drapes, sponges, or falls to the floor. One mathematical model estimated that the recovered portion of RBCs was at 57%, with a 20% variance [70]. It is important to note that the quantity of blood suctioned into the collection reservoir is not the actual EBL because a significant amount of blood is lost in the field and the reservoir also contains saline irrigation and anticoagulant.

There is not a validated formula for estimating the exact volume of lost RBCs that yields an acceptable Hct in the final bag. The volume of RBCs in shed blood can be estimated, however, by considering the volume of whole blood suctioned from the field into the collection reservoir, the anticoagulant solution, and the irrigation fluid, multiplied by the patient's most recent Hct:

$$\begin{aligned}&\text{Volume of RBCs}\left(\text{in shed blood}\right)\\&\quad=\begin{bmatrix}\text{volume in collection reservoir}-\text{anticoagulant solution used}\\-\text{irrigation aspirated from surgical site}\end{bmatrix}\\&\quad\times Hct\left(pre\quad\text{collection}\right)\end{aligned}$$

Applying the above formula, if the collection reservoir holds 1000 mL, of which 400 mL is irrigation and 200 mL is anticoagulant, the resultant volume (whole blood collected) is 400 mL. If the patient's most recent Hct is 31%, the RBC volume available for transfusion is 124 mL (i.e., 400 mL of whole blood × 0.31 = 124 mL RBCs). In small patients, if a 50 mL or 70 mL processing bowl is utilized in a non-continuous mode (see below), a total of 200–300 mL "fill" (consisting of blood plus irrigation fluid) must be in the collection reservoir to produce a target volume (or Hct) of RBCs for administration.

There are now “smart” (e.g., continuous) ICS systems that use an internal scale or infrared optics to detect the RBC contents of the collection reservoir, automatically processing contents when a predetermined quantity of RBCs is detected. These machines obviate the refrain, “There’s not enough here to spin!” These machines are volume independent, operating by continuous centrifugation, processing with bowl sizes as small as 55 mL, and distributing 15–30 mL at times during ongoing blood loss. Some machines have an “autostart” function and will start washing at a preset bowl volume as low as 200 mL, at increments upward of 100 mL.

The quality of salvaged blood has vastly improved over time through use of modern devices and quality standards. The first commercially available devices for ICS were launched in the mid-1970s; prior to that, salvaged blood was grossly filtered (if at all) and readministered unwashed, contributing to reports of poor patient outcomes [14]. Modern ICS systems improve the quality of salvaged RBCs in a variety of ways, including the following:

- ICS now produces fresher RBCs that are comparable to what is already circulating in the patient. They are spared the storage lesions and preservatives associated with banked RBCs.
- ICS RBCs demonstrate a lower degree of hemolysis than banked RBCs when properly collected, washed, and filtered:
  - Proper shed blood collection can lower the shear stress on cell membrane and decrease hemolysis by reducing the surgical suction pressure to (−) 150 mmHg or less and by minimize surface “skimming.” The subsequent cell washing and centrifuging clear the final RBCs from the residual hemolysis byproducts [62, 71, 72].
  - Infusion of hemolyzed blood cells is hazardous as the cell-free hemoglobin scavenges nitric oxide, promotes vasoconstriction, and damages vascular beds including the renal tubules. Per US Food and Drug Administration (FDA) regulations, the maximum allowed hemolysis level for banked blood is 1% of the cells, which typically occurs near the 42 days of storage time for banked RBCs [73].
  - ICS preserves cell membrane deformability which allows RBCs to accommodate and flow through small capillaries, thus maintaining the rheology for oxygen delivery. In contrast, banked RBCs undergo loss of deformability [74, 75]. Over storage time, the stored erythrocyte loses its biconcave disc shape and becomes an echinocyte and then a spherocyte. During this transition, the spicules of the echinocyte get shed and create microparticles which have been implicated in thrombotic complications in patients who have received stored blood.
- Modern ICS preserves levels of 2,3-diphosphoglycerate (2,3-DPG), thus preserving the off-loading of oxygen at the tissue level according to a normal oxygen-hemoglobin dissociation curve, in contrast to the depletion of 2,3-DPG over time with banked RBCs [76, 77].

- Cell salvaged blood has minimal levels of inflammatory mediators, interleukins, tumor necrosis factor, fibrin split products, complement fractions, and fat and stromal components. Banked RBCs have associated acidosis from continued metabolism that increases with longer storage times. There is also an increase in extracellular potassium and free hemoglobin which results from erythrocyte aging during storage.
- ICS RBCs are devoid of citrate which is used as an anticoagulant in banked blood. Citrate toxicity and calcium chelation are concerns when using large volumes of banked blood products, particularly with neonates and small children.
  - The anticoagulant used in the ICS process, typically heparin, is washed off during processing, with clinically insignificant residual amounts being much less than one unit per 100 mL [78, 79].

11.7 What Adverse Effects Are Associated with ICS-Recovered Blood Administration?

11.7.1 Air Embolism

Air embolism can occur with any blood transfusion, whether it is banked, autologous, or ICS-based. During the ICS procedure, air embolism occurs when a unit of blood contains air and is placed under pressure so that the air bolus is not obvious. In ICS administration, an air embolus can also result from connecting the patient to the infusion bag before the infusion bag is filled and clamped off from the processing bowl. This is prevented by using a critical "secondary reinfusion" bag where air is burped into the "primary reinfusion" bag; the blood is then administered via the primary bag (Fig. 11.1). In the modern cell salvage era following best practices and AABB quality standards, this problem is seen less often.

11.7.2 The "Salvaged Blood" Syndrome

Reinfusion of ICS blood has been implicated in disseminated intravascular coagulopathy (DIC), adult respiratory syndrome (ARDS), and hemodynamic instability [80]. In theory, the syndrome is secondary to damaged platelets and activated leukocytes in the centrifugal bowl, causing release of vasoactive procoagulant and leukotactic mediators. A relative coagulopathy may also result because there are technically no platelets or coagulation factors in the returned RBC product or the reinfusion of residual heparin remaining in improperly washed product. Poor management of the cell salvage system has been implicated in these cases. Furthermore, case reports describing poor ICS outcomes have been confounded with comorbid conditions including pre-existing shock, hypothermia, acidosis, and massive transfusions [81]. It is imperative to have standardized policies and procedures for any ICS program, sustained quality monitoring, and, not least of all, properly trained ICS personnel.

11.7.3 Administration of Field Contaminants

Surgical field blood can contain a number of contaminants, both macro-and microparticles, as well as soluble substances that are the byproduct of blood cell activation and physical trauma. These include cellular stroma, free hemoglobin, tissue and field debris, bacteria, fats, activated complement, and anticoagulants [23]. There are case reports of chromium, cobalt, and titanium contamination during hip revisions [82, 83]. The initial, 150-micron filter passing through the ICS machine collection reservoir theoretically removes the solids; the processing bowl "wash out" phase removes much of the soluble contaminants. As stated, it is optional but often recommended to interpose a microaggregate or leukoreduction filter before delivering processed blood to the patient [84].

11.7.4 Febrile Transfusion Reaction

This is the most common adverse reaction using ICS, which is probably the result of cytokine release from RBCs. A febrile, non-hemolytic transfusion reaction is also one of the most common allogeneic transfusion reactions reported in both children and adults [85].

11.7.5 Bacterial Contamination

Almost all bacteria in blood suctioned from the surgical field is removed during the ICS collection, filtration, and washing process [32]. However, improper handling and storage of recovered blood, particularly when ICS units are held for longer than the recommended duration (8 h), will create conditions favorable to bacterial overgrowth. Alternative measures to prevent bacterial contamination include use of a bedside LRF and co-administration of antibiotics [86].

11.7.6 Limitations of ICS

11.7.6.1 Costs

The cost of equipment and staffing are often cited as barriers to ICS use. Comparing the cost of an allogeneic blood unit to an ICS-collected autotransfusion unit is overly simplistic. The cost comparison is not straightforward. The more blood that is produced through autotransfusion per case, the less is the cost per ICS blood unit. ICS programs focus on surgeries where high blood loss is anticipated based on historical data. While many cases may produce insufficient blood for retransfusion, it is important to look at the program as a whole rather than at an individual case. Currently, a disposable setup for autotransfusion costs approximately $100 USD, whereas a unit of allogeneic RBCs costs $225 USD on average [13, 57]. These numbers do not include the cost of acquiring autotransfusion equipment nor do they reconcile the cost of blood bank management, crossmatching, incidental antibody testing, and special blood treatments such as washing and irradiation of allogeneic RBCs.

11.7.6.2 Misinformation Regarding the ICS Setup

A modern ICS setup can be in a "collect only" or "reserve" mode when an anticipated large blood loss does not come to fruition. These preparatory modes may contribute to cost savings with a potential benefit of rapid, full-capacity ICS. For most blood loss procedures, it is reasonable to begin ICS in a reserve mode; here shed blood is aspirated, anticoagulated, and held in a collection reservoir while using minimal consumable equipment. If the volume of RBCs in the shed blood exceeds the volume of the processing chamber, the remaining components of the ICS set up can be assembled to initiate processing. For procedures where considerable blood loss is certain, it is reasonable to have all consumables and the cell salvage device at the ready upon skin incision.

11.7.6.3 Small Patients

While ICS use is widely accepted and commonplace in adult surgeries, its use in children can be somewhat limited. The primary constraint is procuring adequate amounts of blood to process (which is relatively small due to children's reduced total blood volumes) that can be reconciled against the cost expenditure. Continuous systems allow smaller aliquots to be continuously centrifuged and processed and then transfused in a timely manner. Processing bowls smaller than 100 mL are now available.

11.8 Is ICS Recommended by Professional Organizations?

The AABB and other organizations with transfusion policy oversight have published technical and procedural guidelines for ICS [16, 87]. Table 11.2 is an illustration of sample guidelines:

Table 11.2 Clinical recommendations from various professional organizations for ICS

Organization/year	Adults	Level of evidence	Pediatrics	Level of evidence
Society of Thoracic Surgeons/Society for Cardiac Anesthesia (2021) [44]	"Routine use of red cell salvage using centrifugation is helpful for blood conservation in cardiac operations using CPB"	Strong recommendation; High-quality evidence from more than 1 RCT	Not specified	N/A
European Society of Anaesthesiology (2017) [84]	"We recommend the use of red cell salvage, which is helpful for blood conservation in major cardiac and orthopaedic surgery"	Strong recommendation; moderate-quality evidence	Not specified	N/A
	"We recommend that cell salvage is not contraindicated in bowel surgery, provided that the initial evacuation of soiled abdominal contents is undertaken, additional cell washing is performed and that broad-spectrum antibiotics are used"	Strong recommendation; low-quality evidence		
	"We suggest that cell salvage is not contraindicated in cancer surgery, provided that blood aspiration close to the tumor site is avoided and leukodepletion filters are used"	Weak recommendation; low-quality evidence		
Association of Anaesthetists (2018) [3]	"The use of cell salvage is recommended when it can be expected to reduce the likelihood of allogeneic (donor) red cell transfusion and/or severe postoperative anaemia. We support and encourage a continued increase in the appropriate use of peri-operative cell salvage and we recommend that it should be available for immediate use 24 h a day in any hospital undertaking surgery where blood loss is a recognised potential complication (other than minor/day case procedures)"	Expert consensus	"CS should be considered *at least* in 'collect only' mode when blood loss >8 $mL.Kg^{-1}$ (equivalent to approximately >10% of total blood volume) is anticipated *and* the child's weight is >10 kg"	Expert consensus

American Society of Anesthesiologists (2015) [45]	"Meta-analyses of RCTs indicate that intraoperative red blood cell recovery compared with conventional transfusion (i.e., nonblood cell recovery) is effective in reducing the volume of allogeneic blood transfused"	The literature contains a sufficient number of RCTs to conduct meta-analysis; RCTs report comparative findings between clinical interventions; beneficial	Not specified	N/A
Network for the Advancement of PBM (2019) [88]	N/A	N/A	"The authors recommend the use of cell salvage in pediatric cardiac surgery in order to reduce perioperative transfusion" "The authors suggest active salvaging of CPB circuit residual blood as it may decrease the number of transfusions"	Strong recommendation; low-quality evidence Weak recommendation; low-quality evidence
National Blood Authority (2014) [87]	"In adult patients undergoing surgery in which substantial blood loss (blood loss of a volume great enough to induce anaemia that would require therapy) is anticipated, intraoperative cell salvage is recommended"	Body of evidence provides some support for recommendation(s) but care should be taken in its application	N/A	N/A
National Blood Authority (2014) [87]	"Intraoperative cell salvage requires a local procedural guideline that should include patient selection, use of equipment and reinfusion. All staff operating cell salvage devices should receive appropriate training, to ensure knowledge of the technique and proficiency in using it"	Practice points (developed through consensus decision making, when there is no sufficient quality data)	"In paediatric patients undergoing cardiac surgery with cardiopulmonary bypass, intraoperative cell salvage may be considered. If intraoperative cell salvage is used, it requires a local procedural guideline that should include patient selection, use of equipment and reinfusion. All staff operating cell salvage devices should receive appropriate training, to ensure knowledge of the technique and proficiency in using it"	Practice points (developed through consensus decision making, when there is no sufficient quality data)
NICE (NG 24; 2015) [89]	"Do not routinely use cell salvage without tranexamic acid." cell salvage may be considered in adult cases with moderate or > 500 mL blood loss. In cases with very high blood loss, tranexamic acid plus cell salvage should be considered	Expert consensus based on best evidence	"Consider tranexamic acid for children undergoing surgery who are expected to have at least moderate blood loss (greater than 10% blood volume)"	Expert consensus based on best evidence

11.9 Summary of Key Learning Objectives

11.9.1 What Are the Advantages of ICS?

Advantages of an ICS set up in this case include potential avoidance of the side effects known to be associated with allogeneic RBC transfusions and a ready availability of RBCs in a surgical case with potentially high but unpredictable blood loss.

11.9.2 What Are the Indications for ICS?

One professional society recommends ICS use in pediatric patients when the anticipated surgical blood loss is greater than 10% of a patient's EBV and the patient is at least 10 kg in body weight (Table 11.2). ICS is also utilized in procedures requiring at least one RBC unit (approximately 250 mL). Prior to any blood loss procedure, it is important to calculate a patient's allowable blood loss (ABL) based on the preoperative hematocrit and the restrictive transfusion threshold appropriate for this patient. This 20 kg patient has a blood volume of approximately 1400 mL (20 kg × 70 mL/kg for age). Given this patient's starting hematocrit of 39% and an intraoperative transfusion threshold of 24% (e.g., 8 g/dL), the ABL calculation comes to 196 mL. This ABL is 14% of this patient's blood volume. With respect to the specific procedure—a pediatric hepatic resection—blood loss can be significant, up to 250 mL under the best surgical conditions. Both this patient's ABL (196 mL) and the anticipated blood loss associated with pediatric hepatoblastoma resection (250 mL) exceed 10% of this 20 kg patient's EBV. Furthermore, the anticipated RBC transfusion volume is 250 mL, or one adult-sized unit, which is an additional criterion for ICS implementation.

11.9.3 What Are the Absolute and Relative Contraindications to ICS?

In this case, there are no apparent absolute contraindications to ICS because parents have provided informed consent and there should be no loss of bowel integrity leading to frank stool in the field. Prior to incision, the surgeon should be asked to inform you if any hemostatic collagen or tissue adhesive agents are used during the operation. A multidisciplinary planning session with the oncology team will allow for discussion about use of ICS in this cancer surgery, with the understanding that hematogenous spread of cancer cells is common at baseline.

11.9.4 What Is the Quality of RBCs in a Unit of ICS-Recovered Blood?

Compared to allogeneic RBCs, the quality of transfused ICS RBCs is superior with better 2,3-DPG content, no citrate anticoagulant, and absence of RBC storage lesions including high potassium levels.

11.9.5 What Is the Quantity of RBCs in a Unit of ICS-Recovered Blood?

If a 70 mL collection bowl is used (which will require 200–300 mL "fill," consisting of blood plus irrigation fluid), the total blood loss is 250 mL, and 100 mL of irrigation is used, the calculated yield using the manual wash cycle mode is approximately 60 mL (see equation for the estimated volume of RBCs in shed blood, above). A more efficient ICS mode, given the proper machine, is "continuous" processing which can make this volume available in smaller aliquots throughout the case rather than at a late stage of surgery prompting the need for an allogeneic transfusion. A modern, non-volume dependent ICS machine will provide an even more efficient source of RBCs in small aliquots.

11.9.6 Is ICS Cost-Efficient?

If these ICS-recovered cells are the only RBCs administered to this patient, the "cost" of a $250 USD unit of allogeneic RBCs is avoided and is less than the cost of an ICS setup. A banked RBC unit includes indirect labor expense, including the cost splitting the unit into pediatric-sized units (a "pedi pack" equals 80 mL). Given the known adverse effects of allogeneic transfusion as well as patients' mounting concerns over receiving transfusions in general, the potential cost benefit of ICS involves many considerations and must be calculated on a case-by-case basis.

11.9.7 What Adverse Effects, If Any, Are Associated with ICS-Recovered Blood Administration?

During any blood loss surgery using ICS, one must be proactive to avoid potential adverse events. Foremost, one must be vigilant for a potential air embolus due to failure to utilize a primary "burp bag" that extracts free air from the secondary reinfusion line attached to the IV tubing (see Fig. 11.1). Cell salvage "syndrome" can be avoided through meticulous ICS machine management by trained personnel, standardized ICS protocols, as well as frequent point-of-care (POC) evaluation of the patient's coagulation and Hgb values. A microaggregate or leukocyte reduction filter can be interposed at bedside as an extra precaution to remove residual vasoactive or anticoagulant byproducts of RBC processing. Some experts recommend use of a bedside LRF when ICS is utilized during cancer surgery. Although ICS-recovered blood does not contain platelets and other coagulation factors, scrupulous maintenance of body temperature, acid-base status, and perfusion (including keeping pace with RBC deficits) will mitigate the need for administration of allogeneic coagulation factors.

11.9.8 Is ICS Recommended by Professional Organizations?

ICS is recommended by several professional organizations that advocate for PBM. However, only a few organizations have explicit recommendations for pediatric patients, most likely due to the late development of ICS technology such as intrinsic measurements of RBC mass and continuous modes that allow processing of the relatively small total blood volume losses seen in children.

Key Points

- In cases of large volume blood loss, ICS has been shown to be effective in reducing the rate of allogeneic blood transfusions in pediatric patients. The effectiveness increases when ICS is used as part of a PBM program which encompasses preoperative optimization and perioperative strategies for blood conservation.
- A cost-effective "collect-only" mode is available when large blood loss is anticipated but unpredictable.
- Available trained staff and established institutional protocols are essential to the safe implementation of ICS.
- Malignancy is not an absolute contraindication to ICS. The patient may have circulating cancer cells at the time of surgery. Reports of cell salvage blood washed and filtered via leukoreduction filters have shown undetectable cancer cells. The use of ICS blood must be weighed against the use of allogeneic blood and its known immunomodulatory potential.

References

1. Faraoni D, Meier J, New HV, Van der Linden PJ, Hunt BJ. Patient blood Management for Neonates and Children Undergoing Cardiac Surgery: 2019 NATA guidelines. J Cardiothorac Vasc Anesth. 2019;33(12):3249–63.
2. National Blood Authority (NBA). Guidance for the Provision of Intraoperative Cell Salvage. 2014. https://www.blood.gov.au/ics. Accessed 17 Feb 2023.
3. Klein AA, Bailey CR, Charlton AJ, Evans E, Guckian-Fisher M, McCrossan R, et al. Association of Anaesthetists guidelines: cell salvage for peri-operative blood conservation 2018. Anaesthesia. 2018;73(9):1141–50.
4. World Health Organization. Policy brief: the urgent need to implement patient blood management. World Health Organization; 2021. https://www.who.int/publications/i/item/9789240035744. Accessed 3 Jan 2023
5. Widespread KB, Blood Shortages Threaten Global Public Health. JAMA. 2019;322(23):2276.

6. Oakley FD, Woods M, Arnold S, Young PP. Transfusion reactions in pediatric compared with adult patients: a look at rate, reaction type, and associated products. Transfusion. 2015;55(3):563–70.
7. Serious Hazards of Transfusion (SHOT). https://www.shotuk.org/shot-reports/. 2020. Accessed 25 May 2023.
8. Goobie SM, Gallagher T, Gross I, Shander A. Society for the advancement of blood management administrative and clinical standards for patient blood management programs 4th edition (pediatric version). Paediatr Anaesth. 2019;29(3):231–6.
9. Leahy MF, Hofmann A, Towler S, Trentino KM, Burrows SA, Swain SG, et al. Improved outcomes and reduced costs associated with a health-system-wide patient blood management program: a retrospective observational study in four major adult tertiary-care hospitals. Transfusion. 2017;57(6):1347–58.
10. Wan S, Sparring V, Cabrales DA, Jansson K, Wikman A. Clinical and budget impact of treating preoperative anemia in major orthopedic surgery-a retrospective observational study. J Arthroplast. 2020;35(11):3084–8.
11. Trentino KM, Mace HS, Symons K, Sanfilippo FM, Leahy MF, Farmer SL, et al. Screening and treating pre-operative anaemia and suboptimal iron stores in elective colorectal surgery: a cost effectiveness analysis. Anaesthesia. 2021;76(3):357–65.
12. Drabinski T, Zacharowski K, Meybohm P, Rüger AM, Ramirez de Arellano A. Estimating the epidemiological and economic impact of implementing preoperative Anaemia measures in the German healthcare system: the health economic footprint of patient blood management. Adv Ther. 2020;37(8):3515–36.
13. Sikorski RA, Rizkalla NA, Yang WW, Frank SM. Autologous blood salvage in the era of patient blood management. Vox Sang. 2017;112(6):499–510.
14. Frank SM, Waters JH, editors. Patient blood management: multidisciplinary approaches to optimizing care. Bethesda: AABB Press; 2016. p. 29–47, 180–186, 241.
15. Golab HD, Scohy TV, de Jong PL, Takkenberg JJ, Bogers AJ. Intraoperative cell salvage in infants undergoing elective cardiac surgery: a prospective trial. Eur J Cardiothorac Surg. 2008;34(2):354–9.
16. Frank S, Guinn NR. Patient Blood Management. In: Cohn C, Delaney M, Johnson ST, Katz LM, editors. Technical manual. 20th ed. Bethesda, MD: AABB; 2020. p. 592–6.
17. Kuppurao L, Wee M. Perioperative cell salvage. Crit Care Pain Med. 2010;10:104–8.
18. Esper SA, Waters JH. Intra-operative cell salvage: a fresh look at the indications and contraindications. Blood Transfus. 2011;9(2):139–47.
19. Cholette JM, Powers KS, Alfieris GM, Angona R, Henrichs KF, Masel D, et al. Transfusion of cell saver salvaged blood in neonates and infants undergoing open heart surgery significantly reduces RBC and coagulant product transfusions and donor exposures: results of a prospective, randomized, clinical trial. Pediatr Crit Care Med. 2013;14(2):137–47.
20. Trappey AF 3rd, Thompson KM, Kuppermann N, Stephenson JT, Nuno MA, Hewes HA, et al. Development of transfusion guidelines for injured children using a modified Delphi consensus process. J Trauma Acute Care Surg. 2019;87(4):935–43.
21. Neff LP, Cannon JW, Morrison JJ, Edwards MJ, Spinella PC, Borgman MA. Clearly defining pediatric massive transfusion: cutting through the fog and friction with combat data. J Trauma Acute Care Surg. 2015;78(1):22–8; discussion 8–9.
22. Evangelista ME, Gaffley M, Neff LP. Massive transfusion protocols for pediatric patients: current perspectives. J Blood Med. 2020;11:163–72.
23. Waters JH. Intraoperative blood recovery. ASAIO J. 2013;59(1):11–7.
24. Goucher H, Wong CA, Patel SK, Toledo P. Cell salvage in obstetrics. Anesth Analg. 2015;121(2):465–8.
25. The American College of Obstetricians and Gynecologists (ACOG). ACOG Practice Bulletin Number 183. Postpartum Hemorrhage. 2017. https://www.acog.org/clinical/clinical-guidance/practice-bulletin/articles/2017/10/postpartum-hemorrhage. Accessed 1 Jan 2023.
26. Lew E, Tagore S. Implementation of an obstetric cell salvage service in a tertiary women's hospital. Singapore Med J. 2015;56(8):445–9.

27. Waters JH. Intraoperative blood recovery and reinfusion. In: Frank SM, Waters JH, editors. Patient blood management: multidisciplinary approaches to optimizing care. Bethesda: AABB Press; 2016. p. 186.
28. Waters JH, Yazer M, Chen YF, Kloke J. Blood salvage and cancer surgery: a meta-analysis of available studies. Transfusion. 2012;52(10):2167–73.
29. Okunuga A, Skelton VA. Use of cell salvage in patients with sickle cell trait. Int J Obstet Anesth. 2009;18(1):90–1. author reply 1
30. Waters JH, Lukauskiene E, Anderson ME. Intraoperative blood salvage during cesarean delivery in a patient with beta thalassemia intermedia. Anesth Analg. 2003;97(6):1808–9.
31. Perez Ferrer A, Ferrazza V, Gredilla E, de Vicente J, de la Rua A, Larrea A. Bloodless surgery in a patient with thalassemia minor. Usefulness of erythropoietin, preoperative blood donation and intraoperative blood salvage. Minerva Anestesiol. 2007;73(5):323–6.
32. Waters JH, Tuohy MJ, Hobson DF, Procop G. Bacterial reduction by cell salvage washing and leukocyte depletion filtration. Anesthesiology. 2003;99(3):652–5.
33. Frietsch T, Steinbicker AU, Horn A, Metz M, Dietrich G, Weigand MA, et al. Safety of intraoperative cell salvage in cancer surgery: an updated meta-analysis of the current literature. Transfus Med Hemother. 2022;49(3):143–57.
34. Trudeau JD, Waters T, Chipperfield K. Should intraoperative cell-salvaged blood be used in patients with suspected or known malignancy? Can J Anaesth. 2012;59(11):1058–70.
35. Raval JS, Nelson JB, Woldemichael E, Triulzi DJ. Intraoperative cell salvage in radical prostatectomy does not appear to increase long-term biochemical recurrence, metastases, or mortality. Transfusion. 2012;52(12):2590–3.
36. Qureshi H, Massey E, Kirwan D, Davies T, Robson S, White J, et al. BCSH guideline for the use of anti-D immunoglobulin for the prevention of haemolytic disease of the fetus and newborn. Transfus Med. 2014;24(1):8–20.
37. DeAndrade D, Waters JH, Triulzi DJ, Alarcon L, Wisniewski MK, Dyga R, et al. Very low rate of patient-related adverse events associated with the use of intraoperative cell salvage. Transfusion. 2016;56(11):2768–72.
38. Carless PA, Henry DA, Moxey AJ, O'Connell D, Brown T, Fergusson DA. Cell salvage for minimising perioperative allogeneic blood transfusion. Cochrane Database Syst Rev. 2010;3:CD001888.
39. Wang G, Bainbridge D, Martin J, Cheng D. The efficacy of an intraoperative cell saver during cardiac surgery: a meta-analysis of randomized trials. Anesth Analg. 2009;109(2):320–30.
40. Al Khabori M, Al Riyami A, Siddiqi MS, Sarfaraz ZK, Ziadinov E, Al SH. Impact of cell saver during cardiac surgery on blood transfusion requirements: a systematic review and meta-analysis. Vox Sang. 2019;114(6):553–65.
41. van Bodegom-Vos L, Voorn VM, So-Osman C, Vliet Vlieland TP, Dahan A, Koopman-van Gemert AW, et al. Cell salvage in hip and knee arthroplasty: a meta-analysis of randomized controlled trials. J Bone Joint Surg Am. 2015;97(12):1012–21.
42. Hamilton CM, Davenport DL, Bernard AC. Demonstration of a U.S. nationwide reduction in transfusion in general surgery and a review of published transfusion reduction methodologies. Transfusion. 2021;61(11):3119–28.
43. Jones JM, Sapiano MRP, Mowla S, Bota D, Berger JJ, Basavaraju SV. Has the trend of declining blood transfusions in the United States ended? Findings of the 2019 National Blood Collection and utilization survey. Transfusion. 2021;61(Suppl 2(Suppl 2)):S1–S10.
44. Tibi P, McClure RS, Huang J, Baker RA, Fitzgerald D, Mazer CD, et al. STS/SCA/AmSECT/SABM update to the clinical practice guidelines on patient blood management. J Cardiothorac Vasc Anesth. 2021;35(9):2569–91.
45. American Society of Anesthesiologists Task Force on Perioperative Blood M. Practice guidelines for perioperative blood management: an updated report by the American Society

of Anesthesiologists Task Force on perioperative blood management*. Anesthesiology. 2015;122(2):241–75.
46. National Blood Authority. Three pillars of patient blood management. 2023. https://www.blood.gov.au/system/files/documents/pbm-3-pillars.pdf. Accessed 6 June 2023.
47. Bowen RE, Gardner S, Scaduto AA, Eagan M, Beckstead J. Efficacy of intraoperative cell salvage systems in pediatric idiopathic scoliosis patients undergoing posterior spinal fusion with segmental spinal instrumentation. Spine (Phila Pa 1976). 2010;35(2):246–51.
48. Liang J, Shen J, Chua S, Fan Y, Zhai J, Feng B, et al. Does intraoperative cell salvage system effectively decrease the need for allogeneic transfusions in scoliotic patients undergoing posterior spinal fusion? A prospective randomized study. Eur Spine J. 2015;24(2):270–5.
49. Ersen O, Ekinci S, Bilgic S, Kose O, Oguz E, Sehirlioglu A. Posterior spinal fusion in adolescent idiopathic scoliosis with or without intraoperative cell salvage system: a retrospective comparison. Musculoskelet Surg. 2012;96(2):107–10.
50. Dahmani S, Orliaguet GA, Meyer PG, Blanot S, Renier D, Carli PA. Perioperative blood salvage during surgical correction of craniosynostosis in infants. Br J Anaesth. 2000;85(4):550–5.
51. Duncan C, Richardson D, May P, Thiruchelvam J, Shong DC, Potter F, et al. Reducing blood loss in synostosis surgery: the Liverpool experience. J Craniofac Surg. 2008;19(5):1424–30.
52. White N, Bayliss S, Moore D. Systematic review of interventions for minimizing perioperative blood transfusion for surgery for craniosynostosis. J Craniofac Surg. 2015;26(1):26–36.
53. Krajewski K, Ashley RK, Pung N, Wald S, Lazareff J, Kawamoto HK, et al. Successful blood conservation during craniosynostotic correction with dual therapy using procrit and cell saver. J Craniofac Surg. 2008;19(1):101–5.
54. Beethe AB, Spitznagel RA, Kugler JA, Goeller JK, Franzen MH, Hamlin RJ, et al. The road to transfusion-free Craniosynostosis repair in children less than 24 months old: a quality improvement initiative. Pediatr Qual Saf. 2020;5(4):e331.
55. Nathan M, Tishler B, Gauvreau K, Matte GS, Howe RJ, Durham L, et al. A red cell preservation strategy reduces postoperative transfusions in pediatric heart surgery patients. Paediatr Anaesth. 2018;28(5):450–7.
56. Ye L, Lin R, Fan Y, Yang L, Hu J, Shu Q. Effects of circuit residual volume salvage reinfusion on the postoperative clinical outcome for pediatric patients undergoing cardiac surgery. Pediatr Cardiol. 2013;34(5):1088–93.
57. Waters JR, Meier HH, Waters JH. An economic analysis of costs associated with development of a cell salvage program. Anesth Analg. 2007;104(4):869–75.
58. Welsby IJ, Norris PJ, Mauermann WJ, Podgoreanu MV, Conn CM, Meade L, et al. Bedside allogeneic erythrocyte washing with a cell saver to remove cytokines, chemokines, and cell-derived microvesicles. Anesthesiology. 2021;134(3):395–404.
59. Westphal-Varghese B, Erren M, Westphal M, Van Aken H, Ertmer C, Lange M, et al. Processing of stored packed red blood cells using autotransfusion devices decreases potassium and microaggregates: a prospective, randomized, single-blinded in vitro study. Transfus Med. 2007;17(2):89–95.
60. Gruber M, Breu A, Frauendorf M, Seyfried T, Hansen E. Washing of banked blood by three different blood salvage devices. Transfusion. 2013;53(5):1001–9.
61. Lindau S, Kohlhaas M, Nosch M, Choorapoikayil S, Zacharowski K, Meybohm P. Cell salvage using the continuous autotransfusion device CATSmart—an observational bicenter technical evaluation. BMC Anesthesiol. 2018;18(1):189.
62. Waters JH, Williams B, Yazer MH, Kameneva MV. Modification of suction-induced hemolysis during cell salvage. Anesth Analg. 2007;104(3):684–7.
63. Roets M, Sturgess DJ, Obeysekera MP, Tran TV, Wyssusek KH, Punnasseril JEJ, et al. Intraoperative cell salvage as an alternative to allogeneic (donated) blood transfusion:

a prospective observational evaluation of the immune response profile. Cell Transplant. 2020;29:963689720966265.
64. Konig G, Yazer MH, Waters JH. Stored platelet functionality is not decreased after warming with a fluid warmer. Anesth Analg. 2013;117(3):575–8.
65. Diez-Silva M, Dao M, Han J, Lim CT, Suresh S. Shape and biomechanical characteristics of human red blood cells in health and disease. MRS Bull. 2010;35(5):382–8.
66. Haynes SL, Bennett JR, Torella F, McCollum CN. Does washing swabs increase the efficiency of red cell recovery by cell salvage in aortic surgery? Vox Sang. 2005;88(4):244–8.
67. Ronai AK, Glass JJ, Shapiro AS. Improving autologous blood harvest: recovery of red cells from sponges and suction. Anaesth Intensive Care. 1987;15(4):421–4.
68. Perioperative Standards Committee. Sections 1, 5, and 7. In: Standards for perioperative autologous blood collection and administration. 10th ed. Bethesda: AABB; 2023.
69. Mansour A, Decouture B, Roussel M, Lefevre C, Skreko L, Picard V, et al. Combined platelet and erythrocyte salvage: evaluation of a New filtration-based autotransfusion device. Anesthesiology. 2021;135(2):246–57.
70. Waters JH, Lee JS, Karafa MT. A mathematical model of cell salvage efficiency. Anesth Analg. 2002;95(5):1312–7. table of contents.
71. Yazer MH, Waters JH, Elkin KR, Rohrbaugh ME, Kameneva MV. A comparison of hemolysis and red cell mechanical fragility in blood collected with different cell salvage suction devices. Transfusion. 2008;48(6):1188–91.
72. Tinmouth A, Chin-Yee I. The clinical consequences of the red cell storage lesion. Transfus Med Rev. 2001;15(2):91–107.
73. Alquist C, Harm SK. Transfusion service related activities. In: Cohn C, Delaney M, Johnson ST, Katz LM, editors. Technical manual. 20th ed. Bethesda, MD: AABB; 2020. p. 503–504, 510–517, 522.
74. Frank SM, Abazyan B, Ono M, Hogue CW, Cohen DB, Berkowitz DE, et al. Decreased erythrocyte deformability after transfusion and the effects of erythrocyte storage duration. Anesth Analg. 2013;116(5):975–81.
75. Salaria ON, Barodka VM, Hogue CW, Berkowitz DE, Ness PM, Wasey JO, et al. Impaired red blood cell deformability after transfusion of stored allogeneic blood but not autologous salvaged blood in cardiac surgery patients. Anesth Analg. 2014;118(6):1179–87.
76. Scott AV, Nagababu E, Johnson DJ, Kebaish KM, Lipsitz JA, Dwyer IM, et al. 2,3-Diphosphoglycerate concentrations in autologous salvaged versus stored red blood cells and in surgical patients after transfusion. Anesth Analg. 2016;122(3):616–23.
77. Heaton A, Keegan T, Holme S. In vivo regeneration of red cell 2,3-diphosphoglycerate following transfusion of DPG-depleted AS-1, AS-3 and CPDA-1 red cells. Br J Haematol. 1989;71(1):131–6.
78. Sistino JJ, Owitz D, Mongero LB. Heparin washout in the pediatric cell saver bowl. J Extra Corpor Technol. 1992;24(3):94–6.
79. Kling D, Borner U, von Bormann B, Hempelmann G. Heparin elimination and free hemoglobin following cell separation and washing of autologous blood with cell saver 4. Anasth Intensivther Notfallmed. 1988;23(2):88–90.
80. Bull BS, Bull MH. The salvaged blood syndrome: a sequel to mechanochemical activation of platelets and leukocytes? Blood Cells. 1990;16(1):5–20; discussion –3.
81. Tawes RL Jr, Duvall TB. Is the "salvaged-cell syndrome" myth or reality? Am J Surg. 1996;172(2):172–4.
82. Parker LM, Yazer MH, Waters JH. Metallosis identified via intraoperative cell salvage: a case report. A A Case Rep. 2017;8(4):67–9.
83. Simonian PT, Robinson RP. Titanium contamination of recycled cell saver blood in revision hip arthroplasty. J Arthroplast. 1995;10(1):83–6.
84. Kozek-Langenecker SA, Ahmed AB, Afshari A, Albaladejo P, Aldecoa C, Barauskas G, et al. Management of severe perioperative bleeding: guidelines from the European Society of Anaesthesiology: first update 2016. Eur J Anaesthesiol. 2017;34(6):332–95.

85. Kopko PM. Transfusion reactions. 5th ed. Bethesda: AABB Press; 2021. p. 41, 83, 90–92, 98, 102–103, 121, 182, 233–249, 380, 408, 2512–2513.
86. Luque-Oliveros M. Bacteremia in the red blood cells obtained from the cell saver in patients submitted to heart surgery. Rev Lat Am Enfermagem. 2020;28:e3337.
87. National Blood Authority (Australia). Guidance for the Provision of Intraoperative Cell Salvage. https://www.blood.gov.au/ics. Accessed 3 July 2023.
88. Faraoni D, Meier J, New HV, Van der Linden PJ, Hunt BJ. Patient blood Management for Neonates and Children Undergoing Cardiac Surgery: 2019 NATA guidelines. J Cardiothorac Vasc Anesth. 2019;33:3249.
89. NICE: National Institute for Health and Care Excellence. Blood Transfusion. In: NICE guideline [NG24]. 2015. https://www.nice.org.uk/guidance/ng24/chapter/Recommendations#alternatives-to-blood-transfusion-for-patients-having-surgery-2. Accessed 3 July 2023.

Acute Normovolemic Hemodilution (ANH) 12

Destiny F. Chau, Sheri Norton, and Peter Winch

12.1 Case Scenario

A 14-year-old, 49 kg boy with neuromuscular scoliosis (Cobb angle 95°) is scheduled to undergo posterior spine fusion from T6 to L3. He is seen in the spine clinic for perioperative evaluation and planning. The patient's hemoglobin is 12 g/dL. He has a rare blood type (type AB-Rh and -Kell positive, with anti-c antibody), and the blood bank contacts you to say it will have a difficult time procuring sufficient units of blood. To minimize the need for allogeneic transfusion, the plan is to optimize his hemoglobin preoperatively and then perform acute normovolemic hemodilution (ANH). The patient and his parents have provided informed consent for this plan.

Key Learning Objectives

- What are the indications for, advantages of, and contraindications to ANH?
- What is the evidence supporting the rational use of ANH?
- What is the procedure for performing ANH in children?
- What are safety concerns related to ANH?

D. F. Chau (✉)
Department of Anesthesiology and Pain Medicine, University of Arkansas for Medical Sciences, Arkansas Children's Hospital, Little Rock, AK, USA
e-mail: dchau@uams.edu

S. Norton
Perfusion, Arkansas Children's Hospital, Little Rock, AR, USA
e-mail: nortonsa@archildrens.org

P. Winch
Department of Anesthesiology and Pain Medicine, Nationwide Children's Hospital, Columbus, OH, USA
e-mail: peter.winch@nationwidechildrens.org

N. J. Klein (ed.), *Perioperative Pediatric Patient Blood Management and Transfusion Safety*, https://doi.org/10.1007/978-3-031-81666-6_12

- What are current professional guidelines addressing ANH?
- Are there regulatory requirements for intraoperative ANH?

12.2 Discussion

12.2.1 Background

Acute normovolemic hemodilution (ANH) is a form of autologous transfusion, typically performed during the intraoperative period. ANH is based on the principle that blood lost during surgery after autologous blood collection and circulating volume replenishment will have a lower hematocrit (Hct) than the patient's baseline Hct, thus preserving the collected patient's red blood cell (RBC) mass for reinfusion at a later point in the procedure.

Blood is withdrawn from the patient at the beginning of surgery and is replaced with crystalloid solution or colloid suspension. ANH has been pursued in the interest of reducing the need for banked blood products. One of the first published pediatric cases of ANH was described in 1970. According to a Jehovah Witness's publication, the parents of a child needing cardiac surgery refused allogeneic blood products on faith-based grounds [1]. A portion of the patient's blood was withdrawn at the beginning of the case and replaced with Lactated Ringers solution. Severe hemodilution, described as "able to read a paper's headlines through the blood," was the result when the hematocrit dropped from 60% to 10%. The collected blood was reinfused after termination of CPB. The child survived the surgery and reportedly recovered uneventfully.

The practice of ANH gained popularity in the 1980s due to concerns over transfusion-related HIV transmission. It then fell out of favor when blood screening practices improved. Today, restrictive transfusion practices and increased implementation of patient blood management (PBM) programs have standardized blood conservation efforts. Currently, ANH is re-emerging as a blood conservation strategy to minimize the hazards of allogeneic blood product transfusion, improve patient outcomes, and preserve the blood supply. Widespread blood shortages, exacerbated during the COVID-19 pandemic, have reinvigorated these goals [2, 3].

Although ANH has been clinically practiced since the 1970s, the first evidence-based recommendations were published in 2020 with support of the Society for the Advancement of Blood Management [4]. While focused on adult cardiac surgery, this expert consensus identified criteria for incorporating ANH into other clinical settings. Currently, professional guidelines supporting pediatric ANH do not exist largely because the practice lacks supporting evidence in children. The literature reporting successful pediatric ANH practices originates in centers that routinely serve large populations of patients with faith-based refusal of allogeneic blood transfusions. These centers have established ANH protocols and knowledgeable support personnel.

ANH is a strategy that should be reserved for specific patient indications as a complement to a comprehensive PBM program. Additional perioperative PBM strategies include preoperative anemia screening and management, minimization of blood loss, antifibrinolytics, viscoelastic and other point-of-care (POC) testing, and standardized protocols. In the interest of patient safety, practicing institutions must have ANH protocols, equipment, and staff education in place [5]. The Association for the Advancement of Blood and Biotherapies (AABB) standards on autologous blood collection require that the hospital ANH program be overseen by a physician trained or experienced in the procedure [6].

12.2.2 What Are Indications, Advantages, and Contraindications to Intraoperative ANH [4–8]?

12.2.2.1 Indications

- Refusal of allogeneic blood products
- Rare blood types with difficulty securing allogeneic blood products
- Desire to reduce allogeneic donor exposure
- Emergency procedures without time to perform preoperative autologous donation
- Low-resource environments where blood is unavailable, there is no regional blood bank, or transfusion-transmitted infections (TTI) are endemic

12.2.2.2 Advantages

- Reduced exposure to the hazards of allogeneic blood products
- Availability of fresh autologous whole blood with preservation of platelets and clotting factors
- Avoidance of blood storage lesions associated with banked allogeneic blood products
- Preservation of RBC mass because the patient's intraoperative surgical blood loss is relatively hemodiluted (i.e., lower hematocrit than pre-ANH)
- Lower costs
- A theoretically decreased risk of administration error (e.g., ABO incompatible transfusion) when the patient's blood does not leave the operating room

12.2.2.3 Contraindications

- Preoperative anemia (e.g., hemoglobin <8–10 g/dL) in the face of large blood loss or significant end-organ dysfunction
- Patient refusal
- Hemodynamic instability or significant arrhythmia
- Acute infection
- Poor end-organ reserve
- Presence of a coagulation disorder
- Hemoglobinopathy (a relative contraindication)

Current reviews suggest a minimum hemoglobin of 11 g/dL in adult patients before ANH, with a caveat that each patient and procedure enable different thresholds; there is no such guidance in the pediatric literature [4, 5].

12.2.3 What Is the Evidence Supporting the Use of ANH?

Current evidence in support of ANH is primarily found in the adult patient literature. Meta-analyses show high variability in the techniques used and a high degree of heterogeneity in patient selection. In the pediatric population, the literature is even less informative. The following section describes current research findings for both adult and pediatric ANH.

12.2.3.1 Relevant Adult Evidence

Overall, evidence supporting ANH in adults indicates a reduction in the allogeneic perioperative transfusion rate. However, this evidence has been inconsistent due to significant heterogeneity and a lack of standardization in the approach to ANH [4]. A decrease in allogeneic transfusions has been reported when ANH was used in orthopedic, vascular, gynecologic-oncologic, liver transplant, and liver resection procedures [9–13]. Table 12.1 illustrates summary findings of meta-analyses in adult ANH for the period 2015 to 2020:

The evidence suggests that ANH is most effective in reducing allogeneic RBC requirements when larger ANH blood volumes are withdrawn and reinfused. Goldberg et al. analyzed over 13,000 patients in a cardiac surgery registry who were grouped into ANH volumes of 0 mL, <400 mL, 400–799 mL, and >800 mL blood removed. Patients undergoing ANH had associated reductions in allogeneic RBC usage, with the greatest reduction seen in patients receiving ≥800 mL (adjusted relative risk of RBC transfusion, 0.74 vs 0.57) [17]. A recent prospective trial

Table 12.1 Meta-analyses of adult ANH in the literature (years 2015–2020)

First author/ year	Design	Findings	Limitations
Li (2020) [14]	Meta-analysis of 22 randomized controlled trials (RCTs) on coronary artery bypass graft surgeries	Relative risk (RR) 0.65 for the rate of allogeneic blood transfusion; less postoperative blood loss in the ANH vs the control groups	The studies had high levels of heterogeneity
Barile (2017) [15]	Meta-analysis of 27 RCTs on cardiac surgeries	Fewer allogeneic RBC transfusions in the ANH compared to the control group (mean difference of −0.79; 95% CI −1.25 to −0.34), and less postoperative blood loss was reported in the ANH compared to the control group	The studies had high levels of heterogeneity
Zhou (2015) [16]	Meta-analysis of 63 RCTs which included cardiac, vascular, orthopedic, hepatic, maxillofacial, and neurologic surgeries	Reduction in the risk of allogeneic blood transfusion (overall risk reduction = 0.74, 95% CI 0.63–0.88; intraoperative = 0.54, 95% CI 0.38–0.78) between ANH groups compared to control groups. No difference in adverse events and lengths of hospital stay was demonstrated between groups	The authors cautioned regarding the high degree of heterogeneity of the studies

randomized 110 patients undergoing cardiac surgery to medium (M) and large (L) volume ANH (M-ANH 5–8 ml/kg vs L-ANH 12–15 ml/kg collected, to a minimum Hgb 10 mg/dL after collection) [18]. The results found the L-ANH (mean 886 mL) group received reduced allogeneic RBC transfusions compared to the M-ANH (mean 385 mL) group, and the volume of allogeneic RBCs transfused was inversely proportional to the volume of ANH [18].

A current recommendation is that an estimated blood loss of 500–700 mL in adults, equivalent to approximately 10–15% of the average adult total blood volume (i.e., two allogeneic RBC units), should be expected before planning ANH [19, 20]. The 1997 version of the Association for the Advancement of Blood & Biotherapies (AABB) guideline for ANH recommends that the procedure is indicated when the patient is expected to lose >20% of estimated blood volume (EBV) [21].

12.2.3.2 Relevant Pediatric Evidence

To date, there are several small studies and case reports addressing ANH in children, as well as two prospective, randomized, controlled trials (Table 12.2). Most of the case reports involve cardiac surgery in children of Jehovah's Witness parents [29–32].

Table 12.2 Published pediatric ANH studies (2004–2020)

First author/ year	Design	ANH procedure	Findings
Uchida (2022) [22]	Retrospective propensity matched; scoliosis correction surgery; 125 patients (ANH 95; control 30)	Volume collected from central line and calculated to avoid Hgb less than 8 g/dL; volume collected was replaced with equal volume of crystalloid or colloid; phenylephrine or colloid bolus for hypotension during collection	The ANH group had lower intraoperative and postoperative transfusion rates (18% vs 37%) and required less allogeneic blood compared to the control group. No differences were found between groups for other outcomes including adverse events
Harris (2020) [23]	Prospective RCT; cardiopulmonary bypass (CPB) surgery; age 6–36 months; 24 patients (ANH 12, control 12)	The ANH patients had 10 ml/kg autologous blood collected and replaced 1:1 with 5% albumin	No difference between groups for reduced allogeneic transfusion or other postoperative outcomes (blood loss, hematocrit, inotropic agent use, hospital and ICU length of stay)
Nobre (2020) [24]	Retrospective; scoliosis correction surgery; 33 patients (ANH 16 patients, control 17)	Calculated ANH volume was collected via arterial line to target Hct (different for each patient). The first 1 L autologous collected was replaced with colloids/blood 1:1 ratio; above 1 L, 2:1 ratio. All ANH blood was reinfused and furosemide 0.5–1 mg/kg was given	The ANH group had lower rates and volume of allogeneic transfusion (2 vs 12 patients and 86 mL vs 630 mL, respectively) compared to the control group; no other outcome differences were found between groups, including adverse events

(continued)

Table 12.2 (continued)

First author/ year	Design	ANH procedure	Findings
Kaiser (2018) [25]	Retrospective; complex cardiac repair undergoing CPB; weight <10 kg; 36 patients (ANH 18, controls 18)	52 mL autologous blood was collected in a syringe with 8 ml of anticoagulant for each patient; volume replacement was done only if hemodynamically unstable using albumin 5% (1:1); inotropic support as needed	Decreased donor exposure (2.6 vs 6.5 units) without increased postoperative bleeding in the ANH group compared to the control group; the total volume transfused was similar (47 vs 70 mL/kg, $p = 0.07$) between the ANH and control groups
Crescini (2018) [26]	Retrospective; cardiac surgery under CPB; age 0–36 months; 50 patients (ANH 7, control 43)	10 ml/kg autologous blood collected which was replaced 1:1 with 5% albumin. Blood collection duration was 5–15 min	ANH was associated with reduced intraoperative allogeneic blood product use and less blood loss at 6 and 24 h postoperatively; the 48 h postoperative total (mL/kg) plasma and platelet administration also reduced; hospital and ICU length of stay were similar between groups
Naguib (2015) [27]	Retrospective; cardiac surgery under CPB, biventricular; 209 patients <6 kg (ANH 26, no-ANH 47) 6–18 kg (ANH 52, no-ANH 14) >18 kg (ANH 67, no-ANH 3)	Initial Hct and target Hct calculated; in patients <5 kg, 10–20 ml/kg total blood volume removed; if >5 kg, 10–20% of EBV removed; volume replacement limited pre-CPB, vasopressors used to keep hemodynamic stability as guided by spectroscopy and other parameters	Overall, bloodless surgery or no allogeneic blood products received during the hospital stay were: • 0% of <6 kg group; similar hemostatic parameters upon arrival to the ICU; similar ICU and hospital LOS • 36% of 6–18 kg group. Similar hemostatic parameters upon arrival to the ICU; similar transfusion volumes and in ICU; similar ICU and hospital LOS • 81% of ≥18 kg group: no adverse events
Friesen (2006) [28]	Prospective RCT; cardiac surgery under CPB; Wt. 5–12 kg; 32 patients (ANH 16 patients; control 16)	15 mL/kg of blood collected with 15 mL/kg of albumin 5% administered as replacement	The ANH group had improved postoperative coagulation parameters; 24-h postoperative weight-based blood loss was similar

Available evidence for pediatric ANH is inconclusive and insufficient to support its routine use outside of special circumstances. The aforementioned studies report no increase in ANH-related adverse events, but these studies were not adequately powered to detect outcome differences. To date, there is not a published systematic review or meta-analysis on perioperative pediatric ANH.

12.2.4 What Is the Procedure for Performing ANH in Children?

The following discussion will address a suggested initial intraoperative ANH setup, the subsequent blood withdrawal, and the reinfusion procedure.

12.2.4.1 Patient Preparation

(1) Obtain patient and/or guardian *informed consent.*

In addition to the ethical and legal bases for obtaining informed consent before one performs a procedure that carries inherent risk, it is important to keep in mind that ANH, as part of a PBM bundle, has patient-centered underpinnings.

(2) *Determine total blood volume to withdraw*: Prior to initiation of ANH, the amount of whole blood to be collected from the patient should be determined. A good start is to withdraw blood in aliquots equal to 10% of the patient's EBV. In an adult, 10% of EBV is 400–500 ml; in a 50 kg adolescent, 350 ml; and in a 10 kg infant, 80 ml. Also, in children, typical initial aliquots are 10 ml/kg, which can be increased to 20 ml/kg or 20% of EBV as tolerated during close monitoring of end-organ perfusion [27]. In adults with a robust initial Hct who are about to undergo a large blood loss procedure, one may remove 1 to 4 whole blood units as the patient tolerates [20, 33].

(a) In practice, it is suggested to plan a total blood withdrawal volume to achieve a post-ANH Hct 25–30% or Hb 8–9 g/dL [7, 34, 35]. One must leave the patient with a safety margin for surgical blood loss and then maintain the Hct nadir above a critical value. It is also recommended that blood should be reinfused when the Hct is <21% [7].

(b) The target volume of blood to be withdrawn can also be estimated using the following formula [36, 37]:

$$\text{Volume of blood to withdraw} = \text{EBV} \times \left(\text{Hct}_i - \text{Hct}_t\right) / \text{Hct}_{\text{avg}}$$

where Hct_i is the initial hematocrit; Hct_t is the target hematocrit; Hct_{av} is the average hematocrit or $(\text{Hct}_i + \text{Hct}_t)/2$.

Blood volume withdrawal calculations are illustrated below:

For a 10 kg child with initial Hct 35%, a target Hct of 31%, and an EBV of 800 mL (80 mL/kg for age):

$$\text{Volume of blood to withdraw} = \left[\text{EBV}\,800 \times (35 - 31)\right] / \left[35 + 31/2\right] = 97\,\text{mL}$$

If the Hct_f is readjusted to 24% (approximate Hgb 8 g/dL), applying this same formula, the volume to withdraw triples to 290 mL, which is over one-third of the patient's EBV. As stated, the total whole blood withdrawn is best procured in sequential (10 mL/kg) aliquots.

(c) The target hematocrit value is integral to safe ANH practice and must be greater than the patient's "critical" hemoglobin value or when oxygen consumption becomes dependent upon oxygen delivery. This critical hematocrit value may be as low as 15% (e.g., hemoglobin approximately 5 g/dL) in humans, but in practice it varies from patient to patient [38]. A typical target hematocrit for ANH in otherwise healthy adults is 21–30% [20, 34]. A target Hct value for ANH in healthy children has not been determined and will depend on the patient's cardiopulmonary reserve. For instance, children with cyanotic heart disease have been shown through in vitro modeling to require a Hgb greater than 13 g/dL (Hct 39%) to maintain arterial oxygen saturation >70% when cardiac output is fixed at 6 L/min/m^2 [39].

12.2.4.2 The Procedure

VASCULAR ACCESS: There are commercially available ANH kits containing bags with anticoagulation, connectors, and even patient identification bands [20]. An arterial line, central venous line (CVL), or a peripheral intravenous line (PIV) may be used for blood withdrawal (Fig. 12.1).

Since pediatric patients undergoing surgeries with large blood loss are often cannulated for arterial monitoring and large volume administration commensurate with their body weight, those existing lines are sufficient for the ANH process. The larger the line, the greater the success of blood removal and the less risk of hemolysis. The puncture or vascular access site should be prepared in a sterile fashion to minimize bacterial contamination. In general, blood withdrawal is best accomplished in the smallest patients by allowing the blood to freely flow from an arterial line until the desired volume is collected. Due to the pulsatile nature of arterial blood and rate of flow, the rate of removal must be closely monitored. In adolescents and adults, a large bore PIV or a CVL usually provides adequate blood flow to complete blood collection. For fast-flowing or relatively large catheters, the withdrawal rate can be controlled through gently drawing the aliquots into a syringe [32]. It is critical to note that all holding bags or syringes must contain anticoagulant in the appropriate ratios and periodically agitated during collection to ensure admixture [6].

MONITORING: Hemodynamic instability (e.g., hypotension, bradycardia) occurs when blood is withdrawn too quickly. Full hemodynamic monitoring (e.g., blood pressure (BP), heart rate (HR), oxygen saturation, and electrocardiogram (ECG)) is essential. Intermittent pauses in collection are suggested to control the speed of exsanguination and to assess the patient. If using a sole arterial line, continuous beat-to-beat monitoring will be lost during withdrawal. A non-invasive BP cuff on the opposite limb should cycle every minute during the blood removal. Continuous hemodynamic monitoring must be done with a focus on the patient's fluid responsiveness (such as pulse pressure or stroke volume variation). Additional monitoring such as cerebral oximetry with near-infrared spectroscopy (NIRS) and transesophageal echocardiogram may help guide phlebotomy as well as volume

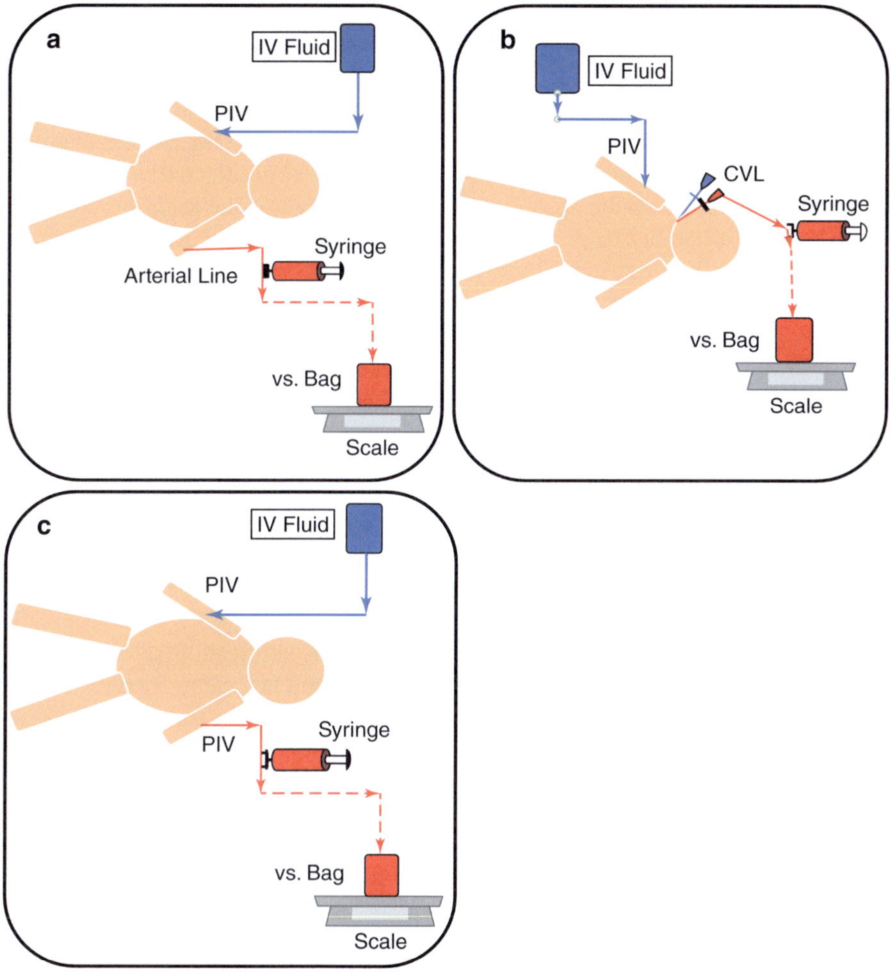

Fig. 12.1 ANH blood can be collected from: (**a**) an arterial line, (**b**) a central venous line (CVL), or (**c**) a large bore peripheral intravenous (IV) catheter (PIV). The collection container can be a graduated syringe or a standardized bag containing anticoagulant. For collection into a bag, use a weighing scale to estimate the volume collected; 1 g is equivalent to 1 ml blood.

replacement. A urethral catheter with a volumetric scale in milliliters is essential to monitor the urine output in small children.

RATE OF BLOOD REMOVAL: The rate of blood collection depends on the patient's ability to tolerate the speed of blood removal during simultaneous volume replacement. If using withdrawal via gravity flow from a CVL or a PIV, a weighing scale should be used to estimate the volume removed. As a rule, 1 g = 1 mL (the density of whole blood is 1.053 g/ml). Adjusting the height difference between the patient and the collection bag will control the speed of blood removal. Blood removal can also be via a syringe, with gentle suction to minimize hemolysis. Allow at least

15–30 min for the entire collection process. Although pediatric standards do not exist, a reasonable withdrawal rate is 10% of EBV over several minutes under continuous hemodynamic monitoring, with a "rest" between aliquots. In adults, the AABB suggests that in adults undergoing autologous donation, an average of 500 mL may be collected in an average time <10 min (e.g., 1.0 ml/kg/min in a 70 kg patient) [20, 40]. The withdrawal rate tolerated by the individual patient may be affected by an underlying condition as well as the vasodilatory effects of the anesthetic. In the event of hemodynamic instability or evidence of end-organ ischemia, the autologous blood may immediately be reinfused to the patient, and the process then terminated.

STORAGE: Institutions using ANH should create a protocol addressing the procedure, blood bag storage, ancillary equipment, and training. The following steps outline the measures to safely preserve the ANH blood prior to reinfusion [6]:

- During blood removal, blood bags should undergo mild agitation to allow the CDPA (citrate-phosphate-dextrose solution with adenine) anticoagulant solution to mix evenly with the whole blood to minimize clot formation. The recommended citrate/blood ratio is 1:7. Agitation is recommended until collection is complete.
- Before storage, all air must be removed from collection bag to avoid air embolization.
- Labeling must comply with specimen and patient verification standards. The blood bag must be labeled with the patient's first and last name, medical record number or birth date, the date and time when collection began, and the time of expiration. Per AABB standards, the label must also include "For Autologous Use Only," "Donor Untested," and "Biohazard."
  - The blood bag may be maintained at room temperature for 8 h or at 1–6 °C in a blood bank-controlled refrigerator or blood cooler for 24 h. This time interval begins at the start of collection. Cold storage must begin within 8 h of the start of the ANH procedure.

REINFUSION:

- Reinfusion should take place when surgical blood loss has ceased, hemoglobin has fallen <7 g/dL, or there is hemodynamic instability, whichever occurs first [41].
- If it is not used within the 8-h room temperature storage period, it should be discarded as with any biohazard waste. Per AABB guidelines, autologous blood should be reinfused *only* to the patient from whom it is collected [6].
- Prior to reinfusion, the standard patient verification process should be followed, as with allogeneic blood from the blood bank.
- Use a standard blood filter (generally150–260 micron) for reinfusion of autologous blood.
- Before administration, a final inspection should be performed checking for the presence of clots, air, or any other abnormalities. If air is seen, remove all air prior to transfusion to prevent air embolism.

- Avoid volume overload; consider diuresis (furosemide) administration as needed.
- Be vigilant for hypocalcemia secondary to calcium chelation during reinfusion because of the presence of citrate preservative in the stored ANH blood.
- The ANH procedure should be documented in the patient's medical record, the same way other blood is documented, including the date, time, volume, pre- and post-transfusion vital signs, and the name of the transfusionist.

If adverse reaction is suspected during reinfusion, stop the transfusion immediately. If the blood has not left the operating room, the most likely causes include citrate toxicity or bacterial contamination. In that case, one should treat the patient and contact blood bank for a transfusion reaction workup at the direction of the blood bank medical director. The event should also be documented in the patient's medical record.

12.2.4.3 Post-ANH Evaluation and Management

There are no generally accepted standards for the postoperative management of patients who have undergone intraoperative ANH. Because ANH can produce a dilutional anemia and coagulopathy from excessive volume replacement, it may be prudent to evaluate the patient's blood count and coagulation parameters following the procedure. There is no data to inform home discharge following surgery; thus the decision to perform ANH in an outpatient should follow the same standards as any blood loss procedure.

Blood collected intraoperatively may be administered in the patient's postoperative location. However, compliance with proper autologous bag labeling and storage regulations is critical to safe patient care and may ultimately impact transfusion service accreditation. The AABB has promulgated perioperative guidelines for autologous collection and administration in the interest of quality care and patient safety [6]. Under the direction of a qualified physician, a process should be in place to standardize the ANH procedure, with monitoring and reporting of quality indicators such as utilization, waste, equipment malfunction, and suspected TTIs. Blood obtained by ANH is intended for the donor patient only and should not be saved for use in another patient; this proscription may be overlooked in low-resource locations with a critical blood shortage [42, 43].

12.2.5 What Are Safety Concerns Related to ANH?

ANH is limited by the amount of blood that may be safely removed at the beginning of the case followed by the patient's ability to tolerate reinfusion when surgical bleeding has ceased. The positive benefit of ANH is directly linked to the amount of collected blood. Anemic patients are unlikely to tolerate removal of a meaningful blood volume. Excessive fluid replacement may produce a dilutional anemia and coagulopathy, impairing hemostasis, as well as compromising end-organ oxygen delivery. Furthermore, small quantities of autologous blood may not justify the burden of collection, including costs, increased intraoperative workload, and the inherent risks associated with any intravascular procedure (e.g., air embolism).

In a retrospective review of 250 adult patients undergoing sagittal split osteotomy, Iwase et al. found that intraoperative blood loss was greatest in patients who had undergone both preoperative autologous donation (PAD) and intraoperative ANH, despite the fact that patients had similar pre- and postoperative Hct values and conventional coagulation parameters [44]. The patients with higher blood loss had more blood withdrawn during ANH (800 ml vs. 660 ml) as well as significantly more volume replacement with low molecular weight hydroxyethyl starch (HES), which has coagulopathic potential in excess quantities. A 2004 meta-analysis of 42 RCTs including 2233 patients undergoing various surgeries (cardiac, thoracic, liver, hip, knee, cranial, and prostate) found that overall, intraoperative and total blood loss was comparable between the ANH and usual care groups, although in the liver resection, aortic bypass, and thoracic surgery subgroups, the intraoperative blood loss was higher in the ANH group by a mean of 380 mL [45]. Fluid replacement type and amount were not described in the meta-analysis. A third study analyzed the hemostatic parameters in 11 adult ANH patients undergoing total hip arthroplasty with spinal anesthesia, using130:0.4 hydroxyethyl starch in a 1:1 replacement volume [46]. Following ANH, rotational thromboelastometry (ROTEM) showed changes consistent with a borderline hypocoagulable state. ROTEM parameters reversed, however, after reinfusion of the patient's autologous blood. Platelet aggregation function was also tested via impedance aggregometry and was not affected by ANH.

There is no data describing a validated or evidence-based blood volume that is appropriate to withdraw in pediatric ANH. The reported volumes have been in the range of 10 mL/kg or 10% total blood volume, expanded to 20 mL/kg or 20% of EBV as tolerated under close monitoring [27]. Successful volumes may be extrapolated from the PAD literature. PAD has been performed in children as young as 6 months and as small as 8 kg, although most reports of smaller children include body weights around 20 kg [47, 48]. Donation volumes documented in the literature range from 6 to 19 ml/kg body weight, most commonly 10 ml/kg per donation event [49]. However, it is important to recognize the additional hemodynamic and stress response effects of ongoing anesthesia and surgery. In children, blood loss equal to approximately 20% of their estimated blood volume (EBV) can occur before hemodynamic instability is evident. Based on the limited data from the adult ANH literature, it may be prudent to employ ANH in pediatric blood loss cases only if the expected procedural blood loss is greater than 10% but less than 20% of the child's EBV.

Since ANH that leads to an effective reduction of allogeneic RBC use is reportedly large volume blood collection, a logical concern is how much blood, and at what rate, can be withdrawn without compromising tissue oxygenation. A prospective investigation of anemia tolerance with profound ANH was conducted in 8 children (mean age 12 years) undergoing scoliosis surgery. Blood was removed (volume not documented) and replaced with NS or 5% albumin to a preoperative target Hgb of 7 g/dL over 45–90 min [50]. The average pre-ANH Hgb was approximately 11 g/dL (the patients had already donated autologous whole blood units before surgery). Although a specific rate of blood withdrawal was not mentioned, central venous and pulmonary capillary wedge pressures were maintained at or above baseline values. Mixed venous oxygenation (SvO_2) was maintained above 60%. The average nadir Hgb was 3.0 g/dL, although one patient fell to 2.1 g/dL which was accompanied by ST-segment depression that reversed when the autologous blood was reinfused. Patient SvO_2 values fell from 90 to 72%, with a 0.09 arterial pH decrease at the Hgb nadir, but the increase in serum lactate (1.2–1.5 mmol/L) was delayed until the completion of surgery. There were no irreversible adverse outcomes reported following the study.

In a 2015 report from a children's hospital practicing PBM for children undergoing congenital cardiac surgery under cardiopulmonary bypass (CPB), a total of 209 children with biventricular defects underwent a highly structured program that included ANH in addition to retrograde arterial, anterograde venous, and moderate ultrafiltration [27]. The volume collected before surgery was 10–20 mL/kg in patients <5 kg body weight and 10–20% of EBV if >5 kg. Rather than replacing autologous blood with crystalloid in a 1:2 or 1:3 ratio, acellular fluids were relatively restricted, and volume replacement was monitored closely with administration of vasopressors as needed. Although all children weighing <6 kg (n = 73) required some allogeneic transfusion, 36% and 57% of children weighing 6–18 kg (n = 66) and >18 kg (n = 70), respectively, required no allogeneic transfusion. The minimum Hct was 15% for the under 6 kg group, 17% in the 6–18 kg group, and 22% in the >18 kg group during CPB. There were five deaths in the <6 kg group and one in the 6–18 kg group, none of which occurred intraoperatively. The minimum Hgb allowed in the PICU was 7 g/dL. No long-term outcome data are available for these patients.

Safety margins for patients undergoing ANH are unknown, particularly with respect to long-term developmental outcomes. In an attempt to determine the lower Hgb limit required to maintain tissue hypoxia, Weiskopf et al. withdrew blood from healthy adult volunteers (450–900 ml/event) to a minimum Hgb 5 g/dl and replaced intravascular volume with albumin and plasma in a 1:1 ratio [51]. In addition to standard cardiovascular monitoring, patients were intensively followed for SvO_2, plasma lactate, and oxygen consumption abnormalities. There was no evidence of critically low O_2 delivery during the 2 ½ h observation period, although 2 ECG abnormalities occurred which the investigators attributed to positioning artifact. The majority of studies testing critically low perioperative Hgb values have been case reports and comparative cohort studies in Jehovah's Witness patients. In an analysis of studies published between 2010 and 2020, patients undergoing "bloodless" cardiac surgery did not have significantly different outcomes compared to patients receiving allogenic transfusions [52]. Postoperative Hbg values in the bloodless group were relatively high (>9 g/dL), which the investigators attributed to multidisciplinary care and a focus on alternative techniques and adjuncts through pharmacologic, autologous blood, surgical, and anesthesia optimization. In another retrospective review of over 2000 adult patients declining perioperative transfusions, no patients with a postoperative Hgb >7 g/dL died (10% experienced at least one adverse event), but over one-third of patients with a Hgb 4–5 g/dL died; the investigators determined that after adjustment for age and illness severity, every 1 g decrease in Hgb ≤8 g/dL in the postoperative period was associated with a 2.5 increased odds of death (95% CI, 1.9–3.2) [53]. In an earlier retrospective study of bloodless surgery outcomes in over 1400 patients (of which 37 were under age 20), mortality was highest for those with a lowest postoperative Hgb to preoperative Hgb ratio ($Hgb_{low\ post}/Hgb_{pre}$) less than 0.5 (10.8%) compared to those with a ratio >0.5 (0.4%; *p* 0.000) [54]. In that review, 4 of 13 patients with a $Hgb_{low\ post}$ of <4 g/dL died. Mortality was noted to be greater in patients >65 years and those with cardiopulmonary disease.

12.2.6 What Are the Current Professional Guidelines Addressing ANH?

Consensus recommendations for ANH were published in 2020 with support of the Society for the Advancement of Blood Management [4]. Other professional society recommendations are illustrated in Table 12.3.

Table 12.3 Acute normovolemic hemodilution (ANH) recommendations by specific professional organizations. Note that the grading system used for evidence and recommendations differs among professional organizations

Organization/year	Adults	Children
Society of Thoracic Surgeons; Society for Cardiac Anesthesia; American Society of Extracorporeal Technology; Society for Advancement of Blood Management (2021) [55]	"Acute normovolemic hemodilution is a reasonable method to reduce bleeding and transfusion" *Moderate strength of recommendation; high-quality evidence from more than one randomized controlled trial*	Not specified
Consensus recommendations for ANH, supported by the Society for the Advancement of Blood Management (2020) [4]	In patients undergoing cardiac surgery with CPB, there are four conditions for which ANH is acceptable: • Pre-autologous donation • Left main stenosis in a stable compensated cardiac patient • Previous cardiac surgery • Anticipated prolonged CPB (>2.5 h) Two conditions for which ANH is not appropriate: • Hemodynamically significant arrhythmia • Acute infection Other conditions: determined by clinical judgment	Not specified

(continued)

Table 12.3 (continued)

Organization/year	Adults	Children
Network for the Advancement of PBM (NATA; 2019) [56]	Not specified	The authors recommend against the use of routine ANH in patients undergoing cardiac surgery with CPB secondary to small sample sizes in limited studies, alternative blood conservation techniques, and overall low-level evidence *Strong recommendation. Low-quality evidence*
European Society of Anaesthesiology (2017) [57]	"We suggest the use of acute normovolaemic haemodilution (ANH) in selected settings" *Weak recommendation. Low-quality evidence* "We recommend against ANH in combination with controlled hypotension" *Strong recommendation. Moderate-quality evidence* "In patients with pre-existing or acquired coagulopathy we suggest that the use of ANH is considered carefully" *Weak recommendation. Low-quality evidence*	Not specified
American Society of Anesthesiologists (2015) [58]	"ANH is effective in reducing the volume of allogeneic blood transfused and the number of patients transfused with allogeneic blood for major cardiac, orthopedic, thoracic, or liver surgery" *Beneficial. Evidence from meta-analysis of RCTs* "ANH combined with intraoperative red blood cell recovery, compared with intraoperative red blood cell recovery alone, is effective in reducing the volume of allogeneic blood transfused" *Beneficial. Evidence from meta-analysis of RCTs* "ANH is equivocal regarding the number of patients transfused with allogeneic blood" *Equivocal. Evidence from meta-analysis of RCTs*	Not specified

(continued)

Table 12.3 (continued)

Organization/year	Adults	Children
Joint United Kington (UK) Blood Transfusion and Tissue Transplantation Services Professional Advisory Committee (JPAC) (2020) [59]	"Mathematical modeling suggests ANH is most effective … in surgery with major blood loss. Systematic reviews of published trials have found no significant reduction in exposure to donor transfusions…the safety of ANH remains unclear"	Not specified
National Blood Authority (2012–2016) [60]	"In adult patients undergoing surgery in which substantial blood loss (blood loss of a volume great enough to induce anaemia that would require therapy) is anticipated, the use of ANH should be considered" "ANH requires a local procedural guideline that addresses patient selection, vascular access, volume of blood withdrawn, choice of replacement fluid, blood storage and handling, and timing of reinfusion"	"In paediatric patients undergoing surgery, the effect of ANH compared with no ANH on transfusion volume and incidence is uncertain" "In pediatric patients, acute normovolemic hemodilution has not been shown to reduce transfusion or improve clinical outcomes. However, if acute normovolemic hemodilution is used, it requires a local procedural guideline that addresses patient selection, vascular access, volume of blood withdrawn, choice of replacement fluid, blood storage and handling, and timing of reinfusion" "There is little evidence on the use of ANH in paediatric surgery; therefore, the effect on transfusion incidence or volume is uncertain. If this technique is used, a local procedural guideline needs to be in place to ensure patient safety"

12.2.7 Are There Regulatory Requirements for Intraoperative ANH?

The US Association for the Advancement of Blood and Biotherapies (AABB) has promulgated standards for perioperative autologous blood collection and administration [6]. The requirements must be followed in AABB-accredited facilities, which include the development of protocols addressing clinical applications, quality control, procedural safety, and informed consent. The American Society of Extracorporeal Technology (AmSECT), a perfusionist advocacy group dedicated to improving the care and safety of patients undergoing extracorporeal circulation technology, has published an ANH guide for perfusionists [61]. However, regulatory oversight for

ANH is uncommon and, when it exists, generally falls under the umbrella of preoperative autologous donation (PAD) safety regulations [59, 62]. Regulatory oversight for ANH is essentially nonexistent in low-resource countries [43, 63].

12.3 Summary of Key Learning Objectives

12.3.1 What Are the Indications for, Advantages of, and Contraindications to ANH?

A major indication for ANH in this case is the fact that the patient has a rare blood type and the blood bank has expressed difficulty in meeting anticipated perioperative blood requirements. Advantages include reduced exposure to the known risks of allogeneic transfusions, cost, and, theoretically, reduced risk of a clerical administration error. This 14-year-old, 49 kg patient has a blood volume close to that of an adult, which will allow ample withdrawal volume (i.e., 350–700 ml) for reinfusion. His preoperative Hgb is 12 g/dl (Hct 36%), which is higher than the minimum Hgb typically used to exclude ANH as an option in a teenager undergoing a blood loss procedure (e.g., 8–10 g/dl). He has no other apparent contraindications to ANH.

12.3.2 What Is the Evidence Supporting the Rational Use of ANH?

Meta-analyses in adult patients and several small, retrospective studies in children suggest that ANH is associated with reduced perioperative allogeneic transfusions, particularly when bundled with other PBM measures including preoperative anemia treatment, cell salvage, appropriate use of antifibrinolytics, meticulous or noninvasive surgical techniques, and maintenance of perioperative normothermia, acid-base status, and hemodynamic stability. In particular, ANH during pediatric scoliosis surgery has been shown to reduce the volume of allogenic transfusions without an increase in adverse outcomes when managed per standardized protocol.

12.3.3 What Is the Procedure for Performing ANH in Children?

1. Determine that the patient is an appropriate candidate for ANH, including a baseline Hgb >8–10 g/dL. The guiding principle is for the patient to have sufficient RBC mass to allow for hemodilution and surgical blood loss.
2. Obtain informed consent.
3. Determine withdrawal volume: 10% of EBV or, in the alternative, apply the formula:

   Maximum volume of blood to withdraw = $[\mathrm{EBV} \times (\mathrm{Hct}_i - \mathrm{Hct}_t)]/[(\mathrm{Hct}_i + \mathrm{Hct}_t)/2]$

   The Hct_t recommended in healthy adults is 21–30%. If this child's EBV is 3.4 L (70 ml/kg × 49 kg) with a preoperative Hct 36% and a target Hct 21%, the volume to withdraw is 1.7 L. This large whole blood volume is best removed in

aliquots of 10% of EBV, or in multiples of 350 mL, under strict monitoring. The rate of withdrawal should be over a minimum of 15 min per 350 mL aliquot.
4. Vascular access: The blood may be withdrawn from several large-bore PIVs, a CVL, or a single intra-arterial line. Use aseptic technique for access placement and blood collection.
5. Volume replacement: Balanced crystalloid solution or albumin 5% in a ratio of 1:1 or 1:2 whole blood: replacement fluid.
6. Monitoring: Standard ASA monitors plus a measure of fluid responsivity, urine output, and, ideally, near intra-red spectroscopy (NIRS).
7. Storage: The whole blood bag must be labeled with the withdrawal start time, and the patient's name plus another identifier (e.g., medical record number or date of birth), and the time of expiration. Initial agitation with the anticoagulant is necessary to prevent clotting. If held at operating room temperature, the autologous blood must be reinfused within 8 h (or, 24 h if held in a cooler validated by the blood bank).

12.3.4 What Are Safety Concerns Related to ANH?

- Hemodynamic instability secondary to an excessive rate of whole blood withdrawal
- Volume overload secondary to excessive fluid replacement
- Misidentification because the bag is not properly labeled and verified
- Bacterial contamination
- Air embolism

12.3.5 What Are Current Professional Guidelines Addressing ANH?

Most ANH guidelines address the adult patient population. At this point in time, the few professional guidelines that address ANH management in children include the Network for the Advancement of PBM (NATA) and the National Blood Authority (Australia).

12.3.6 Are There Regulatory Requirements for Intraoperative ANH?

AABB has promulgated standards for perioperative autologous blood collection and administration. These must be followed in AABB-accredited and, ultimately, US Food and Drug Administration (FDA)-accredited facilities. The standards include oversight by an experienced physician and the development of protocols addressing clinical applications, quality control, procedural safety, and informed consent. However, regulatory oversight for ANH is uncommon and, when it exists, generally falls under the umbrella of preoperative autologous donation (PAD) safety regulations.

Key Points

- In select patients, ANH can preserve the patient's RBC mass, reduce the need for allogeneic blood transfusion, and lower donor exposure when used in conjunction with other blood conservation strategies as part of a robust PBM program.
- ANH is most effective when the surgery is associated with significant blood loss and the patient can tolerate a relatively large amount of blood withdrawal.
- ANH safety concerns include hemodynamic instability due to intolerance of the volume withdrawn, dilutional anemia or coagulopathy, fluid overload, air embolism, and bacterial contamination.
- Performance of ANH is technically involved; thus institutional ANH protocols, education, and experienced pediatric practitioners are crucial for patient safety.

References

1. JW.Org Community Information. OrphanCrow. JW child first pediatric patient to receive normovolemic hemodilution – 1970. 2015. https://www.jehovahs-witness.com/topic/4856993229570048/jw-child-first-pediatric-patient-receive-acute-normovolemic-hemodilution-1970. Accessed 16 June 2023.
2. Al-Riyami AZ, Burnouf T, Wood EM, Devine DV, Oreh A, Apelseth TO, et al. International Society of Blood Transfusion survey of experiences of blood banks and transfusion services during the COVID-19 pandemic. Vox Sang. 2022;117(6):822–30.
3. Riley W, Love K, McCullough J. Public policy impact of the COVID-19 pandemic on blood supply in the United States. Am J Public Health. 2021;111(5):860–6.
4. Shander A, Brown J, Licker M, Mazer DC, Meier J, Ozawa S, et al. Standards and best practice for acute normovolemic hemodilution: evidence-based consensus recommendations. J Cardiothorac Vasc Anesth. 2020;34(7):1755–60.
5. Kopko PM. Transfusion reactions. 5th ed. Bethesda: AABB Press; 2021. p. 41.
6. Perioperative Standards Committee. Sections 1, 5, and 7. In: Standards for perioperative autologous blood collection and administration. 10th ed. Bethesda: AABB; 2023.
7. Henderson RA, Judd M, Strauss ER, Gammie JS, Mazzeffi MA, Taylor BS, et al. Hematologic evaluation of intraoperative autologous blood collection and allogeneic transfusion in cardiac surgery. Transfusion. 2021;61(3):788–98.
8. Kreimeier U, Messmer K. Perioperative hemodilution. Transfus Apher Sci. 2002;27(1):59–72.
9. Bansal N, Kaur G, Garg S, Gombar S. Acute normovolemic hemodilution in major orthopedic surgery. J Clin Orthop Trauma. 2020;11(Suppl 5):S844–8.
10. Droz NM, Lin J, Beach J, Vo C, Morrow K, Lyden SP, et al. Decreased transfusion requirements with use of acute normovolemic hemodilution in open aortic aneurysm repair. J Vasc Surg. 2021;74(6):1885–93.
11. Boerner T, Tanner E, Filippova O, Zhou QC, Iasonos A, Tew WP, et al. Survival outcomes of acute normovolemic hemodilution in patients undergoing primary debulking surgery for advanced ovarian cancer: a Memorial Sloan Kettering Cancer Center Team Ovary study. Gynecol Oncol. 2021;160(1):51–5.
12. Jabbour N, Gagandeep S, Mateo R, Sher L, Strum E, Donovan J, et al. Live donor liver transplantation without blood products: strategies developed for Jehovah's Witnesses offer broad application. Ann Surg. 2004;240(2):350–7.

13. Jarnagin WR, Gonen M, Maithel SK, Fong Y, D'Angelica MI, Dematteo RP, et al. A prospective randomized trial of acute normovolemic hemodilution compared to standard intraoperative management in patients undergoing major hepatic resection. Ann Surg. 2008;248(3):360–9.
14. Li S, Liu Y, Zhu Y. Effect of acute normovolemic hemodilution on coronary artery bypass grafting: a systematic review and meta-analysis of 22 randomized trials. Int J Surg. 2020;83:131–9.
15. Barile L, Fominskiy E, Di Tomasso N, Alpizar Castro LE, Landoni G, De Luca M, et al. Acute normovolemic hemodilution reduces allogeneic red blood cell transfusion in cardiac surgery: a systematic review and meta-analysis of randomized trials. Anesth Analg. 2017;124(3):743–52.
16. Zhou X, Zhang C, Wang Y, Yu L, Yan M. Preoperative acute normovolemic hemodilution for minimizing allogeneic blood transfusion: a meta-analysis. Anesth Analg. 2015;121(6):1443–55.
17. Goldberg J, Paugh TA, Dickinson TA, Fuller J, Paone G, Theurer PF, et al. Greater volume of acute normovolemic hemodilution may aid in reducing blood transfusions after cardiac surgery. Ann Thorac Surg. 2015;100(5):1581–7; discussion 7.
18. Ming Y, Zhang F, Yao Y, Cheng Z, Yu L, Sun D, et al. Large volume acute normovolemic hemodilution in patients undergoing cardiac surgery with intermediate-high risk of transfusion: a randomized controlled trial. J Clin Anesth. 2023;87:111082.
19. Napier JA, Bruce M, Chapman J, Duguid JK, Kelsey PR, Knowles SM, et al. Guidelines for autologous transfusion. II. Perioperative haemodilution and cell salvage. British Committee for Standards in Haematology Blood Transfusion Task Force. Autologous Transfusion Working Party. Br J Anaesth. 1997;78(6):768–71.
20. Shander A. Surgical blood conservation: acute normovolemic hemodilution. UpToDate. 2022. Accessed 27 Feb 2023.
21. Youssef IA, Alredy MM, Attia JZ. Acute normovolemic hemodilution. MJMR. 2021;32:69–70. https://mjmr.journals.ekb.eg/article_220722_97c759028ffb8108c3a827b6079cdba3.pdf.
22. Uchida S, Kinoshita H, Takekawa D, Saito J, Hirota K. Acute normovolemic hemodilution reduced the frequency and amount of perioperative allogeneic blood transfusion in pediatric and adolescent scoliosis surgery: a retrospective observational study. J Anesth. 2022;36(4):484–92.
23. Harris WM, Treggiari MM, LeBlanc A, Giacomuzzi C, You JJ, Muralidaran A, et al. Randomized pilot trial of acute normovolemic hemodilution in pediatric cardiac surgery patients. World J Pediatr Congenit Heart Surg. 2020;11(4):452–8.
24. Nobre LV, Garcia LV. Role of acute hemodilution in blood transfusion rate in patients submmited to scoliosis surgery: observational retrospective study. Braz J Anesthesiol. 2020;70(3):209–14.
25. Kaiser A, Miller K, Tian G, Moore RH, Guzzetta NA. Feasibility of autologous intraoperative blood collection and retransfusion in small children with complex congenital heart defects undergoing cardiopulmonary bypass. Paediatr Anaesth. 2018;28(9):795–802.
26. Crescini WM, Muralidaran A, Shen I, LeBlan A, You J, Giacomuzzi C, et al. The use of acute normovolemic hemodilution in paediatric cardiac surgery. Acta Anaesthesiol Scand. 2018;62(6):756–64.
27. Naguib AN, Winch PD, Tobias JD, Simsic J, Hersey D, Nicol K, et al. A single-center strategy to minimize blood transfusion in neonates and children undergoing cardiac surgery. Paediatr Anaesth. 2015;25(5):477–86.
28. Friesen RH, Perryman KM, Weigers KR, Mitchell MB, Friesen RM. A trial of fresh autologous whole blood to treat dilutional coagulopathy following cardiopulmonary bypass in infants. Paediatr Anaesth. 2006;16(4):429–35.
29. Burnside JL, Ratliff TM, Kelly MN, Naguib AN, Galantowicz M, Hodge A. Bloodless arterial switch operation in a 2.7-kg Jehovah's witness patient. J Extra Corpor Technol. 2020;52(2):142–5.
30. Plancher G, Datt B, Nguyen M, Munro H, DeCampli WM, Pourmoghadam K. Bloodless heart surgery for an 11-kg infant of the Jehovah's witness faith undergoing second repair for complete atrioventricular canal. J Extra Corpor Technol. 2018;50(3):184–6.
31. Karuppiah S, McKee C, Hodge A, Galantowicz M, Tobias J, Naguib A. Perioperative management of a child with hypoplastic left heart syndrome of the Jehovah's witness faith presenting for hybrid comprehensive stage II procedure. J Extra Corpor Technol. 2016;48(3):141–7.

32. Ratliff TM, Hodge AB, Preston TJ, Galantowicz M, Naguib A, Gomez D. Bloodless pediatric cardiopulmonary bypass for a 3.2-kg patient whose parents are of Jehovah's witness faith. J Extra Corpor Technol. 2014;46(2):173–6.
33. Frank S, Guinn NR. Patient blood management. In: Cohn C, Delaney M, Johnson ST, Katz LM, editors. Technical manual. 20th ed. Bethesda: AABB; 2020. p. 592.
34. Jamnicki M, Kocian R, van der Linden P, Zaugg M, Spahn DR. Acute normovolemic hemodilution: physiology, limitations, and clinical use. J Cardiothorac Vasc Anesth. 2003;17(6):747–54.
35. Shander A, Rijhwani TS. Acute normovolemic hemodilution. Transfusion. 2004;44(12 Suppl):26S–34S.
36. Monk TG. Acute normovolemic hemodilution. Surg Infect. 2005;6(1):9–15.
37. Gross JB. Estimating allowable blood loss: corrected for dilution. Anesthesiology. 1983;58(3):277–80.
38. Faraoni D, DiNardo JA. Commentary: Red blood cells transfusion in patients undergoing congenital cardiac surgery: still far from physiology-based practice. J Thorac Cardiovasc Surg. 2022;167(2):e24–6.
39. Ahmed M, Acosta SI, Hoffman GM, Tweddell JS, Ghanayem NS. Mathematical analysis of hemoglobin target in univentricular parallel circulation. J Thorac Cardiovasc Surg. 2022;166(1):214–20.
40. Fung MK. Technical manual. 19th ed. Bethesda: AABB Press; 2017. p. 115.
41. Valentine SL, Bembea MM, Muszynski JA, Cholette JM, Doctor A, Spinella PC, et al. Consensus recommendations for RBC transfusion practice in critically ill children from the pediatric critical care transfusion and anemia expertise initiative. Pediatr Crit Care Med. 2018;19(9):884–98.
42. Osaro E, Charles AT. The challenges of meeting the blood transfusion requirements in Sub-Saharan Africa: the need for the development of alternatives to allogenic blood. J Blood Med. 2011;2:7–21.
43. Jenny HE, Saluja S, Sood R, Raykar N, Kataria R, Tongaonkar R, et al. Access to safe blood in low-income and middle-income countries: lessons from India. BMJ Glob Health. 2017;2(2):e000167.
44. Iwase Y, Kohjitani A, Tohya A, Sugiyama K. Preoperative autologous blood donation and acute normovolemic hemodilution affect intraoperative blood loss during sagittal split ramus osteotomy. Transfus Apher Sci. 2012;46(3):245–51.
45. Segal JB, Blasco-Colmenares E, Norris EJ, Guallar E. Preoperative acute normovolemic hemodilution: a meta-analysis. Transfusion. 2004;44(5):632–44.
46. Shin HJ, Na HS, Do SH. The effects of acute normovolaemic haemodilution on peri-operative coagulation in total hip arthroplasty. Anaesthesia. 2015;70(3):304–9.
47. Lavoie J. Blood transfusion risks and alternative strategies in pediatric patients. Paediatr Anaesth. 2011;21(1):14–24.
48. Vanderlinde ES, Heal JM, Blumberg N. Autologous transfusion. BMJ. 2002;324(7340):772–5.
49. Letts M, Perng R, Luke B, Jarvis J, Lawton L, Hoey S. An analysis of a preoperative pediatric autologous blood donation program. Can J Surg. 2000;43(2):125–9.
50. Fontana JL, Welborn L, Mongan PD, Sturm P, Martin G, Bunger R. Oxygen consumption and cardiovascular function in children during profound intraoperative normovolemic hemodilution. Anesth Analg. 1995;80(2):219–25.
51. Weiskopf RB, Viele MK, Feiner J, Kelley S, Lieberman J, Noorani M, et al. Human cardiovascular and metabolic response to acute, severe isovolemic anemia. JAMA. 1998;279(3):217–21.
52. Chambault AL, Brown LJ, Mellor S, Harky A. Outcomes of cardiac surgery in Jehovah's witness patients: a review. Perfusion. 2021;36(7):661–71.
53. Carson JL, Noveck H, Berlin JA, Gould SA. Mortality and morbidity in patients with very low postoperative Hb levels who decline blood transfusion. Transfusion. 2002;42(7):812–8.
54. Jo KI, Shin JW, Choi TY, Park YJ, Youm W, Kim MJ. Eight-year experience of bloodless surgery at a tertiary care hospital in Korea. Transfusion. 2013;53(5):948–54.

55. Tibi P, McClure RS, Huang J, Baker RA, Fitzgerald D, Mazer CD, et al. STS/SCA/AmSECT/SABM update to the clinical practice guidelines on patient blood management. J Cardiothorac Vasc Anesth. 2021;35(9):2569–91.
56. Faraoni D, Meier J, New HV, Van der Linden PJ, Hunt BJ. Patient blood management for neonates and children undergoing cardiac surgery: 2019 NATA guidelines. J Cardiothorac Vasc Anesth. 2019;33(12):3249–63.
57. Kozek-Langenecker SA, Afshari A, Albaladejo P, Santullano CA, De Robertis E, Filipescu DC, et al. Management of severe perioperative bleeding: guidelines from the European Society of Anaesthesiology. Eur J Anaesthesiol. 2013;30(6):270–382.
58. American Society of Anesthesiologists Task Force on Perioperative Blood M. Practice guidelines for perioperative blood management: an updated report by the American Society of Anesthesiologists Task Force on Perioperative Blood Management. Anesthesiology. 2015;122(2):241–75.
59. Joint United Kington (UK) Blood Transfusion and Tissue Transplantation Services Professional Advisory Committee (JPAC). 6.1: autologous blood transfusion (collection and reinfusion of the patient's own red blood cells). 2020. https://www.transfusionguidelines.org/transfusion-handbook/6-alternatives-and-adjuncts-to-blood-transfusion/6-1-autologous-blood-transfusion-collection-and-reinfusion-of-the-patient-s-own-red-blood-cells. Accessed 19 June 2023.
60. Patient Blood Management Guidelines. 3.6.1. Preoperative autologous donation. National Blood Authority (Australia). https://www.blood.gov.au/system/files/documents/pbm-module-2.pdf. Accessed 16 Mar 2022.
61. Acute Normovolemic Hemodilution, Clinical protocol. American Society of Extracorporeal Technology (AmSECT). 2023. https://www.amsect.org/. Accessed 26 Feb 2023.
62. Canadian Blood Services. Chapter 16: preoperative autologous donation. In: Professional Education/Transfusion. 2021. https://professionaleducation.blood.ca/en/transfusion/clinical-guide/preoperative-autologous-donation. Accessed 19 June 2023.
63. Nnodu OE, Odunukwe N, Odunubi O, Ekanem E, Njoku OS. Cost effectiveness of autologous blood transfusion–a developing country hospital's perspective. West Afr J Med. 2003;22(1):10–2.

Perioperative Adverse Transfusion Reactions

13

Bryce Pasko and Gee Mei Tan

13.1 Case Scenario

You are called to the recovery room to evaluate a 1-year-old male who has undergone cranial vault reconstruction for craniosynostosis. The patient was just transfused an 80 mL aliquot of CPD-A preserved red blood cells (RBCs). Approximately 15 min into the transfusion, the patient's esophageal temperature increases from a baseline of 37.2 °C pre-transfusion to 38.6 °C. His heart rate increased from 98 to 134 bpm; his respiratory rate is stable at 20 breaths/min, oxygen saturation is 99%, and his blood pressure is unchanged at 98/52. You have been asked to manage the fever.

Key Learning Objectives

- Why is it important to report a suspected transfusion reaction?
- What is the differential diagnosis of new-onset fever in a child who has received a blood transfusion in the perioperative period?
- In addition to febrile transfusion reactions, what types of transfusion reactions may present within the perioperative period?
- What is the role of premedication in preventing a transfusion reaction?

B. Pasko (✉)
Medical Director Transfusion Medicine, Apheresis & Coagulation, Department of Pathology and Laboratory Medicine, University of Arizona College of Medicine, Phoenix, AZ, USA
e-mail: bpasko@phoenixchildrens.com

G. M. Tan
Children's Hospital Colorado, School of Medicine, University of Colorado, Aurora, CO, USA
e-mail: geemei.tan@childrenscolorado.org

N. J. Klein (ed.), *Perioperative Pediatric Patient Blood Management and Transfusion Safety*, https://doi.org/10.1007/978-3-031-81666-6_13

- How does one initially approach a suspected transfusion reaction in the perioperative period, including diagnostic evaluation and treatment?

13.2 Discussion

13.2.1 General

An adverse transfusion reaction (ATR) is defined as an adverse patient response to a blood transfusion. An adverse transfusion event (ATE), on the other hand, is an unintended incident that may occur before, during, or following a transfusion [1]. The latter complication is almost always preventable. Examples of ATEs include but are not limited to:

- Wrong-blood-in-tube
- Delays in transfusion
- Administration of the incorrect blood product
- Incorrect patient transfused
- Over-transfusion (in children is usually secondary to incorrect dose calculation)
- Hyperkalemia

A transfusion reaction or event should always be in the differential diagnosis if a patient has an immediate or post-transfusion change in symptoms or vital signs. These reactions include rigors, fever, dyspnea, flank pain, urticaria, pruritis, laryngeal edema, periorbital edema, or localized angioedema [2]. Pediatric patients have been shown to experience a higher rate of transfusion reactions than adult patients, particularly in the neonatal period [3]. This makes it likely that you will oversee at least one transfusion reaction during the perioperative period. With that in mind, it is imperative to know how to identify, manage, and report perioperative transfusion reactions. Diagnosing transfusion reactions can be particularly challenging for patients under anesthesia due to either alterations in consciousness or the myriad effects of anesthetics and fluid shifts [4]. It is particularly important to investigate for signs of hemolysis if the patient has unexpected changes in blood pressure, heart rate, or body temperature during or within the hours following a perioperative transfusion.

When a transfusion reaction is suspected, stop the transfusion, keep the intravenous (IV) line open with fresh normal saline or PlasmaLyte, and then assess the patient. Once you have stopped the transfusion and managed the patient, it is important to decide whether it is safe to restart the transfusion with the suspected unit. *It is appropriate to restart the same transfusion only in cases of a mild allergic transfusion reaction (e.g., urticaria, with or without pruritis), after patient evaluation and possibly treatment* [5, 6]. The following sections will discuss the recognition and management of select adverse transfusion reactions.

13.2.2 Why Is It Important to Report a Suspected Transfusion Reaction?

Standardizing ATR and ATE diagnostic criteria is crucial to facilitating reporting and improving patient outcomes. All suspected transfusions should be reported to the hospital Transfusion Services (i.e., "blood bank") to rule out a transfusion-related event, to identify patients at increased risk of future transfusion reactions, to remove an index blood unit from inventory, or to investigate the unit and the donor for contributing factors. Quality improvements and benchmarking are then possible based on internal ATR or ATE data or participation in a national registry. Furthermore, the hospital Transfusion Services must communicate with bedside practitioners about ongoing incidents to understand gaps in knowledge, guidelines, training, and transfusion safety.

The standard transfusion reaction classification scheme in the United States (US) is the Centers for Disease Control and Prevention National Healthcare Safety Networks (CDC NHSN) Biovigilance component, Hemovigilance Module Surveillance Protocol v2.8 [2]. The purpose of the hemovigilance protocol is to ensure that all transfusion reactions are diagnosed and reported according to standardized criteria. The Hemovigilance Module includes criteria to meet the case definition of a specific transfusion reaction, the severity of the transfusion reaction, and the likelihood of a true transfusion reaction versus a reaction that occurred because of the patient's underlying illness or iatrogenic interventions such as medications. There are also highly developed hemovigilance systems and registries outside the USA, although most do not have a pediatric-specific focus (Fig. 13.1) [7, 8]. Two hemovigilance organizations with online educational tools and consensus updates include the International Society of Blood Transfusion (ISBT; https://www.isbtweb.org/resources/hv-tools.html) and the International Haemovigilance Network (IHN; https://www.ihn-org.com/).

Currently, the most complete database of pediatric ATRs and ATEs is the "SHOT" (Serious Hazards of Transfusion) registry based in the United Kingdom [9, 10].

13.2.3 What Is the Differential Diagnosis of New-Onset Fever in a Child Who Has Received a Blood Transfusion in the Perioperative Period?

Table 13.1 lists commonly encountered transfusion reactions based on presenting signs and symptoms [11]. It is important to note that there can be overlap in the signs or symptoms of the different categories of transfusion reactions. Furthermore, diagnosing a reaction in a patient who is under anesthesia can be particularly difficult, because fever, hypotension, tachycardia, and erythema may have multiple underlying causes, and the patient is unable to self-report symptoms such as pruritis and flank pain.

Note that Table 13.1 groups the febrile nonhemolytic transfusion reaction (FNHTR), the acute hemolytic transfusion reaction (AHR), and bacterial

Fig. 13.1 International hemovigilance organizations. Reprinted with permission from Keir AK, New H, Robitaille N, Crighton GL, Wood EM, Stanworth SJ. Approaches to understanding and interpreting the risks of red blood cell transfusion in neonates. Transfus Med 2019;**29**(4):231-38

Haemovigilance system	Location
SHOT	Manchester, UK
SABRE	London, UK
Portuguese Haemovigilance System	Lisbon, Portugal
Haemovigilance Programme of India – National Institute of Biologicals (NIB)	Mumbai, India
Haemovigilance Malta	Malta
South African National Haemovigilance Program	Johannesburg, South Africa
Norwegian Haemovigilance System (Troll)	Oslo, Norway
Japanese Red Cross Society Blood Service	Japan
US Biovigilance System of the National Healthcare Safety Network (NHSN), Hemovigilance Module	USA
TRIP	Netherlands
Serious Transfusion Incident Reporting (STIR)	Melbourne, Australia
Brazilian Haemovigilance System	Brazil
Systematic Surveillance of Transfusion Treatment	Zagreb, Croatia
Finnish Red Cross Blood Service	Helsinki, Finland
Colombian Haemovigilance Programme	Bogota, Colombia
Danish Registration of Transfusion Risks	Copenhagen, Denmark
The Québec Hemovigilance System	Québec, Canada

contamination (TTI or transfusion-transmitted infection) under the broad category of fever and chills. This categorization is an important starting point, but a fever can be a nonspecific sign in any transfusion reaction. It can also be a sign of physiologic stress in infants and older children and has been associated with drugs, including anesthetics [12–15]. External warming devices commonly used during anesthesia may also masquerade as a febrile transfusion reaction. Thus, it is important to have a basic understanding of the differential diagnosis of transfusion reactions and to maintain a high index of suspicion to forestall and treat the most potentially fatal ones (e.g., acute intravascular hemolysis).

Table 13.1 Presenting signs and symptoms of transfusion reactions

Signs and symptoms	Potential reaction
Abnormal blood product transfusion reactions	
Hives/itching	Mild allergic/allergic
Fever/chills	Febrile nonhemolytic
	Acute hemolytic
	Bacterial contamination
Hypotension	Anaphylaxis
	Transfusion-related acute lung injury (TRALI)
	Acute hemolytic
	Bacterial contamination
Dyspnea	Volume overload (TACO)
	Transfusion-related acute lung injury (TRALI)
	Anaphylaxis
	Transfusion-associated dyspnea (TAD)

Adapted from Centers for Disease Control and Prevention. National Healthcare Safety Network Biovigilance Component Hemovigilance Module Surveillance Protocol v2.8. 2023 [2]. Suddock J.T. & Crookston KP. Transfusion Reactions. StatPearls. Treasure Island (FL): StatPearls Publishing 2022 [11]

13.2.4 Febrile Transfusion Reactions

A febrile transfusion reaction is defined as an oral body temperature ≥38 °C (100.4 °F) *and* an increase in body temperature of ≥1 °C (1.8 °F) above pretransfusion baseline, *or* chills or rigors, during or up to 4 h after completion of a transfusion. The differential diagnosis of fever during transfusion includes but is not limited to AHR, TTI, and FNHTR and the patient's underlying illness. Diagnosis of an FNHTR or attribution of the febrile event to the patient's underlying condition can only occur following a workup in the blood bank that rules out hemolysis or a TTI. The CDC diagnostic criteria for a febrile transfusion reaction specify an oral temperature route; however, a relative rise ≥1 °C (1.8 °F) in an esophageal, skin, or other temperature route is sufficient to trigger suspicion.

13.2.4.1 Febrile Nonhemolytic Transfusion Reaction (FNHTR)

A FNHTR is a diagnosis of exclusion. Once the more serious causes of fever or chills or rigors have been ruled out, a FNHTR can be considered. FNHTR occurs in up to 3% of transfusions; however pre-storage leukoreduction has been associated with a tenfold decrease in FNHTRs [6]. There are multiple proposed mechanisms for FNHTRs, including cytokine release from the leukocytes in the blood product or donor characteristics that produce recipient cytokine activation. Pre-storage leukoreduction reduces the total number of leukocytes in the product minimizing the cytokine levels within the product.

13.2.4.2 Acute Hemolytic Transfusion Reaction (AHR)

An AHR is one of the dreaded adverse outcomes associated with transfusion. It can result from either ABO blood type mismatches or in recipients with underlying antibodies against donor blood cells (e.g., Anti-Jka). Up to 5% of serious transfusion reactions are AHRs [16]. Many hospitals require two blood specimens to evaluate recipient blood type—a primary and confirmatory verification—prior to issuing type-specific blood products. Hemolysis can be divided into two main categories, immune and non-immune. Immune-mediated hemolysis can be further divided into intravascular and extravascular hemolysis. Intravascular hemolysis is typically mediated through IgM isohemaglutinin antibodies, which bind and activate complement, while extravascular hemolysis is initiated by splenic macrophages engulfing RBCs coated with IgG antibodies. Intravascular hemolysis causes the most serious acute reaction. Acute hemolysis usually presents within the first few minutes of transfusion and often includes fever, chills or rigors, back pain, hematuria, pain or oozing at IV sites, DIC, and hypotension [2]. Acute nonimmune hemolysis may result from a variety of causes, including [17]:

- Mechanical hemolysis (e.g., rapid infusers or IV access too small for the rate of transfusion)
- Hypotonic solutions (e.g., D5W)
- Incompatible medications placed into the blood administration catheter
- Underlying hemoglobinopathies in the donor unit with excessive RBC fragility

The most common etiology of fatal AHRs is misidentification of the patient or the blood sample, otherwise known as "wrong-blood-in-tube" [16, 18]. As a result, the Association for the Advancement of Blood and Biotherapies (AABB) has established a clear verification process for both blood samples and patients, which all hospital blood banks must adhere to for certification [19]. Anesthesiologists should be familiar with this verification process because they frequently obtain blood specimens prior to transfusion from unconscious or nonverbal patients, often in a fast-paced environment. As a caveat, although RBCs are the main source of clinically significant AHRs, platelets can also cause hemolysis because they are suspended in donor-compatible plasma when the platelets themselves—due to supply shortages—may not be compatible with the intended recipient [16].

13.2.4.3 Transfusion Transmitted Infection (TTI)

Bacterial contamination of blood products is a major concern when evaluating fevers and occurs in up to 2.5:100,000 transfusions of blood products, although the rate of TTI reporting in children is too low to ascertain age-specific incidence rates [6, 7, 20, 21]. While bacterial contamination can occur with any type of blood product, platelets are most often implicated because they are stored at room temperature. Numerous protocols have been put in place to reduce the likelihood of bacterial contamination, such as sterilization of the venipuncture sites, diversion of the initial donor aliquot, and bacterial screening before blood product release.

13.2.5 In Addition to Febrile Transfusion Reactions, What Types of Transfusion Reactions May Present Within the Perioperative Period?

13.2.5.1 Allergic Transfusion Reaction

Mild allergic transfusion reactions are the most common type of transfusion reactions in both children and adults, occurring up to 3% of all transfused blood products. Plasma-containing products (e.g., fresh frozen plasma (FFP) and platelets) are the most likely products to cause an allergic transfusion reaction, occurring in up to 3% and 0.6%, respectively [5, 6]. Mild allergic transfusion reactions generally present with two or more of the following: cutaneous, nonsystemic symptoms – urticaria, pruritis, or maculopapular rash. These reactions tend to elicit strong concern from clinical teams and families; however, it is important to note that they seldom progress to more severe allergic transfusion reactions, such as anaphylaxis [5]. Thus, while they are uncomfortable for the patient and may cause family distress, mild allergic transfusion reactions do not pose a significant clinical risk. As stated, *it is appropriate to restart the same transfusion only in cases of a mild allergic transfusion reaction (e.g., urticaria, with or without pruritis), after patient evaluation and possibly treatment.*

Unlike mild allergic transfusion reactions, a severe allergic reaction – anaphylaxis—is a rare event, occurring in 1:20,000 to 1:50,000 transfusions, and it is considered a medical emergency [5]. Anaphylactic allergic reactions generally occur within the first 15 min of transfusion and include both cutaneous signs, such as urticaria and/or angioedema, and systemic signs, such as hypotension and bronchospasm [6]. Additional signs and symptoms can be seen that impact one or more organ systems, including the gastrointestinal tract (abdominal pain, nausea, vomiting), the cardiovascular system (hypotension, shock, arrhythmia, or ventricular dysfunction), and the respiratory tract (bronchospasm, stridor, or wheezing) [4, 22].

13.2.5.2 Transfusion-Associated Dyspnea (TAD)

If a patient has new onset dyspnea during or within 24 h following transfusion completion, the differential diagnosis includes anaphylaxis, transfusion-related acute lung injury (TRALI), transfusion-related circulatory overload (TACO), and transfusion-associated dyspnea (TAD). The UK SHOT registry categorizes TAD as pulmonary complications not explained by the patient's underlying condition when TACO, TRALI, and allergic reactions have been excluded within 24 h of a transfusion completion [21]. TAD is difficult (if not impossible) to diagnose during surgery because of the confounding effects of anesthesia on the respiratory system. Dyspnea is also often overlooked in infants because they can compensate for hypoxemia with an increased respiratory rate, albeit for a limited period. Symptoms of hypoxemia in infants can be nonspecific, including nasal flaring, mild chest wall retractions, and increased irritability.

13.2.5.3 Hypotensive Transfusion Reaction

The US CDC NHSN Biovigilance component defines only one pediatric-specific ATR category: the hypotensive reaction. It is a diagnosis of exclusion, defined as a 25% decrease in systolic blood pressure (SBP) in children 1 to <18 years or a 25% decrease in baseline measurement (compared to the measure utilized such as mean arterial pressure or SBP) in children <1 year or any child <12 kg in body weight [2]. Hypotension must occur within 1 h of the end of the transfusion. The 2020 UK SHOT registry reports only a few cases annually, noting that hypotension related to a blood transfusion may be difficult to diagnose because of the many variables in a sick child's environment [23]. Because of these factors, the hypotensive reaction is categorized along with febrile and allergic transfusion reactions (FAHR) in the SHOT registry; FAHRs make up the majority of reported transfusion reactions in children, with an estimated risk of 1:7704–8138 transfusions [10, 24]. Platelets are more likely to be associated with hypotensive reactions in children. It is noteworthy that large volume, rapid transfusions of anticoagulated products (e.g., plasma containing citrate) may produce hypotension secondary to ionized hypocalcemia.

13.2.5.4 Transfusion-Associated Circulatory Overload (TACO)

TACO is becoming one of the most common transfusion reactions, with some estimates suggesting that 1:100 transfusions are complicated by some degree of circulatory overload [4]. It was responsible for over one-third of transfusion-related deaths reported to the US FDA during the period 2016–2020 [18]. TACO is most likely to occur in patients who are very small, older age groups (>70 years carrying the highest risk), and patients with left atrial dysfunction, renal failure, a positive fluid balance, poor cardiac contractility, and chronic anemia [6, 25–27]. TACO usually presents with acute or worsening respiratory distress, radiologic or clinical evidence of acute or worsening pulmonary edema, elevated brain natriuretic peptide (BNP), and evidence of fluid overload occurring within 12 h of transfusion. These patients often have elevated central venous pressure and rales on lung auscultation secondary to cardiogenic pulmonary edema [28]. There are currently no pediatric-specific diagnostic criteria for TACO, although there is an upward trend in the reporting of suspected cases of volume overload [29]. Neonates may develop intraventricular hemorrhage (IVH) [30]. TACO in older infants may present similarly to TAD, manifested by nonspecific signs such as restlessness, irritability, tachypnea, nasal flaring, and marginal oxygen saturation values. Older children may present with a headache and hypertension [31]. With increasing implementation of massive transfusion protocols and use of rapid infusion devices, TACO is a particular risk in all patients resuscitated from hypovolemic shock.

13.2.5.5 Transfusion-Related Acute Lung Injury (TRALI)

TRALI is caused by donor alloantibodies to human lymphocyte antigens (HLA) or human neutrophil antigens (HNA) in the recipient, leading to acute lung injury and pulmonary edema. TRALI is rare with different incidence rates reported in the literature, although a 2023 systematic review found a pooled incidence per 10,000 units transfused of 3.19 for plasma, 0.31 for platelets, and 0.17 for RBCs under active surveillance [6, 32]. A nonimmune mechanism for lung inflammation has been proposed, consisting of polymorphonuclear neutrophils (PMNs) priming by microparticles (e.g., phospholipids) released from RBCs during storage [33]. Between 2016 and 2020, TRALI was responsible for 21% of transfusion-related deaths reported to the US FDA [18]. There were no reports of pediatric TRALI in either the 2020 or 2021 UK SHOT annual summaries [10, 34]. TRALI has become less common since new donor guidelines screen out donors with anti-HLA alloantibodies for plasma and platelet products. The new guidelines restrict ever-pregnant female donors from donating plasma or platelets prior to anti-HLA alloantibody screening because pregnancy has been shown to lead to high levels of anti-HLA alloantibody formation [4, 5]. Diagnostic criteria for TRALI include new onset dyspnea during or within 6 h of the end of transfusion, negative history of acute lung injury in the days prior to transfusion, hypoxemia with oxygen saturations less than 90% on room air or PaO_2/FiO_2 less than or equal to 300, radiologic evidence of bilateral pulmonary infiltrates, and no evidence of left atrial hypertension or cardiogenic pulmonary edema [2].

13.2.5.6 Delayed Hemolytic Transfusion Reactions (DHTR)

DHTRs are usually diagnosed days to weeks following transfusion and are most often mediated by IgG leading to extravascular hemolysis. The known incidence is 1:500 to 1:10,000 transfusions [16]. Most DHTRs are the result of alloimmunization from prior exposure to a foreign RBC antigen when the patient develops a "serologic" reaction; the alloantibody becomes evanescent or undetectable on standardized screening but later resurfaces upon re-exposure to the RBC antigen. At-risk patients include those who have been alloimmunized from a prior transfusion, sickle cell patients, chronically transfused patients, and those receiving emergency release, uncrossmatched RBCs as part of resuscitation [35]. These patients may present to clinic or the emergency department with new onset jaundice, anemia, hyperbilirubinemia, and elevated bilirubin lactate dehydrogenase (LDH) levels. Despite their often subtle and delayed presentation, DHTRs can be fatal if left undetected.

13.2.6 What Is the Role of Premedication in Preventing a Transfusion Reaction?

Many transfusion reactions are idiosyncratic and difficult to predict. Some patients have a history of recurrent febrile or allergic transfusion reactions. However, randomized controlled trials have yet to demonstrate a difference in transfusion reaction rates when patients are pretreated with acetaminophen or antihistamines [36–38]. While acetaminophen can help to control a febrile patient's underlying fever, there is little data showing that it can prevent a transfusion-related fever [6, 39]. Pretreatment is often administered as a comfort measure at the request of the patient, family, or the prescribing physician. The 2021 Annual SHOT report recommends against routine prophylaxis, but in cases of recurrent and product-specific reactions (such as platelets), acetaminophen may be prescribed for an anticipated febrile reaction 1 h prior to transfusion; a combination of special product treatment as determined by Transfusion Services and an antihistamine may be appropriate for recurrent allergic reactions to platelets [21, 40]. A Canadian blood surveillance database report examined over 35,000 transfusions (including more than 4000 children) to ascertain the rate of allergic transfusion reactions to different types of blood products [41]. An allergic reaction was reported in 38 patients, and platelets were involved in 60% of reports. Of the seven patients who experienced recurrent allergic reactions, only one specific type of blood product was involved for each patient, despite these seven patients receiving multiple types of blood products during the surveillance period. The investigators concluded from these results that premedication before a blood product to which the recipient has not had an allergic reaction is not warranted. Fifty-three percent of the children in this study who suffered an allergic reaction had an atopy history, a known risk factor for an allergic transfusion reaction. The single case of anaphylaxis was attributed to albumin [41].

If a patient reports a history of a transfusion-related anaphylaxis, it is best to contact your blood bank to discuss management options. Many blood banks wash platelets or reduce the amount of plasma in platelet products because they are the most likely component to cause an allergic reaction outside of plasma [5, 6, 42]. However, it is important to note that there is one modification that has been shown to reduce the likelihood of most transfusion reactions: a reduced transfusion rate, at approximately 2–4 mL/min or 1 mL/kg/h [4, 19]. While this is not always logistically possible, depending on a patient's blood product needs, this is usually one of the first recommended modifications by Transfusion Services. Slow transfusion rates will not prevent all transfusion reactions, particularly in severe cases such as anaphylaxis. If a patient has a history of transfusion-related anaphylaxis, a presumptive diagnosis of IgA deficiency with an anti-IgA or another plasma protein or preservative allergy is often made in the interest of patient safety, and the blood bank will wash all cellular blood products for that patient. Some centers will continue transfusing unwashed blood products under careful surveillance and with appropriate rescue medications at bedside. Washing cellular blood products requires careful consideration and coordination between the blood bank and the requesting team. The washing process requires at least an hour of preparation time and reduces the expiration time of the blood product to either 4 (open system) or 24 h (closed system) due to removal of preservative solution and increased concern for bacterial contamination.

13.3 How Does One Initially Approach a Suspected Transfusion Reaction in the Perioperative Period, Including Diagnostic Evaluation and Treatment?

13.3.1 General

In all suspected transfusion reactions, immediately stop the transfusion, check the patient's identification (ID) band, and compare it to the implicated blood product to verify the correct patient and the right blood product. If you suspect a transfusion reaction, contact the hospital blood bank, and document what occurred during or following the transfusion. Your local Transfusion Medicine specialist (a physician with subspecialty training in transfusion medicine) will review the reaction and attempt to determine if the implicated transfused unit is responsible for the reaction and if it is safe to transfuse additional units. Sometimes, this includes removing specific donor products from the hospital's inventory and notifying the blood supplier. Some hemovigilance organizations and certain hospitals do not require formal reporting of mild allergic transfusion reactions.

A typical workup performed in the blood bank will begin with a verification of the clerical information and the compatibility of the implicated unit with the patient's information at hand. A repeat blood type of both the patient and the implicated blood product is performed along with a direct antiglobulin test (DAT); the color and clarity of the plasma are also investigated. This workup generally takes 30–60 min to complete and is required prior to the release of additional blood products from the blood bank. If clinical urgency necessitates additional transfusion before the completion of the workup, the requesting clinician can order blood through the hospital's emergency release protocols. These include group O, Rh-negative or Rh-positive RBCs, and group A or AB plasma units for transfusion until the patient's blood type can be re-evaluated. Table 13.2 summarizes the suggested initial management of a suspected transfusion reaction based on presenting signs or symptoms [2].

After stopping the transfusion and initial supportive care, remove all IV tubing down to the patient's IV catheter, and establish an infusion of fresh saline or PlasmaLyte. Further management includes diagnosis-specific treatment and reporting of the suspected transfusion reaction. The Society for Pediatric Anesthesia's Pedi Crisis 2.0 mobile application contains diagnostic criteria and weight-specific management guidelines for transfusion reactions, including anaphylaxis [43]. The following section includes diagnosis-related management of febrile and nonfebrile transfusion reactions seen in the perioperative period.

13.3.2 Transfusion Reactions with Associated Fever

13.3.2.1 Febrile Transfusion Reaction

If the patient's temperature increases ≥1 °C and is ≥38 °C during a transfusion or in the 4 h following the transfusion, the transfusion should be stopped if it was not completed, and the IV line should be kept open with fresh saline or PlasmaLyte. The patient should be evaluated for additional signs or symptoms, such as hypotension, tachycardia, back pain, epistaxis, disseminated intravascular coagulation (DIC), or oozing at the IV site. Following examination and management of the patient, including checking the patient's identification (ID) band with the blood bag label, the remaining blood product and entire tubing should be returned to the blood bank in a hazardous waste bag. All increases in body temperature that meet the CDC threshold should be reported to the blood bank for further guidance.

Table 13.2 Suggested initial management of a suspected transfusion reaction based on presenting signs or symptoms

Transfusion Reaction Type	*Timing*	*Symptoms*	*Immediate Action*	*Appropriate Clinical Workup*	*Symptom Management*
Febrile Non-Hemolytic Transfusion Reaction (FNHTR)	• During or up to 4 hours after transfusion	• Increase in body temperature to ≥1°C *and* ≥38°C *or* chills or rigors	• **Stop the transfusion** • Report to Transfusion Services	• Monitor temperature and blood pressure	• Administer antipyretics and/or meperidine as needed for fever or rigors
Mild Allergic Reaction	• During or up to 4 hours after transfusion	• Hives • Localized rash • Pruritis	• **STOP the transfusion** • Manage symptoms • **Restart the unit if symptoms improve**	• Examine for hives or rash • Measure vital signs	• Administer antihistamines • **Resume transfusion if symptoms improve** • **Stop** if reaction recurs
Severe Allergic Reaction or Anaphylaxis	• During or up to 4 hours after transfusion	• Swelling or hives & airway symptoms • Dyspnea • Cough • Wheezing • Hypotension	• **STOP the transfusion** • Report to Transfusion Service	• Assess airway • Monitor blood pressure	• Provide supportive care • Epinephrine • Blood pressure management
Transfusion-Related Acute Lung Injury (TRALI)	• During or up to 6 hours after transfusion	• Hypoxemia • PaO2/FiO2 ≤ 300 mmHg • O2 Sats < 90% on RA • CXR w/ new BL infiltrates • No evidence of L Atrial HTN	• **STOP the transfusion** • Report to Transfusion Service	• Chest X-ray • Blood cultures	• Treat signs and symptoms, provide respiratory support if needed
Acute Hemolytic Transfusion Reaction (AHTR)	• During or up to 24 hours after transfusion	• Hypotension • Chills • Hemolysis in Catheter bag • Back/chest pain	• **STOP the transfusion** • Report to Transfusion Service	• Assess for pain and hypotension	• Treat symptoms • Administer pain relief and antipyretics as needed
Transfusion-associated circulatory overload (TACO)	• During or up to 12 hours after transfusion	• Dyspnea • Orthopnea • Cough • Tachycardia • Hypertension • Widened pulse pressure • Jugular venous distention • Pulmonary edema	• **STOP the transfusion** • Report to Transfusion Service	• Assess respiratory and cardiovascular status • Perform chest X-ray	• Administer diuretics • Provide O_2 as needed

13.3.2.2 Febrile Nonhemolytic Transfusion Reaction (FNHTR)

A FNHTR is typically managed with acetaminophen. If the patient has moderate to severe rigors, the transfusion should be stopped, and Transfusion Services should be contacted for further guidance. Meperidine (or other narcotic analgesic) and antipyretics may be considered as symptomatic treatment (Table 13.2) [4, 6].

13.3.2.3 Acute Hemolytic Transfusion Reaction (AHR)

If a hemolytic transfusion reaction is suspected, it is imperative that the transfusion is stopped, and the blood bag label is compared to the patient's ID band. Initial management of an AHR is usually supportive, followed by identification of the underlying cause. Supportive management includes vigorous hydration and diuresis to maintain urine output and minimize the effects of free hemoglobin and antibody complexes on the renal tubules [4–6, 16]. Additional laboratory values that can be helpful when trying to rule out an AHR are decreased haptoglobin, elevated bilirubin and LDH, and hemoglobinuria or hemoglobinemia [2, 16]. A transfusion reaction workup must be submitted. The Transfusion Medicine physician will guide additional testing. Key specialty teams should also be consulted, such as nephrology and cardiology, for specific recommendations and the possibility of dialysis if the patient becomes oliguric [4].

13.3.2.4 Transfusion Transmitted Infection (TTI)

The initial presentation of a suspected TTI typically includes fever, hypotension, and tachycardia (particularly with gram-negative bacteria). Management includes antibiotics and supportive care; activation of the sepsis protocol may be necessary [5]. The required initial workup for bacterial contamination includes a gram stain and culture (aerobic and anaerobic) of the blood product and the recipient. The same bacteria must grow in the blood product and the patient cultures to definitively implicate the blood product in the transfusion reaction.

13.3.3 Nonfebrile Transfusion Reactions

13.3.3.1 Allergic Transfusion Reaction

The standard management of an allergic transfusion reaction (after the transfusion has been stopped and the patient assessed) is to administer diphenhydramine or an alternative antihistamine, observation over the next 10–20 minutes, and then slow resumption of the transfusion if symptoms resolve. If symptoms reappear, the transfusion should be stopped, and Transfusion Services should be contacted for further guidance.

13.3.3.2 Anaphylaxis

If an anaphylactic transfusion reaction is suspected, immediate patient management should be initiated following hospital or other best practices protocol [43]. Anaphylaxis management guidelines generally include epinephrine, corticosteroids, H_1 and H_2 receptor antagonists, and bronchodilators [6]. The transfusion should not be restarted. It is also important to discuss this reaction with Transfusion

Services because it may be necessary to modify future transfusions for this patient through either plasma volume reduction or washing of cellular products.

13.3.3.3 Delayed Hemolytic Transfusion Reaction (DHTR)

The management of DHTRs is generally supportive. However, if the patient received large volumes of RBCs with an incompatible antigen, such as during massive transfusion with uncrossmatched blood, an RBC exchange may be considered in consultation with the Transfusion Service. However, these procedures do not remove all incompatible RBCs, so RBC exchange is seldom used in this situation. If a DHTR is suspected, it is critical to notify the blood bank and collect a patient blood sample in an EDTA specimen tube (a "purple top" tube containing ethylenediaminetetraacetic acid, an anticoagulant) for workup of new or anamnestic alloantibodies. Additional labs that are useful in a DHTR workup include a complete blood count (CBC), haptoglobin, LDH, bilirubin, and urinalysis looking for chemical blood without RBCs present [16].

13.3.3.4 Transfusion-Associated Circulatory Overload (TACO)

Management of TACO includes the administration of a diuretic such as furosemide, which is very effective at reducing symptoms within minutes to hours. One of the key diagnostic differences between TACO and TRALI is that TACO will respond briskly to diuretics, whereas TRALI does not; it is critical to ensure the patients have signs and symptoms of circulatory overload prior to treating with a diuretic. Future transfusions in patients with a history of or a risk factor for TACO should be administered slowly at approximately 2–4 mL/min or 1 mL/kg/h [4, 19].

13.3.3.5 TRALI

Management of patients with TRALI is supportive, and most patients recover within 96 h of symptom onset [4]. Although mortality is reported to be approximately 10%, TRALI comprises almost one-quarter of transfusion-related deaths reported to the US FDA [18]. If a patient is suspected of having a TRALI reaction, it is important to notify Transfusion Services as soon as possible so that other blood products from the same donor can be quarantined.

13.4 Summary of Key Learning Objectives

13.4.1 Why Is It Important to Report a Suspected Transfusion Reaction?

Systematic reporting of ATRs and ATEs is essential for improving transfusion-related patient care. Through incident reporting, hospital Transfusion Services can identify patients at increased risk of future transfusion reactions, remove involved blood units from inventory, and implement relevant staff education and guidelines.

13.4.2 What Is the Differential Diagnosis of New-Onset Fever in a Child Who Has Received a Blood Transfusion in the Perioperative Period?

Per standardized diagnostic criteria, a reportable new-onset "fever" is an increase in body temperature ≥1 °C (1.8 °F) and a body temperature ≥38 °C (100.4 °F), or chills or rigors, during or up to 4 h following the transfusion. First, consider the most serious diagnoses to mitigate further deterioration in the patient's condition: an AHR can quickly progress to DIC and renal failure. Patient or specimen misidentification remains the most common cause of an AHR. The blood bank will evaluate further for other possible fever etiologies during or after a transfusion, such as a TTI, FNHTR, or the patient's underlying condition.

13.4.3 In Addition to Febrile Transfusion Reactions, What Types of Transfusion Reactions May Present Within the Perioperative Period?

Acute transfusion reactions (ATRs) include but are not limited to:

- Allergic
- Transfusion-associated dyspnea
- Hypotension
- TACO
- TRALI
- Delayed hemolysis

Acute transfusion events (ATEs) include but are not limited to:

- Wrong-blood-in-tube
- Administration of the incorrect blood product
- Incorrect patient transfused
- Delays in transfusion
- Rapid or high-volume transfusions
  - Over-transfusion: TACO
  - Hyperkalemia
  - Hypothermia
  - Hypocalcemia
  - Mechanical hemolysis
  - Air embolism

13.4.4 What Is the Role of Premedication in Preventing a Transfusion Reaction?

There are no randomized controlled trials that demonstrate a difference in transfusion reaction rates when patients are pretreated with acetaminophen, diphenhydramine, or glucocorticoids. While acetaminophen can help to control a febrile patient's underlying fever, there is little data showing that it can prevent a transfusion-related fever. Patients who undergo repeat transfusions with associated rashes, pruritis, or fevers are often accustomed to pretreatment with acetaminophen or antihistamines, and their expectations must be addressed accordingly. Many institutions have not caught up with the fact that randomized controlled trials have yet to demonstrate a difference in transfusion reaction rates when patients are pretreated with antihistamines, antipyretics, or steroids.

13.4.5 How Does One Initially Approach a Suspected Transfusion Reaction in the Perioperative Period?

This child's esophageal temperature increased ≥1 °C (1.8 °F) and was ≥38 °C (100.4 °F) during the transfusion. This meets the early diagnostic criteria for a potentially catastrophic hemolytic event. Therefore:

- Stop the transfusion, change the IV tubing, keep the line open with fresh saline or PlasmaLyte, and manage the patient's signs and symptoms.
- If the blood bag is still available, verify that the patient's ID band matches the unit(s) information.
- Contact transfusion services for guidance on submitting a transfusion reaction workup. Submit an EDTA "purple top" tube of post-transfusion recipient blood and a urinalysis looking for chemical blood without intact red blood cells.
- The blood bag and all IV tubing used in the index transfusion should also be submitted to the blood bank.

Key Points

- A transfusion reaction or event should always be in the differential diagnosis if a patient has an immediate or post-transfusion change in symptoms or vital signs.
- A febrile transfusion reaction is defined as an oral body temperature ≥38 °C (100.4 °F) *and* an increase in body temperature of ≥1 °C (1.8 °F) above pretransfusion baseline, *or* chills or rigors, during or up to 4 h after completion of a transfusion.
- It is appropriate to resume the same transfusion *only in cases of a mild allergic transfusion reaction* (e.g., urticaria, with or without pruritis), after patient evaluation and a positive response to management.

- All suspected transfusions should be reported to the hospital Transfusion Services (i.e., "blood bank") to rule out a blood-related event, to identify patients at increased risk of future transfusion reactions, to remove an index blood unit from inventory, or to reinvestigate the unit and the donor for contributing factors.
- Randomized controlled trials have yet to demonstrate a difference in transfusion reaction rates when patients are pretreated with antihistamines, antipyretics, or steroids.

References

1. Politis C, Wiersum JC, Richardson C, Robillard P, Jorgensen J, Renaudier P, et al. The international haemovigilance network database for the surveillance of adverse reactions and events in donors and recipients of blood components: technical issues and results. Vox Sang. 2016;111(4):409–17.
2. Centers for Disease Control and Prevention. National Healthcare Safety Network Biovigilance Component Hemovigilance Module Surveillance Protocol v2.8. 2023. https://www.cdc.gov/nhsn/pdfs/biovigilance/bv-hv-protocol-current.pdf. Accessed 26 June 2023.
3. Vossoughi S, Perez G, Whitaker BI, Fung MK, Stotler B. Analysis of pediatric adverse reactions to transfusions. Transfusion. 2018;58(1):60–9.
4. Hod EA, Francis RO. Chapter 22: noninfectious complications of blood transfusion. In: Cohn CS, Delaney M, Johnson ST, Katz LM, editors. Technical manual. 20th ed. Bethesda: American Association of Blood Banks; 2020. p. 627–57.
5. Kopko PM. Transfusion reactions. 5th ed. Bethesda: AABB Press; 2021. p. 41.
6. Delaney M, Wendel S, Bercovitz RS, Cid J, Cohn C, Dunbar NM, et al. Transfusion reactions: prevention, diagnosis, and treatment. Lancet. 2016;388(10061):2825–36.
7. Sostin N, Hendrickson JE. Pediatric hemovigilance and adverse transfusion reactions. Clin Lab Med. 2021;41(1):51–67.
8. Keir AK, New H, Robitaille N, Crighton GL, Wood EM, Stanworth SJ. Approaches to understanding and interpreting the risks of red blood cell transfusion in neonates. Transfus Med. 2019;29(4):231–8.
9. SHOT Bite No. 4: Lessons in Paediatrics (including neonates). Serious Hazards of Transfusion (SHOT). 2018. https://www.shotuk.org/resources/current-resources/shot-bites/. Accessed 4 Dec 2022.
10. Serious Hazards of Transfusion and Medicines and Healthcare Products Regulatory Agency (SHOT). 2020. United Kingdom. https://www.shotuk.org/shot-reports/(2020). Accessed 25 May 2023.
11. Suddock JT, Crookston KP. Transfusion reactions. In: StatPearls. Treasure Island: StatPearls Publishing; 2022. https://www.ncbi.nlm.nih.gov/books/NBK482202/. Accessed 26 June 2023.
12. Barbi E, Marzuillo P, Neri E. Fever in children: pearls and pitfalls. Children. 2017.
13. Chusid MJ. Fever of unknown origin in childhood. Pediatr Clin N Am. 2017;64(1):205–30.
14. Nield LS, Kamat D. Chapter 201: fever. In: Kliegman T, Geme JS, editors. Nelson textbook of pediatrics. 21st ed. Amsterdam: Elsevier; 2019. p. 1386–402.
15. Lerman J, Parness J. Chapter 41: malignant hyperthermia. In: Cote CJ, Lehman J, Anderson BJ, editors. Cote and Lerman's a practice of anesthesia for infants and children. 5th ed. Elsevier: Amsterdam; 2019. p. 921–39.
16. Panch SR, Montemayor-Garcia C, Klein HG. Hemolytic transfusion reactions. N Engl J Med. 2019;381(2):150–62.

17. AABB. Circular of information for the use of human blood and blood components. 2021. https://www.aabb.org/docs/default-source/default-document-library/resources/circular-of-information-watermark.pdf. Accessed 6 July 2023.
18. US Food & Drug Administration. Transfusion/donation fatalities. 2020. https://www.fda.gov/media/160859/download#:~:text=During%20FY%202016%20there%20were,2019%2C%20and%2029%20in%202020. Accessed 15 June 2023.
19. Alquist C, Harm SK. Transfusion service related activities. In: Cohn C, Delaney M, Johnson ST, Katz LM, editors. Technical manual. 20th ed. Bethesda: AABB; 2020. p. 503–4.
20. Moncharmont P. Adverse transfusion reactions in transfused children. Transfus Clin Biol. 2019;26(4):329–35.
21. Serious Hazards of Transfusion and Medicines and Healthcare Products Regulatory Agency (SHOT) annual SHOT report. 2021. https://www.shotuk.org/shot-reports/report-summary-and-supplement-2021/. Accessed 12 September 2023.
22. Triggiani M, Patella V, Staiano RI, Granata F, Marone G. Allergy and the cardiovascular system. Clin Exp Immunol. 2008;153(Suppl 1):7–11.
23. Kelly A, New H. Chapter 22. Paediatric cases n=137. Serious Hazards of Transfusion (SHOT). 2021. https://www.shotuk.org/shot-reports/. Accessed 13 September 2023.
24. Serious Hazards of Transfusion (SHOT). SHOT annual reports and summaries. 2023. https://www.shotuk.org/shot-reports/. Accessed 16 June 2023.
25. De Cloedt L, Emeriaud G, Lefebvre É, Kleiber N, Robitaille N, Jarlot C, et al. Transfusion-associated circulatory overload in a pediatric intensive care unit: different incidences with different diagnostic criteria. Transfusion. 2018;58(4):1037–44.
26. De Cloedt L, Savy N, Gauvin F, Taylor S, Lacroix J, Emeriaud G. Transfusion-associated circulatory overload in ICUs: a scoping review of incidence, risk factors, and outcomes. Crit Care Med. 2019;47(6):849–56.
27. McCormick M, Zullo J, Kalpatthi R. Epidemiology and outcome of TRALI and TACO in the pediatric population: a multi-institutional review. Blood. 2018;132(1):3811. https://doi.org/10.1182/blood-2018-99-113959.
28. U.S. Centers for Disease Control and Prevention. The National Healthcare Safety Network (NHSN) Manual: Biovigilance Component v2.6 Atlanta, GA: Division of Healthcare Quality Promotion, National Center for Emerging and Zoonotic Infectious Diseases; [updated March 2021. V2.6. http://www.cdc.gov/nhsn/PDFs/Biovigilance/BV-HV-protocol-current.pdf.
29. Grey S. Chapter 17a. Transfusion-associated circulatory overload (TACO) n = 131. 2021. https://www.shotuk.org/wp-content/uploads/myimages/17a.-Transfusion-Associated-Circulatory-Overload-TACO-2021.pdf. Accessed 21 September 2022.
30. Späth C, Stoltz Sjöström E, Ågren J, Ahlsson F, Domellöf M. Sodium supply from administered blood products was associated with severe intraventricular haemorrhage in extremely preterm infants. Acta Paediatr. 2022;111(9):1701–8.
31. Wong EC, editor. Pediatric transfusion: a physician's handbook. Bethesda: American Association of Blood Banks; 2015.
32. White SK, Walker BS, Schmidt RL, Metcalf RA. The incidence of transfusion-related acute lung injury using active surveillance: a systematic review and meta-analysis. Transfusion. 2024;64(2):289–300.
33. Yang J, Yang Y, Gao L, Jiang X, Sun J, Wang Z, et al. Adverse effects of microparticles on transfusion of stored red blood cell concentrates. Hematol Transfus Cell Ther. 2024;5(Suppl 5):S48–56.
34. Serious Hazards of Transfusion (SHOT) Annual Report. 2021. https://www.shotuk.org/wp-content/uploads/myimages/SHOT-REPORT-2021-FINAL-bookmarked-V3-November.pdf. Accessed 12 September 2023.
35. US Food and Drug Administration. Fatalities reported to FDA following blood collection and transfusion annual summary for FY2019. 2019. https://www.fda.gov/media/147628/download?attachment. Accessed 12 Apr 2024.
36. Christensen BW, Rubinstein SM, Bastakoty D, Savani BN, Booth GS. A retrospective cost analysis of the frequency and cost of transfusion premedications. Transfusion. 2019;59(8):2523–7.

37. Duran J, Siddique S, Cleary M. Effects of leukoreduction and premedication with acetaminophen and diphenhydramine in minimizing febrile nonhemolytic transfusion reactions and allergic transfusion reactions during and after blood product administration: a literature review with recommendations for practice. J Pediatr Oncol Nurs. 2014;31(4):223–9.
38. Wang SE, Lara PN, Lee-Ow A, Reed J, Wang LR, Palmer P, et al. Acetaminophen and diphenhydramine as premedication for platelet transfusions: a prospective randomized double-blind placebo-controlled trial. Am J Hematol. 2002;70(3):191–4.
39. Sitthi-Amorn J, Denton E, Harper E, Carias D, Hashmi S, Bami S, et al. Improving blood product transfusion premedication plan documentation: a single-institution quality improvement effort. Pediatr Qual Saf. 2022;7(3):e572.
40. Tinegate H, Birchall J, Gray A, Haggas R, Massey E, Norfolk D, et al. Guideline on the investigation and management of acute transfusion reactions. Prepared by the BCSH Blood Transfusion Task Force. Br J Haematol. 2012;159(2):143–53.
41. Bahabri A, Barty R, Li N, Liu Y, Kovalova T, Chan AKC. Do children with an allergic transfusion reaction require premedication for all blood products? J Pediatr Hematol Oncol. 2023;45(5):578–81.
42. Hirayama F. Current understanding of allergic transfusion reactions: incidence, pathogenesis, laboratory tests, prevention and treatment. Br J Haematol. 2013;160(4):434–44.
43. Society for Pediatric Anesthesia. Pedi crisis 2.0 critical events checklists mobile App®. 2021. https://pedsanesthesia.org/pedi-crisis-app/. Accessed 28 June 2023.

The Double Effect of Rapid Transfusions in Children

14

Norma J. Klein and Destiny F. Chau

14.1 Case Scenario

A 6 kg, 8-month-old male is scheduled for an emergency craniotomy to evacuate bilateral subdural hematomas secondary to non-accidental trauma. When he arrives to the operating room (OR), he is intubated and has bilateral antecubital fossae peripheral intravenous catheters (PIVCs) in place. His blood pressure (BP) is 50/25, heart rate (HR) 162, core temperature 35.5 °C, and his initial hemoglobin is 7 g/dL. On admission his pediatric Glasgow Coma Score (pGCS) was 4. The surgeon has not yet opened the dura mater. You consider the available options to rapidly transfuse large volumes of blood in this infant. Only routine monitors are in place and a forced hot air warmer is available.

Key Learning Objectives

- What is meant by a "double effect" in the context of pediatric transfusion?
- What are some of the safety concerns during rapid transfusion in children?

N. J. Klein (✉)
Department of Anesthesiology and Pain Medicine, University of California, Davis, Sacramento, CA, USA
e-mail: nklein@ucdavis.edu

D. F. Chau
Department of Anesthesiology and Pain Medicine, University of Arkansas for Medical Sciences, Arkansas Children's Hospital, Little Rock, AK, USA
e-mail: dchau@uams.edu

N. J. Klein (ed.), *Perioperative Pediatric Patient Blood Management and Transfusion Safety*, https://doi.org/10.1007/978-3-031-81666-6_14

14.2 Discussion

14.2.1 What Is Meant by a "Double Effect" in the Context of Pediatric Transfusion?

The doctrine of double effect is based in medical ethics and occurs when "a harmful effect of treatment … is permissible if it is not intended and occurs as a side effect of a beneficial action" [1]. Stated otherwise, the doctrine of double effect is the dilemma that practitioners experience when life-saving care is associated with patient harm, despite best intentions. According to Beauchamp and Childress, an act that has a double effect is morally permissible if it is good or neutral in character, the act is performed with beneficial intent, the good effect of the act outweighs its bad effects, and the bad effects of the act are incidental in nature [2]. Implementation of a massive transfusion protocol (MTP), for instance, may bring about a number of physiologic derangements, but doing so is often the only management alternative to ensure the preservation of life. Application of the doctrine of double effect to specific medical facts may be controversial, but doing so serves to highlight the conflict between "intended effects and merely foreseen effects…" [2].

Many adverse events can result from the rapid transfusion of blood products to children. At times, they can only be managed and not prevented. The key to safe management is knowledge of potential side effects, an understanding of which patients are at greatest risk, and the presence of a surveillance and mitigation plan. Complications associated with rapid or large volume transfusions in pediatric patients include but are not limited to [3–10]:

- Transfusion-associated hyperkalemia (TAH)
- Transfusion-associated circulatory overload (TACO)
- Hypothermia
- Hypocalcemia
- Hospital-acquired venous thromboembolism (HA-VTE)
- Nonimmune hemolysis
- Venous air embolism (VAE)
- Transfusion-related dyspnea (TAD)
- Transfusion-related acute lung injury (TRALI)
- Dilutional coagulopathy
- Metabolic acidosis
- Release of chemokines and cell-derived particles
- Hypotension
- Rebound hypoglycemia
- Infiltration and extravasation

Some of these adverse events are directly related to the equipment or transfusion techniques used in the perioperative transfusion process. Reporting these adverse events to the hospital transfusion service may be difficult because they do not always meet biovigilance classification criteria as promulgated by the US Centers for Disease Control NHSN Biovigilance Component Protocol [11, 12]. In the alternative, these outcomes may be referred to the hospital quality assurance program for process improvement.

14.2.2 What Are Some of the Safety Concerns During Rapid Transfusion in Children?

The following discussion highlights select adverse transfusion-related events that may occur during a high-volume or rapidly administered blood transfusion. They include transfusion-associated hyperkalemia (TAH), transfusion-associated circulatory overload (TACO), hypothermia, hypocalcemia, hemolysis, hospital-associated venous thromboembolism (HA-VTE), and venous air embolism (VAE). For further information on specific transfusion devices, refer to the chapter entitled "Pediatric Perioperative Transfusion-Related Equipment."

14.2.2.1 Transfusion-Associated Hyperkalemia (TAH)

TAH has been associated with cardiac arrest in patients receiving large volume or rapidly administered red blood cell (RBC) transfusions [13, 14]. Little is known about causative transfusion rates and volumes, although small patient size has been consistently identified as a risk factor. Ultimately, the etiology of TAH is multifactorial, as evidenced by the small number of studies with conflicting results. Risk factors for TAH found in the literature include [3, 8–10, 15, 16]:

Patient factors
- Small patient size
- Acidosis
- Hypothermia
- Hypocalcemia
- High baseline serum potassium level
- Renal insufficiency
- American Society of Anesthesiologists physical classification status > III
- Hypovolemia

Blood product characteristics
- Age of blood >7 days
- Post-red blood cell (RBC) irradiation >6–12 h
- Whole blood versus component RBCs
- Preservative solution: citrate-phosphate-dextrose-adenine (CPDA)

Administration techniques
- Delayed recognition of blood loss
- Short time interval since last RBC transfusion
- Rapid rate of administration

- One blood volume replacement
- Volume >20 mL/kg
- Central venous catheter administration
- Handheld syringing
- Forced manual aspiration from blood bag
- Rapid infusion devices

Table 14.1 illustrates RBC infusion rates that have been associated with TAH:

The Association for the Advancement of Blood and Biotherapies (AABB) notes that a single RBC adult unit (approximately 300 mL) is usually administered over 1–2 h (2.1–4.3 mL/kg/h in a 70 kg adult); in children, a single recommended RBC dose is 10–20 mL/kg, more than twice that of the usual adult RBC infusion bolus or rate [22]. Documented infusion rates that have been associated with TAH vary widely, most likely due to the observational nature of most studies and their heterogenous patient populations [14]. Blood bank and transfusionist efforts to follow recommendations to reduce the transfusion rate, prewash RBCs, or avoid older RBCs may not be feasible when blood is emergently needed for life-threatening bleeding. In an AABB handbook on pediatric transfusions, Roseff et al. state that RBCs do not require washing for the purposes of preventing TAH if the intended volume is ≤20 mL/kg and infusion is 2–4 h in duration [16]. RBC washing is recommended, however, if the storage duration is more than 1 week or if more than 2 days have passed since irradiation.

In a systematic evaluation of TAH in a large population of pediatric patients (*N* = 3777), Yamada et al. performed a multicenter, retrospective review to ascertain the incidence of TAH following an RBC transfusion [23]. Hyperkalemia was defined as a serum potassium level above the age-based institutional reference of normal (e.g., 4.9–5.5 mmol/L) within 12 h of the RBC transfusion. Across 5 age groups, 35 patients developed TAH, with an incidence of 0.93% and a 20% 1-day mortality rate. One-half of affected patients received treatment for TAH. Patients that experienced TAH had a median age of 1.28 years and a median body weight of 9.8 kg. Almost one-half had kidney insufficiency, while approximately one-quarter had anemia, prematurity, or cardiorespiratory disease. The median

Table 14.1 RBC infusion rates associated with TAH

Author (year)	Maximum recommended RBC infusion rate
Brown (1990) [17]	134 mL/kg/4 h whole blood
Miller (2004) [18]	1 mL/kg/h
Barcelona (2005) [10]	1 mL/kg/min
Cote (2008) [19]	1.5–2 mL/kg/min
Strauss (2010) [9]	0.5 mL/kg/min
Vraets (2011) [8]	0.3 mL/kg/min
Papovsky (2011) [20]	0.5 mL/kg/min
Lee (2014) [15]	1 mL/kg/h
Delaney (2016) [21]	0.5 mL/kg/min

transfused volume was 24% of the median estimated blood volume, and the median RBC transfusion rate was 19.6 mL/kg/h. This transfusion rate is mid-way between that found in other reports of pediatric TAH (e.g., 1–30 mL/kg/h) [15, 21]. The median serum potassium level increase was 1.4 mmol/L from baseline. Approximately one-half of TAH events occurred during the transfusion itself. In contrast to prior studies, RBC irradiation status and storage age did not contribute to the development of TAH. In a later study, these same TAH patients were compared to 12 patients in each age group who did not experience TAH within 12 h of transfusion completion [24]. Factors associated with TAH in that comparison were pretransfusion serum creatine (0.7 versus 0.4 mg/dL), a 30 mL/kg total volume of RBCs transfused within 12 h (tV-12), a 30% of estimated blood volume transfused within 12 h, and an RBC age greater than 7.95 days. Neither infusion rate nor RBC irradiation timing were associated with TAH in this relatively small study.

A large, multicenter trial prospectively examined over 1500 children aged 3 days to 16 years who received a RBC transfusion within the first week of intensive care unit admission. Investigators found no difference in mortality, organ failure, or hyperkalemia (serum potassium >5.5 mmol/L) between those that received "fresh" RBCs (median storage age 5 days, IQR 4–6 days) and "standard issue" RBCs (median storage age 18 days, IQR 12–25 days) [25]. Transfusion volumes in this trial were as high as 30 mL/kg (median 17.5 mL/kg in the fresh group and 16.6 mL/kg in the standard issue group). However, investigators noted that the relatively short storage age of the standard issue RBCs precluded analysis of the safety of RBCs dispensed at the end storage life (e.g., >35–42 days). As a matter of protocol, many blood banks dispense RBCs with shorter storage duration when records indicate that the patient is very young.

The free potassium concentration in banked blood increases with storage duration, although definition of "old" packed RBCs in the pediatric literature varies between 3 and 14 days [6, 25, 26]. The potassium ion is maintained within the intracellular compartment by an ATP-dependent pump. As ATP is consumed by the stored but aging RBCs, potassium leaks into the extracellular compartment producing effluent with high potassium levels. The potassium load delivered through an RBC transfusion leads to a less negative cardiomyocyte resting potential, electromechanical instability, and, eventually, myocardial fibrillation. Administered potassium is taken up by potassium-depleted RBCs over several hours, and renal elimination of potassium also requires several hours. However, TAH rarely occur if RBCs are administered at standard infusion doses and rates over 2–4 h [16]. A potassium adsorption filter (PAF) has been shown to reduce an administered potassium load up to 80% in vitro (94–97% in vivo) [27, 28]. Although PAFs may be promising for vulnerable patient populations, current prototypes, including one made for neonatal use (PAF-n), are not designed for rapid transfusions [29]. Currently, these PAFs are not approved for use in the United States.

14.2.2.2 Transfusion-Associated Circulatory Overload (TACO)

TACO is becoming one of the most common transfusion reactions, with an incidence of 1–11% of transfused adults [30–32]. TACO has a high mortality rate and was responsible for 27–36% of transfusion-related deaths reported to the US FDA for the years 2019–2021 [33]. There is very little known about TACO in the perioperative period, including diagnostic criteria and rate of occurrence. Before 2010, there was no disease code for TACO in the ICD (International Classification of Diseases) classification system. Objective diagnostic criteria have since evolved and are now consistent following collaborative work between major international hemovigilance systems. The International Society of Blood Transfusion-International Haemovigilance Network-AABB (ISBT-IHN-AABB) defines adult TACO under the following criteria [34]:

- Worsening respiratory condition or pulmonary edema during or up to 12 h after a blood transfusion
- Cardiovascular system changes not explained by prior medical conditions
- Evidence of fluid overload
- An elevated biomarker (e.g., B-type natriuretic peptide 1.5 times baseline)

With the development of pediatric massive transfusion protocols (MTPs) and the use of rapid infusion devices, children undergoing resuscitation for hypovolemic shock are at a particular risk of TACO. There are currently no pediatric-specific diagnostic criteria for TACO. A pooled incidence of 5.5% has been reported in critically ill children, with the prevalence highly dependent on study diagnostic criteria and the duration of the post-transfusion surveillance [35, 36]. Despite this, there is an upward trend in the number of reported cases [37]. Transfusion-associated dyspnea (TAD) and the hypotensive transfusion reaction, each with specific diagnostic criteria that can be differentiated from TACO, TRALI, and anaphylaxis, may function as surrogate diagnoses for a TACO in children [11].

Both large fluid volumes and a rapid rate of transfusion have been implicated as etiologic agents in TACO, although the specific variables for each are unclear. In a 1982 prospective study of 15 adult patients with severe, chronic anemia (range 2.5–5.2 g/dL), Gupta et al. transfused these anemic patients with RBCs at rates exceeding the recommended rate (9 mL/min versus 2 mL/kg/h) and found the mean pulmonary artery wedge pressure (PAWP)—a surrogate for left ventricular filling pressures (LVFP)—to be significantly elevated [38]. Investigators concluded that although the subjects exhibited no outward signs of pulmonary compromise, the relatively rapid infusion of large volumes of blood creates the setting for development of pulmonary edema and congestive heart failure. When one considers that the usual RBC transfusion volume in a 70 kg adult is 250–500 mL (e.g., 3.5 mL/kg to 7.1 mL/kg) and the recommended RBC transfusion volume in children is 10–15 mL/kg, it is not surprising that small children are at risk of TACO.

Neonates, with a relatively noncompliant myocardium and a cardiac output that is largely rate-dependent, are particularly susceptible to cardiopulmonary compromise from overtransfusion. Diagnosis of pulmonary edema in an infant can be overlooked because signs may be nonspecific, including tachypnea, nasal flaring, restlessness, and even fever; detection requires a high index of suspicion. Neonates may develop intraventricular hemorrhage (IVH) [39]. Older children may present with a headache and hypertension [7]. In a retrospective medical record review of over 400 children who developed hypoxia following an intraoperative blood transfusion, 14 patients met study TACO criteria for an overall incidence of 3.4% [31]. Eleven of those cases were less than 9 years old. Due to the small cohort size, conclusions could not be made regarding subgroups such as surgery type, patient factors, or transfusion rates; however, the median transfusion volume in that review was 18.6 mL/kg (IQR, 9.7–34.7) or 300 mL. In another retrospective review from the Pediatric Health System (PHIS) database, including 45 children's hospitals, investigators found 102 TACO cases in over 380,000 patient encounters for a rate of 2.3/100,000, significantly below expectations based on existing literature. With significant associated mortality (7.8%), hospital costs, and length of stay, investigators concluded that pediatric TACO remains seriously undiagnosed and unreported [31, 40].

Early recognition and treatment of blood loss are critical in exsanguinating pediatric patients to avoid "catch up" infusion of large blood volumes. In the 2007 Pediatric Perioperative Cardiac Arrest Registry (POCA) report, there were 23 deaths secondary to hypovolemia, and almost one-half were attributed to a failure to recognize blood loss [41]. Thus, an important key to prevention is recognition of patients at risk. Known risk factors in children include, but are not limited to, small patient size, young age (i.e., <5 years), and preexisting cardiopulmonary or renal disease [30, 34]. In older patients, risk factors include age >70 years, left atrial dysfunction, a positive fluid balance before transfusion, poor cardiac contractility, and chronic anemia [6, 21, 32]. The UK SHOT hemovigilance registry advises appropriate risk assessment before ordering a transfusion, as well as weight-based dosing for all children [37]. The 2018 Annual SHOT report describes multiple cases of over transfusion, including a triple dose of RBCs in a neonate undergoing an exchange transfusion, a teenager experiencing TACO from a platelet transfusion, and a tenfold miscalculation of a platelet transfusion in a neonate [42].

14.2.3 Hypothermia

Hypothermia is variably defined as a core body temperature <35–36 °C [43–45]. It develops rapidly when large volumes of cold-stored blood products are administered, particularly through centrally placed catheters [15, 44]. Packed RBCs and whole blood are stored at <6 °C, and every full unit administered may reduce the average adult's body temperature by 0.25 °C [46]. Neonates undergoing surgery are at particular risk of transfusion-related hypothermia secondary to heat loss through a large body surface area, immature thermoregulatory capabilities, cold operating room ambient temperatures (<27 °C), anesthesia-induced thermoregulatory inhibition, and inconsistent body temperature monitoring [44]. The downstream metabolic effects of transfusion-induced hypothermia are extensive, including reduced metabolism of citrate preservative (which exacerbates transfusion-induced hypocalcemia), a leftward shift of the oxyhemoglobin-dissociation curve (hampering tissue O_2 delivery), platelet dysfunction, and reduced procoagulant activity [6, 10, 47]. Coagulation factor activity is estimated to decrease by 10% per 1 °C drop in body temperature [48]. Disseminated intravascular coagulopathy (DIC) develops more rapidly in traumatically injured children compared to adults and is associated with a lethal triad: progressive hypothermia, acidosis, and coagulopathy [49]. Other untoward effects of hypothermia include arrhythmias, decreased drug metabolism, apnea, hypoglycemia, and death.

A critical measure in preventing hypothermia and its adverse effects is the use of an effective and validated fluid warming device prior to blood administration. Warming of rapidly administered fluids though a warming device has become a quality standard in pediatric anesthesia.

14.2.4 Hypocalcemia

Hypocalcemia during resuscitation in traumatized pediatric patients has been defined as an ionized calcium (iCa^{2+}) level <1.0–1.1 mmol/L [50]. Blood products are stored using citrate, which is intended to bind calcium and prevent coagulation. Because anticoagulant is present in the effluent of blood products, whole blood and plasma contain more citrate per volume, followed by component RBCs and platelets [3, 7]. Rapid administration of any citrated blood product leads to ionized hypocalcemia, which may be evident on the electrocardiogram (ECG) with prolonged QT-intervals, bradycardia, and predominantly normal T-waves (in contrast to the typical shortened QT-intervals and peaked T-waves of TAH) [19]. Rapid blood administration may also lead to hypocalcemia-related refractory hypotension during anesthesia and surgery [51]. Transfusion-independent ionized hypocalcemia is an important consideration because it may be exacerbated with blood transfusion, particularly during administration of plasma and whole blood [51]. However, evaluation of serum calcium levels is often an afterthought during active bleeding [52]. In one systematic review, pretransfusion ionized hypocalcemia was present in up to 56% of injured adult trauma patients [53]. Studies examining calcium levels in the early resuscitation of traumatized, non-transfused children suggest that the incidence of hypocalcemia following trauma may be less common compared to adults, with reported rates between 5% and 46% [50, 54–56]. A pending systematic review of the prevalence of hypocalcemia in major pediatric trauma may add further clarification to its place in the "lethal diamond" (i.e., hypothermia, coagulopathy, acidosis, and hypocalcemia) [57].

Pediatric patients are susceptible to the development of ionized hypocalcemia during rapid blood transfusions, particularly premature infants who have reduced ability to metabolize citrate, a reduced parathyroid response, and myocardial contraction and relaxation phases that are dependent on ionized calcium levels. Any adverse electrophysiologic effects of hypocalcemia are exacerbated by the addition of halogenated agents which block calcium channels at baseline [3]. The presentation of ionized hypocalcemia in neonates is subtle and may differ from the motor excitability seen in adults, instead manifesting as poor feeding, lethargy, apnea, and cyanosis [7].

Ionized hypocalcemia has been reported to occur when a plasma infusion rate exceeds 1 mL/kg/min [58]. Cote et al. administered plasma to severely burned children at rates up to 2.5 mL/kg/min over 5 min and found that iCa^{2+} decreased significantly with the lowest blood levels between the fourth and fifth minute of infusion [58]. The same investigator administered plasma at 2 mL/kg/min to severely burned children which resulted in significant hypocalcemia without physiologic instability, attributed to the hypermetabolic state associated with burn recovery.

RBC transfusions following adult trauma are independent predictors of hypocalcemia which in turn is associated with increased mortality [51]. There is inadequate data to determine mortality associated with hypocalcemia during pediatric resuscitation, and it is unclear whether treatment improves outcomes during hemostatic resuscitation for shock [3, 50, 55, 59]. In a retrospective review of 457 severely injured children, 5.3% had pretransfusion hypocalcemia on admission which was associated with an increased odds of blood transfusion (OR, odds ratio 5.44; 95% confidence interval 1.44–20.58) [50]. This finding was supported in a retrospective registry review of 142 traumatized children with an iCa^{2+} level <1 mmol/L upon hospital admission [54]. Patients with hypocalcemia (46.5%) had lower systolic BPs, had lower Shock Index Pediatric Adjusted (SIPA) scores, and received more blood at 4 h (65.4 mL/kg versus 32.6 mL/kg; $p = 0.002$) and at 24 h post-admission; in-hospital mortality was unchanged. Because there was no difference in the prehospital transfusion requirement in these hypocalcemic children, investigators theorized that a mechanism other than transfusion-related "citrate toxicity" may influence outcomes [54].

Protocols for infant exchange transfusions include regular calcium supplementation because symptomatic ionized hypocalcemia is a predictable side effect. Although some massive transfusion protocols include empiric calcium administration, it is unclear if acute or empiric calcium administration affects longer-term outcomes in critically ill children [60]. However, it is crucial to monitor iCa^{2+} in susceptible patients during rapid transfusion. Although the typical ECG changes associated with acute citrate toxicity during transfusion and TAH are different, the treatment for each is the same: calcium administration. In children, either calcium chloride or gluconate may be used, although the gluconate form contains less ionizable calcium and dosing must be increased accordingly. Calcium may be administered in bolus or infusion form (10–15 mg/kg/h calcium chloride) through a relatively large peripheral IV or central venous catheter (CVC) separate from the blood infusion line to prevent tissue sclerosing and line clotting [3, 10]. In the event of a persistent arrhythmia during resuscitation with blood products, it is important to note that large volume transfusions also produce low serum magnesium levels; citrate binds magnesium in addition to other divalent cations.

14.2.4.1 Hospital-Associated Venous Thromboembolism (HA-VTE)

The incidence of HA-VTE has increased significantly in hospitalized pediatric patients. Hospitalized children may suffer VTE up to 1000 times more often the general population [61]. In a recent retrospective database review of the American College of Surgeons National Surgical Quality Improvement Project (ACS NSQIP), investigators examined the rate of HA-VTE in over 480,000 hospitalized children who received a perioperative RBC transfusion [61]. All age groups studied had an increased likelihood of HA-VTE, and the risk was transfusion dose-related. Neonates were particularly affected (aOR 4.1; 95% CI 2.5–6.7), followed by infants (aOR 2.4) and older children (aOR 2.2). The authors concluded that their findings must be carefully considered because blood administration in the perioperative period can involve multiple types of blood products, along with multiple confounding variables [62].

The etiology of HA-VTE is multifactorial; however, it is thought that perioperative RBC transfusions induce a proinflammatory state that contributes to the development of thromboses [63]. Stored RBCS have decreased cell membrane deformability, increased aggregability, and endothelial adherence, each of which can theoretically explain an increased risk of VTE formation [61, 64, 65]. VTE is also associated with large PIVC catheter-to-vein ratio (>33% or a 24 G in neonates and >50% or a 22 G in older children), as well as a failure to proactively flush lines and ports when not in use [66]. Prolonged CVC dwelling times and use of the femoral vein are also contributing factors, particularly in traumatized infants and children who are in a hypercoagulable state [67, 68]. In a propensity-matched database review of over 24,000 adult patients who underwent surgery and received both RBCs and plasma, investigators found a 30-day relative increase risk of VTE (1.36, 95% CI, 1.24–1.49) compared to patients who received RBCs only [62].

14.2.4.2 Transfusion-Associated Hemolysis

Non-immune, transfusion-associated hemolysis can occur in pediatric patients through several mechanisms: high infusion rates, RBC irradiation, RBC or platelet washing, small catheter gauge, vigorous suctioning into a cell salvage device, use of one-way valve (e.g., "claves" or needleless ports), overwarming of RBCs >42 °C, and cardiac bypass circuits [32, 69]. Washed RBCs and platelets may be ordered for certain patients, including those with a history of severe allergic reactions to blood products, small patients undergoing large-volume transfusions, and patients with renal failure. Cellular blood products are washed in saline to remove additives (i.e., plasma or preservative solutions) or byproducts (e.g., extracellular potassium). The RBC storage time is shortened to 24 h by washing, and therefore washed RBCs and platelets should be administered near preparation time (e.g., 12 and 4 h, respectively) [70]. RBCs treated with gamma irradiation also have a reduced shelf life (6–12 h) and leak more potassium than untreated RBCs [26]. While high infusion rates and special blood treatments such as irradiation or RBC washing may be unavoidable in some cases, RBC hemolysis may be mitigated by avoiding one-way valves, unsteady and episodic manual syringing, and PIVCs less than 24–22 G [18, 71, 72]. Cold blood products should be warmed only through a validated, US FDA-approved device to avoid heat-related hemolysis, and never by hot water baths, microwave ovens, or any device that does not undergo local quality control [32].

14.2.4.3 Venous Air Embolism (VAE)

VAE can occur with any infusion device because fluid infusion systems contain many potential air entrainment sites. These include loose catheter connections, open stopcocks, catheters left open or not flushed before insertion or removal, upright syringes, and even blood bags [73]. The pathophysiology of a clinically evident VAE is an airlock in the right ventricle, increased afterload, and ventricular failure, as well as massive release of vasoactive substances within the pulmonary circulation [44, 74, 75]. Atmospheric air enters a potential space and then moves down a pressure gradient; thus patients who are hypovolemic with a low right atrial pressure are particularly susceptible to VTE [76]. Furthermore, when cold fluid is warmed, the solubility of gas within the pre-existing bubbles increases, creating the conditions for nitrogen bubble expansion [44]. Most VAEs probably go unreported or are clinically silent. Fatal VAE has been documented in adults with 3–5 mL/kg air volumes but as low as 100 mL [74, 76]. A very small quantity of air can have critical effect if it ends up in blind circulatory beds such as the central nervous system or coronary arteries [75]. A patent foramen ovale (PFO), found in one-quarter of adults and in the majority of newborns, can lead to a paradoxical embolus, air entrainment into the arterial circulation, and stroke or fatal cardiac arrhythmias. Modern infusion devices contain air detection alarms and traps. However, practitioner alarm fatigue and the fact that very large volumes of air may exceed a trap's capacity underscore the importance of vigilance around all infusing devices, particularly those delivering fluids under pressure.

14.3 Summary of Key Learning Objectives

14.3.1 What Is Meant by a "Double Effect" in the Context of Pediatric Transfusion?

The doctrine of double effect is the dilemma that practitioners experience when life-saving care is associated with patient harm, despite best intentions. Implementation of a massive transfusion protocol (MTP), for instance, may cause several physiologic derangements, but the MTP may be the only management alternative to preserve life.

14.3.2 What Are Some Safety Concerns of a Rapid Transfusion in Children?

Many adverse events, including death, can result from the rapid transfusion of blood products to children. Some of these adverse events are directly related to the equipment or transfusion techniques used. Awareness of the following transfusion-related events, an understanding of the equipment at hand, and a knowledge of which patients are at greatest risk are first steps in transfusion safety. At times, these adverse transfusion-related events can only be managed:

- Transfusion-associated hyperkalemia (TAH)
- Transfusion-associated circulatory overload (TACO)
- Hypothermia
- Hypocalcemia
- Hospital-acquired venous thromboembolism (HA-VTE)
- Nonimmune hemolysis
- Venous air embolism (VAE)

14.3.3 Prevention Strategies for a 6 kg, Hypovolemic Patient

Some basic steps can be taken to prevent adverse events secondary to rapid blood administration in this challenging scenario. The patient's initial hypotension, GCS score, and low hemoglobin (Hgb) suggest significant intracranial blood loss which will worsen when the dura mater is opened. With a body temperature of 35.5 °C, it can be assumed he is coagulopathic on arrival. Because close monitoring of his blood pressure and laboratory values is critical, an arterial line and two large-bore peripheral IVs should be inserted if feasible, but not at the expense of timely fluid resuscitation and warming. The following measures may be attempted to achieve an optimal outcome:

- Externally warm the patient and monitor core body temperature with a goal of 36 °C.
- Warm all RBCs and plasma using a validated fluid warming device.
- Maintain a restrictive Hgb threshold goal while remaining vigilant for undiagnosed and occult blood loss.
- Request RBCs with storage age <7–10 days.
- Monitor blood gases, electrolytes, coagulation parameters, and Hgb frequently.
- Consider a calcium infusion.
- Keep up with ongoing blood loss by administering frequent, small RBC aliquots instead of large boluses (>20 mL/kg).
- Prioritize use of secure, large-bore PIVs over a CVC (especially femoral venous lines).
- Prioritize stopcock connectors over clave valves in the infusion set(s).
- Blood can be administered through a hand-held syringe if steady barrel pressure is exerted.
- "Debubble" all infusion lines and syringes; double-check integrity of infusion line connections.
- Suspect TACO if hypotension or hypoxemia occurs mid-transfusion.
- Suspect TAH or hypocalcemia if hypotension and ECG changes occur mid-transfusion.

Key Points

- Many adverse events can result from the rapid transfusion of blood products to children. At times, they can only be managed and not prevented. The key to safe management is knowledge of potential side effects and an understanding of which patients are at greatest risk.

- TAH has been associated with cardiac arrest in patients receiving large volume or rapidly administered RBC transfusions. TAH rarely occur if RBCs are administered at standard infusion doses and rates over 2–4 h.
- Currently, there are not pediatric-specific diagnostic criteria for TACO. Both large fluid volumes and a rapid rate of transfusion have been implicated, although the etiology is usually multifactorial.
- Hypocalcemia is attributed to citrate binding of calcium during rapid transfusion. Ionized calcium levels have an important role in coagulation and cardiovascular stability. Calcium supplementation as guided by point-of-care (POC) calcium monitoring is critical during rapid transfusions.
- The downstream metabolic effects of transfusion-induced hypothermia are extensive, including reduced metabolism of citrate preservative, a leftward shift of the oxyhemoglobin-dissociation curve, platelet dysfunction, and reduced procoagulant activity.
- VAE can occur with any infusion device because fluid infusion systems contain many potential air entrainment sites.

References

1. Kendall CE. At the coalface: medical ethics in practice. A double dose of double effect. J Med Ethics. 2000;26(3):204–5.
2. Beauchamp TL, Childress JF. Principles of biomedical ethics. Oxford: Oxford University Press; 2001. p. 128–32.
3. Cote CJ, Grabowski EF, Stowell CP. Chapter 12: strategies for blood product management, reducing transfusions, and massive blood transfusion. In: Cote CJ, Lehman J, Anderson BJ, editors. Cote and Lerman's a practice of anesthesia for infants and children. 6th ed. Elsevier: Amsterdam; 2019. p. 257–280.e13.
4. Mohamed A, Shah PS. Transfusion associated necrotizing enterocolitis: a meta-analysis of observational data. Pediatrics. 2012;129(3):529–40.
5. SHOT Bite No. 4: Lessons in Paediatrics (including neonates). Serious Hazards of Transfusion (SHOT). 2018. https://www.shotuk.org/resources/current-resources/shot-bites/. Accessed 4 Dec 2022.
6. Kopko PM. Transfusion reactions. 5th ed. Bethesda: AABB Press; 2021. p. 340–341, 476.
7. Roseff SD, Wong EC, editors. Pediatric transfusion: a handbook. Bethesda: AABB; 2020. p. 161–91.
8. Vraets A, Lin Y, Callum JL. Transfusion-associated hyperkalemia. Transfus Med Rev. 2011;25(3):184–96.
9. Strauss RG. RBC storage and avoiding hyperkalemia from transfusions to neonates & infants. Transfusion. 2010;50(9):1862–5.
10. Barcelona SL, Thompson AA, Coté CJ. Intraoperative pediatric blood transfusion therapy: a review of common issues. Part I: hematologic and physiologic differences from adults; metabolic and infectious risks. Paediatr Anaesth. 2005;15(9):716–26.
11. Centers for Disease Control and Prevention. National healthcare safety network biovigilance component hemovigilance module surveillance protocol v2.8. 2023. https://www.cdc.gov/nhsn/pdfs/biovigilance/bv-hv-protocol-current.pdf. Accessed 26 June 2023.

12. Fung MK, AuBuchon JP, Stephens LD. Classification of posttransfusion adverse events using a publicly available artificial intelligence system. Transfusion. 2024;64(4):590–6.
13. Morray JP. Cardiac arrest in anesthetized children: recent advances and challenges for the future. Paediatr Anaesth. 2011;21(7):722–9.
14. Burke M, Sinha P, Luban NLC, Posnack NG. Transfusion-associated hyperkalemic cardiac arrest in neonatal, infant, and pediatric patients. Front Pediatr. 2021;9:765306.
15. Lee AC, Reduque LL, Luban NL, Ness PM, Anton B, Heitmiller ES. Transfusion-associated hyperkalemic cardiac arrest in pediatric patients receiving massive transfusion. Transfusion. 2014;54(1):244–54.
16. Roseff SD, Wong EC. Pediatric transfusion: a handbook. Bethesda: AABB; 2020. p. 225.
17. Brown KA, Bissonnette B, McIntyre B. Hyperkalaemia during rapid blood transfusion and hypovolaemic cardiac arrest in children. Can J Anaesth. 1990;37(7):747–54.
18. Miller MA, Schlueter AJ. Transfusions via hand-held syringes and small-gauge needles as risk factors for hyperkalemia. Transfusion. 2004;44(3):373–81.
19. Cote C, Lerman J, Todres DI. A practice of anesthesia for infants and children. 4th ed. Philadelphia: Saunders; 2008. p. 209.
20. Popovsky MA. Transfusion reactions. 4th ed. Bethesda: AABB; 2011.
21. Delaney M, Wendel S, Bercovitz RS, Cid J, Cohn C, Dunbar NM, et al. Transfusion reactions: prevention, diagnosis, and treatment. Lancet. 2016;388(10061):2825–36.
22. Jorgenson M. Chapter 18: administration of blood components. In: Cohn CS, Delaney M, Johnson ST, Katz LM, editors. Technical manual. 20th ed. Bethesda: AABB; 2020. p. 537.
23. Yamada C, Edelson M, Lee A, Saifee NH, Bahar B, Delaney M. Transfusion-associated hyperkalemia in pediatric population: prevalence, risk factors, survival, infusion rate, and RBC unit features. Transfusion. 2021;61(4):1093–101.
24. Yamada C, Edelson MF, Lee AC, Saifee NH, Dinov ID. Transfusion-associated hyperkalemia in pediatric population: analyses for risk factors and recommendations. Transfusion. 2022;62(12):2503–14.
25. Spinella PC, Tucci M, Fergusson DA, Lacroix J, Hébert PC, Leteurtre S, et al. Effect of fresh vs standard-issue red blood cell transfusions on multiple organ dysfunction syndrome in critically ill pediatric patients: a randomized clinical trial. JAMA. 2019;322(22):2179–90.
26. Roseff SD, Wong EC, editors. Pediatric transfusion: a handbook. Bethesda: AABB; 2020. p. 11–9.
27. Cid J, Villegas V, Carbassé G, Alba C, Perea D, Lozano M. Transfusion of irradiated red blood cell units with a potassium adsorption filter: a randomized controlled trial. Transfusion. 2016;56(5):1046–51.
28. Matsuura H, Akatsuka Y, Muramatsu C, Isogai S, Sugiura Y, Arakawa S, et al. Evaluation of the potassium adsorption capacity of a potassium adsorption filter during rapid blood transfusion. Vox Sang. 2015;108(4):428–31.
29. Ogasawara K, Ohto H, Takano N, Nollet KE, Go H, Sato M, et al. Assessment of a downsized potassium adsorption filter designed to transfuse neonates. Transfusion. 2020;60(11):2494–9.
30. Bulle EB, Klanderman RB, Pendergrast J, Cserti-Gazdewich C, Callum J, Vlaar APJ. The recipe for TACO: a narrative review on the pathophysiology and potential mitigation strategies of transfusion-associated circulatory overload. Blood Rev. 2022;52:100891.
31. Thalji L, Thum D, Weister TJ, Weber WV, Stubbs JR, Kor DJ, et al. Incidence and epidemiology of perioperative transfusion-related pulmonary complications in pediatric noncardiac surgical patients: a single-center, 5-year experience. Anesth Analg. 2018;127(5):1180–8.
32. Hod EA, Francis RO. Chapter 22: noninfectious complications of blood transfusion. In: Cohn CS, Delaney M, Johnson ST, Katz LM, editors. Technical manual. 20th ed. Bethesda: AABB Press; 2020. p. 627–57.
33. US Food and Drug Administration. Transfusion/donation fatalities. 2023. https://www.fda.gov/vaccines-blood-biologics/report-problem-center-biologics-evaluation-research/transfusiondonation-fatalities. Accessed 19 September 2023.

34. Wiersum-Osselton JC, Whitaker B, Grey S, Land K, Perez G, Rajbhandary S, et al. Revised international surveillance case definition of transfusion-associated circulatory overload: a classification agreement validation study. Lancet Haematol. 2019;6(7):350–8.
35. De Cloedt L, Emeriaud G, Lefebvre É, Kleiber N, Robitaille N, Jarlot C, et al. Transfusion-associated circulatory overload in a pediatric intensive care unit: different incidences with different diagnostic criteria. Transfusion. 2018;58(4):1037–44.
36. De Cloedt L, Savy N, Gauvin F, Taylor S, Lacroix J, Emeriaud G. Transfusion-associated circulatory overload in ICUs: a scoping review of incidence, risk factors, and outcomes. Crit Care Med. 2019;47(6):849–56.
37. Grey S. Chapter 17a. Transfusion-associated circulatory overload (TACO) n = 131. 2021. https://www.shotuk.org/wp-content/uploads/myimages/17a.-Transfusion-Associated-Circulatory-Overload-TACO-2021.pdf. Accessed 21 September 2022.
38. Gupta SP, Nand N, Gupta MS. Left ventricular filling pressures after rapid blood transfusion in cases of chronic severe anemia. Angiology. 1982;33(5):343–8.
39. Späth C, Stoltz Sjöström E, Ågren J, Ahlsson F, Domellöf M. Sodium supply from administered blood products was associated with severe intraventricular haemorrhage in extremely preterm infants. Acta Paediatr. 2022;111(9):1701–8.
40. McCormick M, Zullo J, Kalpatthi R. Epidemiology and outcome of TRALI and TACO in the pediatric population: a multi-institutional review. Blood. 2018;132(Supplement 1):3811. https://doi.org/10.1182/blood-2018-99-113959.
41. Bhananker SM, Ramamoorthy C, Geiduschek JM, Posner KL, Domino KB, Haberkern CM, et al. Anesthesia-related cardiac arrest in children: update from the Pediatric Perioperative Cardiac Arrest Registry. Anesth Analg. 2007;105(2):344–50.
42. Serious Hazards of Transfusion (SHOT). Annual SHOT report 2018. Chapter 23. https://www.shotuk.org/wp-content/uploads/myimages/SHOT-Report-2018_Web_Version-1.pdf. Accessed 22 September 2023.
43. Duong H, Patel G. Hypothermia. In: StatPearls. Treasure Island: StatPearls; 2023.
44. Nemeth M, Miller C, Brauer A. Perioperative hypothermia in children. Int J Environ Res Public Health. 2021;18(14):7541.
45. Wright JL, Krug SE. Emergency medicine and critical care. In: Kliegman RM, Blum NJ, Shah SS, editors. Nelson textbook of pediatrics. Philadelphia: Elsevier; 2020. p. 539.
46. Gando S, Hayakawa M. Pathophysiology of trauma-induced coagulopathy and management of critical bleeding requiring massive transfusion. Semin Thromb Hemost. 2016;42(2):155–65.
47. Ireland S, Endacott R, Cameron P, Fitzgerald M, Paul E. The incidence and significance of accidental hypothermia in major trauma–a prospective observational study. Resuscitation. 2011;82(3):300–6.
48. Wolberg AS, Meng ZH, Monroe DM, Hoffman M. A systematic evaluation of the effect of temperature on coagulation enzyme activity and platelet function. J Trauma. 2004;56(6):1221–8.
49. Diab YA, Wong EC, Luban NL. Massive transfusion in children and neonates. Br J Haematol. 2013;161(1):15–26.
50. Epstein D, Ben Lulu H, Raz A, Bahouth H. Admission hypocalcemia in pediatric major trauma patients-An uncommon phenomenon associated with an increased need for urgent blood transfusion. Transfusion. 2022;62(7):1341–6.
51. Byerly S, Inaba K, Biswas S, Wang E, Wong MD, Shulman I, et al. Transfusion-related hypocalcemia after trauma. World J Surg. 2020;44(11):3743–50.
52. DeBot M, Sauaia A, Schaid T, Moore EE. Trauma-induced hypocalcemia. Transfusion. 2022;62(Suppl 1):274–80.
53. Vasudeva M, Mathew JK, Groombridge C, Tee JW, Johnny CS, Maini A, et al. Hypocalcemia in trauma patients: a systematic review. J Trauma Acute Care Surg. 2021;90(2):396–402.
54. Ciaraglia A, Lumbard D, Deschner B, Barry L, Braverman M, Eastridge B, et al. The effects of hypocalcemia in severely injured pediatric trauma patients. J Trauma Acute Care Surg. 2023;95(3):313–8.
55. Cornelius BG, Clark D, Williams B, Rogers A, Popa A, Kilgore P, et al. A retrospective analysis of calcium levels in pediatric trauma patients. Int J Burns Trauma. 2021;11(3):267–74.

56. Gimelraikh Y, Berant R, Stein M, Berzon B, Epstein D, Samuel N. Early hypocalcemia in pediatric major trauma: a retrospective cohort study. Pediatr Emerg Care. 2022;38(10):1637–40.
57. Hibberd O, Price J, Harris T, Barnard EBG. Incidence of admission ionised hypocalcaemia in paediatric major trauma: protocol for a systematic review and meta-analysis. BMJ Open. 2023;13(11):e077429.
58. Cote CJ, Grabowski EF, Stowell CP. Chapter 12: strategies for blood product management, reducing transfusions, and massive blood transfusion. In: Cote CJ, Lehman J, Anderson BJ, editors. Cote and Lerman's a practice of anesthesia for infants and children. 5th ed. Amsterdam: Elsevier; 2019. p. 271.
59. Spinella PC, Holcomb JB. Resuscitation and transfusion principles for traumatic hemorrhagic shock. Blood Rev. 2009;23(6):231–40.
60. Steele T, Kolamunnage-Dona R, Downey C, Toh CH, Welters I. Assessment and clinical course of hypocalcemia in critical illness. Crit Care. 2013;17(3):R106.
61. Goel R, Josephson CD, Patel EU, Petersen MR, Makhani S, Frank SM, et al. Perioperative transfusions and venous thromboembolism. Pediatrics. 2020;145(4):e20192351.
62. Choi UE, Nicholson RC, Frank SM, Cha S, Aziz H, Lester LC, et al. Perioperative plasma in addition to red blood cell transfusions are associated with increased venous thromboembolism risk postoperatively. Anesth Analg. 2024;139(2):254–61.
63. Zallen G, Moore EE, Ciesla DJ, Brown M, Biffl WL, Silliman CC. Stored red blood cells selectively activate human neutrophils to release IL-8 and secretory PLA2. Shock. 2000;13(1):29–33.
64. Relevy H, Koshkaryev A, Manny N, Yedgar S, Barshtein G. Blood banking-induced alteration of red blood cell flow properties. Transfusion. 2008;48(1):136–46.
65. Spinella PC, Sparrow RL, Hess JR, Norris PJ. Properties of stored red blood cells: understanding immune and vascular reactivity. Transfusion. 2011;51(4):894–900.
66. Paterson RS, Chopra V, Brown E, Kleidon TM, Cooke M, Rickard CM, et al. Selection and insertion of vascular access devices in pediatrics: a systematic review. Pediatrics. 2020;145(Suppl 3):243–68.
67. Bhatt MD, Chan AK. Venous thrombosis in neonates. Fac Rev. 2021;10:20.
68. van Ommen CH, Albisetti M, Bhatt M, Bonduel M, Branchford B, Chalmers E, et al. International pediatric thrombosis network to advance pediatric thrombosis research: communication from the ISTH SSC subcommittee on pediatric and neonatal thrombosis and hemostasis. J Thromb Haemost. 2021;19(4):1123–9.
69. O'Leary MF, Szklarski P, Klein TM, Young PP. Hemolysis of red blood cells after cell washing with different automated technologies: clinical implications in a neonatal cardiac surgery population. Transfusion. 2011;51(5):955–60.
70. Crowe EP, Goel R, Al-Mozain N, Josephson CD. Neonatal blood banking practices. Clin Perinatol. 2023;50(4):821–37.
71. Gniadek TJ, Richtsfeld M, Pulkrabek S, Hansen KR, Barnett SL, Joyner N, et al. Mechanical hemolysis in pediatric patients associated with rapid transfusion and one-way valve. Transfusion. 2018;58(5):1228–33.
72. Parker MJ, Manan A. Translating resuscitation guidelines into practice: health care provider attitudes, preferences and beliefs regarding pediatric fluid resuscitation performance. PLoS One. 2013;8(3):e58282.
73. Skelton T, Beno S. Massive transfusion in pediatric trauma: we need to focus more on "how". J Trauma Acute Care Surg. 2017;82(1):211–5.
74. Albin MS, Boyd GL. Chapter 186: Venous air embolism. In: Fleisher LA, Rosenbaum SH, editors. Complications in anesthesia. Philadelphia: Elsevier; 2018. p. 714–7.
75. Kerrigan MJ, Cooper JS. Venous gas embolism. In: StatPearls. 2022. https://pubmed.ncbi.nlm.nih.gov/29489147/. Accessed 22 August 2022.
76. McCarthy CJ, Behravesh S, Naidu SG, Oklu R. Air embolism: practical tips for prevention and treatment. J Clin Med. 2016;5(11):93.

15 Pediatric Massive Transfusion

Krupa D. Desai and Norma J. Klein

15.1 Case Scenario

A 12-year-old, 30 kg female with DiGeorge's syndrome and Tetralogy of Fallot presents with *Staphylococcus aureus* endocarditis. She is status post multiple cardiac surgeries. Chest CT findings upon admission are consistent with an abscess in the anterior mediastinum. The patient has been treated with IV antibiotics. She is now undergoing repeat surgery, and significant bleeding is encountered upon separation from cardiopulmonary bypass (CPB). You consider managing the situation as a massive transfusion (MT) but are unfamiliar with your hospital's massive transfusion protocol (MTP), including the criteria for triggering a pediatric MTP, the blood product composition, and when and how to terminate the MTP.

Key Learning Objectives

- What is the definition of a pediatric massive transfusion (MT)?
- What is a massive transfusion protocol (MTP)?
- What are the components of an MTP?
- How does one dose the components of an MTP?
- When is an MTP activated?
- How does one monitor coagulation during an ongoing MTP?
- How does one deactivate or stop an MTP?

K. D. Desai (✉)
Department of Anesthesiology, Perioperative Care and Pain Medicine, NYU Grossman School of Medicine, New York, NY, USA
e-mail: krupa.desai@nyulangone.org

N. J. Klein
Department of Anesthesiology and Pain Medicine, University of California, Davis, Sacramento, CA, USA
e-mail: nklein@ucdavis.edu

N. J. Klein (ed.), *Perioperative Pediatric Patient Blood Management and Transfusion Safety*, https://doi.org/10.1007/978-3-031-81666-6_15

- What are potential MTP adjuncts for the treatment of massive bleeding?
- What is the role of patient blood management (PBM) in massive bleeding and MTPs?
- What are some of the complications associated with MTP administration to children?

15.2 Discussion

Pediatric massive transfusion protocol (MTP) activation is uncommon [1, 2]. While adult massive transfusion protocols (MTPs) have been of interest for some time, evidence for defined protocols addressing pediatric bleeding has only recently appeared in the literature. The varied physiology and age-related changes in coagulation parameters have further confounded the development of clear guidelines. MTP implementation has been shown to reduce treatment variability, mortality, length of hospital stay, and less blood utilization [3, 4]. Furthermore, an institutional MTP supports faster blood product delivery to the bleeding patient, a crucial advantage since death from hemorrhagic shock typically occurs within several hours of injury [5, 6].

Massive bleeding is associated with the development of a "lethal triad" (hypothermia, acidosis, and coagulopathy) or a "lethal diamond" (when ionized hypocalcemia is added to the triad) [7]. There is a 10% decrease in clotting factor levels for every 1 °C below normothermia [8]. Hypothermia, which may result from shock, exposure, and resuscitation with unwarmed fluids, also inhibits platelet activation and adhesion and leads to coagulation factor dysfunction. Children rapidly become hypothermic with ambient temperature exposure compared to adults due to a larger body surface area to weight ratio. Hemodilution of platelets and coagulation factors exacerbates coagulopathy when there is excessive, unbalanced crystalloid and RBC administration, without replacement of other blood components. Acidosis also worsens coagulopathy by inhibiting clotting factor function [9]. Judicious management of hypovolemia with limited crystalloid resuscitation (e.g., 10–40 mL/kg) and early administration of blood products in the bleeding pediatric trauma patient are now recommended [10, 11]. Excessive fluid resuscitation has been linked to prolonged ICU stays, more ventilator-dependent days, and increased mortality, indicating the importance of further research on the ideal crystalloid and blood volume replacement for pediatric trauma resuscitation [10].

This case-based review aims to explore the current evidence surrounding pediatric massive transfusions, including the definition, activation, suggested monitoring, and complications associated with MT in children.

15.2.1 What Is the Definition of a Pediatric Massive Transfusion (MT)?

Attempts at defining MT in children have been complicated by both the physiologic heterogeneity of pediatric patients and a lack of information about optimal transfusion ratios. An early definition of MT in children is the administration of 50% of a patient's circulating blood volume within 12 h or ≥1 blood volume within 24 h. This MT definition was based on a prospective observation of a mixed population of 55 children over 2 years who required uncrossmatched blood [9]. In that study, the primary trigger for MTP was the development of a coagulopathy as indicated by a partial thromboplastin time (PTT) of 36 s [9]. It is important to note that in institutions providing MTP, the definition of MT often evolves into the "trigger" or MTP activation criteria.

To further define MT in children, Neff et al. studied pediatric combat patients and found that a threshold of 40 mL/kg of all blood products given within 24 h successfully differentiated pediatric patients at increased risk for both early and late death [12]. This was the first study to provide objective evidence that a mortality threshold for blood product administration exists in the pediatric trauma population, determining a potential trigger for balanced-product MTP. Neff's definition for MT has been incorporated into subsequent pediatric MTP research and development. It is important to note Neff's data is derived from pediatric combat trauma. However, the MT definition of 40 mL/kg body weight of blood administration within a 24-h period in children has been incorporated into multiple civilian MTPs across the United States (US) [1].

Massive bleeding in pediatric patients may also occur outside of trauma and instead in the more controlled intraoperative setting with different mechanisms of injury and markers of massive blood loss. In a 2021 prospective, multicenter, observational study of 449 bleeding children (the Massive Transfusion in Children (MATIC) study) who received >40 mL/kg of blood products in 6 h, or who received their institution's MTP, almost 20% of patients had medical bleeding compared to 34.1% surgical- and 46.1% trauma-related bleeding [13]. Twenty-eight-day mortality were greatest in the medically related bleeding group (65.2%) compared to the trauma and operative groups (36.1% and 23.8%, respectively).

15.2.2 What Is a Massive Transfusion Protocol (MTP)?

An MTP is a standardized, fixed-ratio package of RBCs, plasma, and platelets (cryoprecipitate may or may not be included, depending on the institution). The primary objective of an MTP is to provide hemostatic resuscitation as part of damage control resuscitation (DCR) and to avoid coagulopathy development in bleeding patients. Whole blood is of renewed interest in pediatric resuscitation not only because it simplifies the "balanced" approach to hemostatic resuscitation, but it contains a smaller volume of preservatives and anticoagulant (i.e., citrate) and limits donor exposure [14–16]. By design, the MTP must be immediately available and replenished automatically until deactivated. Every 1 min delay in access to balanced product is associated with a 5% mortality increase in the adult trauma population [17, 18]. The initial MTP blood is typically "universal donor" units that are crossmatched once the blood bank receives the patient's first type and screen (T&S) specimen. In many centers, only Rhesus antigen negative blood is supplied to females under a certain age (e.g., 45 or 50 years) and infants [19–21].

Massive hemorrhage and MT in the adult patient population have been studied extensively, with many investigations originating in adult combat trauma populations and subsequent analysis of civilian trauma outcomes [1, 22–24]. The term "Damage Control Resuscitation" (DCR) was derived from these studies and is applied when treating life-threatening bleeding occurs in multiple settings. DCR strategies consist of rapid control of bleeding and hemostasis; avoidance of hemodilution, acidosis, hypocalcemia, and hypothermia; early empiric or balanced ratio-based replacement of blood components or whole blood; and, at times, permissive hypotension. DCR principles are the basis for development of guidelines used to treat all causes of massive hemorrhage (trauma, medical, and surgical), later termed "Massive Transfusion Protocols" (MTPs) [10, 22, 24]. The term "hemorrhage" is often substituted for "transfusion," creating the term "massive hemorrhage protocol (MHP)," because bleeding management rather than transfusion is the priority [18].

Direct extrapolation of adult evidence and MTPs into the pediatric patient populations has been called into question, prompting further investigation [1, 10, 23, 25]. While children often tolerate blood loss better than adults due to a relatively substantial physiologic reserve, they are a heterogeneous group with differing mechanisms of injury compared to adults and different responses to trauma resuscitation [1, 23]. The developmental heterogeneity of the pediatric population and the rapidity at which children spiral into the "lethal triad" make defining DCR and optimal MTP ratios a challenge.

15.2.3 What Are the Components of an MTP?

The optimal ratio of blood components during DCR has been investigated in adults. Two major prospective clinical trials in adults, the Prospective, Observational, Multicenter, Major Trauma Transfusion (PROMMTT) and the Pragmatic, Randomized Optimal Platelet and Plasma Ratios (PROPPR) studies, paved the way for current practice. Finding improved hemostasis and decreased mortality from exsanguination when higher plasma and platelet to RBC ratios were administered, a 1:1:1 ratio of components compared to a lower coagulation factor to RBC ratio was recommended [1, 22, 24].

Multiple studies have examined the relationship between blood product transfusion ratios and mortality in pediatric patients, but evidence is far from definitive [4, 12, 26–30]. In an early retrospective study of 235 children who received RBCs for traumatic injury between 2005 and 2015, 26 were massively transfused (≥40 and ≥80 mL/kg) before MTP implementation, and 17 were massively transfused after MTP implementation [31]. In-hospital mortality was no different between the pre- and post-MTP implementation groups (24% and 19%, respectively), nor was the composite morbidity. However, the post-MTP group did receive a higher ratio of platelets and plasma to RBCs without a difference in overall blood product utilization [31]. Prior to this work, there were no prospective pediatric studies on the subject [32, 33]. A retrospective analysis of 583 patients in the Pediatric Trauma Quality Improvement Program registry found increased survival benefit with a higher plasma/RBC (no less than 1:2) ratio in civilian pediatric trauma with hemorrhagic shock [26]. Survival effects of the optimal platelet ratio in the same study were unclear. Another retrospective study of 110 civilian pediatric trauma subjects found survival benefit with a 1:1 ratio of RBC/plasma compared to ratios ≥2:1, regardless of patient age [28]. In a recent multicenter, prospective, observational study of 191 traumatized children with life-threatening bleeding who received >40 mL/kg of blood products in 6 h, a plasma deficit (calculated as plasma/RBC volume in mL/kg) and a platelet deficit (calculated as plasma/RBC volume in mL/kg) of at least 10% were associated with increased 24-h mortality [29]. In that same study, an adjusted secondary analysis of 449 children found a 12.7% increase in acute kidney injury (AKI) for every 10% increase in the administered platelet/RBC ratio (OR 1.127; 95% CI, 1.025–1.239; $p = 0.013$) [34]. A study of pediatric combat trauma patients from 2001 to 2013, where MT was defined as 40 mL/kg total blood products in 24 h, found practice changes in transfusion ratios with increased plasma/RBC and platelet/RBC ratios over time [4]. Investigators concluded that a more hemostatic management approach had evolved but were unable to define an optimal component ratio. Older review publications have recommended a balanced ratio of plasma/RBC >1:2 with an ideal goal of 1:1 from consensus-based evidence extrapolated from the adult literature [1, 28, 35].

In 2019, consensus guidelines were developed to guide practitioners in managing bleeding in critically ill children. The Transfusion and Anemia Expertise Initiative—Control/Avoidance of Bleeding (TAXI-CAB) recommends a 1:1:1 (RBC/plasma/platelets) or 2:1:1 ratio until bleeding is no longer life threatening [36]. In 2022, a Pediatric Traumatic Hemorrhagic Shock Consensus Conference consisting of 16 pediatric specialists developed evidence-based recommendations for the management of pediatric hemorrhagic shock [25]. While recognizing that high-quality evidence is lacking, a plasma/RBC and a platelet/RBC ratio of 1:1 was recommended, with 100% agreement between specialists. Low titer (≤200 IgG) of type O whole blood was suggested as "might be considered" over individual components when available because of its lower volume of anticoagulant and higher procoagulant content [25]. TAXI-CAB recommends using clinical judgement for platelet transfusion ratios for moderate to severe bleeding [26, 37]. The Traumatic Hemorrhagic Shock Consensus Conference consensus recommends a high platelet/RBC ratio approaching 1:1 [25].

It is important to note that studies and guidelines supporting MTP ratios for bleeding children are largely based on data from the trauma literature and may be subject to survival bias, making recommendations that are not generalizable to the general pediatric population. MTs are also administered to children with medical and intraoperative types of bleeding. Current best evidence for intraoperative MT supports application of trauma-derived, balanced ratios of 1:1 for plasma/RBC (with less clear guidance for platelet ratios) [1, 28]. A recent prospective, multicenter study of 449 patients highlighted the heterogeneous nature of pediatric patients receiving massive transfusions, including the finding that children with traumatic bleeding tended to be older (mean age 10.5 years) than those with intraoperative bleeding (mean age 2.1 years) and have high injury scores [13].

An Initial Pack will be sent regardless of weight with 2 units PRBC's, 1 unit FFP and 1 unit Platelets (pack 0)

	< 20 Kg	21 – 50 Kg	> 50 Kg
PACK 1			
RBC	1 Unit	2 Unit	4 Unit
FFP	1 Unit	2 Unit	4 Unit
PLT	0 Unit	1 Unit	1 Unit
CRYO	As Needed	As Needed	As Needed
PACK 2			
RBC	1 Unit	2 Unit	4 Unit
FFP	1 Unit	2 Unit	4 Unit
PLT	1 Unit	1 Unit	1 Unit
CRYO	2 Unit	5 Unit	10 Unit

Fig. 15.1 A pediatric MTP pack. Reproduced with permission from Dr. Aru Reddy and Dr. Meera Gangadaran, MD, Arkansas Children's Hospital

Furthermore, children with medical or intraoperative bleeding in that study were more likely to have received coagulation factors prior to MTP activation and overall higher volumes of RBCs (35.1 mL/kg versus 17.9 mL/kg) compared to trauma patients [13].

An example of MTP "pack" contents is illustrated in Fig. 15.1.

In conclusion, the optimal ratio for RBCs, plasma, platelets, and coagulation factors in children with massive hemorrhage remains unknown. A large prospective trial from the University of Pittsburgh analyzing bleeding related mortality with whole blood resuscitation, component therapy, and tranexamic acid administration is pending and may help to fill this crucial information gap [38].

15.2.3.1 MTP Implementation Challenges

There are challenges with pediatric MPT implementation beyond the various definitions of MT and MTP product ratios. Pediatric transfusion protocols vary between institutions [2, 25, 39]. Additionally, many institutions face discrepancies in the ratios of blood products actually administered compared to institutional guidelines [2]. One potential factor responsible for observed variability in MT replacement is the extended thawing times required for plasma (which may delay plasma administration and alter the plasma/RBC ratio). Physician discretion in interpretation of the protocols and a lack of knowledge about MT lead to inconsistencies in ratios actually administered [40]. Furthermore, it has been shown that when RBC and coagulation products are released in predetermined MTP "rounds" or packs, overall administration leans toward more balanced product ratios, compared to institutions where products are released separately [2]. Other barriers to consistent MTP execution include lack of EMR functionality and availability of specialty equipment. Finally, variability in MTP activation and hemorrhage management is compounded by the lack of evidence-based data regarding transfusion triggers and critical transfusion thresholds in severely bleeding children [1, 35, 41].

Children experience different mechanisms of injury compared to adults which also differ between age groups. Bleeding pediatric patients also have different physiological responses to trauma, hemorrhage, and treatment. Age-based differences in total blood volume per kilogram of body weight impact the efficacy of hemostatic resuscitation, ranging from 100 mL/kg in preterm neonates, 90 mL/kg in term neonates, and 70–80 mL/kg in adolescents [8]. Given the finding that traumatized children who receive MT tend to be older than their medical or intraoperative counterparts, younger trauma patients may be poorly represented in studies focused on massive transfusion, thus making extrapolation to optimal MTP ratios more challenging.

There are also age-related differences in pediatric hematopathology. Fetal hemoglobin has a relatively low p50 (blood gas tension; 19 vs 27 mmHg in adults), binding oxygen with more affinity, theoretically compromising peripheral oxygen delivery. Additionally, a decrease in 2,3-diphophyglycate (2,3-DPG; which occurs with increased RBC storage duration) may result in a further increase in hemoglobin oxygen affinity and theoretically reduce peripheral oxygen delivery [42, 43]. Oxygen carrying capacity and the physiologic response to bleeding are also affected by age-related normal hemoglobin values: children experience a compensated but physiologic hemoglobin nadir of 9 g/dL at 10–12 weeks of age (and as low as 7 g/dL at 4–6 weeks in preterm infants) [44]. These normal hemoglobin values may be interpreted as critical anemia during massive bleeding and prompt over-transfusion in a situation where pediatric MTP is seldom implemented.

The coagulation profiles of children also vary with age. At birth, children have low levels of both anticoagulant and procoagulant proteins. Procoagulant factors do not cross the placenta and factors II, V, VII, IX, X, XI, and XII are lower in infants compared to older children and adults; differences also exist in levels of protein C, protein S, and antithrombin [8, 45, 46]. Absolute platelet counts generally are elevated compared to adults, but platelets are often qualitatively dysfunctional, particularly in newborns and infants [8]. A newborn's coagulation system takes approximately 6 months to mature to adult levels. Children are also at high risk for rapid-onset coagulopathy following traumatic bleeding, especially in the face of traumatic brain injury (TBI), with reported rates ranging from 10–77% [13, 47].

15.2.4 How Does One Dose the Components of an MTP?

Unlike MTP dosing in the adult patient population, pediatric MTPs apply weight-based product dosing for smaller patients (e.g., less than approximately 50 kg). This is crucial because small patients are easily over-transfused [48]. The recommended transfusion aliquot of 10–20 mL/kg results in a volume proportionally larger than that recommended for adults. Ten mL/kg in a 70 kg adult is 700 mL of blood;

however, the recommended incremental dose in the adult patient population is one-third at 250 mL. In its 2020 summary, the UK's Serious Hazards of Transfusion (SHOT) received nine reports of pediatric over-transfusion, prompting recommendations that all bedside providers involved in pediatric transfusions receive specific training in weight-based administration [48, 49]. In the case of infants, transfusion services should dispense blood bags in age- and weight-appropriate aliquots (e.g., 40 mL or 80 mL) rather than "adult" units that are typically 250 mL in volume [48]. Examples of "balanced" weight-based dosing recommendations for RBC/plasma/platelet ratios include 20:10:5 mL/kg; 20:20:10 mL/kg; and 30:20:0 mL/kg [50–52].

Figures 15.2 illustrates a weight-based, color-coded table that facilitates quick dosing identification and management for a range of pediatric age groups [52].

There is recent evidence when children who have life-threatening bleeding of any cause are resuscitated under an MTP; females may receive a higher volume of blood products compared to their male counterparts. In a secondary adjusted analysis of 449 children from the MATIC study, females received 76 mL/kg (range 40–150 mL/kg) total blood volume compared to 53 mL/kg (range 24–100 mL/kg) in their male counterparts ($p < 0.001$) [29]. Children over 11 years received 48% less blood volume than those 0–11 years in that same secondary analysis ($p < 0.001$) [29].

15.2.5 When Is an MTP Activated?

Specific pediatric patient populations at high risk of coagulopathy associated with massive bleeding include neonates and infants, traumatic brain injury, sepsis, and those presenting with an elevated partial thromboplastin time (PT) [53–55]. Because survival in exsanguinating patients is related to the early administration of blood products, a successful MTP response requires clearly defined activation or trigger criteria. In a recent multicenter observational study of 449 children (median age 7.3

Broselow™-based Transfusion Guide				
		20 mL/kg	10 mL/kg	5 mL/kg
		PRBC	FFP	Platelets
Pink	6–7 kg	120	60	30
Red	8–9 kg	160	80	40
Purple	10–11 kg	200	100	50
Yellow	12–14 kg	260	130	65
White	15–18 kg	320	160	80
Blue	19–23 kg	400	200	100
Orange	24–29 kg	500	250	125
Green	30–36 kg	600	300	150

Fig. 15.2 A color-coded guide to drive weight-based pediatric massive transfusion decisions. Reprinted with permission from Trappey AF, 3rd, Thompson KM, Kuppermann N, Stephenson JT, Nuno MA, Hewes HA, et al. Development of transfusion guidelines for injured children using a Modified Delphi Consensus Process. J Trauma Acute Care Surg. 2019;87 (4):935-43

years), the death rate was 2–3 times that reported in the adult literature, and in many cases, plasma and platelets—if administered—were often delayed by 30 min [13].

Pediatric MTP activation is an uncommon event, which may contribute to arbitrary hemostatic resuscitation and overutilization of precious universal donor blood products [1]. A 2014 survey of 50 pediatric hospitals in the USA and Canada found the median MTP activation rate to be only 5–6 times per year [2]. The classic trigger has been an actual or potential volume of blood loss (e.g., one-half of total blood volume in 1 h) [11]. To avoid arbitrary ordering practices, the decision to trigger an MTP requires clinical judgment that is best guided through decision aides and the patient's clinical course, not isolated physiologic or hematologic values. Specific MTP activation criteria for bleeding patients that have evolved as more institutions develop their own protocols include [2, 18, 52, 55–58]:

- 1/2 total blood volume in 1 h
- 20–40 mL/kg transfusion requirement within 2 h
- ≥3 units of crossmatched blood required in 1 h in adult patients
- SIPA (shock index pediatric adjusted) >1.4 plus systolic BP <100
- Assessment of blood consumption (ABC) score ≥2 in adult patients
- Trauma protocol activation
- Penetrating injury
- Intracranial bleed in a child <2 years going to the operating room
- Bleeding in an anticoagulated patient
- Persistent hemodynamic instability
- An immediate need to acquire blood products
- Acidosis
- Coagulopathy

Figure 15.3 is an example of a level 1 trauma center pediatric massive transfusion algorithm [52]. Note that after failing to achieve clinical stability following administration of 20 mL/kg crystalloid and at least 20 mL/kg of RBC, the MTP is activated if more than 40 mL/kg of any blood product has been given or is anticipated.

Figure 15.4 illustrates pediatric MTP activation based on a range of physiologic parameters: hemodynamic stability, tachycardia, or hemodynamic instability.

There are multiple scoring systems designed to predict MTP activation in the adult trauma population; however, validated prediction models are unavailable for traumatized pediatric patients. Mortality rates, rather than predictive models, tend to be used as surrogates for bleeding assessment and MTP activation in critically ill children [59, 60]. Nellis et al. conducted a survey of pediatric intensivists' criteria for determination of critical bleeding, citing patient characteristics such as >5 mL/kg/h of active bleeding, a decrease in BP or an increase in HR >20%, and bleeding into major body cavities [61]. However, this survey was not intended to assess intraoperative management or MTP activation criteria.

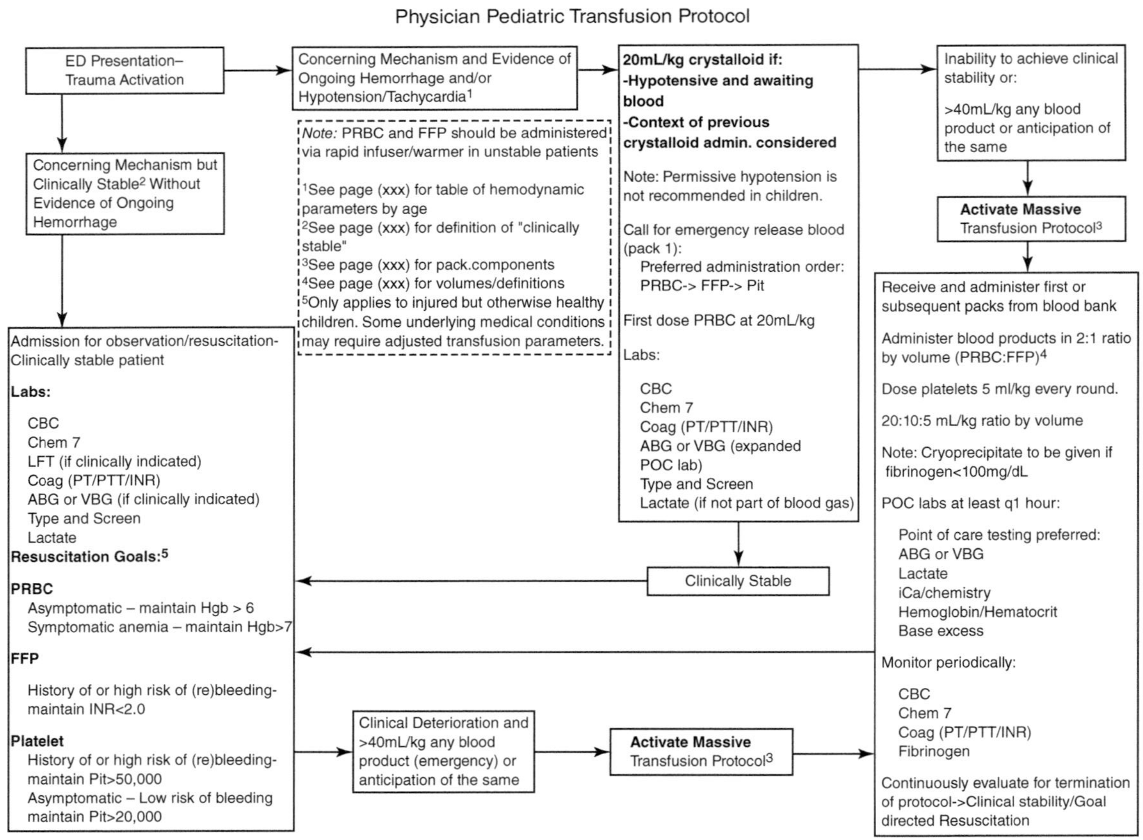

Fig. 15.3 A pediatric-focused MTP algorithm. Reprinted with permission from Trappey AF, 3rd, Thompson KM, Kuppermann N, Stephenson JT, Nuno MA, Hewes HA, et al. Development of transfusion guidelines for injured children using a Modified Delphi Consensus Process. J Trauma Acute Care Surg. 2019;87 (4):935-43

Ongoing bleeding

Clinical signs	Stable	Tachycardia*	Haemodynamic instability			
Blood loss	0–10 ml/kg	10–20 ml/kg	20–40 ml/kg	1 BV lost	2 BV lost	For every BV lost
Crystalloid **	10 ml/kg	0	0	0	0	0
RBC	0	10 ml/kg	20 ml/kg	20 ml/kg	20 ml/kg	20 ml/kg
FFP ***	0	10 ml/kg	20 ml/kg	20 ml/kg	20 ml/kg	20 ml/kg
Platelet concentrate	0	0	10 ml/kg	10 ml/kg	10 ml/kg	10 ml/kg
TEG®/ROTEM®	+	+	+	+	+	+
Cryoprecipitate, Fibrinogen, Tranexamic Acid etc. used goal-directed according to concurrent TEG®/ROTEM® monitoring						

Fig. 15.4 MTP activation using physiologic parameters as triggers. Reprinted from Nystrup KB, Stensballe J, Bottger M, Johansson PI, Ostrowski SR. Transfusion therapy in paediatric trauma patients: a review of the literature. Scand J Trauma Resusc Emerg Med. 2015;23:21, under Creative Commons Attribution License (http://creativecommons.org/licenses/by/2.0)

15.2.5.1 Hematologic MTP Activation Thresholds

In the past, RBCs were recommended for initial resuscitation in massive hemorrhage. Modern pediatric MTPs now incorporate plasma along with RBCs as initial therapy. However, platelets are usually protocolled into the second or later rounds unless there is severe hemodynamic instability. Similarly, pediatric MTPs supply cryoprecipitate under various conditions, including a specific fibrinogen level, after several MTP rounds, or only according to viscoelastic testing results. It is important to note that many patients—adults and children—can undergo significant blood loss with RBC replacement (up to 3–5 units in the average size adult) during surgery if other parameters remain stable, including body temperature, acid-base status, and perfusion pressures.

It is not necessary to obtain a hemoglobin value to guide transfusion in the face of life-threatening hemorrhage [62]. Children have been shown to tolerate lower hemoglobin than adults, but there is controversy regarding acceptable levels of severe anemia relative to outcomes [8]. There is some consensus that stable but critically ill, acyanotic children who are under careful observation (e.g., managed in alternative ways such as iron administration) do not require an RBC transfusion for hemoglobin levels less than 5 g/dL [8, 63]. The Transfusion and Anemia Expertise Initiative (TAXI) consensus recommends a post-transfusion Hgb in the range 7–9.5 g/dL in hemodynamically stable, critically ill children (level of evidence 2C, low quality) [64].

Children with cyanotic heart disease traditionally have been thought to require higher hemoglobin thresholds. This has been called into question with recent guidelines and studies dedicated to this specific patient population. The 2019 Network for the Advancement of Patient Blood Management, Haemostasis, and Thrombosis (NATA) guidelines recommend a postoperative hemoglobin threshold for RBC transfusion of 8 g/dL in children with congenital heart disease who are symptomatic and 7 g/dL for those who are asymptomatic [65]. For stable children with cyanotic heart disease, NATA recommends a postoperative hemoglobin threshold of 9 g/dL for symptomatic anemia. A recent study found that a hematocrit greater than 42% in cyanotic patients (38% in acyanotic patients) upon arrival to ICU after undergoing operative correction of congenital heart disease is associated with higher rate of complications and mortality [66].

Normal platelet levels range from 250 to 450 × 10^9/L in children. Platelet transfusion thresholds in pediatrics are typically extrapolated from the adult population and assume that no other coagulation abnormality is present. Perioperatively, suggested platelet transfusion thresholds tend to be procedure specific. Low-risk procedures such as central lines and airway management may be managed with platelet counts of 20 × 10^9/L or greater [67]. Platelet transfusion thresholds for high-risk procedures, neurosurgery, and major bleeding range from 50 to 100 × 10^9/L [67, 68]. TAXI-CAB recommends evaluation of the clinical etiology (e.g., mechanical injury, Von Willebrand disease, antiplatelet medications, renal insufficiency), as well as timing and type of surgery. A platelet transfusion threshold of ≤20 × 10^9/L for absent or minimal bleeding around noncardiac surgery and a threshold of ≤50 × 10^9/L for moderate bleeding peri-noncardiac surgery may be considered on balance with the clinical context (96% agreement of the TAXI-CAB Expert Consensus Panel) [36].

Plasma fibrinogen levels fall earlier than other coagulation factors during massive hemorrhage [18]. Fibrinogen deficiency increases bleeding due to a reduction in fibrin production and compromised platelet aggregation. The critical fibrinogen level and appropriate monitoring are debatable due to variations in measurement tools and interpatient physiological variation [69]. Cryoprecipitate, or alternatively fibrinogen concentrate which provides an equivalent dose of fibrinogen in a smaller volume, has been shown to effectively restore fibrinogen levels [70–73]. Of note, fibrinogen concentrate lacks procoagulant proteins C and S which naturally function to prevent hypercoagulation in the face of injury. Fibrinogen concentrate is not readily available in all US clinical settings. Critical hypofibrinogenemia is defined as 50–200 mg/dL based on the International Council for Standardization in Hematology; however there is overlap with normal reference ranges as clinical context is necessary for critical level determination [70, 71, 74]. An increased risk in perioperative bleeding has been noted in the adult surgical setting with a fibrinogen levels <150–200 mg/dL [71]. In addition, it has been shown that children undergoing cardiac surgery have increased rates of postoperative bleeding when the fibrinogen level is less than 150 mg/dL [71]. In a recent retrospective study of 1948 traumatically injured, propensity matched children, those treated with cryoprecipitate upon admission had a lower mortality rate [75].

In the absence of heavy perioperative bleeding and other contributing factors, a prothrombin time (PT), partial thromboplastin time (PTT), and international normalized ratio (INR) ≤2 times the patient's baseline upper limits of normal are unlikely to require treatment with either plasma, cryoprecipitate, or fibrinogen [36].

15.2.6 How Does One Monitor Coagulation During an Ongoing MTP?

Early resuscitation of children with massive hemorrhage may require empirically based administration of blood products in an RBC/plasma/platelet 1:1:1: or 2:1:1 ratio. Once vital signs and clinical bleeding have stabilized, transition from an MTP to goal directed management with coagulation testing is necessary to avoid blood product overuse or wastage. Either version of VET—thromboelastography (TEG) or rotational thromboelastography (ROTEM)—may be used in children to follow traumatically induced bleeding [76, 77]. Viscoelastic testing (VET) has been shown to correlate with conventional laboratory tests of coagulation in children and can be performed at the bedside with more rapid results [25]. However, during ongoing, rapid bleeding, no test of coagulation can produce timely feedback in sync with blood loss [78]. Thus, it has been suggested that the empirically based MTP should be followed until hemostasis can be evaluated in a timely manner; opponents of this approach cite unnecessary blood administration and wastage, instead suggesting ongoing VET monitoring during active bleeding [18, 79–81].

Viscoelastic testing uses whole blood samples and thus gives information about the adequacy and interplay of factors in the entire coagulation system. The use of these technologies is now recommended by both American and European transfusion guidelines [18, 25, 81–86]. A 2007 study comparing variations in 100 healthy children age 1 month to 16 years and 25 adults found no age-related differences in the major TEG parameters [87]. Healthy young infants, however, have demonstrated accelerated clot formation (TEG) and propagation times (ROTEM), despite the fact that coagulation factor levels are reduced until 6–12 months of age [45, 46, 88, 89]. In a recent prospective study of 100 healthy children, adult ROTEM reference ranges were adopted for children over 11 years, but younger children especially neonates and infants demonstrated significant age variation with stronger clot formation [90]. Viscoelastic assays cannot give accurate information about pharmaceutical anticoagulation or congenital bleeding diatheses [91]. Point-of-care (POC) VET (i.e., TEG®6s, Quantra®) is now available at the anesthesia workstation to provide rapid feedback during active bleeding [92, 93]. A newer POC device, the Quantra, analyzes whole blood clot formation using ultrasound technology. It has been validated against ROTEM and TEG, and reference values have been established in 50 children aged 2–17 years [94].

Viscoelastic analysis can also inform transition to crossmatched blood products after MTP activation, often called MTP "deactivation." Deng et al. retrospectively reviewed ROTEM goal directed management in 332 traumatically injured children (and 332 matched controls) and found decreased plasma transfusions and hospital length of stay compared to children managed with conventional coagulation studies [77]. However, further research is necessary to validate the clinical efficacy of TEG and ROTEM hemorrhage management in massively bleeding children [42].

15.2.7 How Does One Stop or Deactivate an MTP?

When a massively bleeding patient is hemodynamically stable and bleeding is controlled, the MTP should be deactivated. This is an active communication process; the hospital Transfusion Service must be asked to stop automatic delivery of MTP "packs" or "rounds." At that point in DCR, goal-directed product administration can replace empiric, fixed-ratio MTP dosing through POC or conventional laboratory assessment of hemoglobin, coagulation, and acid base status. Deactivation is crucial to avoid over-transfusion as well as preservation of the scarce supply of universally compatible blood [95]. A substantial percentage of activated MTPs are not utilized, and, although they may be returned to the issuing blood bank if properly handled, MTP activation in and of itself places blood products at risk of wastage and consumes significant hospital resources.

15.2.8 What Are Potential MTP Adjuncts for the Treatment of Massive Bleeding?

Most literature concerning MT and MTP in children focuses on balanced resuscitation and optimal MTP component ratios. Very limited data exists regarding the use of the adjuncts, such as tranexamic acid, recombinant factor VIIa, fibrinogen, and prothrombin concentrate in pediatric MT.

Tranexamic acid (TXA) is a lysine analogue with antifibrinolytic properties that prevents fibrinolysis by inhibiting plasminogen activation. A reduction in plasminogen activation inhibits plasmin formation and fibrin breakdown (which is a normal mechanism leading to clot disruption). There is strong evidence that TXA use in adult trauma decreases mortality, and it is recommended in postpartum hemorrhage to minimize blood loss [10, 96, 97]. TXA use in pediatrics was at one time controversial since data came from trauma studies (PEDTRAX) in children with blast and penetrating injuries (rather than blunt injury which is most common in civilian trauma), as well as rarely reported side effects including anaphylaxis and seizures [8, 98]. In a secondary analysis from the MATIC study, 6- and 24-h survival was examined in children (median age 7 years) with life-threatening bleeding who either received >40 mL/kg of blood or were treated under an MTP [99]. Twelve percent received an antifibrinolytic (i.e., TXA, epsilon aminocaproic acid, or both), and those patients had improved short-term survival compared to hemorrhaging children who did not receive an antifibrinolytic. The median TXA dose of was 20 mL/kg and there were no seizures reported in that group. There are an increasing number of pediatric studies that demonstrate relative efficacy and safety of fibrinolytics when administered in the perioperative setting [8, 80, 98, 100]. Seizures have been associated with higher doses of TXA, but lower doses (e.g., a loading dose of 10 mg/kg and maintenance infusion of 5 mg/kg/h) have been recently shown to be effective in preventing blood loss in pediatric patients undergoing craniosynostosis surgery [101]. The doses recommended in trauma settings are lower than the published doses for pediatric cardiac, spinal, and craniofacial surgery, although the optimal dosing for traumatized children remains unclear [59]. Perioperative loading doses as high as 50 mg/kg with continuous infusions up to 20 mg/kg are found in the literature, although a typical loading dose for trauma is 15 mg/kg followed by 1–2 mg/kg/h over 8 h [102]. In a 2022 update review on perioperative TXA, Patel et al. 10–30 mg/kg IV load (maximum loading dose 2 g) followed by 5–10 mg/kg/h infusion as a typical dose for children undergoing surgery [80]. Although acute thromboembolism and consumption coagulopathy are absolute contraindications to TXA administration, the same update noted that a history of seizures is not a contraindication to TXA administration in high blood loss cases. Outcomes are optimal when TXA is administered within the first 3 h of injury or active bleeding [25, 103]. TXA may be administered through either intravenous (IV) or intraosseous (IO) routes and should be considered in all severely bleeding pediatric patients [1]. The Pediatric Traumatic Hemorrhagic Shock Consensus Conference recommends TXA over aminocaproic acid due to insufficient trauma-related comparison data with a suggestion of increased renal injury using aminocaproic acid [25].

The Pediatric Traumatic Hemorrhagic Shock Consensus Conference recommends fibrinogen replacement during massive bleeding using either cryoprecipitate or fibrinogen concentrate [25]. Although outcomes are unclear, replacement thresholds as part of massive hemorrhage protocols are typically at 150 mg/dL. The most recent TAXI-CAB consensus does not specify fibrinogen thresholds but recognizes fibrinogen level evaluation as essential to hemostasis management and suggests that it be done in conjunction with overall coagulation monitoring (e.g., conventional coagulation parameters, VET, and platelet number and function) [36]. Cryoprecipitate is routinely used in a setting of congenital heart operations to minimize bleeding with most given intraoperatively [104].

A 2019 retrospective analysis of 468 severely injured adult trauma patients found that four-factor prothrombin complex concentrate (4-PCC) along with plasma over plasma alone is associated with improved survival and reduction in transfusion requirements [105]. However, a 2023 randomized clinical trial, early administration of prothrombin concentrate complex in patients with acute hemorrhage following severe trauma (PROCOAG), found an increased risk of thromboembolic events in patients at risk of MT [106]. In the PROCOAG study, there was no difference in the 24-h blood product consumption after 4-PCC administration compared to patients that did not receive the 4-PCC. Based on these findings, 4-PCC is not recommended in patients who are potential candidates for MT. There is inadequate evidence to establish the efficacy and safety of use of prothrombin complex concentrates in bleeding pediatric patients, including those with hemorrhagic shock [25, 107].

Routine use of recombinant FVIIa (rFVIIa) in treatment of pediatric bleeding is not supported in the literature [23]. Recombinant FVIIa use is off-label in pediatric patients, but some studies have shown a decrease in amount of blood products administered following rFIIa administration [23, 108]. Use of rFVIIa in MT and hemostatic resuscitation is controversial due to a concern over past reports of thromboembolism [1, 8].

Deliberate or permissive hypotension has been used in adults to minimize blood loss, but it is not recommended in bleeding children [8, 25]. To date, there is not a clear definition of permissive hypotension in the pediatric literature. Baseline blood pressures in children are close to the limits of cerebral autoregulation. Children with traumatic brain injury (TBI) are at exceptional risk of secondary brain injury when mean blood pressure is less than intracranial pressure. Furthermore, children tolerate significant volumes of blood loss (e.g., 30%) before systolic hypotension is evident [25]. Although the American College of Surgeons Committee on Trauma (ACSCT) classification scheme in adults recommends crystalloid resuscitation until greater than 30% of total blood volume is lost or hypotension ensues, delaying transfusion until these thresholds are met places children, especially infants, at high risk of acidosis and coagulopathy [109].

15.2.9 What Is the Role of Patient Blood Management (PBM) in Massive Bleeding and MTPs?

Patient blood management (PBM) is "… a patient-centered, systematic, evidence-based approach to improve patient outcomes by managing and preserving a patient's own blood, while promoting patient safety and empowerment" [110]. An MTP will optimize patient outcomes by standardizing certain blood management practices, specifically, preservation of the patient's hemoglobin level, prevention of coagulopathy, and nonarbitrary pediatric MT practices [111]. Select PBM measures that advance the safety and efficiency of MTPs include:

- Management algorithms and crisis checklists to reduce variability in management
- Bedside POC hemoglobin, viscoelastic, and blood gas capability
- Adherence to evidence-based restrictive transfusion thresholds with concomitant monitoring of global oxygenation and coagulation
- Access to readily available thawed plasma, in accordance with the American College of Surgeons (ACS) best practice advisory for initial balanced product availability in under 15 min [17]
- Early administration of antifibrinolytics in cases of life-threatening bleeding
- Strict attention to hypothermia prevention in the perioperative environment
- Autotransfusion (cell salvage) support
- Staff education regarding age- and weight-based transfusion management in children
- Regular quality assurance reviews of all massively transfused patients for guideline compliance and patient outcome

With recognition that an institution's response to critical bleeding is complex and difficult to implement effectively in the best of circumstances, a Canadian group developed a cognitive aide entitled "The 7 T's of massive hemorrhage protocol (MHP)" [18, 40]. The seven steps include:

- Trigger the protocol
- Team preparation and performance

- Tranexamic acid
- Test hourly
- Transfuse to target
- Temperature management
- Terminate the protocol

A critical 8th "T" might include "transport": communication from the first responders, emergency department, or intensive care unit concerning blood products already administered to support continuity of care as the patient is received in the operating room. Furthermore, sending a patient specimen for blood type and antibody screen (T&S) as soon as possible is critical to allow type-specific blood product administration once hemostatic damage control resuscitation is no longer necessary.

15.2.10 What Are Some of the Complications Associated with MTP Administration to Children?

Metabolic disturbances are a common risk of massive transfusion, particularly in very small patients. Hyperkalemia has been associated with rapid RBC administration; blood product extracellular potassium levels increase with duration of RBC storage. Unrecognized and untreated, elevated effluent potassium levels can lead to fatal cardiac arrhythmias [112–114]. Concomitant intravenous calcium gluconate administration, as well as a decreased rate of transfusion, may be used empirically to mitigate this unavoidable side effect [115]. Frequent potassium level monitoring, administration of RBC via largest catheter possible, and the use of "fresh" blood in neonates are preventive measures currently recommended. "Fresh" blood has been defined as RBCs stored for less than 1 week [116]. In a 2019 randomized controlled trial of over 1500 critically ill children, administration of fresh rather than standard issue RBCs was not associated with multiple organ dysfunction (MOD) or mortality [116]. Although all children were transfused within a week of admission to the pediatric ICU, the infusion rates of the fresh and standard RBCs were not clear. In a secondary analysis of 257 patients from the TRIPICU (Transfusion Strategies for Patients in Pediatric Intensive Care Units) randomized trial, receipt of a single, leukoreduced RBC unit stored for more than 35 days was associated with a significant increase in hospital-acquired infections compared to patients transfused with RBCs stored for 11–20 days [117].

Hypothermia (core body temperature <35–36 °C) develops rapidly when large volumes of cold-stored blood products are administered. Neonates undergoing surgery are at particular risk of transfusion-related hypothermia secondary to heat loss through a large body surface area, immature thermoregulatory capabilities, cold operating room ambient temperatures (<27 °C), anesthesia-induced thermoregulatory inhibition, and inconsistent body temperature monitoring. The collateral effects of hypothermia include reduced metabolism of citrate preservative, a leftward shift of the oxyhemoglobin-dissociation curve (theoretically hampering tissue O_2

delivery), platelet dysfunction, and reduced procoagulant activity [115, 118, 119]. Disseminated intravascular coagulopathy (DIC) develops more rapidly in cold, traumatically injured children compared to adults [13]. Other untoward effects of hypothermia include arrhythmias, decreased drug metabolism, apnea, hypoglycemia, and death. Administering rapidly transfused fluids through a warming device has become a quality standard in pediatric anesthesia.

While severe injury and hemorrhage carry inherent coagulation dysregulation, transfusion-induced coagulopathy is iatrogenic and can be attributed to delivery of blood products in an unbalanced fashion [1]. This has been the driving force behind the quest to define the optimal component blood product transfusion ratio in hemorrhaging patients. As discussed previously, judicious use of blood products in a 1:1 ratio (RBC/plasma) and possibly 1:1:1 ratio (RBC/plasma/platelet) is recommended to minimize coagulopathy.

Volume overload can result in transfusion-associated circulatory overload (TACO). It presents with clinical features similar to TRALI, but in TACO, pulmonary infiltrates develop due to increased hydrostatic pressure or "cardiogenic" pulmonary edema secondary to volume overload. Symptoms must occur within 12 h of transfusion per CDC guidelines [120]. Diagnosis in children is challenging and is likely evidenced by tachypnea and grunting or nasal flaring, before pulse oximetry changes are seen [121]. Bedside clinical acumen to detect circulatory overload in children is necessary, particularly when transfusing infants. Echocardiography and a trial of diuretic therapy may be helpful in the differentiation of TACO from TRALI. A gold standard pediatric textbook lists TACO as a risk of transfusion under "respiratory symptoms" [122, 123].

Pediatric patients are susceptible to the development of ionized hypocalcemia during rapid blood transfusions, particularly premature infants who have reduced ability to metabolize citrate. Hypocalcemia during resuscitation in traumatized pediatric patients has been defined as an ionized calcium (iCa^{2+}) level <1.0–1.1 mmol/L [124]. Blood products are stored using citrate, which is intended to bind calcium and prevent coagulation. Because anticoagulant is present in the effluent of blood products, whole blood and plasma contain more citrate per volume, followed by component RBCs and platelets. Signs of ionized hypocalcemia during transfusion include bradycardia, prolonged QT-intervals, and refractory hypotension. The importance of routine calcium measurement and administration during massive transfusion is becoming increasingly recognized.

Immunologic reactions can also result during massive transfusion, but febrile nonhemolytic hemolytic reactions (FNHTRs) and allergic urticaria are the most common transfusion-related complications in children. Although MTPs contain "universal" donor products, Rh-antigen, blood type B antibody, or non-type-specific platelets may be administered per institutional protocol. These incompatibilities uncommonly result in acute hemolysis and are more likely, albeit rarely, to produce delayed hemolysis [120, 123, 125].

Transfusion-related immunomodulation (TRIM) occurs secondary to the suppression of transfusion recipient's cell-mediated immunity. While the exact mechanism is unclear, it is hypothesized that donor WBCs present in transfused blood are involved, leading to immunosuppression and increased inflammation in the recipient. Most blood banks in resource-rich countries practice universal leukoreduction (LR) post-donation, which has been shown to reduce the likelihood of TRIM [126]. Transfusion-associated-graft-versus-host-disease (TA-GVHD) has also been described when family members donate to their children; HLA-antigen similarity between the donor and recipient leads to donor leukocytes engrafting in the recipient, with typically fatal outcomes.

Transfusion-related acute lung injury (TRALI) rarely occurs in the setting of MT. TRALI mimics adult respiratory distress syndrome (ARDS) and should be diagnosed within 6 h of transfusion [120]. The pulmonary infiltrates associated with TRALI are caused by increased vascular permeability in the absence of clinical signs of volume overload. Plasma, RBCs, and apheresis platelets have all been implicated [127].

15.3 Summary of Key Learning Objectives

15.3.1 What Is the Definition of a Pediatric Massive Transfusion (MT)?

A MT definition of 40 mL/kg body weight of blood administration within a 24-h period in children has been incorporated into multiple civilian MTPs across the USA.

15.3.2 What Is a Massive Transfusion Protocol (MTP)?

An MTP is a standardized, fixed-ratio package of RBCs, plasma, and platelets (and sometimes cryoprecipitate) along with adjuncts such as tranexamic acid (TXA). The primary objective of an MTP is to replicate the blood component ratios in whole blood, to provide hemostatic resuscitation as part of damage control resuscitation (DCR), and to avoid coagulopathy development in bleeding patients.

15.3.3 What Are the Components of an MTP?

Review publications suggest a component ratio extrapolated from the adult literature, supporting a balanced plasma/RBC ≥1:2 with an ideal ratio of 1:1. The Transfusion and Anemia Expertise Initiative—Control/Avoidance of Bleeding (TAXI-CAB) recommends a 1:1:1 (RBC/plasma/platelet) or 2:1:1 ratio until bleeding is no longer life threatening. The Traumatic Hemorrhagic Shock Consensus recommends a plasma/RBC and a platelet/RBC ratio of 1:1. There is insufficient evidence to definitively establish an ideal MTP in bleeding children.

15.3.4 How Does One Dose the Components of an MTP?

Unlike MTP dosing in the adult patient population, pediatric MTPs apply weight-based product dosing for smaller patients (e.g., less than approximately 50 kg). Examples of "balanced" weight-based (mL/kg body weight) dosing recommendations for RBC/plasma/platelet ratios include 20:10:5 mL/kg, 20:20:10 mL/kg, and 30:20:0 mL/kg.

15.3.5 When Is an MTP Activated?

A classic MTP trigger is an actual or potential volume of blood loss, such as 1/2 of total blood volume in 1 h. A decision to trigger an MTP requires clinical judgment that is best guided through standardized decision aides and the patient's overall clinical profile, and not isolated physiologic or hematologic variables. Examples of MTP activation criteria for bleeding pediatric patients include:

- 20–40 mL/kg transfusion requirement within 2 h
- SIPA (Shock Index Pediatric Adjusted) >1.4 plus systolic BP <100
- Trauma protocol activation
- Penetrating injury
- Intracranial bleed in a child <2 years going to the operating room
- Bleeding in an anticoagulated patient
- Persistent hemodynamic instability
- An immediate need to acquire blood products
- Acidosis
- Coagulopathy

15.3.6 How Does One Monitor Coagulation Status During an Ongoing MTP?

During ongoing and rapid bleeding, no coagulation test can produce timely feedback in sync with blood loss. Either version of viscoelastic testing (VET)—thromboelastography (TEG) or rotational thromboelastography (ROTEM)—may be used in children to follow traumatically induced bleeding. VET has been shown to correlate with conventional laboratory tests of coagulation in children and can be performed at the bedside with more rapid results.

Thus, it is recommended that the empirically based MTP should be followed until hemostasis can be evaluated in a timely manner; opponents of this approach recommend ongoing viscoelastic testing (VET) during active bleeding to avoid unnecessary blood administration and wastage.

15.3.7 How Does One Deactivate or Stop an MTP?

MTP deactivation is an active communication process that should be performed to preserve the blood supply and prevent over-transfusion. The hospital Transfusion Service must be asked to stop automatic delivery of MTP "packs" or "rounds."

15.3.8 What Are Potential MTP Adjuncts for the Treatment of Massive Bleeding?

Fibrinogen level monitoring and replacement during massive bleeding are critical and can be replaced with either cryoprecipitate or fibrinogen concentrate. Fibrinogen administration should be performed in conjunction with overall coagulation monitoring (e.g., conventional coagulation parameters, VET, and platelet number and function). An increasing number of pediatric studies demonstrate relative efficacy and safety of fibrinolytics (e.g., tranexamic acid, TXA) when administered in both the perioperative and trauma settings. Prothrombin complex concentrates (PCC), factor VII (rFVII), and permissive hypotension are *not* recommended as routine MTP adjuncts for bleeding children.

15.3.9 What Is the Role of Patient Blood Management (PBM) in Massive Bleeding and MTPs?

An MTP optimizes patient outcomes by standardizing blood resuscitation practices. This includes preservation of the patient's hemoglobin level, prevention of coagulopathy, and nonarbitrary pediatric transfusion practices.

15.3.10 What Are Some Complications Associated with MTP Administration?

- Hyperkalemia
- Hypocalcemia
- Hypothermia
- Coagulopathy
- Transfusion-associated circulatory overload (TACO)

Key Points

- Massive transfusion protocol (MTP) implementation has been shown to reduce treatment variability, patient mortality, length of hospital stays, and blood utilization.
- The primary objective of an MTP is to avoid coagulopathy development in bleeding patients through the administration of blood products in a standardized, empirically driven manner.

- Current best evidence for intraoperative massive transfusion supports application of trauma-derived, balanced ratios of 1:1 for RBC/plasma (with less clear guidance for platelet ratios).
- Unlike MTP dosing in the adult patient population, pediatric MTPs apply weight-based product dosing for smaller patients. This is crucial because small patients are easily over-transfused.
- Once vital signs and clinical bleeding have stabilized, transition from an MTP to goal-directed management with coagulation testing is necessary to avoid blood product overuse or wastage.
- When a massively bleeding patient is hemodynamically stable and bleeding is controlled, the MTP should be deactivated. This is an active communication process.
- An increasing number of pediatric studies demonstrate relative efficacy and safety of fibrinolytics when administered in the perioperative setting, and they are now a standard element of the MTP.

References

1. Evangelista ME, Gaffley M, Neff LP. Massive transfusion protocols for pediatric patients: current perspectives. J Blood Med. 2020;11:163–72.
2. Horst J, Leonard JC, Vogel A, Jacobs R, Spinella PC. A survey of US and Canadian hospitals' paediatric massive transfusion protocol policies. Transfus Med. 2016;26(1):49–56.
3. Dente CJ, Shaz BH, Nicholas JM, Harris RS, Wyrzykowski AD, Patel S, et al. Improvements in early mortality and coagulopathy are sustained better in patients with blunt trauma after institution of a massive transfusion protocol in a civilian level I trauma center. J Trauma. 2009;66(6):1616–24.
4. Cannon JW, Neff LP, Pidcoke HF, Aden JK, Spinella PC, Johnson MA, et al. The evolution of pediatric transfusion practice during combat operations 2001-2013. J Trauma Acute Care Surg. 2018;84(6S):S69–76.
5. Demetriades D, Murray J, Charalambides K, Alo K, Velmahos G, Rhee P, Chan L. Trauma fatalities: time and location of hospital deaths. J Am Coll Surg. 2004;198(1):20–6.
6. Camazine MN, Hemmila MR, Leonard JC, Jacobs RA, Horst JA, Kozar RA, et al. Massive transfusion policies at trauma centers participating in the American College of Surgeons Trauma Quality Improvement Program. J Trauma Acute Care Surg. 2015;78(6):48–53.
7. Ciaraglia A, Lumbard D, Deschner B, Barry L, Braverman M, Eastridge B, et al. The effects of hypocalcemia in severely injured pediatric trauma patients. J Trauma Acute Care Surg. 2023;95(3):313–8.
8. Clebone A. Pediatric trauma transfusion and cognitive aids. Curr Opin Anaesthesiol. 2018;31(2):201–6.
9. Chidester SJ, Williams N, Wang W, Groner JI. A pediatric massive transfusion protocol. J Trauma Acute Care Surg. 2012;73(5):1273–7.
10. Gilley M, Beno S. Damage control resuscitation in pediatric trauma. Curr Opin Pediatr. 2018;30(3):338–43.
11. Society for Pediatric Anesthesia. Pedi crisis critical events checklist. 2023. https://pedsanesthesia.org/wp-content/uploads/2023/04/SPAPediCrisisChecklistsMarch2023.pdf. Accessed 1 December 2023.
12. Neff LP, Cannon JW, Morrison JJ, Edwards MJ, Spinella PC, Borgman MA. Clearly defining pediatric massive transfusion: cutting through the fog and friction with combat data. J Trauma Acute Care Surg. 2015;78(1):22–8; discussion 8–9.

13. Leonard JC, Josephson CD, Luther JF, Wisniewski SR, Allen C, Chiusolo F, et al. Life-threatening bleeding in children: a prospective observational study. Crit Care Med. 2021;49(11):1943–54.
14. McCoy CC, Brenner M, Duchesne J, Roberts D, Ferrada P, Horer T, et al. Back to the future: whole blood resuscitation of the severely injured trauma patient. Shock. 2021;56(1S):9–15.
15. Shea SM, Staudt AM, Thomas KA, Schuerer D, Mielke JE, Folkerts D, et al. The use of low-titer group O whole blood is independently associated with improved survival compared to component therapy in adults with severe traumatic hemorrhage. Transfusion. 2020;60(3):2–9.
16. Leeper CM, Yazer MH, Cladis FP, Saladino R, Triulzi DJ, Gaines BA. Use of uncross-matched cold-stored whole blood in injured children with hemorrhagic shock. JAMA Pediatr. 2018;172(5):491–2.
17. Meyer DE, Vincent LE, Fox EE, O'Keeffe T, Inaba K, Bulger E, et al. Every minute counts: time to delivery of initial massive transfusion cooler and its impact on mortality. J Trauma Acute Care Surg. 2017;83(1):19–24.
18. Petrosoniak A, Pavenski K, da Luz LT, Callum J. Massive hemorrhage protocol: a practical approach to the bleeding trauma patient. Emerg Med Clin North Am. 2023;41(1):51–69.
19. Yazer MH, Dunbar NM, Delaney M, Collaborative BEfST. Survey of the RhD selection and issuing practices for uncrossmatched blood products at pediatric trauma hospitals in the United States: The BEST collaborative study. Transfusion. 2021;61(12):3328–34.
20. Yazer MH, Waters JH, Spinella PC. Use of uncrossmatched erythrocytes in emergency bleeding situations. Anesthesiology. 2018;128(3):650–6.
21. Kolodziej JH, Leonard JC, Josephson CD, Gaines BA, Wisniewski SR, Yazer MH, Spinella PC. Survey to inform trial of low-titer group O whole-blood compared to conventional blood components for children with severe traumatic bleeding. Transfusion. 2021;61(Suppl 1):S43–S8.
22. Holcomb JB, Fox EE, Wade CE, Group PS. The PRospective observational multicenter major trauma transfusion (PROMMTT) study. J Trauma Acute Care Surg. 2013;75(1 Suppl):S1–2.
23. Maw G, Furyk C. Pediatric massive transfusion: a systematic review. Pediatr Emerg Care. 2018;34(8):594–8.
24. Holcomb JB, Tilley BC, Baraniuk S, Fox EE, Wade CE, Podbielski JM, et al. Transfusion of plasma, platelets, and red blood cells in a 1:1:1 vs a 1:1:2 ratio and mortality in patients with severe trauma: the PROPPR randomized clinical trial. JAMA. 2015;313(5):471–82.
25. Russell RT, Esparaz JR, Beckwith MA, Abraham PJ, Bembea MM, Borgman MA, et al. Pediatric traumatic hemorrhagic shock consensus conference recommendations. J Trauma Acute Care Surg. 2023;94(1S):S2–S10.
26. Butler EK, Mills BM, Arbabi S, Bulger EM, Vavilala MS, Groner JI, et al. Association of blood component ratios with 24-h mortality in injured children receiving massive transfusion. Crit Care Med. 2019;47(7):975–83.
27. Cunningham ME, Rosenfeld EH, Zhu H, Naik-Mathuria BJ, Russell RT, Vogel AM. A high ratio of plasma: RBC improves survival in massively transfused injured children. J Surg Res. 2019;233:213–20.
28. Noland DK, Apelt N, Greenwell C, Tweed J, Notrica DM, Garcia NM, et al. Massive transfusion in pediatric trauma: an ATOMAC perspective. J Pediatr Surg. 2019;54(2):345–9.
29. Spinella PC, Leonard JC, Marshall C, Luther JF, Wisniewski SR, Josephson CD, et al. Transfusion ratios and deficits in injured children with life-threatening bleeding. Pediatr Crit Care Med. 2022;23(4):235–44.
30. Valentine SL, Cholette JM, Goobie SM. Transfusion strategies for hemostatic blood products in critically ill children: a narrative review and update on expert consensus guidelines. Anesth Analg. 2022;135(3):545–57.
31. Hwu RS, Spinella PC, Keller MS, Baker D, Wallendorf M, Leonard JC. The effect of massive transfusion protocol implementation on pediatric trauma care. Transfusion. 2016;56(11):2712–9.

32. Nosanov L, Inaba K, Okoye O, Resnick S, Upperman J, Shulman I, et al. The impact of blood product ratios in massively transfused pediatric trauma patients. Am J Surg. 2013;206(5):655–60.
33. Edwards MJ, Lustik MB, Clark ME, Creamer KM, Tuggle D. The effects of balanced blood component resuscitation and crystalloid administration in pediatric trauma patients requiring transfusion in Afghanistan and Iraq 2002 to 2012. J Trauma Acute Care Surg. 2015;78(2):330–5.
34. Vaizer R, Leeper CM, Lu L, Josephson CD, Leonard JC, Brown JB, Spinella PC. Increased platelet to red blood cell transfusion ratio associated with acute kidney injury in children with life-threatening bleeding. Transfusion. 2024;64(Suppl 2):S62–71.
35. Kinslow K, McKenney M, Boneva D, Elkbuli A. Massive transfusion protocols in paediatric trauma population: a systematic review. Transfus Med. 2020;30(5):333–42.
36. Nellis ME, Karam O, Valentine SL, Bateman ST, Remy KE, Lacroix J, et al. Executive summary of recommendations and expert consensus for plasma and platelet transfusion practice in critically ill children: from the transfusion and anemia EXpertise initiative-control/avoidance of bleeding (TAXI-CAB). Pediatr Crit Care Med. 2022;23(1):34–51.
37. Pagano MB, Allen ES, Chou ST, Dunbar NM, Gniadek T, Goel R, et al. Current advances in transfusion medicine: a 2019 review of selected topics from the AABB Clinical Transfusion Medicine Committee. Transfusion. 2020;60(7):1614–23.
38. Pitt launches trial tackling the leading cause of death in kids. UPMC. 2024. https://www.upmc.com/media/news/092123-ped-trauma-blood. Accessed 5 April 2024.
39. Arsenault V, Lieberman L, Akbari P, Murto K, Canadian Obstetrical Pediatric Transfusion N. Canadian tertiary care pediatric massive hemorrhage protocols: a survey and comprehensive national review. Can J Anaesth. 2023;71(4):453–64.
40. Chin V, Cope S, Yeh CH, Thompson T, Nascimento B, Pavenski K, et al. Massive hemorrhage protocol survey: marked variability and absent in one-third of hospitals in Ontario, Canada. Injury. 2019;50(1):46–53.
41. Kamyszek RW, Leraas HJ, Reed C, Ray CM, Nag UP, Poisson JL, Tracy ET. Massive transfusion in the pediatric population: a systematic review and summary of best-evidence practice strategies. J Trauma Acute Care Surg. 2019;86(4):744–54.
42. Markham C, Small S, Hovmand P, Doctor A. Transfusion decision making in pediatric critical illness. Pediatr Clin N Am. 2017;64(5):991–1015.
43. Dumbill R, Rabcuka J, Fallon J, Knight S, Hunter J, Voyce D, et al. Impaired O_2 unloading from stored blood results in diffusion-limited O_2 release at tissues: evidence from human kidneys. Blood. 2023;143(8):721–33.
44. Grossman BJ, Hillyer C, Westhoff C. Technical manual. Bethesda: American Association of Blood Banks (AABB); 2014. p. 545.
45. Khizroeva J, Makatsariya A, Vorobev A, Bitsadze V, Elalamy I, Lazarchuk A, et al. The hemostatic system in newborns and the risk of neonatal thrombosis. Int J Mol Sci. 2023;24(18):13864.
46. Toulon P, Berruyer M, Brionne-Francois M, Grand F, Lasne D, Telion C, et al. Age dependency for coagulation parameters in paediatric populations. Results of a multicentre study aimed at defining the age-specific reference ranges. Thromb Haemost. 2016;116(1):9–16.
47. Christiaans SC, Duhachek-Stapelman AL, Russell RT, Lisco SJ, Kerby JD, Pittet JF. Coagulopathy after severe pediatric trauma. Shock. 2014;41(6):476–90.
48. SHOT Bite No. 4: lessons in paediatrics (including neonates). Serious Hazards of Transfusion (SHOT). 2018. https://www.shotuk.org/resources/current-resources/shot-bites/. Accessed 4 December 2022.
49. Serious Hazards of Transfusion and Medicines and Healthcare Products Regulatory Agency, SHOT Bite No. 4: lessons in Pediatrics. 2018. https://www.shotuk.org/wp-content/uploads/myimages/SHOT-Bite-No-4-Lessons-in-Paediatrics-July-2018.pdf. Accessed 29 July 2023.
50. Nystrup KB, Stensballe J, Bottger M, Johansson PI, Ostrowski SR. Transfusion therapy in paediatric trauma patients: a review of the literature. Scand J Trauma Resusc Emerg Med. 2015;23:21.

51. Dehmer JJ, Adamson WT. Massive transfusion and blood product use in the pediatric trauma patient. Semin Pediatr Surg. 2010;19(4):286–91.
52. Trappey AF, Thompson KM, Kuppermann N, Stephenson JT, Nuno MA, Hewes HA, et al. Development of transfusion guidelines for injured children using a Modified Delphi Consensus Process. J Trauma Acute Care Surg. 2019;87(4):935–43.
53. Talving P, Lustenberger T, Lam L, Inaba K, Mohseni S, Plurad D, et al. Coagulopathy after isolated severe traumatic brain injury in children. J Trauma. 2011;71(5):1205–10.
54. Jhang WK, Park SJ. Evaluation of sepsis-induced coagulopathy in critically ill pediatric patients with septic shock. Thromb Haemost. 2021;121(4):457–63.
55. Hendrickson JE, Shaz BH, Pereira G, Parker PM, Jessup P, Atwell F, et al. Implementation of a pediatric trauma massive transfusion protocol: one institution's experience. Transfusion. 2012;52(6):1228–36.
56. Savage SA, Zarzaur BL, Croce MA, Fabian TC. Redefining massive transfusion when every second counts. J Trauma Acute Care Surg. 2013;74(2):396–400; discussion 2.
57. American College of Surgeons ACS TQIP Massive Transfusion in Trauma Guidelines. 2014. https://www.facs.org/media/zcjdtrd1/transfusion_guildelines.pdf. Accessed 28 November 2023.
58. Phillips R, Shahi N, Acker SN, Meier M, Shirek G, Stevens J, et al. Not as simple as ABC: tools to trigger massive transfusion in pediatric trauma. J Trauma Acute Care Surg. 2022;92(2):422–7.
59. Borgman MA, Maegele M, Wade CE, Blackbourne LH, Spinella PC. Pediatric trauma BIG score: predicting mortality in children after military and civilian trauma. Pediatrics. 2011;127(4):892–7.
60. Venkatesh V, Curley A, Khan R, Clarke P, Watts T, Josephson C, et al. A novel approach to standardised recording of bleeding in a high risk neonatal population. Arch Dis Child Fetal Neonatal Ed. 2013;98(3):260–3.
61. Nellis ME, Tucci M, Lacroix J, Spinella PC, Haque KD, Stock A, et al. Bleeding assessment scale in critically ill children (BASIC): physician-driven diagnostic criteria for bleeding severity. Crit Care Med. 2019;47(12):1766–72.
62. Doctor A, Cholette JM, Remy KE, Argent A, Carson JL, Valentine SL, et al. Recommendations on RBC transfusion in general critically ill children based on hemoglobin and/or physiologic thresholds from the pediatric critical care transfusion and anemia expertise initiative. Pediatr Crit Care Med. 2018;19(Suppl 1):S98–S113.
63. Lacroix J, Tucci M, Du Pont-Thibodeau G. Red blood cell transfusion decision making in critically ill children. Curr Opin Pediatr. 2015;27(3):286–91.
64. Valentine SL, Bembea MM, Muszynski JA, Cholette JM, Doctor A, Spinella PC, et al. Consensus recommendations for RBC transfusion practice in critically ill children from the pediatric critical care transfusion and anemia expertise initiative. Pediatr Crit Care Med. 2018;19(9):884–98.
65. Faraoni D, Meier J, New HV, Van der Linden PJ, Hunt BJ. Patient blood management for neonates and children undergoing cardiac surgery: 2019 NATA guidelines. J Cardiothorac Vasc Anesth. 2019;33(12):3249–63.
66. Long JB, Engorn BM, Hill KD, Feng L, Chiswell K, Jacobs ML, et al. Postoperative hematocrit and adverse outcomes in pediatric cardiac surgery patients: a cross-sectional study from the Society of Thoracic Surgeons and Congenital Cardiac Anesthesia Society Database Collaboration. Anesth Analg. 2021;133(5):1077–88.
67. Hess AS, Ramamoorthy J, Hess JR. Perioperative platelet transfusions. Anesthesiology. 2021;134(3):471–9.
68. Alsheikh B, Chegondi M, Totapally B. Platelet transfusion thresholds among children admitted to a pediatric intensive care unit. Cureus. 2017;9(10):e1797.
69. Huisman EJ, Crighton GL. Pediatric fibrinogen PART I-pitfalls in fibrinogen evaluation and use of fibrinogen replacement products in children. Front Pediatr. 2021;9:617500.

70. Gautam NK, Cai C, Pawelek O, Rafique MB, Cattano D, Pivalizza EG. Performance of functional fibrinogen thromboelastography in children undergoing congenital heart surgery. Paediatr Anaesth. 2017;27(2):181–9.
71. Crighton GL, Huisman EJ. Pediatric fibrinogen PART II-overview of indications for fibrinogen use in critically ill children. Front Pediatr. 2021;9:647680.
72. Solomon C, Pichlmaier U, Schoechl H, Hagl C, Raymondos K, Scheinichen D, et al. Recovery of fibrinogen after administration of fibrinogen concentrate to patients with severe bleeding after cardiopulmonary bypass surgery. Br J Anaesth. 2010;104(5):555–62.
73. Galas FR, de Almeida JP, Fukushima JT, Vincent JL, Osawa EA, Zeferino S, et al. Hemostatic effects of fibrinogen concentrate compared with cryoprecipitate in children after cardiac surgery: a randomized pilot trial. J Thorac Cardiovasc Surg. 2014;148(4):1647–55.
74. Gosselin RC, Adcock D, Dorgalaleh A, Favaloro EJ, Lippi G, Pego JM, et al. International Council for Standardization in Haematology recommendations for hemostasis critical values, tests, and reporting. Semin Thromb Hemost. 2020;46(4):398–409.
75. Tama MA, Stone ME Jr, Blumberg SM, Reddy SH, Conway EE, Meltzer JA. Association of cryoprecipitate use with survival after major trauma in children receiving massive transfusion. JAMA Surg. 2021;156(5):453–60.
76. Cunningham AJ, Condron M, Schreiber MA, Azarow K, Hamilton NA, Downie K, et al. Rotational thromboelastometry predicts transfusion and disability in pediatric trauma. J Trauma Acute Care Surg. 2020;88(1):134–40.
77. Deng Q, Hao F, Wang Y, Guo C. Rotation thromboelastometry (ROTEM) enables improved outcomes in the pediatric trauma population. J Int Med Res. 2018;46(12):5195–204.
78. Baksaas-Aasen K, Gall LS, Stensballe J, Juffermans NP, Curry N, Maegele M, et al. Viscoelastic haemostatic assay augmented protocols for major trauma haemorrhage (ITACTIC): a randomized, controlled trial. Intensive Care Med. 2021;47(1):49–59.
79. Blaine KP, Dudaryk R. Pro-con debate: viscoelastic hemostatic assays should replace fixed ratio massive transfusion protocols in trauma. Anesth Analg. 2022;134(1):21–31.
80. Patel PA, Wyrobek JA, Butwick AJ, Pivalizza EG, Hare GMT, Mazer CD, Goobie SM. Update on applications and limitations of perioperative tranexamic acid. Anesth Analg. 2022;135(3):460–73.
81. Rossaint R, Afshari A, Bouillon B, Cerny V, Cimpoesu D, Curry N, et al. The European guideline on management of major bleeding and coagulopathy following trauma: sixth edition. Crit Care. 2023;27(1):80.
82. Spahn DR, Bouillon B, Cerny V, Coats TJ, Duranteau J, Fernandez-Mondejar E, et al. Management of bleeding and coagulopathy following major trauma: an updated European guideline. Crit Care. 2013;17(2):R76.
83. American Society of Anesthesiologists Task Force on Perioperative Blood M. Practice guidelines for perioperative blood management: an updated report by the American Society of Anesthesiologists Task Force on Perioperative Blood Management. Anesthesiology. 2015;122(2):241–75.
84. Galvagno SM, Nahmias JT, Young DA. Advanced trauma life support. Anesthesiol Clin. 2019;37(1):13–32.
85. Kozek-Langenecker SA, Afshari A, Albaladejo P, Santullano CA, De Robertis E, Filipescu DC, et al. Management of severe perioperative bleeding: guidelines from the European Society of Anaesthesiology. Eur J Anaesthesiol. 2013;30(6):270–382.
86. Kietaibl S, Ahmed A, Afshari A, Albaladejo P, Aldecoa C, Barauskas G, et al. Management of severe peri-operative bleeding: guidelines from the European Society of Anaesthesiology and Intensive Care: second update 2022. Eur J Anaesthesiol. 2023;40(4):226–304.
87. Chan KL, Summerhayes RG, Ignjatovic V, Horton SB, Monagle PT. Reference values for kaolin-activated thromboelastography in healthy children. Anesth Analg. 2007;105(6):1610–3.
88. Regan I, Cox D, McMahon C. PB2641 thromboelastography (TEG) reference ranges in a healthy paediatric cohort show accelerated coagulation and clot formation time. HemaSphere. 2023;7:e9020579.

89. Oswald E, Stalzer B, Heitz E, Weiss M, Schmugge M, Strasak A, et al. Thromboelastometry (ROTEM) in children: age-related reference ranges and correlations with standard coagulation tests. Br J Anaesth. 2010;105(6):827–35.
90. Goodhue Meyer EK, Uffman J, Townsend S, Rice-Weimer J, Tobias J, Nicol K. Establishing pediatric reference ranges for rotational thromboelastometry. Am J Clin Pathol. 2023;160(1):72–7.
91. Haas T, Faraoni D. Viscoelastic testing in pediatric patients. Transfusion. 2020;60(Suppl 6):S75–85.
92. Hemostasis Management. Haemonetics corporation. Hospital. 2023. https://hospital.haemonetics.com/hemostasis-management/teg-6s. Accessed 10 December 2023.
93. Faraoni D, DiNardo JA. Viscoelastic hemostatic assays: update on technology and clinical applications. Am J Hematol. 2021;96(10):1331–7.
94. Tumber S, Stondell C, Wilson M, Yang NT, Tafoya S. Reference values in healthy children using the Quantra Hemostasis Analyzer, a novel point of care viscoelastic testing device. Paediatr Anaesth. 2022;32(12):1370–1.
95. Murphy M, Ben AD. Recommendations on the use of group O red blood cells. Bethesda: AABB; 2019. https://www.aabb.org/docs/default-source/default-document-library/resources/association-bulletins/ab19-02.pdf. Accessed 21 July 2023.
96. Ferrari FA, Garzon S, Raffaelli R, Cromi A, Casarin J, Ghezzi F, et al. Tranexamic acid for the prevention and the treatment of primary postpartum haemorrhage: a systematic review. J Obstet Gynaecol. 2022;42(5):734–46.
97. Godbey EA, Schwartz J. Massive transfusion protocols and the use of tranexamic acid. Curr Opin Hematol. 2018;25(6):482–5.
98. Eckert MJ, Wertin TM, Tyner SD, Nelson DW, Izenberg S, Martin MJ. Tranexamic acid administration to pediatric trauma patients in a combat setting: the pediatric trauma and tranexamic acid study (PED-TRAX). J Trauma Acute Care Surg. 2014;77(6):852–8.
99. Spinella PC, Leonard JC, Gaines BA, Luther JF, Wisniewski SR, Josephson CD, et al. Use of antifibrinolytics in pediatric life-threatening hemorrhage: a prospective observational multicenter study. Crit Care Med. 2022;50(4):e382–e92.
100. Goobie SM, Zurakowski D, Glotzbecker MP, McCann ME, Hedequist D, Brustowicz RM, et al. Tranexamic acid is efficacious at decreasing the rate of blood loss in adolescent scoliosis surgery: a randomized placebo-controlled trial. J Bone Joint Surg Am. 2018;100(23):2024–32.
101. Goobie SM, Staffa SJ, Meara JG, Proctor MR, Tumolo M, Cangemi G, Disma N. High-dose versus low-dose tranexamic acid for paediatric craniosynostosis surgery: a double-blind randomised controlled non-inferiority trial. Br J Anaesth. 2020;125(3):336–45.
102. Wei Y, Zhang Y, Jin T, Wang H, Li J, Zhang D. Effects of tranexamic acid on bleeding in pediatric surgeries: a systematic review and meta-analysis. Front Surg. 2021;8:759937.
103. Beno S, Ackery AD, Callum J, Rizoli S. Tranexamic acid in pediatric trauma: why not? Crit Care. 2014;18(4):313.
104. Hanson SJ, Karam O, Birch R, Goel R, Patel RM, Sola-Visner M, et al. Transfusion practices in pediatric cardiac surgery requiring cardiopulmonary bypass: a secondary analysis of a clinical database. Pediatr Crit Care Med. 2021;22(11):978–87.
105. Zeeshan M, Hamidi M, Feinstein AJ, Gries L, Jehan F, Sakran J, et al. Four-factor prothrombin complex concentrate is associated with improved survival in trauma-related hemorrhage: a nationwide propensity-matched analysis. J Trauma Acute Care Surg. 2019;87(2):274–81.
106. Bouzat P, Charbit J, Abback PS, Huet-Garrigue D, Delhaye N, Leone M, et al. Efficacy and safety of early administration of 4-factor prothrombin complex concentrate in patients with trauma at risk of massive transfusion: the PROCOAG randomized clinical trial. JAMA. 2023;329(16):1367–75.
107. Karube T, Andersen C, Tobias JD. Single-center use of prothrombin complex concentrate in pediatric patients. J Pediatr Intensive Care. 2020;9(2):106–12.
108. Stinger HK, Spinella PC, Perkins JG, Grathwohl KW, Salinas J, Martini WZ, et al. The ratio of fibrinogen to red cells transfused affects survival in casualties receiving massive transfusions at an army combat support hospital. J Trauma. 2008;64(2):79–85.

109. Parks J, Vasileiou G, Parreco J, Pust GD, Rattan R, Zakrison T, et al. Validating the ATLS shock classification for predicting death, transfusion, or urgent intervention. J Surg Res. 2020;245:163–7.
110. Shander A, Hardy JF, Ozawa S, Farmer SL, Hofmann A, Frank SM, et al. A global definition of patient blood management. Anesth Analg. 2022;135(3):476–88.
111. Frank SM, Waters JH, editors. Patient blood management: multidisciplinary approaches to optimizing care. Bethesda: AABB Press; 2016. p. 6.
112. Lee AC, Reduque LL, Luban NL, Ness PM, Anton B, Heitmiller ES. Transfusion-associated hyperkalemic cardiac arrest in pediatric patients receiving massive transfusion. Transfusion. 2014;54(1):244–54.
113. Ramamoorthy C, Haberkern CM, Bhananker SM, Domino KB, Posner KL, Campos JS, Morray JP. Anesthesia-related cardiac arrest in children with heart disease: data from the Pediatric Perioperative Cardiac Arrest (POCA) registry. Anesth Analg. 2010;110(5):1376–82.
114. Bhananker SM, Ramamoorthy C, Geiduschek JM, Posner KL, Domino KB, Haberkern CM, et al. Anesthesia-related cardiac arrest in children: update from the Pediatric Perioperative Cardiac Arrest Registry. Anesth Analg. 2007;105(2):344–50.
115. Barcelona SL, Thompson AA, Coté CJ. Intraoperative pediatric blood transfusion therapy: a review of common issues. Part I: hematologic and physiologic differences from adults; metabolic and infectious risks. Paediatr Anaesth. 2005;15(9):716–26.
116. Spinella PC, Tucci M, Fergusson DA, Lacroix J, Hébert PC, Leteurtre S, et al. Effect of fresh vs standard-issue red blood cell transfusions on multiple organ dysfunction syndrome in critically ill pediatric patients: a randomized clinical trial. JAMA. 2019;322(22):2179–90.
117. Flatman LK, Fergusson DA, Lacroix J, Ducruet T, Papenburg J, Fontela PS. Association between the length of storage of transfused leukoreduced red blood cell units and hospital-acquired infections in critically ill children: a secondary analysis of the TRIPICU study. Transfus Med. 2021;31(6):467–73.
118. Kopko PM. Transfusion reactions. 5th ed. Bethesda: AABB Press; 2021. p. 41.
119. Ireland S, Endacott R, Cameron P, Fitzgerald M, Paul E. The incidence and significance of accidental hypothermia in major trauma–a prospective observational study. Resuscitation. 2011;82(3):300–6.
120. Centers for Disease Control and Prevention. National healthcare safety network biovigilance component hemovigilance module surveillance protocol v2.8. 2023. https://www.cdc.gov/nhsn/pdfs/biovigilance/bv-hv-protocol-current.pdf. Accessed 26 June 2023.
121. De Cloedt L, Emeriaud G, Lefebvre É, Kleiber N, Robitaille N, Jarlot C, et al. Transfusion-associated circulatory overload in a pediatric intensive care unit: different incidences with different diagnostic criteria. Transfusion. 2018;58(4):1037–44.
122. Josephson CD, Strauss RG. Chapter 497: red blood cell transfusions and erythropoietin therapy. In: Kliegman RM, Geme JS, editors. Nelson textbook of pediatrics E-book. 21st ed. Elsevier: Amsterdam; 2019. p. 2581–7.
123. Serious Hazards of Transfusion (SHOT). 2020. https://www.shotuk.org/shot-reports/. Accessed 25 May 2023.
124. Epstein D, Ben Lulu H, Raz A, Bahouth H. Admission hypocalcemia in pediatric major trauma patients-An uncommon phenomenon associated with an increased need for urgent blood transfusion. Transfusion. 2022;62(7):1341–6.
125. Roseff SD, Wong EC, editors. Pediatric transfusion: a handbook. Bethesda: AABB; 2020. p. 161–91.
126. Oldebecken S, Jankowska AE. Chapter 15: blood conservation in cardiac surgery. In: Awad AS, editor. Cardiac anesthesia: the basics of evaluation and management. Cham: Springer; 2021.
127. US Food and Drug Administration. Transfusion/donation fatalities. 2021. https://www.fda.gov/media/172382/download?attachment. Accessed 11 December 2023.

Noninvasive Assessment of Blood Loss 16

Abigail Smith, Niroop Ravula, and Norma J. Klein

16.1 Case Scenario

A 4-year-old boy with Hirschsprung's disease is scheduled for a pull-through procedure. He was scheduled for surgery 3 days ago. He has a growth delay, with a body weight of 12 kg (i.e., 5% for age). There is no patient or family history of excessive bleeding or coagulopathy. His hemoglobin (Hgb) level is 13 g/dL and hematocrit (Hct) is 39%; coagulation parameters have not been assessed. During the procedure, you find yourself turning down the anesthetic due to frequent low blood pressure readings. You assess blood loss to be 90 mL or 10% of his estimated blood volume (EBV; 70 mL/kg or 840 mL). Monitors include the ASA recommended standard, an indwelling bladder catheter, and an invasive radial arterial line. You have administered 40 mL/kg of crystalloid solution. However, the bleeding and the relative hypotension continue. The surgeon overhears you ordering red blood cells (RBCs) and states "Let me know when you decide to transfuse."

Key Learning Objectives

- What tools are available to quantify perioperative blood loss?
- What are some physical exam findings indicative of clinically significant blood loss?

A. Smith
Department of Anesthesiology and Pain Medicine, University of California, Davis, Sacramento, CA, USA

Anesthesiology and Intensive Care, Saint Joseph Mercy Hospital, Saint Joseph Mercy Hospital, Ann Arbor, Michigan, USA
e-mail: Asmit136@hfhs.org

N. Ravula · N. J. Klein (✉)
Department of Anesthesiology and Pain Medicine, University of California, Davis, Sacramento, CA, USA
e-mail: nrravula@ucdavis.edu; nklein@ucdavis.edu

N. J. Klein (ed.), *Perioperative Pediatric Patient Blood Management and Transfusion Safety*, https://doi.org/10.1007/978-3-031-81666-6_16

- Do conventional pediatric vital signs reliably indicate perioperative blood loss?
- How is circulatory function monitored using pulse wave form analysis?
- Do near infrared spectroscopy (NIRS) and Hgb co-oximetry (SpHb) reliably guide perioperative RBC transfusion decisions?

16.2 Discussion

16.2.1 General

Altering an anesthetic to maintain hemodynamic stability is a familiar conundrum for anesthesiologists. In children, blood loss-related anemia has unique physiologic implications. When considering Hgb transfusion thresholds in the perioperative period, it is important to understand that existing studies in children typically pertain to the pre- and postoperative, not the intraoperative, phases of care. The following discussion addresses noninvasive diagnostic tools available to anesthesiologists and other pediatric intensivists to manage RBC transfusions in children. The Hgb level still receives priority in driving RBC transfusion decisions in most patient groups, even under "restrictive" standards [1]. Because the decision to administer RBCs during surgery is complex and should not be a function of a single test, Hgb transfusion triggers based solely on laboratory values are mentioned but not discussed in detail [2–5]. The following discussion addresses noninvasive diagnostic tools available to anesthesiologists and other pediatric intensivists to manage perioperative RBC transfusions in children.

16.3 What Tools Are Available to Quantify Perioperative Blood Loss?

16.3.1 Blood Loss Assessment

16.3.1.1 Calculations

Blood loss should be regularly assessed during active bleeding. Recommendations to guide initiation of blood replacement often include an assessment of the percentage of estimated blood volume (EBV) lost. The adult-based Ottawa criteria recommends an estimated blood loss >1500 mL (i.e., ~30% of an average adult's EBV) as a threshold for RBC transfusion [2, 6]. The American College of Surgeons Advanced Trauma Life Support (ATLS) guideline advises blood product administration based on a percentage of EBV as reflected in decreased blood pressure (BP) and urine output (UO), along with an increase in heart rate (HR) and base deficit [7–9] (Table 16.1). According to ATLS guidelines, changes in BP, lactate, and base deficit are signs of "moderate" (31–40%) blood loss. However, children are unique compared to adults: up to 30% of blood loss can occur before changes in BP are evident due to reflexively increased sympathetic tone [10]. Because of the significant risks associated with underestimating intraoperative blood loss in small children, awaiting a 30% loss of EBV along with changes in BP, UO, HR, and base deficit before

Table 16.1 ATLS shock classifications of hypovolemia based on percentage of blood volume lost

Indices of blood loss	EBV loss <15%	15–30% EBV loss (mild)	31–40% EBV loss (moderate)	>40% EBV loss (severe)
HR	↔	↔/↑	↑	↑↑
BP	↔	↔	↔/↓	↓
PP	↔	↓	↓	↓
UO	↔	↔	↓	↓↓
BD (mEq/L)	0 to −2	−2 to −6	−6 to −10	≥−10

EBV estimated blood volume, *HR* heart rate, *BP* blood pressure, *PP* pulse pressure, *UO* urine output, *BD* base deficit

Adapted from Henry S. ATLS 10th edition offers new insights into managing trauma patients. 2018, found online at https://bulletin.facs.org/2018/06/atls-10th-edition-offers-new-insights-into-managing-trauma-patients/#printpreview

making a transfusion decision may be a delayed response [11]. Other experts suggest initiating a blood transfusion at a lower estimated blood loss (e.g., 15% of EBV) when there is ongoing bleeding or symptomatic anemia including evidence of end-organ hypoxia [12].

Estimating the maximum volume of blood loss that a patient can tolerate should be made prior to any blood loss surgery. There are several formulae available to calculate the maximum allowable blood loss (MABL) prior to surgery, including calculation of RBC mass, logarithmic equations, and modified (simple) formulae. A commonly used formula calculates the ratio of Hct change during surgery to the child's initial Hct [13]:

$$\text{MABL} = \text{EBV} \times \left(\text{Hct}_I - \text{Hct}_{\text{min}}\right) / \text{Hct}_I$$

where Hct_I is the starting Hct and Hct_{min} is the target Hct. Under this calculation, the MABL for a 4-year-old, 12 kg child with an EBV of 70 mL/kg (840 mL), a preoperative Hct of 39%, and a minimum allowable Hct of 25% is 300 mL. However, the minimum Hct tolerated depends on the rate of blood loss (rapid blood loss does not allow time for physiologic compensation) and any comorbidities that may impact tissue oxygenation (such as cyanotic heart disease). During the course of surgery, the Hct_I and the Hct_{min} have an algorithmic (versus linear) relationship secondary to hemodilution; hence the Hct of lost blood decreases as the surgery progresses [14]. The MABL formula has therefore been modified (i.e., entitled the Gross formula) to reflect the average of the Hct_I and Hct_{min} at any point in time:

$$\text{MABL} = \text{EBV} \times \left(\text{Hct}_\text{I} - \text{Hct}_{\text{min}}\right) / \left[\text{Hct}_\text{I} + \text{Hct}_{\text{min}}\right) / 2\right]$$

There are also many formulae to calculate blood loss after-the-fact [15]. These calculations are more complicated than the Gross formula that is based on the patient's Hct and a weight-based EBV. These formulae incorporate multiple patient variables, including height, body surface area, sex, amount of blood received during surgery, and the postoperative day [16]. A 2021 systematic review found that these more complex formulae tend to overestimate blood loss, and none are precise enough to serve as a gold standard for estimating perioperative blood loss [17].

Online calculators, available as an application or a web site, can conveniently estimate MABL. The popular MD+CALC program uses the Gross formula and does not incorporate prior transfusions [18].

16.3.1.2 Observation of the Surgical Field

The ASA Task Force on Perioperative Blood Transfusion and Adjuvant Therapies (2015) advises "visual assessment of the surgical field, including the extent of blood present, presence of microvascular bleeding, surgical sponges, clot size and shape, and volume in suction canister" to prevent undiagnosed exsanguination and development of a blood loss-associated coagulopathy (consensus (N = 72): 72% of experts strongly agreed, 8.3% were uncertain, and 0% disagreed) [2, 19]. Regular, systematic assessment of blood loss is particularly important when small patients undergo blood loss surgeries; the Pediatric Perioperative Cardiac Arrest Registry found that one-half of the events reported were secondary to failure to recognize blood loss [20]. Over 88% of anesthesiologists surveyed (n = 26) in the 2015 ASA guidelines agreed that there should be regular communication with the surgeon regarding excessive microvascular bleeding [19].

In an effort to establish objective criteria defining the severity of bleeding, Nellis et al. surveyed 24 pediatric experts about clinical signs that may indicate clinically relevant bleeding (i.e., bleeding associated with organ dysfunction or hemodynamic instability) in sick children [21]. Some of the responses included bleeding in critical body compartments (such as the brain and chest) and 5 mL/kg/h blood loss for longer than 1 h. The definitions were later applied to 40 bleeding children with an inter-rater reliability of 0.74 (95% CI, 0.61–0.86). The resulting bleeding scale (BASIC) was tied to blood loss but not to treatments such as the need for a blood transfusion. Also, the bleeding severity categories (mild, moderate, and severe) applied to postoperative, but not intraoperative, surgical interventions [22, 23]. Severe, clinically relevant bleeding under the BASIC scale includes a >20% decrease in BP from baseline; there is no decrease in BP described for minimal or moderate bleeding [21] (Table 16.2). Anesthetics that produce hypotension secondary to vasodilation may complicate the ability to accurately apply these diagnostic categories when trying to assess clinically relevant bleeding during surgery.

Significant volumes of blood loss can be hidden inside drapes, aprons, the patient's bed, and even the floor. In children, the smallest surgical sponges can absorb significant blood volumes. Visual estimation of blood loss alone, the historical and still the most used standard, is inaccurate [16, 17, 24]. A systematic review of available estimation techniques (visual, gravimetric before-and-after weighing of sponges, direct weighing, and colorimetric technology) determined that colorimetric technology had the highest degree of correlation with reference samples and the greatest degree of accuracy [17]. In colorimetric assessment, photographs are processed to determine blood versus non-Hgb contents in a given sample. However, other techniques to estimate blood loss, such the Gross formula, direct weighing of blood bags, and gravimetric technology, are more likely to be available for general perioperative use.

Gravimetric weighing of surgical sponges and other materials used to soak up blood on the surgical field are commonly used in pediatric surgeries, whereby 1 gram weight is equivalent to 1 mL of blood loss. The amount each sponge type can

Table 16.2 The BASIC scale

Bleeding severity	Any of these	All of these
Consensus definition for bleeding assessment scale in critically ill children (BASIC)		
Minimal	• Bleeding <1 mL/kg/h • Endotracheal or nasogastric tube blood streaks • Hematuria/≤1+ RBC on urine dipstick • Blood-stained dressings <1 mL/kg/h or change necessary ≥6 h intervals • Subcutaneous bleeding <5 cm diameter	
Moderate		• Bleeding not associated with hemodynamic instability or organ dysfunction • ≤20% decrease in Hgb • Blood loss 1–5 mL/kg/h
Severe	• Bleeding-related hemodynamic instability or organ dysfunction • >20% decrease in Hgb • Blood loss ≥5 mL/kg/h for ≥1 h • Intraspinal, intra-articular, or intra-ocular bleeding with associated reduction in function	

Adapted from Nellis ME, Tucci M, Lacroix J, Spinella PC, Haque KD, Stock A, et al. Bleeding Assessment Scale in Critically Ill Children (BASIC): Physician-Driven Diagnostic Criteria for Bleeding Severity. Crit Care Med. 2019;47(12):1766-72

Table 16.3 In vitro estimates of fluid held by various types of surgical sponges and gauze

Material (cm)	25% saturation	50% saturation	100% saturation
Fluid retained by surgical sponges and gauze			
45 × 45 lap sponge	25 mL blood	80 mL blood	160 mL blood
30 × 30 lap sponge	12.5 mL saline	23.3 mL saline	61 mL saline
	25 mL blood	50 mL blood	100 mL blood
35 × 5 lap sponge	7 mL saline	12.2 mL saline	18.9 mL saline
4 × 4 Raytec	6.1 mL saline	9.7 mL saline	13.5 mL saline
	3 mL blood	6 mL blood	12 mL blood
2 × 2 cottonoid pattie	0.3 mL saline	0.6 mL saline	1 mL saline
2 × 2 gauze pad	n/a	n/a	2–4.5 mL saline
Peanut	n/a	n/a	1 mL saline

Adapted from Hughes K, Chang YC, Sedrak J, Torres A. A clinically practical way to estimate surgical blood loss. Dermatol Online J. 2007;13(4):17; Ali Algadiem E, Aleisa AA, Alsubaie HI, Buhlaiqah NR, Algadeeb JB, Alsneini HA. Blood Loss Estimation Using Gauze Visual Analogue. Trauma Mon. 2016 May 3;21(2):e34131. doi: 10.5812/traumamon.34131. PMID: 27626017; PMCID: PMC5003499

hold varies. In vitro experiments using surgical gauze soaked in saline or blood demonstrate that a substantial quantity of blood may be hidden in sponges, although dilution effect with irrigation and other body fluids can affect accuracy [17, 25]. Table 16.3 illustrates the combined findings of several in vitro studies analyzing gravimetric estimation of blood loss [25, 26].

In conclusion, available methods to estimate blood loss during surgery are imprecise but necessary. A best practice to prevent the consequences of undiagnosed blood loss, including cardiac arrest, is to estimate MABL *before* surgery, consistently monitor ongoing blood loss by available means, and close observation of physiologic and laboratory changes throughout the intra- and postoperative periods.

16.4 What Are Some Physical Exam Findings Indicative of Clinically Significant Blood Loss?

16.4.1 Physiologic Indicators of Volume Status

A decision to transfuse RBCs should not be guided by a single vital sign, lab result, monitor reading, or estimated blood loss. A 2021 systematic review of guideline triggers for intraoperative RBC transfusions found that Hgb, Hct, BP, HR, electrocardiogram (ECG), estimated blood loss (EBL), and signs of altered end-organ perfusion[1] are commonly incorporated into the complex decision to administer RBCs during surgery [2]. Only one of the ten guidelines that met study inclusion criteria addressed children; that study emphasized physiologic changes and lab results (including Hgb level) as appropriate determinants of an intraoperative RBC transfusion [27]. The following is a discussion of select physiologic assessment tools available during an anesthetic to guide a pediatric patient's need for an RBC transfusion.

These include:

- Physical exam
- Basic oxygen (O_2) delivery and extraction
- Blood pressure
- Heart rate
- Electrocardiogram
- End-tidal carbon dioxide
- Urine output
- Monitors of tissue oxygenation
- Monitors of circulatory function

16.4.1.1 Physical Exam

Monitors that assess physiologic derangements and trends during blood loss often lack validation, appropriate proprietary algorithms, or body size adaptations for children and infants. However, physical exam findings during blood loss are readily available, do not require special monitoring, and may be seen early in hypovolemia before vital sign changes are evident [28–30]. An understanding of these basic tools is particularly relevant in low-resource environments where recommended monitoring devices may not be available [31]. The following is a discussion of physical assessment tools available during anesthesia to assess intraoperative volume depletion.

[1] Altered end organ perfusion was assessed using urine output, blood gases including lactate, cerebral oximetry, echocardiography, and mixed venous oxygen saturation.

Capillary Refill Time (CRT)

CRT is defined as the time required for color to return to the skin when pressure is applied [30]. CRT in healthy children is less than 2–3 s but lasts up to 5 s in adults [32]. Prolongation of CRT may be evident before decreases in BP secondary to an early neurohumoral response to bleeding. Because the definition of a normal CRT is controversial, including the applied technique, serial determinations should be used to follow trends during volume loss and treatment. A patient's baseline CRT may be affected by many factors, including age (CRT is most variable in infants), ambient temperature (CRT is inversely related to external temperature), body temperature (CRT is prolonged with low body temperatures), location tested (extremities tend to have a longer CRT than head or chest), duration of applied pressure (shorter pressure times create shorter CRT's), and interobserver variability [29, 30, 32–35]. A CRT that remains prolonged beyond the resuscitation period is associated with worse outcomes in both children and adults [28, 30]. Table 16.4 is an example of a standardized technique to assess CRT in children as determined in one systematic review [30].

Skin Mottling

Mottling is irregular "lace-like" blotching of the skin caused by hypoperfusion and patchy capillary vasoconstriction. In the context of blood loss, mottling may occur when the carotid baroreceptors sense a fall in BP, leading to an increase in sympathetic nervous system activity and shunting of blood from the periphery to the vital central organs. Skin mottling during intraoperative blood loss reflects decompensated hypovolemia and is likely to be associated with a CRT >3–4 s [36]. Mottling that is persistent despite resuscitation efforts may be a negative prognostic indicator in shock states [28]. Ambient light may be inadequate during surgery to properly evaluate for the presence or absence of skin mottling.

Body Temperature Gradients

Peripheral vasoconstriction associated with volume loss may produce a lowered skin temperature as blood flows away from the periphery to the central circulation. If the ambient temperature is constant, this will result in a temperature differential (Tskin-diff) between the patient's finger and core, arm, or rectal temperature. Thus, a Tskin-diff may indicate volume depletion or hemodynamic compromise and may be used to

Table 16.4 A uniform approach to determining CRT

Location	Patient's fingertip is preferred
Standardized measurement of capillary refill time (CRT)	
Duration of pressure	5 s
Amount of pressure	Moderate
Ideal ambient temperature	20–25 °C
Timing	Use stopwatch or timer
Normal value	Age 7 days to 18 years, <2 s Age <7 days, <3 s

Adapted from Fleming S, Gill P, Jones C, Taylor JA, Van den Bruel A, Heneghan C, et al. The Diagnostic Value of Capillary Refill Time for Detecting Serious Illness in Children: A Systematic Review and Meta-Analysis. PLoS One. 2015;10(9):e0138155 follow resuscitation efforts. On average, a forehead skin temperature is 2 °C lower than core temperature but has been shown to track with changes in the latter [37, 38]. On physical exam, hydration status can be assessed by tactile assessment of a temperature difference between the patient's hands, forearm, and upper arm; a patient that is cold to the touch above the elbow may have >10–15% dehydration or volume depletion [39].

Pulse Amplitude and Heart Sounds

Peripheral pulse intensity decreases during volume depletion or blood loss and may be evident prior to a decrease in BP [40]. Pulse amplitude may be graded on a scale (0–4) and followed during fluid replacement: 0 = pulseless; 1+ = faint amplitude; 2+ = diminished; 3+ = normal; 4+ = bounding. Hypothermia may produce a diminished pulse amplitude; hyperthermia, "warm" sepsis, or the vasodilation associated with volatile anesthetics may produce a bounding pulse amplitude. Heart sounds are audibly diminished prior to the onset of hypotension during volume loss and are best assessed continuously with a precordial stethoscope utilized from the onset of anesthesia and surgery.

16.5 Do Conventional Pediatric Vital Signs Reliably Indicate Perioperative Blood Loss?

The American Society of Anesthesiologists recommends basic monitors for patients undergoing a general anesthetic which include BP, HR, oxygen saturation (SaO_2), body temperature, inspired oxygen concentration (FiO_2), expired carbon dioxide concentration ($ETCO_2$), electrocardiogram (ECG), and adequacy of "circulatory function" [41]. The following discussion addresses the basics of oxygen delivery, BP, HR, urine output (UO), ECG, $ETCO_2$, and specialized monitors of circulatory function and tissue oxygenation. Pulse oximetry (SaO_2) is not discussed in detail because it is a ubiquitous gold standard that is often relied upon as the primary assessment tool for oxygenation status, but may remain relatively normal despite decreases in Hgb levels when administering FiO_2 >21% under anesthesia.

16.5.1 Basic Oxygen Delivery

A primary objective of an intraoperative RBC transfusion is to increase peripheral and end-organ oxygenation. Hypotension during blood loss is most likely due to a decrease in either preload or cardiac output [42]. Reducing the anesthetic with the intent to increase cardiac contractility is a common approach to the latter source of hypotension; administration of fluid is often a reflexive response to the former. The effect of bleeding on tissue oxygenation, however, is complex and is best gauged using different indices of oxygenation: arterial oxygen content (CaO_2), cardiac output (CO), oxygen content difference between the arterial and venous sides of the circulation (a-v DO_2), and mixed venous oxygen (SvO_2). It is important to appreciate that these measures of oxygenation are interrelated and should not be used in isolation to initiate an RBC transfusion. At best, they are a guide to a patient's response to anemia or to treatment of bleeding-related hypotension.

16.5.1.1 Arterial Oxygen Content (CaO_2)

CaO_2 is highly dependent on Hgb level and SaO_2. Under static conditions, only a minor fraction (0.003) of CaO_2 is based on the partial pressure of oxygen (PaO_2):

$$CaO_2 = (1.34 \times Hgb \times SaO_2) + (0.003 \times PaO_2)$$

Increasing the FiO_2 during blood loss will significantly improve CaO_2 only in a case of profound anemia. Take the example of a patient with a Hgb of 5 g/dL, SaO_2 100%, and PaO_2 250 mmHg. Applying the abovementioned oxygen content formula while the patient is receiving FiO_2 1.0, increasing the patient's PaO_2 from 250 mmHg to 500 mmHg will increase the CaO_2 by 0.75 mL/dl (CaO_2 7.45 to 8.2 mL/dl). However, if the FiO_2 (100%) or PaO_2 (250 mmHg) remain constant, but the patient receives an RBC transfusion to increase the Hgb level from 5 g/dL to 8 g/dL, the CaO_2 now increases by >4 mL/dL (i.e., CaO_2 7.45 to 11.47 mL/dL). It is important to note that these calculations apply only when oxygen consumption, systemic vascular resistance (SVR), cardiac contractility, and rhythm are unchanged.

16.5.1.2 Cardiac Output (CO)

Delivery of oxygen (DO_2) to the tissues depends on the CO as well as the CaO_2, according to the oxygen delivery equation [43]:

$$\text{Oxygen delivery} = DO_2 = CaO_2 \times CO;$$

and,

$$CO = SV \times HR;$$

therefore,

$$DO_2 = CaO_2 \times (SV \times HR)$$

where SV is stroke volume which may be a function of preload. Because oxygen in the blood is carried primarily by Hgb, a reduction in systemic oxygenation attributable to *active* bleeding is most likely due to a decrease in CaO_2 (i.e., the Hgb content) or CO (SV or HR). To improve systemic oxygenation during active bleeding, then, there must be an increase in Hgb, SV, HR, or all three. The relationship between SV and CO may be assessed noninvasively using a variety of surrogate markers of "fluid responsiveness." These indices are discussed in the section entitled "How is circulatory function monitored using wave form analysis?"

16.5.1.3 Arterial-Venous Oxygen Difference (a-v DO_2)

Another method to determine the clinical significance of blood loss is the oxygen content difference between the arterial and venous sides of the circulation (a-v DO_2) [44]:

$$a - vDO_2 = CaO_2 - CvO_2$$

where CvO_2 is the oxygen content of venous blood. A-v DO_2 is normally 4–8 mL/100 mL [43]. In anemia, oxygen extraction is increased at the tissue level, thereby decreasing the value of CvO_2 as it returns to the central circulation. The effect may be an increase in a-vDO_2. In an observational study of 177 anemic adult ICU patients (mean Hgb 8.3, range 7–9 g/dL), investigators found reduced 90-day mortality and AKI in the cohort that was transfused with RBCs when the a-v DO_2 was >3.7 mL, compared to those transfused with an a-v DO_2 ≤3.7 mL. The overall mean post-transfusion Hgb was 9.0 g/dL (range 7.7–11.3 g/dL) [45]. The a-v DO_2 may also be reduced by non-blood fluid administration, vasopressors, and, in cases of extreme anemia, increasing the FiO_2. The European Society of Anaesthesiology and Intensive Care (ESAIC) recommends using the a-vDO_2 to individualize RBC transfusion decisions if a superior vena cava catheter is in place where central venous blood can be sampled [44].

16.5.1.4 Mixed Venous Oxygen Saturation (SvO_2)

SvO_2 is the saturation of blood in the pulmonary artery, obtained via a pulmonary artery catheter (PAC), where there is mixing of venous blood from both the upper and lower body. SvO_2 is a function of oxygen delivery to the tissues (DO_2) in relation to oxygen consumption (VO_2). Because DO_2 is affected by CO, Hgb, and SaO_2, a decrease in SvO_2 may occur when there is a decrease in either of those variables. As a consequence, the SvO_2 is sometimes used to assess a patient's anemia tolerance, a response to an RBC transfusion, or response to measures intended to increase CO (e.g., volume administration or vasopressors) [40, 46]. SvO_2 may be paradoxically elevated in cases of abnormal oxygen extraction, such as sepsis or cyanide toxicity.

Unlike the SaO_2 which is obtained noninvasively using a standard pulse oximeter probe, SvO_2 requires a venous blood gas drawn from the central circulation. In the absence of a PAC, a venous saturation from a central venous line at the right atrium-superior vena cava junction ($ScvO_2$) is often used as a surrogate for SvO_2 from the pulmonary artery. Under normal conditions, the $ScvO_2$ (normal value approximately 70–80%) is approximately 5% less than an SvO_2; the SvO_2 represents true mixing of deoxygenated blood returning from the inferior vena cava (IVC) with the less deoxygenated blood returning from the superior vena cava (SVC) [40].

16.5.2 Blood Pressure (BP)

Hypotension during anesthesia triggers a concern that DO_2 to the tissues is inadequate to meet metabolic demand. However, as aptly stated, "the numeric blood pressure is not a divine dimension" [47]. Multiple factors affect the systolic blood pressure (SBP) during anesthesia and surgery, including all the variables contributing to cardiac output (CO):

$$\mathrm{CO} = \mathrm{SV} \times \mathrm{HR} = \mathrm{DO_2} / \mathrm{CaO_2} = \mathrm{SBP} / \mathrm{SVR}$$

where SVR is systemic vascular resistance. Thus, peripheral DO_2 is not simply a function of SBP or MAP, but is also dependent on CaO_2 (i.e., Hgb level, SaO_2, PaO_2), HR, SVR, and even body temperature [48]. Oxygen consumption increases approximately 10% for every 1 °C increase in body temperature [43]. For this reason, BP readings under anesthesia are a surrogate measure of end-organ oxygenation at best. Hypotension under anesthesia in a blood loss case may not necessarily be related to inadequate SV (i.e., preload) because other causes of reduced CO must be ruled out: cardiogenic (as in excessive vapor), distributive (including excessive vasodilation), and obstructive (e.g., a pneumothorax).

16.5.2.1 Noninvasive Blood Pressure Measurements

Most blood pressures are obtained indirectly during pediatric surgery (i.e., noninvasive BP; NIBP). Noninvasive oscillometer device measurements are based on proprietary algorithms; the amplitude of oscillations determines the SBP and the diastolic blood pressure (DBP), from which the mean arterial pressure (MAP)—a primary factor in peripheral perfusion—is calculated [49]. NIBP cuffs may produce readings that vary with a patient's extremity size (an oversized cuff will produce an erroneously low BP), patient positioning (the "up" arm will have a lower systolic NIBP than the dependent arm), and extremity (a leg calf NIBP will be higher than an arm NIBP). Furthermore, oxygen transfer at the capillary level results from diffusion across a pre- and post-capillary partial pressure gradient and not SBP per se [47, 50].

There are several reasons that isolated BP readings should not be used to diagnose significant intraoperative blood loss in children. Pediatric patients can lose a significant percentage of their total blood volume (e.g., 20–30%) before BP changes are evident. The hemodynamic response to early and clinically significant blood loss may instead be an *increase* in the DBP secondary to a compensatory generalized sympathetic response, resulting in a decrease in the pulse pressure (PP; the difference between SBP and DBP) [9, 10]. According to the ATLS bleeding severity classifications, the PP begins to change in hypovolemic shock before a decrease in SBP is evident [36, 51].

16.5.2.2 Normal Blood Pressures

Blood pressure reference ranges in healthy children in the *unanesthetized* state are based on hypertensive values for age and sex [52]. Table 16.5 illustrates "normal" 90th percentile weight- and height-based BP reference values for boys; normative values for girls vary slightly but are similar in these age groups [53].

Table 16.5 The 90th percentile weight- and height-based blood pressure reference values for boys (not under anesthesia) from birth to age 13 years

Age (years)	Birth	1	2	3	4	5	6	7	8	9	10	11	12	13
90th percentile age-specific blood pressures in children														
SBP (mmHg)	87	105	106	107	108	109	111	112	114	115	117	119	121	124
DBP (mmHg)	68	69	68	68	69	69	70	71	73	74	75	76	77	79
Weight (kg)	4	11	14	16	18	22	25	29	34	39	44	50	55	62

DBP diastolic blood pressure, *SBP* systolic blood pressure
Adapted from Nelson Textbook of Pediatrics E-Book, 21st ed, p. 2346–2350

Although various pediatric societies have set thresholds for intraoperative hypotension, anesthesiologists continue to vary widely in practice, with goals usually set between 20 and 30% of baseline [54–56]. During normal sleep, SBP and HR decrease approximately 20% without untoward consequences, but the clinical relevance of similar decreases in blood pressure during an uneventful anesthetic is not known [57]. In the GAS (general anesthesia or awake-regional anesthesia in infancy) trial, a noninvasively obtained MAP less than 35 mmHg was observed in one-third of infants undergoing general anesthesia (mean duration 54 min) [58]. However, Wechsler Full Intelligence scores at 5 years of age were not different than those receiving awake regional analgesia (mean difference 0.23; 95% CI, 2.59–3.06). Postoperative encephalopathy has been reported in infants maintained in the NIBP MAP range <35 mmHg for an extended period under anesthesia, prompting consideration of other intraoperative conditions including hypoglycemia and hypocapnea [59].

16.5.2.3 Intraoperative Blood Pressure Norms

Normal intraoperative blood pressure values have been retrospectively studied in several recent studies [52, 60, 61]. Hillgruber et al. examined the records of over 20,000 children <19 years old (median age 7 years) to identify median BPs during inhalation (IHA), total intravenous (TIVA), and mostly intravenous anesthesia (MIVA) [60]. The median actionable BP values are found in Table 16.6. The 5th percentile of MAP and SBP was chosen as clinically relevant based on other studies incorporating that benchmark for treatment [62].

In the Hillgruber study, there was an age-related increase in mean noninvasive MAP readings under anesthesia, but there was not a difference in those readings based on type of anesthesia except in neonates. For children <1 year, the median MAP was 3.8 mmHg higher during TIVA compared to IHA ($p < 0.001$). There was also no difference in median MAPs based on patient sex. Of interest, the Hillgruber findings are comparable to a 2009 Society for Pediatric Anesthesia (SPA) survey on age-related definitions of hypotension, but are lower than the actionable values in the 2000 Pediatric Advanced Life Support (PALS) guidelines which are focused on unanesthetized children [55, 63, 64].

Hillgruber et al. devised a formula based on their study findings to determine an age-appropriate noninvasive MAP under general anesthesia (with slightly higher thresholds for TIVA):

- Children ≤1 year: 46 mmHg + 1 mmHg/month
- Children >1 year: 61 mmHg + 0.5 mmHg/year

Another retrospective review examined noninvasive BPs from a perioperative outcome dataset (2007–2014) during the pre- and intraoperative phases of anesthesia in 116,362 children [52]. Although outcomes were not evaluated, this multicenter study demonstrated real clinical practice patterns. The low noninvasive SBP cutoff (2 standard deviations below the 50% percentile) was chosen to reflect an actionable pressure thought to risk end-organ hypoperfusion. The cutoffs for actionable noninvasive SBP values during the surgical phase of anesthesia were

Table 16.6 Actionable 5th percentile MAPs in children under anesthesia

	Age category[a]	Total intravenous anesthesia (TIVA)			Inhalational anesthesia (IHA)			Mostly intravenous anesthesia (MIVA)		
		Median [IQR]	5th centile	*n*	Median [IQR]	5th centile	*n*	Median [IQR]	5th centile	*n*
MAP	<1 month	48 [44–55]	34	53	45 [39–52]	32	116	41 [37–45]	34	39
	1–12 months	57 [51–63]	42	430	51 [46–57]	38	682	57 [51–63]	40	401
	1–2 years	59 [55–64]	49	816	58 [53–63]	45	346	59 [54–63]	49	626
	2–5 years	63 [58–69]	52	4013	62 [57–67]	49	859	64 [58–70]	52	1344
	6–11 years	65 [60–71]	53	3665	64 [59–70]	52	1093	64 [59–71]	52	1103
	12–18 years	66 [60–73]	52	2842	67[61–73]	54	1656	66 [61–73]	52	529
SBP	<1 month	68 [62–77]	47	53	66 [57–76]	46	116	58 [52–68]	43	39
	1–12 months	85 [76–94]	63	430	77 [67–87]	54	682	83 [74–93]	61	401
	1–2 years	85 [79–93]	70	816	84 [76–93]	66	346	85 [78–94]	70	626
	2–5 years	88 [81–97]	72	4013	88 [80–96]	70	859	90 [83–101]	72	1344
	6–11 years	90 [83–101]	73	3665	90 [83–101]	73	1093	90 [83–101]	72	1103
	12–18 years	93 [84–105]	73	2842	94 [84–105]	73	1656	93 [83–104]	71	529

IQR interquartile range.

Reprinted with permission from Hillgruber RJ, Lutskov P, West NC, Whyte S, Görges M. Blood pressure nomograms for children undergoing general anesthesia, stratified by age and anesthetic type, using data from a retrospective cohort at a tertiary pediatric center. J Clin Monit Comput. 2022;36(6):1667-77

[a]Age categories from the National Institute of Child Health and Human Development

approximately 32 mmHg at birth, 62 mmHg at 4 years, and 70 mmHg at 15 years for both boys and girls [52]. These findings did not include children with an ASA physical status ≥III.

Thus far, there are no validated NIBP reference ranges for children undergoing anesthesia. The absence of reference values during anesthesia continues to cause a wide variation in diagnosis and potential treatments. Adding to the complexity of using SBP to follow volume loss is the myriad of intraoperative events during surgery, including painful stimulation, surgical manipulation, and a multitude of medications, all of which can affect BP independent of blood loss. As a rule, hypotension secondary to blood loss in a child is a late event and will be accompanied by other signs of hypoperfusion such as lactic acidosis.

16.5.3 Heart Rate (HR)

An increase in HR is a physiologic response to hypotension but may be nonspecific for blood loss. Intraoperative tachycardia has a multitude of etiologies, including painful stimulation, hypercapnia, fever, excessive anesthetic, anticholinergic administration, and hypovolemia. Ascertaining the cause is complicated by the fact that reference heart rates in children are age-related. Table 16.7 lists normal pediatric HR ranges [65].

The neonatal baseline HR is tachycardic relative to older children and adults. Neonates have limited stroke volume variability with a CO is largely HR-dependent. Furthermore, neonates may develop paradoxical responses (e.g., bradycardia) to stressful stimuli such as blood loss-related hypotension. Anesthesia practitioners often set a HR goal during surgery that is within 20–30% of baseline [36]. As with initial BP changes, tachycardia in an infant may not be apparent early in blood loss as peripheral blood flow is shunted to the central circulation through compensatory vasoconstriction.

The age-adjusted shock index (SIPA) has been validated as one measure to predict the need for an early blood transfusion in traumatically injured children [66]. SIPA is a coefficient of HR divided by systolic blood pressure (SBP). Abnormal

Table 16.7 Normal HR by age

Age	Heart rate (beats per minute)
Premature	120–170
0–3 months	100–150
3–6 months	90–120
6–12 months	80–120
1–3 years	70–110
3–6 years	65–110
6–12 years	60–95
>12 years	55–85

Adapted from Marciniak, B. Growth and Development. In: Coté CJ, Lerman J, Anderson B, editors. A Practice of Anesthesia for Infants and Children. 5th ed. Philadelphia: Elsevier Inc.; 2013. p. 7–20

SIPA values for children are 1–6 years, >1.2; 6–12 years, >1.0; and >12 years, >0.9 [66, 67]. Zhu et al. examined over 2000 children who received a massive transfusion (i.e., >40 mL/kg blood products) in the first 24 h after admission [68]. For all forms of traumatic injury studied, a combination of SBP < 100 mmHg and SIPA > 1.4 demonstrated a 94% specificity and 45% sensitivity for early massive transfusion requirement. Children meeting both criteria were seven times more likely to require early massive transfusion protocol activation [68].

16.5.4 Electrocardiogram (ECG)

ECG waveform changes consistent with hemodynamic instability are often used to guide RBC transfusion decisions in adults and children during cardiac surgery [2]. ECG changes associated with severe anemia or hypovolemia in children, particularly infants, are more likely to be rate-rhythm related (e.g., bradycardia or supraventricular tachycardia). In adult patients, ECG changes related to severe anemia, hypotension, or altered end-organ oxygenation tend to be reflected in waveform changes (e.g., ST depression).

16.5.5 End-Tidal Carbon Dioxide ($ETCO_2$)

Continuous capnography, or $ETCO_2$ monitoring, serves several vital functions during anesthesia, including assessment of ventilation, endotracheal tube placement, and perfusion. A key indicator of hemodynamically significant blood loss is the physiologic dead space (V_D). V_D describes a condition in which the patient's airways are ventilated but inadequately perfused, leading to a decreases in CO_2 elimination from the venous circulation. Applying the Bohr equation, V_D can be calculated by multiplying the patient's tidal volume (V_T) by the difference between arterial ($PaCO_2$) and alveolar CO_2 ($PETCO_2$) concentrations:

$$V_D = V_T \times \left(\mathrm{PaCO_2} - \mathrm{PETCO_2}\right) / \mathrm{PaCO_2}$$

In patients with mild lung disease, $PaCO_2$ has been found to approximate $PETCO_2$ when the PaO_2/FiO_2 ratio is >200 [69]. However, sudden decreases in CO or hypotension due to blood loss may create significant V_D secondary to a decrease in blood return to the heart, a decrease in alveolar CO_2, and a large gap between $PaCO_2$ (which increases) and $PETCO_2$ (which is diminished) [70, 71]. The 2020 American Heart Association Pediatric Advanced Life Support (AHA PALS) guidelines recommend that $ETCO_2$ be used to assess the quality of resuscitation efforts in children who have experienced cardiac arrest with decreased pulmonary blood flow [62]. In a successful resuscitation, a rise in $ETCO_2$ may be seen prior to normalization of blood pressure or cardiac rhythm. To obviate the need for invasive laboratory testing, $ETCO_2$ has been studied as a surrogate measure of serum bicarbonate levels in diabetic ketoacidosis and severe dehydration, as well $PaCO_2$ in critically ill patients [69, 72, 73].

16.5.6 Urine Output

Urine output is a crude measure of hypovolemia during surgery. Intraoperative stress responses including a release of antidiuretic hormone (ADH), fluid sifts, and electrolyte changes may reduce urine output up to 20% of nonoperative levels [74]. Assessing blood loss using urine volume as a guide may be further complicated by the fact that renal function in children does not reach adult levels until 2 years of age [75]. Acute kidney injury (AKI) is a concern when urine output is diminished in the perioperative period and has been associated with intraoperative fluid restriction [76, 77]. A typical recommendation when using urine output to assess the quality of fluid resuscitation is 1–2 mL/kg/h in infants and 0.5–1 mL/kg/h in older children, but there is a lack of evidence to support this guideline [36, 78, 79]. Administering fluids with those output goals in mind may lead to relative fluid overload and poor outcomes, particularly in certain patient populations and procedures (e.g., right ventricular failure or colorectal surgery) [80]. In a retrospective review, 689 pediatric patients undergoing major abdominal surgery were stratified by high and low urine output (10.81 versus 3.23 mL/kg/h, respectively). The low urine output group received less intravenous (IV) fluid overall, with similar untoward outcomes including postoperative AKI [74]. In a prospective study, adults undergoing major abdominal surgery were randomized to a low urine output group (i.e., 0.2 mL/kg/h); they received less IV fluid, but outcomes were similar to patients treated with a 0.5 mL/kg/h urine output goal, including AKI [81]. Perfusion in the microcirculation is dependent on blood flow between the afferent and efferent arterioles. However, urine production is dependent on the hydrostatic pressure in the glomeruli (approximately 55 mmHg). A recent retrospective review of over 4500 children who underwent noncardiac surgery did not find an association between intraoperative hypotension and AKI; in that study, a mean preoperative Hgb of 12.1 g/dL was speculated to offer a protective effect compared to the mean Hgb of 10.6 g/dL in the group that developed AKI (OR 0.77, 95% CI 0.74–0.81; $p < 0.001$) [82]. The optimal urine output rate management for children in the perioperative period remains unknown.

16.6 How Is Circulatory Function Monitored Using Pulse Wave Form Analysis?

16.6.1 Monitors of Circulatory Function

Hypotension secondary to surgery-related volume loss is most likely due to inadequate preload or a decrease in CO. Once the anesthetic dosing is reduced, assessment of the patient's response to fluid administration or an RBC transfusion is crucial to identify those patients that may benefit from fluid replacement and those that may benefit from alternative measures [56]. Both inadequate and excessive fluid resuscitation may be harmful [42]. Perioperatively, noninvasive measures of CO are increasingly used to assess the patient's response to fluid administration (e.g., perfusion indices and bioreactance).

The gold standard to measure cardiac output (CO) in critically ill patients has been the pulmonary artery catheter (PAC), an invasive monitor that requires expert management, has associated complications, and inconsistently predicts CO [83]. In an effort to quickly and safely assess a patient's CO response to fluid resuscitation at the bedside, surrogate measures of CO have been adopted. These measures rely on the fact that during normal respiration there is an increase in intrathoracic pressure with a decrease in venous return, followed by a decrease in stroke volume (SV), with each respiratory cycle. The changes in SV with fluid administration can be continuously followed using an arterial catheter or pulse oximeter waveform. These functionalities are called "pulse waveform analysis." Accurate pulse wave analysis requires stable intrathoracic compliance, hence the recommendation to assess parameters only during controlled ventilation without patient movement or breakthrough breathing [84].

Studies supporting bedside pulse waveform analysis to guild fluid therapy in children tend to be small in cohort size or manufacturer sponsored [85, 86]. Currently, there are no large randomized trials of arterial or pulse wave form analysis in children undergoing anesthesia. Continuous (dynamic) and automated pulse waveform analysis is possible through proprietary algorithms comparing a patient's variables to "normal" hemodynamic parameters [83]. Original data underlying wave form reference values were obtained in adults. At this point in time, there is not a consistent definition of fluid responsiveness in children; it may vary from 10% to over 25%, depending on the study, the patient population, and the particular monitor [83, 84, 87, 88]. As a result, practitioners are not always prepared to evaluate the validity or clinical relevance of a monitor purported to assess fluid responsiveness [83, 84]. Furthermore, it is not always evident that a device operates from an algorithm adapted to pediatric patients.

The following discussion addresses surrogate measures of CO and fluid responsiveness in children.

Invasive Assessment of CO

- Stroke volume variation (SVV)
- Pulse pressure variation (PPV)
- Central venous pressure (CVP)

Noninvasive Assessment of CO

- Inferior vena cava distensibility (ΔIVC)
- Plethysmographically derived wave amplitude (ΔPOP)
- Peripheral perfusion index (PI)
- Plethysmographic variability index (PVI)
- Respiratory variation in peak aortic flow (ΔV_{peak})
- Passive leg raise
- Bioimpedance and bioreactance

16.6.1.1 Invasive Assessment of CO

Stroke Volume Variation (SVV)

SVV is defined as the change in stroke volume (SV) during one respiratory cycle following volume loading in patients who are mechanically ventilated. An increase in CO in response to fluid administration reflects an increase in myocardial fiber tension and the patient's position on the Frank–Starling (F–S) curve. If a patient is volume dependent (i.e., a "responder") or on the steep portion of the F–S curve,

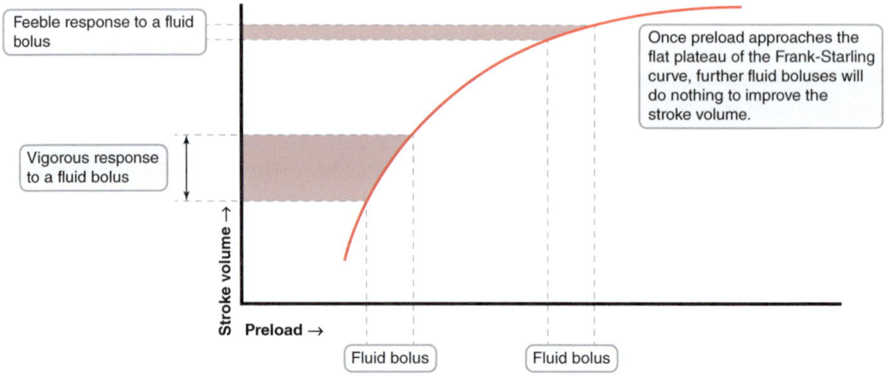

Fig. 16.1 The Frank–Starling mechanism whereby an increase in left ventricular preload increases stroke volume (SV) and thereby CO, until left ventricular stretch is maximal. Found online at https://derangedphysiology.com/main/required-reading/equipment-and-procedures/Chapter%20 2411/fluid-resuscitation-and-assessment-fluid-responsiveness

there may be a large increase in SV as represented by a percentage change in SVV. If a patient has a baseline SVV of <10–12%, she may be on the flat portion of the F–S curve and will not respond to bolus fluid administration (i.e., she is a "nonresponder") (Fig. 16.1).

Pulse Pressure Variation (PPV)

PPV is defined as a change in pulse pressure as read through an arterial catheter during one respiratory cycle following volume loading in patients who are mechanically ventilated. Like SVV, PVV indicates a patient's position on the F–S curve but is not necessarily indicative of overall volume status [89]. A large increase in PPV after fluid administration indicates the patient is on the steep portion of the F–S curve and is predicted to show improvement in CO with further fluid loading. Reportedly, changes in vasomotor tone affect PPV more than SVV [83, 90]. A PPV >13% may reflect fluid responsiveness in children [83, 85].

In adults, the ability of SVV or PPV to predict fluid responsivity is generally accepted [85, 91, 92]. However, neither parameter has been consistently shown to predict fluid responsiveness in children [87, 90, 93, 94]. Both SVV and PPV continue to be used to follow hemodynamic trends during pediatric resuscitation, including transfusion. However, there are several limitations when extrapolating arterial catheter-derived reference values from adult studies to children. These limitations include the following [90, 95]:

- Children vary in age, size, and body weight more than adults.
- Children have greater thoracic cage compliance compared to adults.
- Children tend to have lower systolic and higher diastolic blood pressures compared to adults.
- Children have smaller blood volumes, smaller tidal volumes, and faster heart rates than adults.

- The neonatal myocardium is immature with less contractile elements, making it more sensitive to preload and afterload challenges. This physiology requires higher preload volumes to achieve an increase in SV.

Both SVV and PPV monitoring require the presence of an indwelling arterial catheter and controlled ventilation. Furthermore, increases of 10–15% are typically considered to be positive responses to fluid administration (thereby identifying fluid responders), although there is no consensus on this reference value. Both SVV and PPV will be inaccurate if the patient has right heart failure, arrhythmias, rapid respiratory rates, low tidal volumes, intracardiac shunts, and the presence of an intra-aortic balloon pump [83, 85, 90, 92, 96].

Central Venous Pressure (CVP)

A CVP indwelling line has been shown to be a poor monitor of fluid responsiveness; at best, it is a static measure of central blood volume.

However, patients with high CVP values may be at the flat portion of the F–S curve and susceptible to volume overload with excessive fluid challenges [97].

16.6.1.2 Noninvasive Assessment of CO

Inferior Vena Cava Distensibility (ΔIVC)

ΔIVC is the change in the IVC diameter as assessed by ultrasound during a respiratory cycle. A >50% variation in IVC diameter under ultrasound in spontaneously breathing patients may indicate fluid responsivity [36]. The nonresponder cutoff threshold may be as high as 23% in children [98]. High tidal volumes may impede venous return and produce inaccurate ΔIVC readings [85]. An IVC to abdominal aorta diameter ratio (IV/Ao) <0.6–0.8 has been found to correlate with a SV increase >10% in both mechanically ventilated and spontaneously breathing children [99]. Because the Ao should not change during blood loss, the IV/Ao ratio may reflect fluid responsiveness as well as clinically significant dehydration [36, 99].

Plethysmographically Derived Wave Amplitude (ΔPOP)

ΔPOP is a measure of respiratory variations in the pulse oximeter wave form amplitude. Because the pulse oximeter probe site is placed on peripheral skin rather than intra-arterial, readings are not as severely affected by changes in arterial compliance as seen in shock states or anesthesia [85]. In a study of 43 adult cardiac surgery patients, Westphal et al. found that ΔPOP correlated with PPV under controlled ventilation within 3 h post surgery. The ΔPOP threshold cutoff for nonresponders was 11%, with 90% sensitivity and 100% specificity [91]. However, in a prospective observational study of 30 children, age 0–14 years, scheduled for neurosurgery under general anesthesia, the ΔPOP immediately post-induction did not vary significantly between responders and nonresponders during three respiratory cycles following a fluid bolus 20 mL/kg [87].

Peripheral Perfusion Index (PI)

The PI is a calculated, algorithm-based ratio of the strength of the arterial pulsation (AC) to venous and capillary nonpulsatile flow (DC) during a respiratory cycle as detected by the infrared pulse oximeter signal [85]. The PI is calculated as a percentage:

$$\mathrm{PI} = \left(\mathrm{AC} / \mathrm{DC}\right) \times 100$$

According to the pulse oximeter manufacturer of this derived index, the "normal" PI value varies between 0.02% and 20% depending on the clinical context and patient comorbidity [86]. The PI is thought to reflect peripheral perfusion, and therefore sensor placement site may affect readings. Vasomotor tone in hypoperfusion states may be more labile in the periphery than the central circulation (e.g., finger versus the earlobe) [86, 100, 101]. In a 2013 prospective, controlled study, 25 adult volunteers were subjected to lower body negative pressure (creating central hypovolemia) [102]. In that study, PI decreased from 2.2% to 1.2% ($p = 0.007$) before the onset of detectable hypotension, a rise in heartrate, or a decrease in SV. The investigators thereby concluded that PI may be useful in the early diagnosis of hypovolemia [102]. The PI has been used in children to detect onset of epidural analgesia, illness severity, and postoperative pain [103–105]. In an effort to explore a potential relationship between intraoperative PI values and postoperative outcomes, secondary data in 741 adults undergoing hip and abdominal surgery was used to determine postoperative complications, 90-day mortality, and RBC transfusion requirements [106]. Patients with a mean PI ≤ 1.5 and a minimum intraoperative Hgb of $\leq$9.7 g/dL received significantly more RBC transfusions and had more postoperative complications than those with higher mean PI values plus anemia. However, there was not an independent association between mean PI and RBC requirements, as 40% of patients with a low PI and 50% of those with a high PI received a transfusion despite both groups being anemic [106].

In an effort to establish normal reference ranges in newborns, a cohort that benefits from reliable noninvasive hemodynamic monitoring, Hu et al. examined over 3800 healthy newborns, gestational age 35–41 weeks, to establish PI reference ranges during the first 2 days of life [94]. Investigators found that both pre- and post-ductal PI increased with gestational and post-conceptual ages (Fig. 16.2).

Plethysmographic Variability Index (PVI)

PVI is an algorithmically based calculation of variations in the PI during a complete respiratory cycle:

$$\mathrm{PVI} = \left(\mathrm{PI}_{\mathrm{max}} - \mathrm{PI}_{\mathrm{min}} / \mathrm{PI}_{\mathrm{max}}\right) \times 100$$

PVI cutoff values found in the literature for fluid responders versus nonresponders vary from 28% in shocked neonates to 8% in adults undergoing spine surgery [107, 108]. The ability of PVI to predict fluid responsiveness and shock-related mortality in adult patients has been shown in a number of studies [102, 109]. Studies of PVI efficacy in assessing fluid responsiveness in pediatric patients, however, have

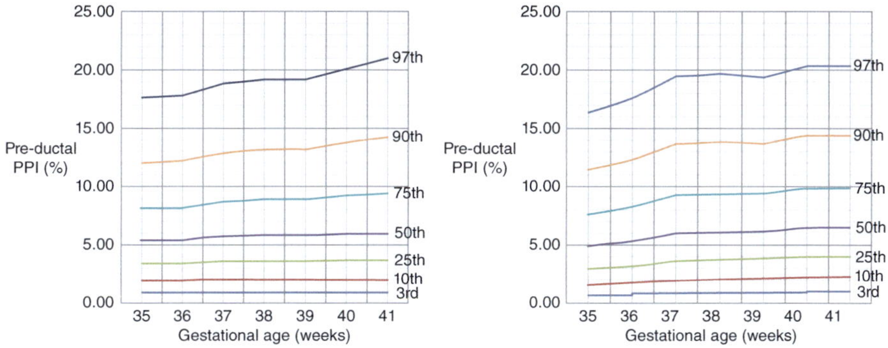

Fig. 16.2 Percentile curves of PI in over 3800 newborns less than 48 h old: the left graph depicts preductal and the right graph depicts postductal PPI values. Reprinted from: Hu X. Peripheral perfusion index percentiles for healthy newborns by gestational age and sex in China. Scientific Reports: Nature Research (2020)10:4213 under Creative Commons Attributions License 4.0 International

produced conflicting results. In a 2012 Canadian study applying Bland-Altman analysis in 33 operating room and PICU patients, ages 0–12 years, there was a strong correlation between PVI and PPV ($r = 0.7049$, 95% CI, 0.4771–0.844; $p < 0.0001$) and PVI and ΔPOP ($r = 0.715$, 95% CI, 0.4926–0.8497; $r < 0.0001$) [96]. The mean PI was 3.8% (standard deviation 2.3), with a mean PVI of 15% (range 4–41%). In another study of anesthetized children, over one-third of PVI readings fell into what is termed the "gray zone" for which reference values are inconclusive; in this study, PVI gray zones were 10–17% and >22% [110].

A 2016 meta-analysis was unable to conclude that PVI is a reliable predictor of fluid responsiveness in children undergoing intraoperative procedures [88]. In that study, only four publications met review criteria, with a mean PVI 14% (SD 3%) cutoff for nonresponders. The investigators concluded that PVI could be a useful predictor of fluid responsiveness in children undergoing surgery but that more studies were needed. In a follow up meta-analysis 7 years later, there were eight pediatric studies that met inclusion criteria (n = 283 patients) analyzing the ability of digital (finger probe) PVI to predict fluid responsiveness in the perioperative period [101]. There was significant heterogeneity between studies, with a pooled sensitivity and specificity of 72% and 66%, respectively. The sensitivity and specificity were less than those found in the adult patient population, leading investigators to conclude that PVI is unlikely to predict fluid responsivity in children as reliably as with adults. The definition of fluid responsiveness used for analysis in the eight studies was >10% (2 studies) and >15% (6 studies). The cutoff range in the meta-analysis for fluid responders was 5–16%, with an odds ratio 9.26 for positivity (95% CI; 5.31–16.16) for responders diagnosed in that PVI range. Bolus fluid challenges ranged from 10 mL/kg to 20 mL/kg. Investigators concluded that PVI could reliably predict fluid responsivity in children undergoing surgery, but it should not be used in isolation to monitor intraoperative hemodynamics unless direct measures of CO such as echocardiography are not available [101].

Respiratory Variation in Peak Aortic Flow (ΔV_{peak})

ΔV_{peak} is an ultrasound-guided estimation of blood flow velocity at the level of the aortic annulus during a respiratory cycle.

The cutoff for nonresponders to fluid administration was 12.2% in one prospective study of children ages 1–14 years who received a crystalloid bolus 10 mL/kg under general anesthesia [98]. In another pediatric study, ΔV_{peak} was compared with PPV, ΔPOP, and PVI and was found to be the only measure to accurately predict fluid responsiveness in 30 children under general anesthesia (age 0–14 years); the nonresponder ΔV_{peak} cutoff point was 15% when assessed post-induction [87]. Of all the aforementioned pulse waveform assessment tools, only the ΔV_{peak} has consistently been shown to reliably predict fluid responsiveness in children [84, 93, 98, 110].

Two of the noninvasive techniques to assess fluid responsiveness (ΔV_{peak} and ΔIVC) require expert sonography skills, whereas the other three (PI, PVI, and ΔPOP) suffer from the same factors affecting pulse oximetry in general: patient movement, peripheral vasoconstriction, pressure produced by the probe, extremity temperature, and site of probe placement (e.g., fingers, toes, nose, foot, forehead, and earlobe, each of which may produce a different reading) [85]. Further studies and clinical experience hold a promise of enhanced algorithm accuracy for pediatric patients in different clinical contexts.

16.6.2 A Note About the PVI

With its bedside convenience, noninvasive nature, and robust marketing, the PVI obtained from a pulse oximeter has been studied in several clinical situations involving both children and adults. Peripheral vasoconstriction leading to reduced skin blood flow is an early response to hypovolemia, resulting from sympathetic nervous system, endothelial, and platelet activation [109]. The pulse oximeter probe is sensitive to clinically significant alterations in peripheral perfusion and vasomotor tone; thus the PI and PVI readings may reflect early hypovolemia and shock states. As a result, pulse wave analysis using PVI has expanded from an assessment tool for fluid responsiveness to the assessment of overall health. The following paragraphs describe the application of PVI or PI in specific clinical situations:

16.6.2.1 Dehydration

Dehydration is a significant cause of childhood mortality. The presentation of dehydration in children can be nonspecific and complicated by paradoxical vital signs and difficult intravenous access, both of which result in treatment delay. In a prospective study of adults presenting to an emergency room with a diagnosis of gastroenteritis, patients with moderate to severe dehydration ($n = 81$) demonstrated improvements in PI and PVI (1.8–2% and 33–28%, respectively; $p < 0.001$) after fluid resuscitation [111]. Future PI studies that include children offer a potential solution to the timely treatment of severe pediatric dehydration.

16.6.2.2 Asthma

In a prospective study of 138 children admitted to an emergency department with asthma, PVI was correlated with the severity of asthma before and after bronchodilator therapy [112]. The physiologic connection between PVI and asthma is *pulsus paradoxus*: a >10% fall in systolic blood pressure with inspiration in the setting of obstructive lung disease. Because PVI scores were significantly higher in children with severe (versus mild or moderate) asthma, the investigators concluded that PVI may have a place in the diagnosis and management of emergency room asthma.

16.6.2.3 Surgery in the Prone Position

Venous return to the central circulation (i.e., preload) may fall when a patient is placed in the prone position during surgery. Two pediatric studies found no change in either PVI or the invasively obtained PPV in the prone position, nor was there a correlation between PVI and PPV [113, 114]. Both investigations concluded that PVI should not replace PPV in children undergoing surgery in the prone position.

16.6.2.4 Neonatal Shock

In a recent observational study of 37 premature infants in early shock, the mean PVI at diagnosis was 28% (±5%) [107]. Following treatment (87% received fluid resuscitation; most received vasopressors), approximately 97% of patients had a decrease in PVI, with an average decrease of 11% (±5%) and a mean of 17% ($p < 0.001$). One interesting finding was that systolic and diastolic blood pressures did not change during this phase of early shock. The investigators emphasized the importance of obtaining a baseline PVI prior to initiating therapy for neonatal shock, given the relatively high PVI values at diagnosis.

16.6.2.5 Detection of Anesthesia Onset

As discussed, the PI and PVI are sensitive to peripheral vasomotor tone. The PVI has been used to gauze the onset of anesthesia in several studies. In 1 study of 40 children undergoing single-shot epidural anesthesia for inguinal hernia repair, PI increased from baseline and was also greater than the PI of both unanesthetized upper extremities at 5 min ($p < 0.05$) [103]. PVI has also been shown to increase following the induction of propofol anesthesia, with a cutoff of 15% associated with a 25% decrease in MAP [115].

16.6.2.6 Substitute for Serum Lactate in Shock States

Both serum lactate and urine output are indices of severe hypovolemia and shock but may not be immediately apparent for timely resuscitation. In a prospective study of 50 patients (age 1 month to 15 years) admitted to the emergency room in shock, admission serum lactate level (>5.7 mmol/L) and PI (≤0.18) demonstrated similar sensitivity in predicting mortality (70% and 74%, respectively) [116]. Investigators concluded that PVI may be used to diagnose early shock because it can detect shock-related changes in the microcirculation before serum lactate increases to critical levels.

16.6.2.7 Early Diagnosis of Patent Ductus Arteriosus (PDA)

It is standard to screen for a patent ductus arteriosus (PDA) in premature neonates using echocardiography. However, ultrasonography expertise is not readily available in some low resource communities. Pulse oximetry, however, is often available in neonatal units. In a sample of 27 premature infants, gestational age <34 weeks, a PI difference of 0.85% between pre-ductal and post-ductal PI values had good sensitivity and specificity to diagnosis symptomatic disease requiring early intervention [117]. The results of this study suggest that the PI may offer a simple method to distinguish infants with a PDA who may require treatment.

16.6.3 Other Noninvasive Measures of CO or Fluid Responsiveness

16.6.3.1 Passive Leg Raise

The passive leg raise (PLR) is a relatively old technique for autotransfusion that has recently been systematically studied as a test of fluid responsivity. With the patient supine, the legs are raised 45° to the horizontal. As blood flows with gravity from the legs to the central circulation, direct or surrogate measures of CO are made continuously over several minutes. Significant changes in hemodynamics following PLR are then interpreted as evidence that the patient will be responsive to fluid administration.

Patients who at the far right end of the preload-SV relationship on the Frank-Starling curve may respond negatively to fluid administration with respiratory distress or congestive heart failure (CHF) [118]. The ability of PLR to predict fluid responsivity has been studied in a variety of clinical conditions. Recognizing its relative simplicity, the ESICM suggests that PLR may be a useful bedside tool to prevent unnecessary and potentially harmful excessive fluid administration [42]. Observational studies in adults have found $ETCO_2$ changes greater than 5% of baseline or 2 mmHg following PLR to be correlated with fluid responsiveness [119, 120]. Some patients, such as those with abdominal compartment syndrome or increased intracranial pressure, should not undergo a PLR trial.

A 2010 meta-analysis of 9 clinical trials including 353 adult patients examined the relationship between PLR and changes in CO and determined that PLR can reliably affect changes in CO in both mechanically ventilated and spontaneously breathing patients (pooled sensitivity and specificity 89.4% and 91.4%, respectively) [121]. The PLR correlation to an increase in CO after fluid loading was 0.81 ($r = 0.75$–0.86). In a later systematic review of 21 studies ($n = 991$ adults in circulatory failure), PLR-related changes in CO ≥10% as well as a 12% change in pulse pressure (PP) demonstrated a greater than 80% specificity [122]. Based on their findings, however, the authors cautioned against using PP to gauge fluid responsivity following PLR because its pooled sensitivity was poor (0.56; 95% CI, 0.49–0.53) [122].

One of the first studies to examine the ability of PLR to predict fluid responsivity in children was conducted in 2012 [123]. Investigators measured HR, BP, SBP, SV, and cardiac index (CI) using transthoracic echocardiography in a mixed cohort of

40 PICU patients (ages 1–8 years). PLR predicted fluid responsivity only when CI changed at least 5% from baseline. However, the sensitivity and specificity (both 70%) were lower than those found in adult studies. When the PLR-related CO threshold was increased to $\geq$10%, the corresponding sensitivity and specificity were 55% and 85%, respectively. Consistent with prior adult studies, HR and SBP were not significantly affected by PLR [123]. One-half of patients in this study were initially assessed as nonresponders, also in agreement with prior studies [118, 122, 123]. In another study of 57 critically ill children, age 1 month to 5 years, a change in both SV >10% and CI >8.7% following PLR predicted fluid responsivity as assessed by echocardiography [124]. Again, the specificity (>90%) of the PLR test was greater than the sensitivity, giving further support for PLR testing in critically ill patients that may not tolerate or respond to a fluid challenge. In a third study using standard hemodynamic parameters in 39 children (49% with sepsis, 59% in hypovolemic shock) using electrical cardiometry, only FTc (flow time, corrected) and LVET (left ventricular ejection time) measured at 5 min after PLR were affected [125]. In conclusion, the few studies in children combined with many confounders including varied outcome measures (HR, SBP, SV, CO, CI, PP, $ETCO_2$, etc.), different assessment tools (e.g., echocardiography, bioreactance, thermodilution, pulse contour analysis, and vein diameter), the increased compliance of the child's vascular system, and the hemodynamic depressant effects of anesthetics currently make PLR an uncertain assessment tool of fluid responsiveness in children during blood loss surgery [119, 126].

16.6.3.2 Bioimpedance and Bioreactance CO Monitoring

Noninvasive cardiac output (NiCO) evaluation using bioreactance and bioimpedance has been performed in adults for years but only recently in children. Most NiCO studies in children involve bioimpedance (electrical cardiometry; EC), whereby a high frequency current is transmitted across the thorax between sensor electrodes. As blood flows through the aorta, a change in voltage (resistance) occurs that is then used to calculate cardiac output according to an algorithm [127]. Bioreactance (BR), on the other hand, relies on phase shifts in voltage between sensors in proportion to stroke volume (SV) changes with heart beats [128]. BR sensors are placed on both the right and left sides of the thorax (or, in the case of infants, body trunk), and the phase shifts are averaged together to calculate SV (Fig. 16.3). Because CO = SV × HR, CO is calculated based on the SV at a given heart beat [127, 128].

Most NiCO studies use transthoracic echocardiography (TTE) as the gold standard for comparison, a noninvasive technique requiring expertise and which has limited precision (e.g., approximately 30%) [128]. NiCO has been used in infants to evaluate CO changes at delivery, with position changes, sedation, umbilical cord clamping, and during anesthesia induction. Vergnaud et al. examined 30 sedated and mechanically ventilated children, ages 0–16 years, in the immediate postoperative period and determined that although BR (NICOM®, Cheetah Medical, Tel Aviv, Israel) was predictive in determining fluid responsivity at a SVV cutoff of 10% within 6 hours of surgery, it demonstrated wide limits of agreement compared to

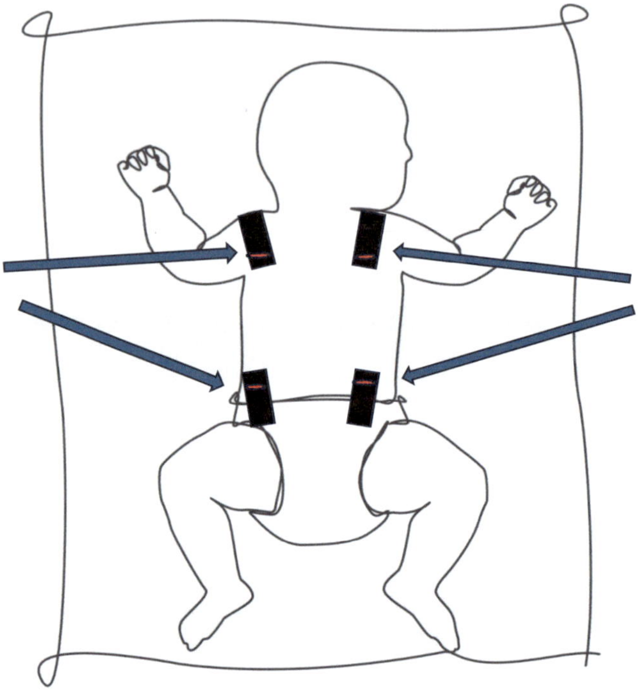

Fig. 16.3 Bioreactance lead placement on an infant

TTE (−0.11; −1.4 to 1.2) and had low precision (45%) [129]. A more recent retrospective review attempted to correlate EC findings with low CO state (as determined by TTE) in 61 children with shock or respiratory failure [130]. Of 41 qualifying patients, a low CO state was not consistently identified through EC.

Although studies are inconsistent as to whether EC or BR is interchangeable with TTE to evaluate CO, studies demonstrate that BR readings for CO tend to be lower than the ultrasound comparisons [127, 131]. NiCO limitations include the size and placement capabilities of the sensors on the small infant trunk, as well as the fact that certain conditions such as intracardiac shunts and high-frequency oscillation may create over- or underestimation of CO [132]. So far, NiCO research is limited to observations of CO changes during or shortly after transfusion, but not for general outcomes or the determination of which patients best benefit from NiCO guidance [128, 132, 133]. In conclusion, EC and BR demonstrate reasonable correlation compared to a gold-standard TTE determination of CO but are best used as trend monitors. There is currently insufficient evidence to support making blood management decisions based on EC or BR values alone [128, 134, 135].

The development of noninvasive monitors of CO and fluid responsivity in children will continue. Scientific exploration for the ideal monitor—noninvasive, continuous, noncalibrated, validated across different age groups and patient types—is fraught with limitations. Reassuring data on pediatric reference values and outcomes is lacking. However, marketing pressures, analytics, and algorithms continue to evolve outside the reach of the busy practitioner [136–138]. A 2020 meta-analysis of 24 studies (16 involving the operating room) determined that finger blood cuff BP measurements in adult surgical patients are not interchangeable with invasive BP reference values [139]. The enticement to employ a finger BP cuff in a healthy child under anesthesia may be great when one considers the difficulty in placing an arterial line in a small child combined with the lack of vascular disease in that population [140]. Still, safety concerns underscore the importance of knowing the basic technology, validation data, study quality, and pediatric-based algorithms behind a developing monitor before using it to make management decisions [139, 141].

16.7 Do Near-Infrared Spectroscopy (NIRS) and Hgb Co-oximetry (SpHb) Reliably Guide Perioperative RBC Transfusion Decisions?

Emerging tools to assess and guide oxygenation management include hemoglobin co-oximetry (SpHb) and near-infrared spectroscopy (NIRS) [142]. These noninvasive monitors provide continuous observation of Hgb levels and regional oxygen saturation (rSO_2), respectively, with the potential to guide blood management. Peripheral pulse oximetry readings (SpO_2) may remain relatively normal despite decreases in Hgb levels or end-organ oxygenation when administering FiO_2 >21% under anesthesia. Trends in SpHb and rSO_2 may signal early changes during blood loss, thus allowing more timely diagnosis and treatment [143]. The following discussion addresses the basics of NIRS and Hgb co-oximetry, with a focus on their utility and limitations in guiding RBC transfusions.

16.7.1 Near-Infrared Spectroscopy (NIRS)

Since the first demonstration in 1977, near-infrared spectroscopy (NIRS) has been increasingly used as a management tool to prevent hypoxemia and subsequent end-organ injury in hospitalized children and adults [144]. The clinical application has expanded beyond direct assessment of regional oxygenation and is now used to guide a variety of clinical situations, particularly in the neonatal patient population. NIRS has become a standard in many institutions to guide clinical management of premature infant care, including patient ductus arteriosus (PDA) treatment, apnea and bradycardia, use of vasopressors, hyperoxia, ventilator management, and hypoxic ischemic encephalopathy [145, 146]. NIRS has also been used to follow ventilation and hemodynamic management during a variety of procedures, including trauma resuscitation, pyloric stenosis repair, and congenital heart surgery [144, 146–148].

NIRS monitors tissue oxygenation through a skin sensor probe that emits near infrared light to a tissue depth of 1–3 cm [149, 150]. The light is absorbed differentially by oxygenated and deoxygenated hemoglobin passing through the underlying arterial-capillary-venous system. Hemoglobin flowing beneath the NIRS probe is sensed by superficial and deep photodetectors in an arc pattern and is then represented as a ratio (percentage) of oxygenated hemoglobin to total hemoglobin (rSO_2) exiting the area underneath the probe [151, 152] (Fig. 16.4). The information

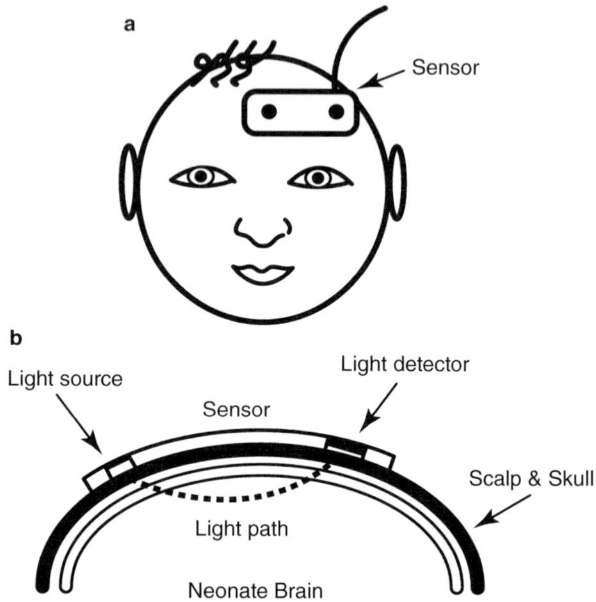

Fig. 16.4 Placement and infrared light path of a neonatal cerebral oximeter. (**a**) Placement of sensor containing light source and sensor. (**b**) Light path from source to detector through scalp, skull, and brain tissue layers. Reprinted with permission from Rais-Bahrami K, Rivera O, Short BL. Validation of a noninvasive neonatal optical cerebral oximeter in veno-venous ECMO patients with a cephalad catheter. J Perinatol. 2006;26(10):628-35

gleaned from the "shallow" skin or scalp layer is extracted from the deeper cortical infrared data.

The rSO_2 value is an algorithmic calculation (which may vary between device manufacturers) with an arterial: venous saturation contribution of approximately 30:70 due to the preponderance of venous circulation underlying the probe [145, 153, 154]. Different NIRS devices may express tissue oxygenation values as either a saturation percentage (rSO_2), a tissue oxygenation index (TOI), or, when factored against systemic arterial saturation, as fractional tissue oxygen extraction (FTOE) [146, 154, 155]. Cortical rSO_2 has been shown to correlate with jugular and central venous oxygen saturations, and the latter are often used for comparison because the ideal tissue oxygen saturation is unknown; jugular venous blood is located more proximal to blood leaving the NIRS-monitored cortical tissue [156–158]. Although a low rSO_2 suggests high oxygen extraction, it can also indicate a low flow state or severe anemia. Ongoing clinical experience and NIRS research have established that clinical interpretation is complex and should be based on trend patterns rather than individual values. The patient's baseline rSO_2 must be obtained as a reference point before interpreting rSO_2 results.

Although NIRS is most commonly used to monitor cerebral cortex oxygenation, it has been used to follow rSO_2 in the renal, splanchnic, and musculoskeletal vascular beds [146, 149]. The accuracy of readings is affected by several factors, including dark skin, pressure placement, scalp tissue, and body hair [159]. It is important to use age-appropriate probes; adult-sized NIRS probes may have an upper limit rSO_2 of 95%, therefore not sensing neonatal rSO_2 values that are approximately 10% higher than adult values. According to manufacturer data, the baseline rSO_2 of dark-pigmented individuals may range from 55 to 82 [160]. The proprietary algorithms of the various device manufacturers can also influence rSO_2 readings and may vary up to 15% [154, 161].

The ideal NIRS rSO_2 value(s) for currently used clinical applications are unknown, particularly in the non-neonatal patient population [161]. Numerous small studies have been performed in the neonatal ICU and congenital heart surgery patient populations, with particular focus on cerebral rSO_2 lower limits that may be associated with poor neurologic outcomes. Healthy infants have an rSO_2 between 40 and 55% at birth which increases to approximately 75% during the first few postnatal days and then falls into the range of 55–85% during childhood. Thereafter, NIRS values progressively increase until approximately age 65 years when the mean rSO_2 drops to 63% (range 54.7–70.8%) [162]. There is significant interpatient variability in baseline rSO_2 values. A critically low rSO_2 value in children is approximately 40% but cannot be interpreted in isolation [146, 163]. A 20% decrease in rSO_2 from baseline has been associated with altered neurologic outcomes in children undergoing cardiac surgery [164, 165]. In premature infants, a population for which the critically low mean blood pressure is uncertain, the amount of time spent with a low rSO_2 relative to baseline may influence neurodevelopmental outcome more than hypotension alone [166]. When two sites are monitored simultaneously, a difference in rSO_2 greater than >20% is considered actionable [150, 161, 167] (Fig. 16.5).

Many of the normative NIRS values used in sick children have been extrapolated from adult experience. Most studies before 2012 were performed using adult probes [161]. Furthermore, many studies of cerebral oximetry use unilateral (versus bilateral) probe placement, but rSO_2 differences of more than 10% between the right and left cerebral hemisphere are common in severely ill patients [161]. In a prospective

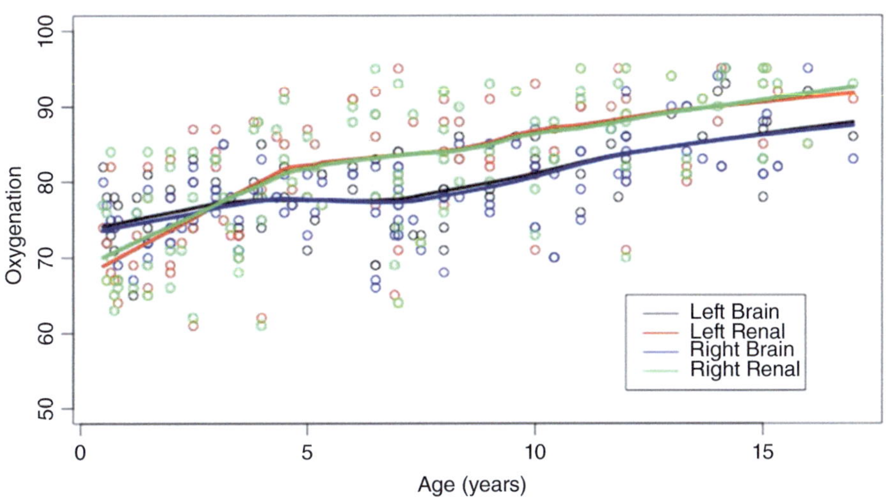

Fig. 16.5 Age-related differences in cerebral and renal NIRS values in healthy children. Reprinted with permission from Ozturk NY, Aygun B, Uyar E, Girgin FI. Comparison of Bilateral Cerebro-Renal Tissue Oxygenations in Healthy Children. Indian J Pediatr. 2020;87(2):99-104

observational study of 124 extremely low birthweight (ELBW) premature infants whose cerebral and mesenteric FTOE were monitored in the first week of life, anemia, a lower Hgb RBC transfusion threshold, and greater prematurity were associated with increased FTOE, with the brain preferentially extracting more oxygen compared to the gut [143]. The clinical relevance of this relationship was not determined, but the authors suggest it may one day inform protective brain and feeding practices.

Our ability to understand the ability of NIRS to gauze safe Hgb levels and to guide RBC transfusions is in its infancy [154]. Most studies exploring NIRS for RBC transfusions are observational and document rSO_2 changes during or shortly after transfusion [145, 149, 168–173]. The correlation of NIRS with Hgb levels also varies between studies [154, 170]. Because tissue oxygen extraction increases with systemic hypoxemia or anemia, an increased cerebral FTOE (e.g., >0.4) may prompt a change in perioperative management, such as altered ventilation, an increase in FiO_2, addition of vasopressors, or, when all other contributing factors are considered, an increase in the patient's hemoglobin [150]. A prospective randomized trial assessed rSO_2 FTOE from skeletal muscle sensors (i.e., forearm, rather than brain), but investigators did not find FTOE to be predictive of the need for an RBC transfusion [174]. In another small trial of preterm neonates, FTOE did not vary with hypotension or levels of hemoglobin F (HgbF), prompting investigators to conclude that the findings were confounded by autoregulation changes in cerebral blood flow [175]. In an observational study of 53 critically ill children with a mean baseline hemoglobin of 6.3 g/dL, median age 11 months, a RBC transfusion (15 mL/kg) was correlated with an improvement in cerebral rSO_2, a decrease in FTOE, and reduced rSO_2 variability up to 7 h post-transfusion [176]. In addition, decreases in rSO_2 were associated with active bleeding and decreases in Hgb levels. However, the overall data in that study was deemed inadequate to support general use of NIRS to guide blood transfusions [153]. With an understanding that the ideal Hgb transfusion trigger in neonates is unknown, a prospective observational study of premature neonates found that a NIRS splanchnic-cerebral oxygenation ratio ($\leq$0.73) predicted which patients would benefit from an RBC transfusion 15 mL/kg over 4 h [177]. The Hgb threshold for transfusion in the included cohort ($n = 34$) was $\leq$11 g/dL.

The clinical interpretation of a low cerebral rSO_2 and a high FTOE is complicated and should be based on multiple considerations. Pain, light anesthesia, and seizure activity may lead to increased oxygen consumption with altered cerebral blood flow, resulting in an increase in FTOE and a decrease in cerebral rSO_2 ($rScO_2$) [150]. A low blood pressure has been associated with a 15% decrease in rSO_2 in children undergoing scoliosis surgery [147]. During mechanical ventilation, an anemic patient may have a sudden decrease in cerebral rSO_2, prompting the assumption that an increase in FiO_2, administration of a vasopressor, or an RBC transfusion is necessary to improve cerebral perfusion and oxygen delivery. In fact, hyperventilation may produce a decrease in cerebral rSO_2 secondary to cerebral vasoconstriction and a concomitant decrease in cerebral blood flow. The relationship between end-tidal CO_2 and neonatal cerebral rSO_2 is illustrated in Fig. 16.6 [146]. The appropriate solution to a decrease in cerebral rSO_2 may be ventilator adjustment rather than

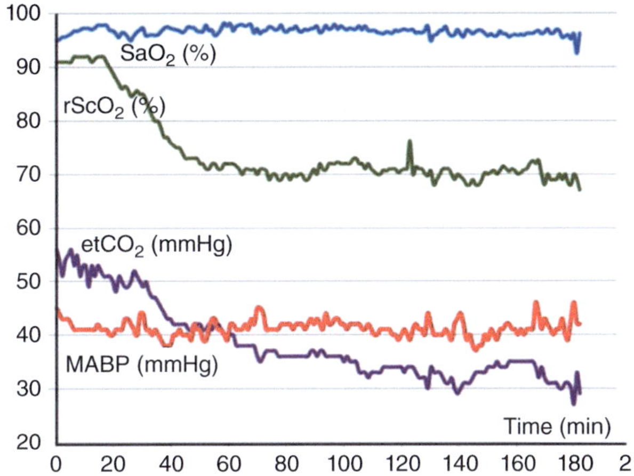

Fig. 16.6 An illustration of how an acute decrease in $etCO_2$ may relate to a decrease in regional cerebral oxygen saturation (rScO2), when MAP and peripheral SaO_2 remain stable. The effects of hyperventilation on cerebral perfusion. Reprinted from Dix LM, van Bel F, Lemmers PM. Monitoring Cerebral Oxygenation in Neonates: An Update. Front Pediatr. 2017;5:160 under Creative Commons License Attribution (CC BY)

unnecessary treatment such as hyperoxia, vasopressor therapy, or an RBC transfusion.

Systematic reviews have failed to conclude that NIRS is appropriate for routine patient oxygenation assessment [144, 153, 178]. Evidence that NIRS-guided patient management improves pediatric patient outcomes is inconsistent and confounded by multiple variables including small study size, bias, excessive heterogeneity, and implementation of multiple device brands (there are at least 10 on the market) [153, 154, 157]. However, widespread NIRS usage during surgery and anesthesia is likely to continue, paving the way for large-scale studies addressing accuracy and outcomes in specific management situations [157]. In one small study, a 20% decrease in baseline rSO_2 (a degree of change considered actionable) occurred in one-fifth of infants under general anesthesia [179]. In an editorial review addressing NIRS in adult cardiovascular surgery, it was emphasized that the lack of definitive evidence that NIRS can improve patient outcomes neither precludes nor supports its routine use in monitoring cerebral oxygenation during cardiac surgery [159]. Standardized protocols based on what is generally accepted can minimize variability in both application and interpretation. A pragmatically based guideline for children without cyanotic heart disease from the Scottish National Health Service advises management changes with the following NIRS values [150]:

- An rSO_2 <60%
- A >20% difference in rSO_2 between two sites that are monitored simultaneously (e.g., right and left cerebral hemispheres, renal-cerebral, or cerebral-mesenteric)

- A >20% decrease in rSO_2 from baseline
- A persistently elevated rSO_2 (i.e., >95%)

A persistently elevated rSO_2 may indicate reduced oxygen extraction, consistent with hypoxic encephalopathy. Large interhemispheric differences in rSO_2 may be seen in shock states or during a cerebrovascular accident.

In conclusion, the data supporting NIRS to guide RBC transfusion is inconclusive. However, NIRS has been shown to be associated with slight improvements in rSO_2 following transfusion in the short term. The longer-term clinical significance of this relationship is unknown. Although it is not recommended as a routine monitor of cerebral oxygenation, NIRS may be a useful adjunct in overall assessment of children with concerning perfusion and oxygenation profiles [180].

16.7.2 Continuous Hgb Co-oximetry

A transfusion decision should not be made based on a single diagnostic variable [3, 5, 181, 182]. Despite this evidence-based principle, the Hgb level as an RBC transfusion trigger continues to be a focus in clinical practice and academic research. In both children and adults, there is now a debate over whether to advocate a disease-specific versus a one-size-fits-all restrictive Hgb trigger (e.g., 7 g/dL) [183–185]. There is a tendency to perform serial testing with a goal to maintain the Hgb within a narrow range during perioperative blood loss. Frequent testing is invasive and contributes to iatrogenic anemia, and results are often not in step with actual blood loss. The Hgb co-oximeter is a logical solution to noninvasive, continuous Hgb monitoring of critically ill patients who are at risk of serial phlebotomy.

Clinically available noninvasive Hgb monitors calculate the Hgb level based on its variable absorption of different light wavelengths during pulsatile flow, using spectrophotometry or photoplethysmography, in a continuous or spot-check fashion [186]. The noninvasively obtained Hgb is designated as SpHb and can be monitored continuously using a probe similar to that used for SpO_2 or monitored intermittently using a hand-held co-oximeter [187, 188]. A commonly used brand of co-oximeter has additional functions for continuous monitoring including carboxyhemoglobin, methemoglobin, and a variety of peripheral perfusion indices [189].

There are numerous small studies and several systematic reviews examining the accuracy of clinically available SpHb devices used in pediatric patients. Although SpHb has demonstrated good correlation with invasively obtained laboratory Hgb results, devices continue to demonstrate wide levels of agreement under

Bland-Altman analysis, creating concern that noninvasive Hgb monitoring cannot be relied upon to make sound transfusion decisions based on SpHb values alone [188, 190–195]. In general, SpHb values seen during surgery may deviate from the corresponding conventional laboratory value by 1–3 g/dL [186–188, 192, 196, 197]. Many prior studies compare SpHb measurements—which are the result of averaging over minutes—to single laboratory measurements obtained at single point in time [195, 198]. The sensor probe size can also contribute to variable readings based on placement location, patient size, and device brand [187, 199, 200]. In one observational study, SpHb overestimated corresponding laboratory Hgb values <12 g/dL and underestimated laboratory results ≥12 g/dL [186]. This lack of precision is most evident with severe anemia (e.g., 6.5–8 g/dL), which is the range that is often used as a transfusion trigger [44, 194, 201]. In a meta-analysis of 32 adult and pediatric studies (13 performed in the operating room), the mean difference and standard deviation between the various SpHb monitors and laboratory analyzers were 0.39 ± 1.32 g/dL and (−2.21 to 2.98) [188]. There was also significant heterogeneity in accuracy between locations (e.g., OR, ICU, or emergency department). Investigators in this meta-analysis estimated that if a patient has a laboratory Hgb of 10 g/dL during surgery, the SpHb is predicted to fall between 7.8 and 13.0 g/dL [188]. They concluded that a SpHb <8.69 g/dL should be confirmed with a laboratory sample because there is a 2.5% chance that the invasively obtained Hgb will be <6 g/dL. Park et al. compared accuracy of SpHb during preoperative evaluation in 100 patients and found the median accuracy to be significantly greater in children compared to the adult cohort (bias −1.2 ± 1.5 g/dL and −2.6 ± 2.2 g/dL, respectively; $p < 0.001$) [199].

Despite the fact that there is not an accepted SpHb threshold for RBC transfusion, interest in noninvasive SpHb monitoring is likely to continue. Its greatest value is as a trend monitor to alert the practitioner to real-time changes in the Hgb tracing, persistent downward trends, or patient responses to volume resuscitation [195]. Recognizing its limitations, the SpHb monitor continues to be recommended for blood loss cases to reduce phlebotomy and supplement overall hemodynamic assessment [44, 181]. Because of its moderately good specificity and negative predictive value, spot checks using the handheld SpHb monitor in the preoperative setting may be used to screen for anemia and avoid unnecessary venipuncture [202].

A conventional laboratory Hgb level should be obtained before making an RBC transfusion decision based on SpHb values, when feasible [200, 201, 203]. Figure 16.7 illustrates the relationship between spot and continuous Hgb measurements with conventional laboratory Hgb values during surgery [195].

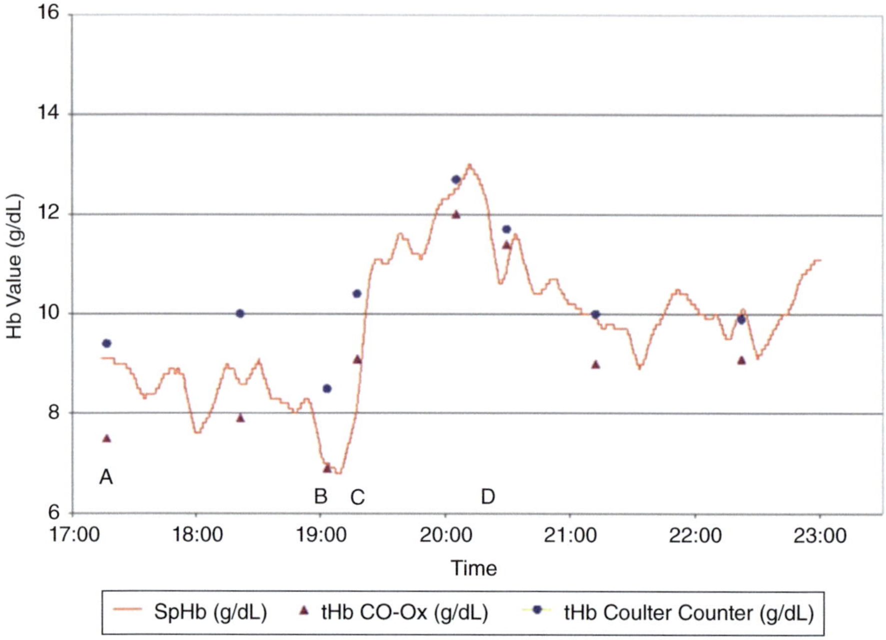

Fig. 16.7 The relationship between continuous SpHb (orange line) to spot co-oximeter (red triangles) and laboratory Hgb values (blue dots) during surgery. Note the varied relationship between the co-oximeter and laboratory values. Reprinted from Barker SJ, Shander A, Ramsay MA. Continuous Noninvasive Hemoglobin Monitoring: A Measured Response to a Critical Review. Anesth Analg. 2016;122(2):565-72 under Creative Commons Attribution License (CCBY-NC-ND)

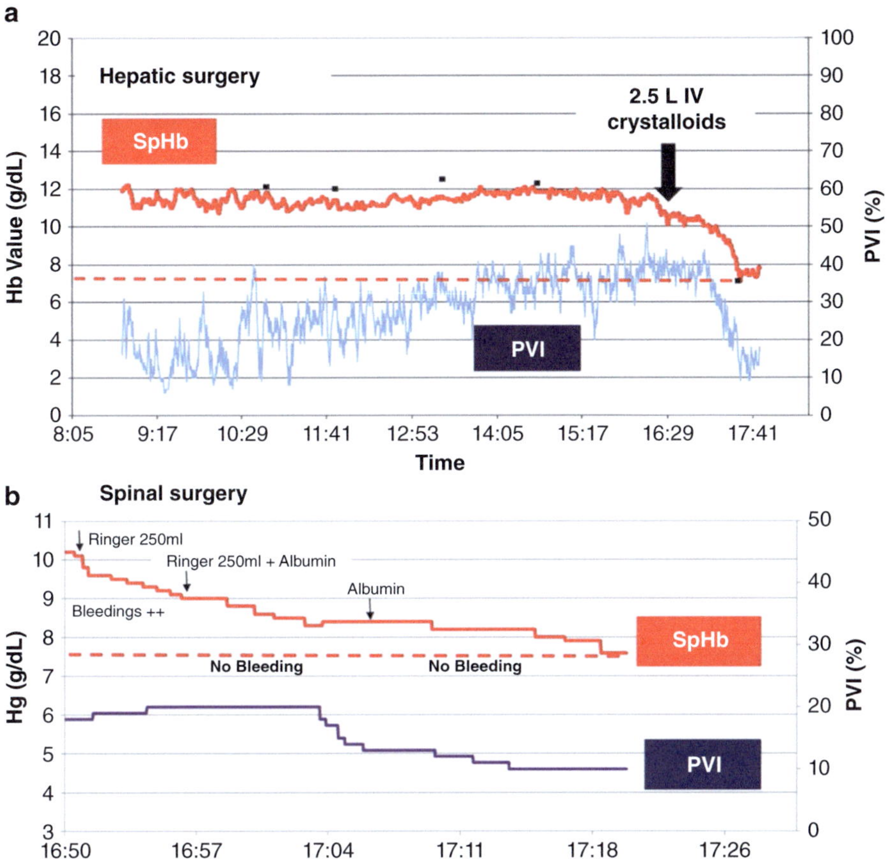

Fig. 16.8 Hemodilution secondary to colloid and crystalloid administration in (**a**) posthepatic resection and (**b**) spine surgery in the absence of intraoperative blood loss (red dotted line) as denoted by decreases in both SpHb and PVI. Reprinted from Perel A. Iatrogenic hemodilution: a possible cause for avoidable blood transfusions? Crit Care. 2017;21(1):291 under Creative Commons Attribution License 4.0

SpHb monitoring may also be used in conjunction with PVI to uncover hemodilution that may occur with goal-directed fluid therapy in the absence of blood loss (Fig. 16.8) [204].

16.8 Summary of Key Learning Objectives

16.8.1 What Tools Are Available to Quantify Perioperative Blood Loss?

Available tools to assess perioperative blood loss include visual observation of the surgical field, gravimetric before-and-after weighing of sponges, direct weighing, and colorimetric technology. Visual estimation of blood loss alone, the historical standard, is inaccurate. In general, available methods to estimate blood loss during surgery are imprecise but necessary. A maximal allowable blood loss (MABL) should be calculated before all blood loss surgeries to support safe and rational transfusion decision-making.

16.8.2 What Are Some Physical Exam Findings Indicative of Clinically Significant Blood Loss?

Readily available physical findings during clinically significant blood loss include:

- Capillary refill time: the time required for color to return to the skin when pressure is applied.
- Skin mottling: the irregular "lace-like" blotching of the skin caused by hypoperfusion and patchy capillary vasoconstriction.
- Body temperature gradients: peripheral vasoconstriction associated with volume loss leading to a lowered skin temperature as blood flows away from the periphery to the central circulation.
- Pulse amplitude and heart sounds: peripheral pulse intensity decreases during volume depletion or blood loss and may be evident prior to a decrease in SBP.
- Skin color observation: ambient light may be inadequate during surgery to properly evaluate for the presence or absence of skin color changes.

16.8.3 Do Conventional Pediatric Vital Signs Reliably Indicate Perioperative Blood Loss

The decision to transfuse a patient due to clinically significant blood loss may not be apparent early in surgery because children compensate with intense vasoconstriction and a rapid heart rate that may have other causes. Thus, the determination of clinically significant blood loss requires utilization of all conventional vital signs (BP, HR, body temperature, ECG), indices of oxygenation and cardiac output (SaO_2 and $ETCO_2$), and, when possible, CaO_2, surrogates of CO, a-v DO_2, and SvO_2, as well as conventional laboratory values. The SBP is often a focus of intraoperative transfusion decision-making. Blood pressure reference ranges in healthy children in the *unanesthetized* state are based on hypertensive values for age and sex. Although normal intraoperative blood pressures have been retrospectively studied, there are yet no validated NIBP reference ranges for children undergoing anesthesia.

16.8.4 How Is Circulatory Function Monitored Using Wave Form Analysis?

The gold standard to measure cardiac output (CO) in critically ill patients has been the pulmonary artery catheter (PAC), an invasive monitor that requires expert management, has associated complications, and inconsistently predicts CO. To quickly and safely assess a patient's CO response to fluid resuscitation at the bedside, surrogate measures of CO have been adopted. These measures rely on the fact that during normal respiration there is an increase in intrathoracic pressure with a decrease in venous return, followed by a decrease in stroke volume (SV), with each respiratory cycle. The changes in SV with fluid administration can be continuously followed using an arterial catheter or pulse oximeter through "pulse waveform analysis." At this point in time, there is not a consistent definition of fluid responsiveness in children; it may vary from 10% to over 25%, depending on the study, the patient population, and the monitor utilized.

16.8.5 Do Hgb Co-oximetry (SpHb) and Near-Infrared Spectroscopy (NIRS) Accurately Guide Perioperative RBC Transfusion Decisions?

Emerging tools to guide oxygenation management include hemoglobin co-oximetry (SpHb) and near-infrared spectroscopy (NIRS). These noninvasive monitors provide continuous observation of Hgb levels and regional oxygen saturation (rSO_2), respectively. NIRS is increasingly used as a management tool to assess hypoxemia and subsequent end-organ injury in hospitalized children and adults. The ideal NIRS rSO_2 value(s) for currently used clinical applications are unknown, particularly in the non-neonatal patient population. Our ability to understand the ability of NIRS to gauze Hgb levels and to guide RBC transfusions is in its infancy. The clinical interpretation of a low cerebral rSO_2 is complicated and should be based on multiple considerations. Systematic reviews have failed to conclude that NIRS is appropriate for routine patient oxygenation assessment. However, NIRS may be a useful adjunct in overall assessment of children with concerning perfusion and oxygenation profiles.

The Hgb level as an RBC transfusion trigger continues to be a focus in clinical practice and academic research. Although SpHb has demonstrated good correlation with invasively obtained laboratory Hgb results, devices continue to demonstrate wide levels of agreement. Recognizing its limitations, the SpHb monitor continues to be recommended for blood loss cases to reduce phlebotomy and supplement overall hemodynamic assessment. A conventional laboratory Hgb level should be obtained before making an RBC transfusion decision based on SpHb values, when feasible.

References

1. Fasano RM, Doctor A, Stowell SR, Spinella PC, Carson JL, Maier CL, et al. Optimizing RBC transfusion outcomes in patients with acute illness and in the chronic transfusion setting. Transfus Med Rev. 2023;37(4):150758.
2. Baker L, Park L, Gilbert R, Ahn H, Martel A, Lenet T, et al. Intraoperative red blood cell transfusion decision-making: a systematic review of guidelines. Ann Surg. 2021;274(1):86–96.
3. Valentine SL, Bembea MM, Muszynski JA, Cholette JM, Doctor A, Spinella PC, et al. Consensus recommendations for RBC transfusion practice in critically ill children from the pediatric critical care transfusion and anemia expertise initiative. Pediatr Crit Care Med. 2018;19(9):884–98.
4. Faraoni D, Meier J, New HV, Van der Linden PJ, Hunt BJ. Patient blood management for neonates and children undergoing cardiac surgery: 2019 NATA guidelines. J Cardiothorac Vasc Anesth. 2019;33(12):3249–63.
5. Russell RT, Esparaz JR, Beckwith MA, Abraham PJ, Bembea MM, Borgman MA, et al. Pediatric traumatic hemorrhagic shock consensus conference recommendations. J Trauma Acute Care Surg. 2023;94(1S):S2–S10.
6. Bennett S, Baker LK, Martel G, Shorr R, Pawlik TM, Tinmouth A, et al. The impact of perioperative red blood cell transfusions in patients undergoing liver resection: a systematic review. HPB. 2017;19(4):321–30.
7. Mutschler M, Nienaber U, Brockamp T, Wafaisade A, Wyen H, Peiniger S, et al. A critical reappraisal of the ATLS classification of hypovolaemic shock: does it really reflect clinical reality? Resuscitation. 2013;84(3):309–13.
8. Guly HR, Bouamra O, Spiers M, Dark P, Coats T, Lecky FE, et al. Vital signs and estimated blood loss in patients with major trauma: testing the validity of the ATLS classification of hypovolaemic shock. Resuscitation. 2011;82(5):556–9.
9. Henry S. ATLS 10th edition offers new insights into managing trauma patients. 2018. https://bulletin.facs.org/2018/06/atls-10th-edition-offers-new-insights-into-managing-trauma-patients/#printpreview. Accessed 21 March 2023.
10. Galvagno SM, Nahmias JT, Young DA. Advanced trauma life support. Anesthesiol Clin. 2019;37(1):13–32.
11. Ramamoorthy C, Haberkern CM, Bhananker SM, Domino KB, Posner KL, Campos JS, et al. Anesthesia-related cardiac arrest in children with heart disease: data from the Pediatric Perioperative Cardiac Arrest (POCA) registry. Anesth Analg. 2010;110(5):1376–82.
12. Teruya J. Red blood cell transfusion in infants and children: indications. In: UpToDate Pathways. 2023. www.uptodate.com. Accessed 20 February 2023.
13. Cote CJ, Grabowski EF, Stowell CP. Chapter 12: strategies for blood product management, reducing transfusions, and massive blood transfusion. In: Cote CJ, ehman J, Anderson BJ, editors. Cote and Lerman's a practice of anesthesia for infants and children. 6th ed. Elsevier: Amsterdam; 2019. p. 257–80.e13.
14. Gross JB. Estimating allowable blood loss: corrected for dilution. Anesthesiology. 1983;58(3):277–80.
15. Gibon E, Courpied JP, Hamadouche M. Total joint replacement and blood loss: what is the best equation? Int Orthop. 2013;37(4):735–9.
16. Lopez-Picado A, Albinarrate A, Barrachina B. Determination of perioperative blood loss: accuracy or approximation? Anesth Analg. 2017;125(1):280–6.
17. Gerdessen L, Meybohm P, Choorapoikayil S, Herrmann E, Taeuber I, Neef V, et al. Comparison of common perioperative blood loss estimation techniques: a systematic review and meta-analysis. J Clin Monit Comput. 2021;35(2):245–58.
18. Gross JB. Maximum allowable blood loss (ABL) without transfusion. MD+Calc. 2023. https://www.mdcalc.com/calc/3905/maximum-allowable-blood-loss-abl-without-transfusion. Accessed 18 October 2023.

19. American Society of Anesthesiologists Task Force on Perioperative Blood M. Practice guidelines for perioperative blood management: an updated report by the American Society of Anesthesiologists Task Force on Perioperative Blood Management. Anesthesiology. 2015;122(2):241–75.
20. Bhananker SM, Ramamoorthy C, Geiduschek JM, Posner KL, Domino KB, Haberkern CM, et al. Anesthesia-related cardiac arrest in children: update from the Pediatric Perioperative Cardiac Arrest Registry. Anesth Analg. 2007;105(2):344–50.
21. Nellis ME, Tucci M, Lacroix J, Spinella PC, Haque KD, Stock A, et al. Bleeding assessment scale in critically ill children (BASIC): physician-driven diagnostic criteria for bleeding severity. Crit Care Med. 2019;47(12):1766–72.
22. Nellis ME, Karam O, Valentine SL, Bateman ST, Remy KE, Lacroix J, et al. Executive summary of recommendations and expert consensus for plasma and platelet transfusion practice in critically ill children: from the transfusion and anemia EXpertise initiative-control/avoidance of bleeding (TAXI-CAB). Pediatr Crit Care Med. 2022;23(1):34–51.
23. Karam O, Nellis ME, Zantek ND, Lacroix J, Faustino EV. Criteria for clinically relevant bleeding in critically ill children: an international survey. Pediatr Crit Care Med. 2019;20(3):137–44.
24. Piekarski F, Gerdessen L, Schmitt E, Friedrichson B, Neef V, Meybohm P, et al. Quantification of intraoperative blood loss in a simulated scenario using a novel device. Shock. 2021;55(6):759–65.
25. Ali Algadiem E, Aleisa AA, Alsubaie HI, Buhlaiqah NR, Algadeeb JB, Alsneini HA. Blood loss estimation using gauze visual analogue. Trauma. 2016;21(2):e34131. https://doi.org/10.5812/traumamon.34131.
26. Hughes K, Chang YC, Sedrak J, Torres A. A clinically practical way to estimate surgical blood loss. Dermatol Online J. 2007;13(4):17.
27. Cholette JM, Willems A, Valentine SL, Bateman ST, Schwartz SM, et al. Recommendations on RBC transfusion in infants and children with acquired and congenital heart disease from the pediatric critical care transfusion and anemia expertise initiative. Pediatr Crit Care Med. 2018;19(9S):S137–48.
28. Lima A, Bakker J. Clinical assessment of peripheral circulation. Curr Opin Crit Care. 2015;21(3):226–31.
29. Eisenhut M. Factors influencing capillary refill time. J Pediatr. 2007;151(5):e17.
30. Fleming S, Gill P, Jones C, Taylor JA, Van den Bruel A, Heneghan C, et al. The diagnostic value of capillary refill time for detecting serious illness in children: a systematic review and meta-analysis. PLoS One. 2015;10(9):e0138155.
31. Atandi BO, Chokwe TM, Sulemanji DS. Challenges of anesthetic monitoring in low- and middle-income countries: availability of equipment in major referral hospitals in Kenya. Anesth Analg. 2023;137(3):648–55.
32. Pickard A, Karlen W, Ansermino JM. Capillary refill time: is it still a useful clinical sign? Anesth Analg. 2011;113(1):120–3.
33. Van de Voorde P, Turner NM, Djakow J, de Lucas N, Martinez-Mejias A, Biarent D, et al. European resuscitation council guidelines 2021: paediatric life support. Resuscitation. 2021;161:327–87.
34. Atkins DL, Berger S, Duff JP, Gonzales JC, Hunt EA, Joyner BL, et al. Part 11: pediatric basic life support and cardiopulmonary resuscitation quality: 2015 American Heart Association Guidelines update for cardiopulmonary resuscitation and emergency cardiovascular care. Circulation. 2015;132(18 Suppl 2):S519–25.
35. Duff JP, Topjian AA, Berg MD, Chan M, Haskell SE, Joyner BL, et al. 2019 American Heart Association focused update on pediatric basic life support: an update to the American Heart Association guidelines for cardiopulmonary resuscitation and emergency cardiovascular care. Circulation. 2019;140(24):915–21.
36. Balamuth F, Fitzgerald JC, Weiss SL. Chapter 10: shock. In: Bachur RG, Shaw KN, editors. Fleisher & Ludwig's textbook of pediatric emergency medicine. 8th ed. Philadelphia: Lippincott and Wilkins; 2021.

37. Sessler DI. Temperature monitoring and perioperative thermoregulation. Anesthesiology. 2008;109(2):318–38.
38. Burgess GE, Cooper JR, Marino RJ, Peuler MJ. Continuous monitoring of skin temperature using a liquid-crystal thermometer during anesthesia. South Med J. 1978;71(5):516–8.
39. Greenbaum LA. Deficit therapy. In: Kliegman RM, Geme J, editors. Nelson textbook of pediatrics. 21st ed. Philadelphia: Elsevier; 2020. p. 429.
40. Pfeiffer S, Wong HR. Circulatory failure/shock. In: Lucking SE, Maffei FA, Tamburro RF, editors. Pediatric critical care study guide. 2nd ed. Springer: Cham; 2021. p. 479–82.
41. American Society of Anesthesiologists. Standards for basic anesthetic monitoring. 2020. https://www.asahq.org/standards-and-practice-parameters/standards-for-basic-anesthetic-monitoring. Accessed 7 February 2024.
42. Cecconi M, De Backer D, Antonelli M, Beale R, Bakker J, Hofer C, et al. Consensus on circulatory shock and hemodynamic monitoring. Task force of the European Society of Intensive Care Medicine. Intensive Care Med. 2014;40(12):1795–815.
43. Gutierrez JA, Theodorou AA. Oxygen delivery and oxygen consumption in pediatric critical care. In: Lucking SE, Maffei FA, Tamburro RF, editors. Pediatric critical care study guide. 2nd ed. Cham: Springer; 2021. p. 17.
44. Kietaibl S, Ahmed A, Afshari A, Albaladejo P, Aldecoa C, Barauskas G, et al. Management of severe peri-operative bleeding: guidelines from the European Society of Anaesthesiology and Intensive Care: second update 2022. Eur J Anaesthesiol. 2023;40(4):226–304.
45. Fogagnolo A, Taccone FS, Vincent JL, Benetto G, Cavalcante E, Marangoni E, et al. Using arterial-venous oxygen difference to guide red blood cell transfusion strategy. Crit Care. 2020;24(1):160.
46. Vallet B, Adamczyk S, Barreau O, Lebuffe G. Physiologic transfusion triggers. Best Pract Res Clin Anaesthesiol. 2007;21(2):173–81. https://doi.org/10.1016/j.bpa.2007.02.003.
47. Karlsson J, Lönnqvist PA. Blood pressure and flow in pediatric anesthesia: an educational review. Paediatr Anaesth. 2022;32(1):10–6.
48. Scott MJ. Perioperative patients with hemodynamic instability: consensus recommendations of the anesthesia patient safety foundation. Anesth Analg. 2024;138(4):713–24.
49. Papaioannou TG, Karageorgopoulou TD, Sergentanis TN, Protogerou AD, Psaltopoulou T, Sharman JE, et al. Accuracy of commercial devices and methods for noninvasive estimation of aortic systolic blood pressure a systematic review and meta-analysis of invasive validation studies. J Hypertens. 2016;34(7):1237–48.
50. Joffe R, Duff J, Garcia Guerra G, Pugh J, Joffe AR. The accuracy of blood pressure measured by arterial line and non-invasive cuff in critically ill children. Crit Care. 2016;20(1):177.
51. Galvagno SM, Nahmias JT, Young DA. Advanced Trauma Life Support((R)) update 2019: management and applications for adults and special populations. Anesthesiol Clin. 2019;37(1):13–32.
52. de Graaff JC, Pasma W, van Buuren S, Duijghuisen JJ, Nafiu OO, Kheterpal S, et al. Reference values for noninvasive blood pressure in children during anesthesia: a multicentered retrospective observational cohort study. Anesthesiology. 2016;125(5):904–13.
53. Bernstein D. History and physical examination in cardiac evaluation. In: Kliegman RM, Geme J, editors. Nelson textbook of pediatrics. 21st ed. Philadelphia: Elsevier; 2020. p. 2351–58.
54. Wani TM, Hakim M, Ramesh A, Rehman S, Majid Y, Miller R, et al. Risk factors for post-induction hypotension in children presenting for surgery. Pediatr Surg Int. 2018;34(12):1333–8.
55. Nafiu OO, Voepel-Lewis T, Morris M, Chimbira WT, Malviya S, Reynolds PI, et al. How do pediatric anesthesiologists define intraoperative hypotension? Paediatr Anaesth. 2009;19(11):1048–53.
56. Society for Pediatric Anesthesia. Pedi crisis critical events checklist. 2023. https://pedsanesthesia.org/wp-content/uploads/2023/04/SPAPediCrisisChecklistsMarch2023.pdf. Accessed 1 December 2023.
57. Karlsson J, Lonnqvist PA. Blood pressure and flow in pediatric anesthesia: an educational review. Paediatr Anaesth. 2022;32(1):10–6.

58. McCann ME, de Graaff JC, Dorris L, Disma N, Withington D, Bell G, et al. Neurodevelopmental outcome at 5 years of age after general anaesthesia or awake-regional anaesthesia in infancy (GAS): an international, multicentre, randomised, controlled equivalence trial. Lancet. 2019;393(10172):664–77.
59. McCann ME, Schouten AN. Beyond survival; influences of blood pressure, cerebral perfusion and anesthesia on neurodevelopment. Paediatr Anaesth. 2014;24(1):68–73.
60. Hillgruber RJ, Lutskov P, West NC, Whyte S, Görges M. Blood pressure nomograms for children undergoing general anesthesia, stratified by age and anesthetic type, using data from a retrospective cohort at a tertiary pediatric center. J Clin Monit Comput. 2022;36(6):1667–77.
61. Sottas CE, Cumin D, Anderson BJ. Blood pressure and heart rates in neonates and preschool children: an analysis from 10 years of electronic recording. Paediatr Anaesth. 2016;26(11):1064–70.
62. Topjian AA, Raymond TT, Atkins D, Chan M, Duff JP, Joyner BL, et al. Part 4: pediatric basic and advanced life support 2020 American Heart Association guidelines for cardiopulmonary resuscitation and emergency cardiovascular care. Pediatrics. 2021;147(Suppl 1):S469–523.
63. Topjian AA, Raymond TT, Atkins D, Chan M, Duff JP, Joyner BL, et al. Part 4: pediatric basic and advanced life support: 2020 American Heart Association guidelines for cardiopulmonary resuscitation and emergency cardiovascular care. Circulation. 2020;142(suppl 2):S469–523.
64. European Resuscitation Council. Part 10: pediatric advanced life support. Resuscitation. 2000;46(1-3):343–99.
65. Marciniak B. Growth and development. In: Coté CJ, Lerman J, Anderson B, editors. A practice of anesthesia for infants and children. 5th ed. Philadelphia: Elsevier; 2013. p. 7–20.
66. Nordin A, Shi J, Wheeler K, Xiang H, Kenney B. Age-adjusted shock index: from injury to arrival. J Pediatr Surg. 2019;54(5):984–8.
67. Acker SN, Bredbeck B, Partrick DA, Kulungowski AM, Barnett CC, Bensard DD. Shock index, pediatric age-adjusted (SIPA) is more accurate than age-adjusted hypotension for trauma team activation. Surgery. 2017;161(3):803–7.
68. Zhu CS, Braverman M, Goddard S, McGinity AC, Pokorny D, Cotner-Pouncy T, et al. Prehospital shock index and systolic blood pressure are highly specific for pediatric massive transfusion. J Trauma Acute Care Surg. 2021;91(4):579–83.
69. Mehta H, Kashyap R, Trivedi S. Correlation of end-tidal and arterial carbon-dioxide levels in critically ill neonates and children. Indian J Crit Care Med. 2014;18(12):833–4.
70. Intagliata S, Rizzo A, Gossman W. Physiology, lung dead space. In: StatPearls. Treasure Island: StatPearls Publishing; 2024. https://www.ncbi.nlm.nih.gov/books/NBK482501/. Accessed 8 February 2024.
71. Kozek-Langenecker SA, Ahmed AB, Afshari A, Albaladejo P, Aldecoa C, Barauskas G, et al. Management of severe perioperative bleeding: guidelines from the European Society of Anaesthesiology: first update 2016. Eur J Anaesthesiol. 2017;34(6):332–95.
72. Yang HW, Jeon W, Min YG, Lee JS. Usefulness of end-tidal carbon dioxide as an indicator of dehydration in pediatric emergency departments: a retrospective observational study. Medicine. 2017;96(35):e7881.
73. Fearon DM, Steele DW. End-tidal carbon dioxide predicts the presence and severity of acidosis in children with diabetes. Acad Emerg Med. 2002;9(12):1373–8.
74. Zheng C, Guo C. Intraoperative urine output is associated with postoperative outcome in pediatric population undergone major abdominal operations. Ther Clin Risk Manag. 2019;15:1453–60.
75. Nehus EJ. Glomerular filtration. In: Kliegman RM, Geme J, editors. Nelson textbook of pediatrics. 21st ed. Philadelphia: Elsevier; 2020. p. 2716.
76. Myles PS, Bellomo R, Corcoran T, Forbes A, Peyton P, Story D, et al. Restrictive versus liberal fluid therapy for major abdominal surgery. N Engl J Med. 2018;378(24):2263–74.
77. Wingert T, Grogan T, Cannesson M, Sapru A, Ren W, Hofer I. Acute kidney injury and outcomes in children undergoing noncardiac surgery: a propensity-matched analysis. Anesth Analg. 2021;132(2):332–40.

78. Centers for Disease Control and Prevention. Hydration status. https://www.cdc.gov/dengue/training/cme/ccm/Hydration%20Status_F.pdf. Accessed 6 May 2024.
79. Greenbaum LA. Maintenance and replacement therapy. In: Kliegman RM, Geme J, editors. Nelson textbook of pediatrics. 21st ed. Philadelphia: Elsevier; 2020. p. 425–8.
80. Thiele RH, Raghunathan K, Brudney CS, Lobo DN, Martin D, Senagore A, et al. American Society for Enhanced Recovery (ASER) and perioperative quality initiative (POQI) joint consensus statement on perioperative fluid management within an enhanced recovery pathway for colorectal surgery. Perioper Med. 2016;5:24.
81. Puckett JR, Pickering JW, Palmer SC, McCall JL, Kluger MT, De Zoysa J, et al. Low versus standard urine output targets in patients undergoing major abdominal surgery: a randomized noninferiority trial. Ann Surg. 2017;265(5):874–81.
82. Schacham NY, Chhabada S, Efune PN, Pu X, Liu L, Yang D, et al. Intraoperative hypotension and acute kidney injury after noncardiac surgery in infants and children: a retrospective cohort analysis. Anesthesiology. 2022;136(1):93–103.
83. Hofer CK, Cecconi M, Marx G, della Rocca G. Minimally invasive haemodynamic monitoring. Eur J Anaesthesiol. 2009;26(12):996–1002.
84. Weber F, Rashmi BK, Karaoz-Bulut G, Dogger J, de Heer IJ, Prasser C. The predictive value of the pleth variability index on fluid responsiveness in spontaneously breathing anaesthetized children-a prospective observational study. Paediatr Anaesth. 2020;30(10):1124–31.
85. Lee JH, Kim EH, Jang YE, Kim HS, Kim JT. Fluid responsiveness in the pediatric population. Korean J Anesthesiol. 2019;72(5):429–40.
86. Masimo Corporation. Clinical application of perfusion index. 2007. https://digivet.corecommerce.com/uploads/file/pi%20white%20paper.pdf. Accessed 25 October 2023.
87. de Souza P, Neto E, Grousson S, Duflo F, Ducreux C, Joly H, Convert J, et al. Predicting fluid responsiveness in mechanically ventilated children under general anaesthesia using dynamic parameters and transthoracic echocardiography. Br J Anaesth. 2011;106(6):856–64.
88. Desgranges FP, Evain JN, de Souza P, Neto E, Raphael D, Desebbe O, Chassard D. Does the plethysmographic variability index predict fluid responsiveness in mechanically ventilated children? A meta-analysis. Br J Anaesth. 2016;117(3):409–10.
89. Michard F, Lopes MR, Auler JO. Pulse pressure variation: beyond the fluid management of patients with shock. Crit Care. 2007;11(3):131.
90. Cannesson M. Pulse pressure variation in children. Society for Pediatric Anesthesia. 2012. http://www2.pedsanesthesia.org/meetings/2012winter/syllabus/ccas/submissions/Pulse%20Pressie%20Analysis%20in%20Children_Past_Present%20and%20Future.pdf. Accessed 1 May 2023.
91. Westphal GA, Silva E, Gonçalves AR, Caldeira Filho M, Poli-de-Figueiredo LF. Pulse oximetry wave variation as a noninvasive tool to assess volume status in cardiac surgery. Clinics. 2009;64(4):337–43.
92. Cannesson M, Slieker J, Desebbe O, Bauer C, Chiari P, Hénaine R, et al. The ability of a novel algorithm for automatic estimation of the respiratory variations in arterial pulse pressure to monitor fluid responsiveness in the operating room. Anesth Analg. 2008;106(4):1195–200.
93. Gan H, Cannesson M, Chandler JR, Ansermino JM. Predicting fluid responsiveness in children: a systematic review. Anesth Analg. 2013;117(6):1380–92.
94. Hu XJ, Ding JX, Wang Y, Niu C, Zhang Y, Zhao QM, et al. Peripheral perfusion index percentiles for healthy newborns by gestational age and sex in China. Sci Rep. 2020;10(1):4213.
95. Durand P, Chevret L, Essouri S, Haas V, Devictor D. Respiratory variations in aortic blood flow predict fluid responsiveness in ventilated children. Intensive Care Med. 2008;34(5):888–94.
96. Chandler JR, Cooke E, Petersen C, Karlen W, Froese N, Lim J, et al. Pulse oximeter plethysmograph variation and its relationship to the arterial waveform in mechanically ventilated children. J Clin Monit Comput. 2012;26(3):145–51.
97. De Backer D, Vincent JL. Should we measure the central venous pressure to guide fluid management? Ten answers to 10 questions. Crit Care. 2018;22(1):43.

98. Achar SK, Sagar MS, Shetty R, Kini G, Samanth J, Nayak C, et al. Respiratory variation in aortic flow peak velocity and inferior vena cava distensibility as indices of fluid responsiveness in anaesthetised and mechanically ventilated children. Indian J Anaesth. 2016;60(2):121–6.
99. Kusumastuti NP, Latief A, Pudjiadi AH. Inferior vena cava/abdominal aorta ratio as a guide for fluid resuscitation. J Emerg Trauma Shock. 2021;14(4):211–5.
100. Fidan S, Zengin SU, Orhon M, Umuroglu T. Comparative efficacy of finger versus forehead plethysmographic variability index monitoring in pediatric surgical patients. Paediatr Anaesth. 2023;33(1):52–8.
101. Desgranges FP, Bouvet L, de Souza P, Neto E, Evain JN, Terrisse H, Joosten A, et al. Non-invasive measurement of digital plethysmographic variability index to predict fluid responsiveness in mechanically ventilated children: a systematic review and meta-analysis of diagnostic test accuracy studies. Anaesth Crit Care Pain Med. 2023;42(3):101194.
102. van Genderen ME, Bartels SA, Lima A, Bezemer R, Ince C, Bakker J, et al. Peripheral perfusion index as an early predictor for central hypovolemia in awake healthy volunteers. Anesth Analg. 2013;116(2):351–6.
103. Uemura A, Yagihara M, Miyabe M. Pulse oxymeter perfusion index as a predictor for the effect of pediatric epidural block. Anesthesiology. 2006;105:A1354.
104. De Felice C, Latini G, Vacca P, Kopotic RJ. The pulse oximeter perfusion index as a predictor for high illness severity in neonates. Eur J Pediatr. 2002;161(10):561–2.
105. Ahmed A, Lotfy A, Elkholy J, Abdelhamid B, Ollaek M. Perfusion index as an objective measure of postoperative pain in children undergoing adenotonsillectomy: a cohort study. J Clin Monit Comput. 2022;36(3):795–801.
106. Lau FF, Agerskov M, Thusholdt ANW, Hojlund J, Meyhoff CS, Jans O, et al. Peripheral perfusion index stratifies risk in patients with intraoperative anemia: a multicentre cohort study. J Clin Anesth. 2024;95:111472.
107. Pawale D, Murki S, Kulkarni D, Vardhelli V, Sharma D, Oleti T, et al. Plethysmography variability index (PVI) changes in preterm neonates with shock-an observational study. Eur J Pediatr. 2021;180(2):379–85.
108. Kim DH, Shin S, Kim JY, Kim SH, Jo M, Choi YS. Pulse pressure variation and pleth variability index as predictors of fluid responsiveness in patients undergoing spinal surgery in the prone position. Ther Clin Risk Manag. 2018;14:1175–83.
109. Hariri G, Joffre J, Leblanc G, Bonsey M, Lavillegrand JR, Urbina T, et al. Narrative review: clinical assessment of peripheral tissue perfusion in septic shock. Ann Intensive Care. 2019;9(1):37.
110. Julien F, Hilly J, Sallah TB, Skhiri A, Michelet D, Brasher C, et al. Plethysmographic variability index (PVI) accuracy in predicting fluid responsiveness in anesthetized children. Paediatr Anaesth. 2013;23(6):536–46.
111. Emektar E. The role of perfusion index and plethysmography variability index for predicting dehydration severity in patients with gastroenteritis. Hong Kong J Emerg Med. 2022;29:78–83.
112. Demir G, Berksoy E, Bardak Ş, Elibol P, Çiçek A, Özön A, et al. Use of the pleth variability index in children with obstructive respiratory disease. Am J Emerg Med. 2022;56:28–32.
113. Ji SH, Song IK, Jang YE, Kim EH, Lee JH, Kim JT, et al. Comparison of pulse pressure variation and pleth variability index in the prone position in pediatric patients under 2 years old. Korean J Anesthesiol. 2019;72(5):466–71.
114. Feldman JM, Sussman E, Singh D, Friedman BJ. Is the pleth variability index a surrogate for pulse pressure variation in a pediatric population undergoing spine fusion? Paediatr Anaesth. 2012;22(3):250–5.
115. Tsuchiya M, Yamada T, Asada A. Pleth variability index predicts hypotension during anesthesia induction. Acta Anaesthesiol Scand. 2010;54(5):596–602.
116. Bazaraa H, Roby S, Salah E, Algebaly H. Assessment of tissue perfusion using the peripheral perfusion index and lactate clearance in shock in pediatric patients. Shock. 2021;56(6):933–8.
117. Balla KC, John V, Rao Pn S, Varghese K. Perfusion index-bedside diagnosis of hemodynamically significant patent ductus arteriosus. J Trop Pediatr. 2016;62(4):263–8.

118. Ismail J, Bansal A. Passive leg raising for fluid responsiveness in children: is it reliable? Indian J Crit Care Med. 2020;24(5):291–2.
119. Toupin F, Clairoux A, Deschamps A, Lebon JS, Lamarche Y, Lambert J, et al. Assessment of fluid responsiveness with end-tidal carbon dioxide using a simplified passive leg raising maneuver: a prospective observational study. Can J Anaesth. 2016;63(9):1033–41.
120. Huang H, Wu C, Shen Q, Fang Y, Xu H. Value of variation of end-tidal carbon dioxide for predicting fluid responsiveness during the passive leg raising test in patients with mechanical ventilation: a systematic review and meta-analysis. Crit Care. 2022;26(1):20.
121. Cavallaro F, Sandroni C, Marano C, La Torre G, Mannocci A, De Waure C, et al. Diagnostic accuracy of passive leg raising for prediction of fluid responsiveness in adults: systematic review and meta-analysis of clinical studies. Intensive Care Med. 2010;36(9):1475–83.
122. Monnet X, Marik P, Teboul JL. Passive leg raising for predicting fluid responsiveness: a systematic review and meta-analysis. Intensive Care Med. 2016;42(12):1935–47.
123. Lukito V, Djer MM, Pudjiadi AH, Munasir Z. The role of passive leg raising to predict fluid responsiveness in pediatric intensive care unit patients. Pediatr Crit Care Med. 2012;13(3):e155–60.
124. El-Nawawy AA, Farghaly PM, Hassouna HM. Accuracy of passive leg raising test in prediction of fluid responsiveness in children. Indian J Crit Care Med. 2020;24(5):344–9.
125. Pham A, Chandran S, Shah N, et al. Assessing passive leg raising test in pediatric shock using electrical cardiometry. Crit Care Med. 2023;1:51.
126. Macaskill J, Emadi R, Zhao MY, Barbour-Tuck E, Walker ME, Valcke PM, et al. A randomized controlled trial of passive leg raise to facilitate pediatric peripheral intravenous access. Can J Anaesth. 2023;70(11):1848–50.
127. McCarthy KN, Pavel A, Garvey AA, Hawke AL, Levins C, Livingstone V, et al. Feasibility of non-invasive cardiac output monitoring at birth using electrical bioreactance in term infants. Arch Dis Child Fetal Neonatal Ed. 2021;106(4):431–4.
128. O'Neill R, Dempsey EM, Garvey AA, Schwarz CE. Non-invasive cardiac output monitoring in neonates. Front Pediatr. 2020;8:614585.
129. Vergnaud E, Vidal C, Verchere JM, Taright H, Meyer PG, Carli PA, et al. Noninvasive cardiac output measurement using bioreactance in postoperative pediatric patients. Paediatr Anaesth. 2015;25(2):160–6.
130. Sumbel L, Annamalai MR, Wats A, Salameh M, Agarwal A, Bhalala U. Noninvasive cardiac output monitoring using electrical cardiometry and outcomes in critically ill children. J Pediatr Intensive Care. 2022;11(2):114–9.
131. Ballestero Y, Lopez-Herce J, Urbano J, Solana MJ, Botran M, Bellon JM, et al. Measurement of cardiac output in children by bioreactance. Pediatr Cardiol. 2011;32(4):469–72.
132. Sun Y, Wu C, Wu JZ, Wang SS, Bai J, Zhu M, et al. Noninvasive cardiac output monitoring using bioreactance-based technique in pediatric patients with or without ventricular septal defect during anesthesia: in comparison with echocardiography. Paediatr Anaesth. 2015;25(2):167–73.
133. Weisz DE, Jain A, Ting J, McNamara PJ, El-Khuffash A. Non-invasive cardiac output monitoring in preterm infants undergoing patent ductus arteriosus ligation: a comparison with echocardiography. Neonatology. 2014;106(4):330–6.
134. Weaver B, Guerreso K, Conner EA, Russell K, Vogel R, Rodriguez M. Hemodynamics and perfusion in premature infants during transfusion. AACN Adv Crit Care. 2018;29(2):126–37.
135. Van Wyk L, Gupta S, Lawrenson J, de Boode WP. Accuracy and trending ability of electrical biosensing technology for non-invasive cardiac output monitoring in neonates: a systematic qualitative review. Front Pediatr. 2022;10:851850.
136. Romagnoli S, Bevilacqua S, Lazzeri C, Ciappi F, Dini D, Pratesi C, et al. Most care: a minimally invasive system for hemodynamic monitoring powered by the Pressure Recording Analytical Method (PRAM). HSR Proc Intensive Care Cardiovasc Anesth. 2009;1(2):20–7.
137. Kouz K, Scheeren TWL, de Backer D, Saugel B. Pulse wave analysis to estimate cardiac output. Anesthesiology. 2021;134(1):119–26.

138. Nasr VG, Friedman K. Importance of noninvasive cardiac output measurement in children: feasibility or applicability? J Cardiothorac Vasc Anesth. 2021;35(5):1358–9.
139. Saugel B, Hoppe P, Nicklas JY, Kouz K, Korner A, Hempel JC, et al. Continuous noninvasive pulse wave analysis using finger cuff technologies for arterial blood pressure and cardiac output monitoring in perioperative and intensive care medicine: a systematic review and meta-analysis. Br J Anaesth. 2020;125(1):25–37.
140. Heeney ND, Habib F, Brar GK, Krahn G, Campbell DA, Sanatani S, et al. Validation of finger blood pressure monitoring in children. Blood Press Monit. 2019;24(3):137–45.
141. Saugel B, Hoppe P, Khanna AK. Automated continuous noninvasive ward monitoring: validation of measurement systems is the real challenge. Anesthesiology. 2020;132(3):407–10.
142. Harer MW, Rumpel JA, Stoops C, Slagle CL, Liberio B, Daniel J, et al. Current state of renal NIRS monitoring in the NICU: results from a CHNC survey. J Perinatol. 2023;43(8):1047–9.
143. Chock VY, Smith E, Tan S, Ball MB, Das A, Hintz SR, et al. Early brain and abdominal oxygenation in extremely low birth weight infants. Pediatr Res. 2022;92(4):1034–41.
144. Hansen ML, Hyttel-Sorensen S, Jakobsen JC, Gluud C, Kooi EMW, Mintzer J, et al. Cerebral near-infrared spectroscopy monitoring (NIRS) in children and adults: a systematic review with meta-analysis. Pediatr Res. 2022;96(4):856–67.
145. El-Dib M, Soul JS. Monitoring and management of brain hemodynamics and oxygenation. Handb Clin Neurol. 2019;162:295–314.
146. Dix LM, van Bel F, Lemmers PM. Monitoring cerebral oxygenation in neonates: an update. Front Pediatr. 2017;5:46.
147. Liu L, Qiang Z, Zhang J, Ren Y, Zhao X, Fu W, et al. Effect of hemoglobin content on cerebral oxygen saturation during surgery for scoliosis in pediatric patients. BMC Anesthesiol. 2021;21(1):165.
148. Austin EH, Edmonds HL, Auden SM, Seremet V, Niznik G, Sehic A, et al. Benefit of neurophysiologic monitoring for pediatric cardiac surgery. J Thorac Cardiovasc Surg. 1997;114(5):707–15.
149. Balegar KK, Stark MJ, Briggs N, Andersen CC. Early cerebral oxygen extraction and the risk of death or sonographic brain injury in very preterm infants. J Pediatr. 2014;164(3):475–80.
150. National Health Service. Near infrared spectroscopy (NIRS) guideline. 2023. https://www.clinicalguidelines.scot.nhs.uk/nhsggc-guidelines/nhsggc-guidelines/intensive-and-critical-care/near-infrared-spectroscopy-nirs-guideline/. Accessed 4 October 2023.
151. Calderone A, Jarry S, Couture EJ, Brassard P, Beaubien-Souligny W, Momeni M, et al. Early detection and correction of cerebral desaturation with noninvasive oxy-hemoglobin, deoxy-hemoglobin, and total hemoglobin in cardiac surgery: a case series. Anesth Analg. 2022;135(6):1304–14.
152. Rais-Bahrami K, Rivera O, Short BL. Validation of a noninvasive neonatal optical cerebral oximeter in veno-venous ECMO patients with a cephalad catheter. J Perinatol. 2006;26(10):628–35.
153. Crispin P, Forwood K. Near infrared spectroscopy in anemia detection and management: a systematic review. Transfus Med Rev. 2021;35(1):22–8.
154. Bailey SM, Mally PV. Near-infrared spectroscopy to guide and understand effects of red blood cell transfusion. Clin Perinatol. 2023;50(4):895–910.
155. Balegar V, Low GK, Nanan RK. Regional tissue oxygenation and conventional indicators of red blood cell transfusion in anaemic preterm infants. EClinicalMedicine. 2022;46:101365.
156. Gil-Anton J, Redondo S, Garcia Urabayen D, Nieto Faza M, Sanz I, Pilar J. Combined cerebral and renal near-infrared spectroscopy after congenital heart surgery. Pediatr Cardiol. 2015;36(6):1173–8.
157. Kasman N, Brady K. Cerebral oximetry for pediatric anesthesia: why do intelligent clinicians disagree? Paediatr Anaesth. 2011;21(5):473–8.
158. Bhutta AT, Ford JW, Parker JG, Prodhan P, Fontenot EE, Seib PM, et al. Noninvasive cerebral oximeter as a surrogate for mixed venous saturation in children. Pediatr Cardiol. 2007;28(1):34–41.

159. Hogue CW, Levine A, Hudson A, Lewis C. Clinical applications of near-infrared spectroscopy monitoring in cardiovascular surgery. Anesthesiology. 2021;134(5):784–91.
160. Medtronic. Invos-technology-difference-information-sheet.pdf. 2021. https://www.medtronic.com/content/dam/covidien/library/us/en/product/cerebral-somatic-oximetry/invos-technology-difference-information-sheet.pdf. Accessed 24 October 2023.
161. Ozturk NY, Aygun B, Uyar E, Girgin FI. Comparison of bilateral cerebro-renal tissue oxygenations in healthy children. Indian J Pediatr. 2020;87(2):99–104.
162. Lian C, Li P, Wang N, Lu Y, Shangguan W. Comparison of basic regional cerebral oxygen saturation values in patients of different ages: a pilot study. J Int Med Res. 2020;48(8):300060520936868.
163. Hou X, Ding H, Teng Y, Zhou C, Tang X, Li S, et al. Research on the relationship between brain anoxia at different regional oxygen saturations and brain damage using near-infrared spectroscopy. Physiol Meas. 2007;28(10):1251–65.
164. Kussman BD, Wypij D, Laussen PC, Soul JS, Bellinger DC, DiNardo JA, et al. Relationship of intraoperative cerebral oxygen saturation to neurodevelopmental outcome and brain magnetic resonance imaging at 1 year of age in infants undergoing biventricular repair. Circulation. 2010;122(3):245–54.
165. Conforti A, Giliberti P, Landolfo F, Valfre L, Columbo C, Mondi V, et al. Effects of ventilation modalities on near-infrared spectroscopy in surgically corrected CDH infants. J Pediatr Surg. 2016;51(3):349–53.
166. Alderliesten T, Lemmers PM, van Haastert IC, de Vries LS, Bonestroo HJ, Baerts W, et al. Hypotension in preterm neonates: low blood pressure alone does not affect neurodevelopmental outcome. J Pediatr. 2014;164(5):986–91.
167. Kurth CD, Levy WJ, McCann J. Near-infrared spectroscopy cerebral oxygen saturation thresholds for hypoxia-ischemia in piglets. J Cereb Blood Flow Metab. 2002;22(3):335–41.
168. Seidel D, Blaser A, Gebauer C, Pulzer F, Thome U, Knupfer M. Changes in regional tissue oxygenation saturation and desaturations after red blood cell transfusion in preterm infants. J Perinatol. 2013;33(4):282–7.
169. Sandal G, Oguz SS, Erdeve O, Akar M, Uras N, Dilmen U. Assessment of red blood cell transfusion and transfusion duration on cerebral and mesenteric oxygenation using near-infrared spectroscopy in preterm infants with symptomatic anemia. Transfusion. 2014;54(4):1100–5.
170. Mintzer JP, Parvez B, Chelala M, Alpan G, LaGamma EF. Monitoring regional tissue oxygen extraction in neonates <1250 g helps identify transfusion thresholds independent of hematocrit. J Neonatal-Perinatal Med. 2014;7(2):89–100.
171. Vretzakis G, Georgopoulou S, Stamoulis K, Tassoudis V, Mikroulis D, Giannoukas A, et al. Monitoring of brain oxygen saturation (INVOS) in a protocol to direct blood transfusions during cardiac surgery: a prospective randomized clinical trial. J Cardiothorac Surg. 2013;8:145.
172. van Hoften JC, Verhagen EA, Keating P, ter Horst HJ, Bos AF. Cerebral tissue oxygen saturation and extraction in preterm infants before and after blood transfusion. Arch Dis Child Fetal Neonatal Ed. 2010;95(5):F352–8.
173. Dani C, Pratesi S, Fontanelli G, Barp J, Bertini G. Blood transfusions increase cerebral, splanchnic, and renal oxygenation in anemic preterm infants. Transfusion. 2010;50(6):1220–6.
174. Wardle SP, Garr R, Yoxall CW, Weindling AM. A pilot randomised controlled trial of peripheral fractional oxygen extraction to guide blood transfusions in preterm infants. Arch Dis Child Fetal Neonatal Ed. 2002;86(1):F22–7.
175. Wardle SP, Yoxall CW, Weindling AM. Determinants of cerebral fractional oxygen extraction using near infrared spectroscopy in preterm neonates. J Cereb Blood Flow Metab. 2000;20(2):272–9.
176. Ceylan G, Sandal O, Sari F, Atakul G, Topal S, Colak M, et al. Monitoring of near-infrared spectrum values during packed red blood cell transfusion in pediatric intensive care unit. Transfus Clin Biol. 2021;28(3):234–8.
177. Bailey SM, Hendricks-Munoz KD, Wells JT, Mally P. Packed red blood cell transfusion increases regional cerebral and splanchnic tissue oxygen saturation in anemic symptomatic preterm infants. Am J Perinatol. 2010;27(6):445–53.

178. Yu Y, Zhang K, Zhang L, Zong H, Meng L, Han R. Cerebral near-infrared spectroscopy (NIRS) for perioperative monitoring of brain oxygenation in children and adults. Cochrane Database Syst Rev. 2018;1(1):CD010947.
179. Razlevice I, Rugyte DC, Strumylaite L, Macas A. Assessment of risk factors for cerebral oxygen desaturation during neonatal and infant general anesthesia: an observational, prospective study. BMC Anesthesiol. 2016;16(1):107.
180. DiNardo JA. Cerebral oximetry in children: so NIRS yet so far. Anesth Analg. 2019;128(4):605–6.
181. Shander A, Corwin HL, Meier J, Auerbach M, Bisbe E, Blitz J, et al. Recommendations from the international consensus conference on anemia management in surgical patients (ICCAMS). Ann Surg. 2023;277(4):581–90.
182. Faraoni D, DiNardo JA. Commentary: Red blood cells transfusion in patients undergoing congenital cardiac surgery: still far from physiology-based practice. J Thorac Cardiovasc Surg. 2022;167(2):e24–6.
183. Stanworth SJ, Carson JL. AABB RBC transfusion guidelines debate: which restrictive hemoglobin threshold? AM23-ST-05-L. Oct. 14, 2023. AABB Annual Meeting. Nashville, TN.
184. Warner MA, Shore-Lesserson L, Shander A, Patel SY, Perelman SI, Guinn NR. Perioperative anemia: prevention, diagnosis, and management throughout the spectrum of perioperative care. Anesth Analg. 2020;130(5):1364–80.
185. Warner MA, Hanson AC, Plimier C, Lee C, Liu VX, Richards T, et al. Association between anaemia and hospital readmissions in patients undergoing major surgery requiring postoperative intensive care. Anaesthesia. 2023;78(1):45–54.
186. Joseph B, Haider A, Rhee P. Non-invasive hemoglobin monitoring. Int J Surg. 2016;33(Pt B):254–7.
187. Hiscock R, Kumar D, Simmons SW. Systematic review and meta-analysis of method comparison studies of Masimo pulse co-oximeters (radical-7 or pronto-7) and HemoCue(R) absorption spectrometers (B-Hemoglobin or 201+) with laboratory haemoglobin estimation. Anaesth Intensive Care. 2015;43(3):341–50.
188. Kim SH, Lilot M, Murphy LS, Sidhu KS, Yu Z, Rinehart J, et al. Accuracy of continuous noninvasive hemoglobin monitoring: a systematic review and meta-analysis. Anesth Analg. 2014;119(2):332–46.
189. Masimo. European Society of Anaesthesiology and Intensive Care (ESAIC) recommends noninvasive, continuous hemoglobin monitoring. 2023. https://investor.masimo.com/news/news-details/2023/European-Society-of-Anaesthesiology-and-Intensive-Care-ESAIC-Recommends-Noninvasive-Continuous-Hemoglobin-Monitoring/default.aspx. Accessed 25 October 2023.
190. Kazanasmaz H, Demir M. The comparison of hemoglobin values measured by blood and continuous non-invasive monitoring (SpHb) in newborn infants. J Trop Pediatr. 2021;67(3):50.
191. Garcia-Soler P, Camacho Alonso JM, Gonzalez-Gomez JM, Milano-Manso G. Noninvasive hemoglobin monitoring in critically ill pediatric patients at risk of bleeding. Med Intensiva. 2017;41(4):209–15.
192. Wittenmeier E, Bellosevich S, Mauff S, Schmidtmann I, Eli M, Pestel G, et al. Comparison of the gold standard of hemoglobin measurement with the clinical standard (BGA) and noninvasive hemoglobin measurement (SpHb) in small children: a prospective diagnostic observational study. Paediatr Anaesth. 2015;25(10):1046–53.
193. Bhat A, Upadhyay A, Jaiswal V, Chawla D, Singh D, Kumar M, et al. Validity of non-invasive point-of-care hemoglobin estimation in healthy and sick children-a method comparison study. Eur J Pediatr. 2016;175(2):171–9.
194. Patino M, Schultz L, Hossain M, Moeller J, Mahmoud M, Gunter J, et al. Trending and accuracy of noninvasive hemoglobin monitoring in pediatric perioperative patients. Anesth Analg. 2014;119(4):920–5.
195. Barker SJ, Shander A, Ramsay MA. Continuous noninvasive hemoglobin monitoring: a measured response to a critical review. Anesth Analg. 2016;122(2):565–72.

196. Knutson T, Della-Giustina D, Tomich E, Wills B, Luerssen E, Reynolds P. Evaluation of a new noninvasive device in determining hemoglobin levels in emergency department patients. West J Emerg Med. 2013;14(3):283–6.
197. Skelton VA, Wijayasinghe N, Sharafudeen S, Sange A, Parry NS, Junghans C. Evaluation of point-of-care haemoglobin measuring devices: a comparison of Radical-7 pulse co-oximetry, HemoCue((R)) and laboratory haemoglobin measurements in obstetric patients. Anaesthesia. 2013;68(1):40–5.
198. Man J, Zielinski MD, Das D, Wutthisirisart P, Pasupathy KS. Improving non-invasive hemoglobin measurement accuracy using nonparametric models. J Biomed Inform. 2022;126:103975.
199. Park YH, Lim S, Kang H, Shin HY, Baek CW, Woo YC. Comparison of the accuracy of noninvasive hemoglobin monitoring for preoperative evaluation between adult and pediatric patients: a retrospective study. J Clin Monit Comput. 2018;32(5):863–9.
200. Wittenmeier E, Paumen Y, Mildenberger P, Smetiprach J, Pirlich N, Griemert EV, et al. Non-invasive haemoglobin measurement as an index test to detect pre-operative anaemia in elective surgery patients - a prospective study. Anaesthesia. 2021;76(5):647–54.
201. Park YH, Lee JH, Song HG, Byon HJ, Kim HS, Kim JT. The accuracy of noninvasive hemoglobin monitoring using the radical-7 pulse CO-Oximeter in children undergoing neurosurgery. Anesth Analg. 2012;115(6):1302–7.
202. Hornedo-González KD, Jacob AK, Burt JM, Higgins AA, Engel EM, Hanson AC, et al. Non-invasive hemoglobin estimation for preoperative anemia screening. Transfusion. 2023;63(2):315–22.
203. Masimo. Total hemoglobin (SpHb). 2024. https://professional.masimo.com/evidence/pulse-co-oximetry/sphb/. Accessed 17 February 2024.
204. Perel A. Iatrogenic hemodilution: a possible cause for avoidable blood transfusions? Crit Care. 2017;21(1):291.

Part III

Intraoperative Phase of Care

Postoperative Anemia

17

Norma J. Klein and Destiny F. Chau

17.1 Case Scenario

You are covering the pediatric intensive care unit (PICU) in your hospital. During morning rounds, it was determined that several patients were ready for discharge to the general inpatient hospital unit. From experience, you know that patients on the general unit are unlikely to undergo laboratory testing before discharge to home. You decide to check the hemoglobin (Hgb) of the postoperative patients before they leave your PICU, but the senior intensivist physician says that will be unnecessary laboratory testing.

Key Point Objectives

- *What is the definition of postoperative anemia in children?*
- *What are the known consequences of postoperative anemia?*
- *What is the prevalence of pediatric postoperative anemia?*
- *What factors contribute to the development of pediatric postoperative anemia?*
- *What are recommended solutions to the management of pediatric postoperative anemia?*

N. J. Klein (✉)
Department of Anesthesiology and Pain Medicine, University of California, Davis, Sacramento, CA, USA
e-mail: nklein@ucdavis.edu

D. F. Chau
Department of Anesthesiology and Pain Medicine, University of Arkansas for Medical Sciences, Arkansas Children's Hospital, Little Rock, AK, USA
e-mail: dchau@uams.edu

N. J. Klein (ed.), *Perioperative Pediatric Patient Blood Management and Transfusion Safety*, https://doi.org/10.1007/978-3-031-81666-6_17

17.2 Discussion

17.2.1 What Is the Definition of Postoperative Anemia in Children?

There is not a definition of *postoperative* anemia per se in either children or adults [1]. Otherwise, red blood cell (RBC) anemia is defined as a Hgb that is two standard deviations below the mean (i.e., the lowest 2.5% of samples) taken from a large, representative general population[1] [2–4]. Normal Hgb values are further defined according to age, gender, pregnancy status, habitat altitude, and smoking status [5, 6]. Neonates and infants, who exhibit the widest range of Hgb values, are usually differentiated from older children and adults when classifying anemia status [7, 8]. Neonatal Hgb values are not derived from general, population-based means but instead are based on "reference ranges" between 5th and 95th percentile values measured in large convenience samples obtained for clinical indications [8]. Children residing in resource-limited countries or food-insecure settings often fall out of these normative definitions with significantly lower mean Hgb values [1, 9–11]. Hemoglobin cutoff values for women, which tend to be lower than men, have recently been questioned. Furthermore, the optimal Hgb for proper growth and development during childhood is unknown [12]. An anemia diagnosis in children is further complicated by the fact that normal Hgb values are age-related. As a result, there is not a global definition of anemia, and postoperative anemia diagnosis and treatment decisions must be made on a case-by-case basis [3, 12–14].

Iron deficiency anemia (IDA) is the most common form of anemia, affecting up to 50% of children worldwide [15–17]. Consequently, a postoperative anemia diagnosis entails determination of the patient's iron indices. Total body iron deficiency (ID) can occur without evidence of anemia as defined by a reduction in Hgb value; ID is significantly advanced by the time a patient is diagnosed with anemia [12, 18]. Once IDA manifests, the iron stores are already depleted as the body preferentially uses iron for RBC production.

17.2.2 What Are the Known Consequences of Postoperative Anemia?

Anemia in adults has been associated with multiple untoward outcomes, including decreased survival, fatigue, dementia, increased hospital readmission rates, postoperative acute kidney injury (AKI), heart failure, and a reduction in health-related quality of life (HRQoL) [14, 19–22]. Neonates, infants, and children introduce additional concerns related to growth and development, such as neurodevelopmental maturation and school performance [23–27]. Children who remain severely anemic following surgery have been shown to have higher mortality and readmission

[1] Published age-related hemoglobin normal values can be found in the Chap. 4.

rates than children with milder forms of anemia [20, 28]. The long-term effects of postoperative anemia in children have not been studied.

The last trimester of pregnancy is a vulnerable period because both anemia and ID are independent variables affecting neurodevelopment. Anemia adversely impacts white matter myelination and hippocampus development during a critical period of brain development [29]. Brain oxygen consumption, which is partly dependent on circulating Hgb levels, is 60% of the total body oxygen consumption in newborns (compared to 20% in adults) [29]. Brain iron is a cofactor in dopamine and serotonin synthesis pathways and remains essential to the early childhood myelination process [30]. Many small observational studies of infants and toddlers have found associations of anemia, ID, or both, with an array of neurodevelopmental disorders including attention deficit hyperactivity disorder (ADHD), cognitive delay, academic underperformance, externalizing behaviors (e.g., aggression), and poor recognition memory [23, 30–35]. In a 2017 controlled study of 14 young adults who were iron deficient as infants, differences in functional brain connectivity were found on functional magnetic resonance imaging (fMRI) compared to 17 adult controls [36]. However, the underlying mechanisms of these observed aberrations, as well as the associated Hgb levels at different developmental stages, remain unknown [29]. The picture is further complicated by the fact that the origin of IDA is often multifactorial and is inextricably tied to nutritional status [25]. Several early studies of anemic children with a Hgb ≤10 g/dL during infancy who lived in areas where food insecurity and economic stress are endemic found a relationship between anemia and reduced developmental scores that was not found in their non-iron-deficient counterparts [23, 26, 27, 37–39]. Later, systematic reviews, however, have not been able to establish a definitive relationship between iron therapy in preschoolers with ID and developmental scores [40, 41]. A recent systematic review of the role of iron interventions in ID and IDA in the cognitive function of teenagers was similarly inconclusive due to a lack of quality studies [31]. In a large population-based survey of children age 36–59 months living in nine low- and middle-income countries, family wealth and involvement with an early childhood education program, but not anemia (i.e., Hgb ≤11 g/dL), were consistently associated with delayed developmental benchmarks ($p < 0.05$) [42]. Specific weaknesses in the available data on anemia, growth, development, and cognitive function in children include the variety of tests used to measure intelligence and cognition, along with confounding variables such as age differences, socioeconomic status, baseline nutrition, and dietary interventions [31].

Despite shortcomings in the pediatric literature, existing evidence that postoperative anemia in adult patients is associated with significant morbidity and mortality begs the conclusion that growing children are at least as vulnerable to the untoward effects of anemia following surgery. There is now an appreciation that outcome studies for restrictive versus liberal RBC transfusion thresholds should focus on quality-of-life outcomes as well as mortality and transfusion risk [43–46]. There are no randomized controlled trials (RCTs) of functional outcomes, including health-related quality of life (HRQoL), for the different RBC transfusion thresholds in children [43]. Defining quality of life in a growing child who is dependent and an extension of a family unit, with age-related Hgb values, makes evaluating HRQoL outcomes difficult [46–48].

17.2.3 What Is the Prevalence of Pediatric Postoperative Anemia?

The known rates of postoperative anemia in children are currently based on mixed cohort studies in the pediatric intensive care unit (PICU) literature. Up to 41% of children have been shown to develop anemia during an intensive care hospitalization; however, the actual rate is unclear since restrictive RBC transfusion thresholds are increasingly implemented [1, 3, 6, 13, 49]. In observational studies of children surviving to PICU discharge, the rate of discharge anemia based on Hgb levels has been found to range from 8.3% to 58.9% [1, 13, 50–52]. The contribution of postoperative patients to these numbers may be disproportionately large, reported to be as high as 70% [6]. In a 2019 retrospective review of over 2900 PICU patients, children admitted for medical reasons had a reduced risk of discharge anemia compared to surgical patients (adjusted odds ratio 0.75; 95% CI, 0.61–0.91; $p = 0.004$) [1]. An earlier prospective observational study of 679 children in a tertiary children's hospital found that children admitted to the PICU for noncardiac surgery had an unadjusted rate of anemia at discharge more than two times that of children admitted for cardiac surgery [13]. This discrepancy may be partially explained by the application of higher RBC transfusion thresholds in children with heart disease, particularly the cyanotic cohorts [6, 53–55]. Adult studies of posthospitalization anemia cite a prevalence from 27% to 90% [12, 14, 56–58]. Adult patients have more chronic disease and experience more operative procedures than children on average and thus are more susceptible to a persistent decline in perioperative Hgb levels. Preteens and adolescents (particularly females) are reported to be disproportionately affected, but other patient populations at risk of worsened anemia during hospitalization include neonates and patients who are not transfused, a diagnosis of respiratory disease on admission, and high injury severity scores [1, 3, 6, 13, 51]. When ID alone is taken into consideration, children with the most rapid growth needs are at greatest risk, including infants, those less than 5 years, and women in the third trimester of pregnancy [17]. Individuals who may have inadequate iron intake (e.g., menstruating teens and vegetarians) are also at elevated risk of ID as well as IDA during hospitalization [15, 59].

At present, there are no studies of postoperative anemia in children who have been discharged to home on the day of surgery, thus creating an information gap for that population who may benefit from follow-up.

17.2.4 What Factors Contribute to the Development of Pediatric Postoperative Anemia?

17.2.4.1 Hospital-Acquired Anemia

All surgical patients are at risk of hospital-acquired anemia (HAA).[2] The main contributors to postoperative anemia in both children and adults are preoperative anemia, surgical procedures, phlebotomy, and anemia upon hospital admission [1, 12, 60–62]. Preoperative anemia is a major cause of postoperative anemia [12, 18, 22, 51, 62–64]. Furthermore, anemia before surgery increases the likelihood of a perioperative transfusion, which introduces further risks for the hospitalized child [1, 6, 52, 65].

17.2.4.2 Restrictive RBC Transfusion Thresholds

Anemia in a stable, hospitalized pediatric patient is often managed under a restrictive RBC transfusion standard, with fewer RBC transfusions administered and a focus on supporting patients through anemia tolerance [52, 53, 66, 67]. Following the landmark TRICC (Transfusion Requirements in Critical Care) trial in critically ill adults establishing the noninferiority of a lower Hgb transfusion threshold (i.e., 7 g/dL) compared to a higher threshold (i.e., 9 g/dL), both adult and pediatric practitioners have at least partially adopted a reduction in the standard RBC transfusion threshold [68–72]. The 2018 TAXI (Transfusion and Anemia Expertise Initiative) consensus recommends a postoperative Hgb threshold for RBC transfusion of <7 g/dL in critically ill children who are stable and not bleeding [73]. TAXI further emphasizes clinical judgment and suggests that nonoperative pediatric patients should not be transfused while hemodynamically stable if the Hgb is >5 g/dL. The TAXI guidelines also provide recommendations for a restrictive RBC transfusion threshold in various subpopulations but lack follow-up recommendations including posthospitalization surveillance or therapy for hemodynamically stable anemia [73–75]. As such, there is a notable gap in the appropriate management of all patients, including children, who become anemic with surgery [13, 22, 29, 61].

17.2.4.3 Awareness Gaps

When surveyed about transfusion practices in a French pediatric ICU, pediatric intensivist physicians "frequently" measured Hgb levels at discharge less than 40% of the time, and fewer than 20% were aware that the prevalence of anemia at discharge may be as high as 50–70% [54]. In the same study, physicians tended to manage Hgb values at discharge similar to Hgb management during the acute phase of illness. As patient acuity and survival increase with advances in care, the rates of postoperative anemia are unlikely to improve without the necessary research and practitioner education.

---

[2] For further discussion regarding HAA, refer to the chapter entitled "Hospital-Acquired Anemia and Blood Conservation."

17.2.4.4 Intensive Care Status

Iatrogenic anemia is a particular concern in small patients when undergoing acute care because of their relatively small blood volumes in the face of frequent phlebotomy, overdraw, invasive procedures, indwelling catheter placement, inconsistent microtube technology use, and the difficulty assessing small blood loss. In a prospective, multicenter study of approximately 1000 children admitted to a PICU, the mean phlebotomy volume was 2.7 ± 2.3 mL/draw, with a mean of 3 draws per day [3]. This represents a 1% daily blood volume loss from phlebotomy alone in an 8-kg infant with an estimated blood volume of 80 mL/kg. In observational study of PICU patients, mean phlebotomy losses were 7.1 ± 5.3 mL/day, including 3.8 ± 3.6 mL/day discarded as waste [76]. In adults, Hgb levels decrease by approximately 0.7 g/dL for every 100 mL of blood removed [77]. In a prospective animal study, phlebotomy to a hematocrit less than 25% during the first 2 weeks of life decreased hippocampal iron content in mice pups by 40% [78].

17.2.4.5 Acute and Chronic Illness

Hemoglobin recovery is hampered by a systemic inflammatory state that occurs following trauma and surgery. Also called "functional anemia," a rise in many inflammatory mediators following surgery, including interleukin 6 (IL-6), C-reactive protein (CRP), and hepcidin, hinders iron adsorption and transport [4, 17, 52, 79]. Hepcidin is a peptide hormone synthesized in the liver that inhibits ferroportin on membrane surfaces of enterocytes and macrophages [80]. Ferroportin is the primary exporter of iron from these cells into the plasma where it becomes available for erythropoiesis. When hepcidin levels increases, ferroportin is inhibited, and therefore less iron is available for Hgb synthesis. Iron that may be available through diet or oral supplementation is therefore poorly absorbed, and iron scavenged by macrophages from senescent red blood cells is not recovered [81]. Serum ferritin levels also increase in response to systemic inflammation and thus can lead to a missed diagnosis of iron deficiency or anemia in the postoperative period when relied upon in the absence of more definitive iron studies. This postoperative inflammatory state may help explain why, in addition to other factors such as socioeconomic status, diet, and chronic illness, over one-half of critically ill adults with posthospitalization anemia may not recover iron stores or Hgb levels for months after surgery [22, 57]. In a post-PICU follow-up of 19 patients discharged with a Hgb $<$ 10 g/dL, over one half remained anemic at 6 months, and the average time to recovery was 11 weeks (range 9–26) [52]. In that same study, all anemic patients were deemed to be non-iron-deficient, with a serum ferritin concentration $>$ 12 μg/L, although 12 (63%) of patients had elevated CRP and IL-6 levels at week 13. Surgical and hospital-associated blood loss leading to anemia in the preterm or small-for-gestational-age (SGA) neonate is particularly burdensome because of reduced iron stores, a shorter RBC lifespan (35–50 days versus 60–90 days in adults), blunted erythropoietin responses, and increased growth requirements [81].

Other factors contributing to postoperative anemia in children include:

- Occult postoperative blood loss, including unmonitored surgical drains

- Female sex [12, 29]
- Equipment-related hemolysis (e.g., clave catheter connectors and extracorporeal perfusion devices [82–86]
- Medications (e.g., herbals, H2-blockers, inappropriate anticoagulation bridging) [87]
- Malnutrition (including folate, iron, and vitamin B_{12} deficiencies) in the face of rapid growth needs [24]
- Low iron and ferritin body stores (particularly premature neonates)
- Absent pediatric-specific guidelines on perioperative anemia surveillance and iron replacement [54]
- Age group (especially premature infants, preschool-aged, and adolescents) [6, 17]
- Noncardiac surgery [6]
- Hemodilution and volume overload [12, 81]
- Invasive monitoring allowing convenient laboratory testing [1]

17.2.5 What Are Recommended Solutions to the Management of Pediatric Postoperative Anemia?

Solutions to postoperative anemia and its untoward effects may be found in the basic tenants of patient blood management (PBM)[3] [88]:

- Anemia management
- Minimizing blood loss through blood conservation techniques
- Optimization of coagulation status
- Consideration of the patient's unique physiologic reserve and stated goals

17.2.5.1 Anemia: Early Diagnosis

Preoperative anemia significantly increases the surgical patient's risk of leaving the hospital in an anemic state as well as receiving an allogeneic RBC transfusion [1, 3, 12, 18, 62, 64, 65, 89]. Prevention of postoperative anemia requires evaluation of the surgical patient's Hgb level before surgery and again prior to hospital or surgical center discharge [12, 61]. An international consortium recommends that all patients undergoing *major* surgery should be screened for anemia as soon as possible in both elective and urgent procedures and screening should extend into the postoperative period [61]. An earlier consensus recommends evaluating all adult patients for postoperative anemia if they have preoperative anemia and lose more than 500 mL of blood during major surgery [12]. This blood loss constitutes 7–10% of a 70-kg adult's 5–7 estimated total blood volume. There are no such guidelines addressing how and when to screen pediatric patients [53, 54].

A crucial first step in managing postoperative anemia is a better understanding of the pediatric patient's iron profile before blood loss surgery [90–94]. A significant

[3] Pediatric blood conservation strategies and preoperative anemia management are discussed further in the chapter "Hospital-Acquired Anemia and Blood Conservation."

portion of children are anemic in the preoperative period (at least one quarter), and many are unlikely to be screened for anemia before surgery [94]. Iron deficiency is often present without laboratory evidence of anemia (up to 20%, although the true prevalence is unknown) [15]. Currently, management of postoperative anemia in children is likely to be based partly on recommendations for adults or in pediatric disease states where iron treatment has received the most focus (e.g., inflammatory bowel disease (IBD), chronic renal disease, and the pediatric intensive care unit (PICU)) [53, 54, 93].

17.2.5.2 Anemia: Initial Screening

Anemia screening prior to major blood loss surgeries may begin with a capillary sample for Hgb and hematocrit (Hct) with addition of RBC indices, reticulocyte count, and serum ferritin if the Hgb and Hct are abnormal for age [93]. When available, a noninvasive Hgb trend (e.g., pulse co-oximetry) may be utilized for initial anemia screening, but all treatment decisions and further iron studies should be based on conventional laboratory tests [51, 95]. In search for the optimal biomarker to facilitate ID diagnosis before it progresses to anemia, a number of laboratory parameters have been investigated [1, 16, 22, 29]. Serum ferritin (SF) is the primary protein harboring intracellular iron stores and is commonly used to diagnose ID and IDA [15].

If the serum ferritin is elevated for age, additional iron studies may be necessary to rule out an inflammatory condition, as directed by a hematologist [61, 92, 93]. A new test, the reticulocyte hemoglobin concentration (CHr), may be more sensitive for diagnosing early iron deficiency than serum ferritin [15, 93]. ID with and without anemia is also diagnosed using transferrin saturation, total iron-binding capacity (TIBC), free erythrocyte protoporphyrin, and hepcidin, alone or in combination [12, 29, 38, 51, 63, 93]. These assays are not usually necessary in the majority of pediatric ID cases. An early postoperative diagnosis of anemia based on mean corpuscular volume (MCV) is not realistic because acute blood loss is normochromic and normocytic on blood smear [1, 3, 16].

Serum ferritin should be evaluated within the first postoperative day before levels rise with the inflammatory response to surgery [12]. Preexisting acute or chronic illness may require additional testing (e.g., serum hepcidin or reticulocyte Hgb concentration) to differentiate anemia of inflammation or chronic disease from absolute ID [61, 93].

17.2.5.3 Intravenous Iron Therapy: General

Most literature addressing preoperative anemia treatment emphasizes iron therapy. In the past, anemic children were presumed to have iron deficiency, and oral iron was empirically prescribed [96]. Today, iron studies are recommended in anemic patients before initiating iron therapy.

Intravenous (IV) iron therapy has received increased attention as a more efficient treatment alternative for perioperative anemia, particularly single-dose regimens [93, 97–99]. IV iron has been shown to improve both hemoglobin levels and iron stores in anemic patients in single studies and at least one meta-analysis [51, 93, 97, 98, 100, 101]. However, there are conflicting data about its effectiveness in treating preoperative ID and IDA [99, 102]. A 2021 Cochran review of six randomized controlled trials (RCTs) comparing IV iron with standard or placebo therapy given to anemic adults before surgery found insufficient evidence (specifically, too small sample sizes) to conclude that IV management reduces allogeneic transfusions [103]. A second meta-analysis of eleven RCTs that compared IV iron to placebo in adults with nonanemic iron deficiency was also unable to conclude that IV iron was beneficial in that population due to insufficient evidence [99]. A more recent systematic review of eight observational studies examining postoperative outcomes in nonanemic, iron-deficient adults undergoing cardiac surgery found that the iron-deficient cohort required more RBC transfusions (odds ratio 1.39; 95% CI, 1.16–1.68), but other outcomes including length of stay (LOS), postoperative complications, and readmission were indeterminate due to limited study quality [104]. Despite these systematic reviews, individual studies have shown improved iron profiles as well as a reduction in allogenic RBC transfusions and postoperative anemia rates in adult patients with perioperative anemia [105–107].

Successful prevention and treatment of postoperative anemia is ideally based on the best available evidence and practices. However, treatment targets for Hgb and iron indices after surgery is uncertain, and it is not known which patients are most likely to benefit from diagnosis and treatment [29, 89, 108, 109]. The ideal time to begin postoperative anemia treatment is also unknown [12].

17.2.5.4 Intravenous Iron Therapy: Children

IV iron is used in children for different ID etiologies, but administration is not standardized, and an assortment of formulations are used [93, 97, 98]. Perioperative IV iron therapy remains an off-label use in children unless there is severe, symptomatic anemia with ongoing blood loss [93, 97]. Currently, there are four IV formulations approved by the US Food and Drug Administration (US FDA) for pediatric anemia treatment, but only low molecular weight iron dextran is approved for general use in children (who are less than 1 year) [97]. Other formulations are approved for pediatric use in non-US countries; however, regulatory approval is often narrow [93]. In a retrospective analysis of 194 pediatric, non-nephrology patients in a US children's hospital who received IV iron for a variety of conditions (mean age 10.2 ± 6.5 years), the mean elemental iron dose was less than 3 mg/kg body weight, and the mean infusion time was approximately 1.5 h per administration [98]. There was a wide range in the number of doses required per patient (i.e., 1–12). Only 2.6% ($n = 5$) patients received IV iron for surgically related anemia; all but one administrations were with iron sucrose. There were 20 minor but no severe reactions reported. Approximately 10% of administrations ($n = 113$) received premedication with diphenhydramine, hydrocortisone, acetaminophen, and hydroxyzine, alone or in combination; none of the 20 children with minor reactions were premedicated [98]. In a retrospective record review of 72 children who were refractory to a course of oral iron therapy, single-dose ferric carboxymaltose (approved in the United States for IV administration to iron-deficient children over 1 year old who have failed a course of oral iron) was associated with an increase in a median Hgb 9.1 g/dL to 12.3 g/dL [110]. There was a positive response rate of 72% at 1–3 months following a single IV dose. It is not clear from that data, however, what the oral iron dosing was prior to IV carboxymaltose administration, but the median serum ferritin levels increased from 3.4 ng/mL (range 1–35) to 114.7 ng/mL (range 2.3–407.5) during that same follow-up period [110].

The maximum approved dose for IV iron varies widely (e.g., 100–1000 mg), depending on country of use and formulation [97]. There are standardized formulae available to calculate both total body iron content and IV iron dosing [93, 97, 111]. An example of a standardized total body iron deficiency formula in children is shown below [93]:

Total body iron deficiency in milligrams = Body weight (kg) × (target Hgb – measured Hgb g/dL) × 2.4 + iron reserves (mg)[4]

A gold standard general pediatric text advises a maximum daily supplemental iron dose of 200 mg, but higher IV iron doses in a single setting have been reported with rare serious side effects [97, 98, 110, 112, 113].

17.2.5.5 Iron Therapy: Follow-Up

Both IV and oral iron therapy produce a reticulocytosis within 1 week of treatment, but the IV formulation produces a more rapid replenishment of iron and ferritin stores [97]. The circulation half-life of IV iron is approximately 2 weeks in adults [113]. Because ferritin is the primary storage protein for iron, an early increase in serum ferritin levels is central to recovering usable iron and mobilizing iron stores acquired through iron therapy. Initially, IV iron produces an increase of serum ferritin to approximately 125% of normal within 1–2 weeks, followed by a normalization of Hgb within 1 month (in mild anemia) or 2 months (severe anemia) in nonbleeding patients [97]. Serum ferritin levels vary with age, inflammatory state, and laboratory assay; thus, a hematologist should be consulted for monitoring during and after IV iron therapy. The World Health Organization (WHO) and the American Academy of Pediatrics (AAP) define iron deficiency as a serum ferritin below 10–30 μg/L for older children [5, 91, 93, 96, 97]. However, in adult patients at high risk of severe postoperative anemia, a consortium of international experts advises iron therapy (orally, initially, when feasible) for an isolated serum ferritin <100 μg/L (or ferritin <30 μg/L plus a transferrin saturation <20% or a CRP >5 mg/L) [12, 114]. The goal of this higher ferritin treatment threshold is to maximize iron stores prior to blood loss surgery [115].

Diagnosing IGA with serum ferritin levels in children is complicated because "normal" serum ferritin levels for newborns and infants less than 3 months range from approximately 150 to 1000 μg/L [Table 17.1]. The short- and long-term effects of supranormal ferritin levels associated with iron therapy are unknown [93, 116].

If iron therapy is initiated, Hgb and serum ferritin levels should be monitored for several days and iron studies for at least 1 month under the guidance of a qualified

[4] Iron reserves: target Hgb 13 g/dL and body weight <35 kg = 15 mg/kg; target Hgb 15 g/dL and body weight ≥35 kg = 500 mg

Table 17.1 Normal serum ferritin levels by age

Age	Serum ferritin (μg/L)
Cord blood	Range 45–636
Preterm	20 weeks after birth: Mean 37.8
	55 weeks after birth: Mean 15.9
Term	20 weeks after birth: Mean 71.7
	55 weeks after birth: Mean 21.5
0–7 days	Range 153–1092
8–30 days	Range 247–692
1–3 months	Range 148–744
4–9 months	Range 21–240
9–24 months	Range 10–168
2–16 years	Range 10–99
Females >16 years	Range 18–103
Males >16 years	Range 16–213

Adapted from Mattiello et al. [93]; Brugnara [4]

pediatrician or hematologist [93]. A reticulocyte response will not be evident for at least 1 week [12]. If serum ferritin is added to these studies to follow iron therapy, a minimum of 1 mL is required, although in some laboratories the test can be performed with capillary sample (i.e., 0.1 mL). A full iron study panel may require 1–3 mL per venipuncture using pediatric-sized "microtubes"; a standard specimen tube requires up to 5 mL per sample. It is important to investigate each hospital's specimen requirements because not all institutions use microtube analyzers on a consistent basis [93, 117–119].

17.2.5.6 Iron Therapy: Side Effects

Untoward reactions occur with all iron preparations. Oral therapy has a high rate of gastric upset, constipation, and noncompliance, and good regimen compliance requires 1–3 months for a 2 g/dL Hgb increase [15, 92, 120]. Minor side effects associated with IV therapy have been reported in approximately 10–15% of pediatric patients [97, 98, 110, 116]. These include, but are not limited to, pruritis, urticaria, fever, skin staining at the infusion site, headache, nausea, and arthralgias [93]. IV iron has been reported to exacerbate rheumatoid arthritis and lupus [121]. Because of its potential effect on neutrophil and T-cell function, adult studies have raised concerns that supplemental iron increases infection risk, but this finding is debated and not generally accepted [89, 101, 113, 116, 122]. A dreaded adverse reaction is anaphylaxis that was historically linked to early dextran formulations, leading to its removal from the market in 1991 [92]. IV iron preparations are iron-carbohydrate complexes which vary in formulation between manufacturers [121, 123]. Newer preparations allow delayed release of elemental iron and are rarely associated with serious events such as hypotension, dyspnea, and anaphylaxis [97, 124]. It is not known if these reactions are immune-mediated or complement-activated. In a 2022 retrospective review of adults receiving Medicare part D insurance coverage (n = 167,925), the rate of anaphylaxis requiring cardiopulmonary resuscitation was 0.4/100,000 for first time administrations of ferric carboxymaltose and 1/100,000 for iron sucrose [125]. An earlier retrospective review of adult Medicare beneficiaries found an anaphylaxis-like event rate of 24/100,000 administrations for non-dextran formulations compared to 67/100,000 for both old and new dextran formulations [123]. Because IV-iron-associated anaphylaxis-like events are rare, the true incidence in children receiving their first dose of IV iron is unknown. In two retrospective studies analyzing a combined total of 266 children treated with IV iron for iron deficiency, there was only 1 severe reaction (dyspnea) in an adolescent which resolved without incident [98, 110]. Although iron dextran preparations may come with manufacturer recommendations for a "test" dose (e.g., 25-mg elemental iron in adults) under close cardiovascular monitoring, the practice is falling out of favor, and non-dextran formulations are often given to children without a test dose [121, 126].

There is a general agreement that despite established safety, IV infusions should be administered in a controlled environment under a standardized protocol with trained staff and readily available emergency resuscitation equipment [12, 93, 98, 121]. A 2014 literature review of articles addressing anaphylaxis-like reactions associated with IV iron therapy found certain predisposing factors for hypersensitivity: a prior reaction to IV iron, atopy, mastocytosis, old age, beta blockade or angiotensin-converting enzyme (ACE) inhibitor therapy, severe cardiopulmonary disease, and caregiver anxiety over IV iron administration [121]. IV iron is contraindicated during the first trimester of pregnancy (due to a lack of safety data) and during active infections [93, 121]. Some experts recommend against IV iron in preterm infants due to concerns over oxidative stress, iron overload, and a lack of evidence-based dosing guidelines [127, 128]. The complexity of the issue is magnified when one considers that newborns and preterm infants typically have high serum ferritin levels at baseline, and many preterm infants receive multiple RBC transfusions resulting in excess total body iron [91, 127, 128]. A 2014 publication outlines IV iron administration guidelines for adults with iron deficiency anemia, but there are no such guidelines for children [121].

Insurance coverage for anemia treatment is varied, and government-funded or third-party insurance plans may pay for iron therapy only for specific conditions (e.g., IBD or chronic renal insufficiency) [93, 97]. Intravenous iron therapy is more expensive than oral therapy, but cost savings may be achieved when anemia-related postoperative morbidity and mortality are reduced in the long term or extended follow-up requiring repeat blood draws and clinic visits is avoided [93, 98, 129]. In the US, insurance coverage for IV iron therapy is often unavailable unless the patient cannot tolerate a course of oral iron, there is an inadequate response with oral treatment, or the patient is unable to take medications by mouth.

In conclusion, IV iron can mitigate the known effects of postoperative anemia by increasing iron stores and Hgb levels in anemic patients. IV iron is becoming increasingly recognized as an alternative treatment to rapidly replace iron stores in adults with preoperative or blood loss-associated postoperative anemia. It has been safely administered in children when administered under controlled conditions. However, there is a paucity of information available to guide pediatric IV iron dosing, management, and long-term monitoring in the perioperative period.

17.2.5.7 Erythropoietin (EPO)

EPO levels and the response to exogenous therapy are reduced in critically ill patients and premature neonates [51]. Supplemental erythropoietin-stimulating agents (ESAs) have been used successfully to treat anemia in patients with cancer and chronic kidney disease on hemodialysis [12, 45, 89]. ESAs have also been administered to critically ill adults and children on a research basis to address anemia and RBC transfusion requirements [130, 131]. However, ESAs are contraindicated for acute anemia treatment, partly because of its delayed effect; a positive reticulocyte response is not evident for up to 1 week of therapy. There are also lingering concerns over thromboembolism and seizures in patients with epilepsy [132]. If an ESA is administered to treat preoperative anemia, one expert consensus recommends simultaneous iron therapy and possibly thromboembolism prophylaxis [61]. There is no data available to guide its safe use in pediatric perioperative anemia [51]. Although ESAs are off-label for the management of postoperative anemia in adults, they may be considered in cases of severe, symptomatic anemia in the face of transfusion refusal [12, 61].

17.2.5.8 RBC Transfusions

RBC transfusions are an appropriate treatment for postoperative anemia when the patient is hemodynamically unstable in the face of continuing blood loss and there is no other alternative to achieve clinical stability [12, 51, 61, 73]. The Choosing Wisely campaign advises against treating IDA with an RBC transfusion if the child has no symptoms [133]. In the absence of active bleeding and unstable physiologic and laboratory indices, a Hgb of 5–7 g/dL in most critically ill children is acceptable in the short term, provided anemia and iron reserves are addressed, anemia treatment begins prior to hospital discharge, and there is a postoperative surveillance plan [73].

17.2.5.9 Education and Research

Physicians and other practitioners should be educated about the potential consequences of anemia as well as surveillance and management strategies that can be implemented prior to hospital discharge. Families may benefit from nutrition counseling, particularly if the child undergoes iron therapy which should eventually be supplanted with a micronutrient-rich diet. Despite the growing acceptance of IV iron as a safe and effective alternative to an RBC transfusion for perioperative anemia, a recent systematic review found that most guidelines for IV iron were outdated, with a significant deficiency in guidelines addressing IV iron therapy in children [2, 110, 134]. Research on postoperative anemia is in its infancy, with many questions that must be answered through large, high-quality studies, including [18, 135, 136]:

- The true incidence of postoperative anemia
- Target laboratory and physiologic parameters for therapy
- Patient populations most likely to benefit from diagnosis and treatment
- The best nutritional and pharmacologic therapies
- The optimal time to begin treatment

- Development effects of postoperative anemia in children of all age groups
- Outcomes measure that include quality-of-life measures
- Cost-benefit analyses of treatment

17.3 Summary of Key Learning Objectives

17.3.1 What Is the Definition of Postoperative Anemia in Children?

There is not a definition of postoperative anemia per se in either children or adults. A postoperative anemia diagnosis and treatment plan must therefore be made on a case-by-case basis, taking into consideration the patient's clinical situation, physiologic ability to tolerate anemia, and support system upon hospital discharge.

17.3.2 What Are the Known Consequences of Postoperative Anemia?

Anemia in adults has been associated with multiple untoward outcomes, including decreased survival, fatigue, dementia, increased hospital readmission rates, postoperative acute kidney injury (AKI), heart failure, and a reduction in health-related quality of life. Many small observational studies of infants and toddlers have associated anemia, ID, or both, with an array of neurodevelopmental disorders including attention deficit hyperactivity disorder (ADHD), cognitive delay, academic underperformance, externalizing behaviors (e.g., aggression), and poor recognition memory. Children who remain severely anemic following surgery may have higher mortality and readmission rates compared to children with milder forms of anemia. The long-term effects of postoperative anemia in children have not been studied.

17.3.3 What Is the Prevalence of Pediatric Postoperative Anemia?

In observational studies of children surviving to PICU discharge, the rate of discharge anemia based on Hgb levels has been found to range from 8.3% to 58.9%. The contribution of postoperative patients to these numbers may be disproportionately large, reported to be as high as 70%.

17.3.4 What Factors Contribute to the Development of Pediatric Postoperative Anemia?

In both children and adults, the main contributors to postoperative anemia are preoperative anemia, surgical procedures, phlebotomy, and anemia upon hospital admission. Other important risk factors for postoperative anemia include small body size, convenience blood sampling through indwelling catheters, and possibly the standardization of restrictive RBC transfusion thresholds without follow up before discharge.

17.3.5 What Are Recommended Solutions to the Management of Pediatric Postoperative Anemia?

In addition to adherence to the basic tenants of PBM (i.e., minimizing blood loss through blood conservation techniques, optimized coagulation status, and consideration of the patient's unique physiologic reserve), the best practice to prevent postoperative anemia is to diagnose and treat *preoperative* anemia. All patients undergoing blood loss surgery and those at risk for anemia should undergo hemoglobin testing preoperatively. Iron studies and therapy should be initiated in consultation with a qualified pediatrician or hematologist once surgery is scheduled. In emergency and urgent procedures, IV iron may be an option if there is severe anemia in the face of ongoing bleeding, again under the direction of a hematologist. However, currrently in the US, both IV iron and ESA administrations are off-label in children undergoing surgery. A hemoglobin level should be measured at hospital discharge in all children who were anemic before surgery, those who have undergone blood loss surgery, and those who are receiving iron therapy. Continuity with the child's pediatrician or a hematologist should be arranged for follow-up over the first postoperative months to ensure recovery of hemoglobin and iron stores.

Key Points

- There is not a definition of postoperative anemia per se in either children or adults.
- There are numerous untoward effects associated with childhood anemia and iron deficiency, but the prevalence of postoperative anemia has only recently been investigated. The long-term effects of postoperative anemia in children have not been studied.
- The best practice to prevent postoperative anemia is to diagnose and treat *preoperative* anemia.
- A high percentage of children and adults with postoperative anemia do not recover for weeks to months after surgery.
- Children who were anemic before surgery or who have undergoing major blood loss should have a hemoglobin level measured before hospital discharge and managed accordingly to support anemia recovery.

Bibliography

1. Demaret P, Valla FV, Behal H, Mimouni Y, Baudelet JB, Karam O, et al. Anemia at discharge from the PICU: a Bicenter descriptive study. Pediatr Crit Care Med. 2019;20(9):e400–e9.
2. Numan S, Kaluza K. Systematic review of guidelines for the diagnosis and treatment of iron deficiency anemia using intravenous iron across multiple indications. Curr Med Res Opin. 2020;36(11):1769–82.
3. Bateman ST, Lacroix J, Boven K, Forbes P, Barton R, Thomas NJ, et al. Anemia, blood loss, and blood transfusions in north American children in the intensive care unit. Am J Respir Crit Care Med. 2008;178(1):26–33.
4. Brugnara C, Oski F, Nathan DG. Diagnostic Approach to the Anemic Patient. Orkin SH, Nathan DG, Ginsburg D. editors. In: Nathan and Oski's Hematology and Oncology of Infancy and Childhood. 2015. Philadelphia: Elsevier Saunders. p. 293–307.
5. World Health Organization. Haemoglobin concentrations for the diagnosis of anaemia and assessment of severity: vitamin and mineral nutrition information system. 2011. https://www.who.int/publications/i/item/WHO-NMH-NHD-MNM-11.1. Accessed 2 Feb 2024.
6. Jutras C, Sauthier M, Tucci M, Trottier H, Lacroix J, Robitaille N, et al. Prevalence and determinants of anemia at discharge in pediatric intensive care survivors. Transfusion. 2023;63(5):973–81.
7. Thornburg CD. The Anemias. In: Kliegman RM, Geme JS, editors. Nelson Textbook of Pediatrics E-book. 21st ed. 2019. Elsevier-OHCE; 2019. p. 2505–2506.
8. Henry E, Christensen RD. Reference intervals in neonatal hematology. In: Christensen RD, Juul SE, Del Veccio A, editors. Clinics in perinatology. Neonatal hematology and transfusion medicine, vol. 42. Philadelphia: Elsevier; 2015.483-497. p. 483.
9. Meyer HM, Torborg A, Cronje L, Thomas J, Bhettay A, Diedericks J, et al. The association between preoperative anemia and postoperative morbidity in pediatric surgical patients: a secondary analysis of a prospective observational cohort study. Paediatr Anaesth. 2020;30(7):759–65.
10. Stevens GA, Finucane MM, De-Regil LM, Paciorek CJ, Flaxman SR, Branca F, et al. Global, regional, and national trends in haemoglobin concentration and prevalence of total and severe anaemia in children and pregnant and non-pregnant women for 1995-2011: a systematic analysis of population-representative data. Lancet Glob Health. 2013;1(1):e16–25.
11. Hassan NE, Reischman DE, Fitzgerald RK, Faustino EVS. Prophylaxis against thrombosis practice study I, the pediatric acute lung I, sepsis investigators /BloodNet I. Hemoglobin levels across the pediatric critical care Spectrum: a point prevalence study. Pediatr Crit Care Med. 2018;19(5):e227–e34.
12. Muñoz M, Acheson AG, Bisbe E, Butcher A, Gómez-Ramírez S, Khalafallah AA, et al. An international consensus statement on the management of postoperative anaemia after major surgical procedures. Anaesthesia. 2018;73(11):1418–31.
13. Demaret P, Karam O, Tucci M, Lacroix J, Behal H, Duhamel A, et al. Anemia at pediatric intensive care unit discharge: prevalence and risk markers. Ann Intensive Care. 2017;7(1):107.
14. Gomez-Ramirez S, Jerico C, Munoz M. Perioperative anemia: prevalence, consequences and pathophysiology. Transfus Apher Sci. 2019;58(4):369–74.
15. Tong S, Vichinsky E. Iron deficiency: implications before anemia. Pediatr Rev. 2021;42(1):11–20.
16. Wang M. Iron deficiency and other types of anemia in infants and children. Am Fam Physician. 2016;93(4):270–8.
17. Camaschella C. Iron deficiency. Blood. 2019;133(1):30–9.
18. Shander A, Roy RC. Postoperative anemia: a sign of treatment failure. Anesth Analg. 2016;122(6):1755–9.
19. Mirski MA, Frank SM, Kor DJ, Vincent JL, Holmes DR Jr. Restrictive and liberal red cell transfusion strategies in adult patients: reconciling clinical data with best practice. Crit Care. 2015;19(1):202.

20. Khanna R, Harris DA, McDevitt JL, Fessler RG, Carabini LM, Lam SK, et al. Impact of anemia and transfusion on readmission and length of stay after spinal surgery: a single-center study of 1187 operations. Clin Spine Surg. 2017;30(10):E1338–E42.
21. Choi YJ, Kim SO, Sim JH, Hahm KD. Postoperative anemia is associated with acute kidney injury in patients undergoing Total hip replacement arthroplasty: a retrospective study. Anesth Analg. 2016;122(6):1923–8.
22. Warner MA, Hanson AC, Frank RD, Schulte PJ, Go RS, Storlie CB, Kor DJ. Prevalence of and recovery from anemia following hospitalization for critical illness among adults. JAMA Netw Open. 2020;3(9):e2017843.
23. Ai Y, Zhao SR, Zhou G, Ma X, Liu J. Hemoglobin status associated with performance IQ but not verbal IQ in Chinese preschool children. Pediatr Int. 2012;54(5):669–75.
24. Das BK, Kaushik JS. Cognitive development in children with malnutrition: a 50-year tale. Indian Pediatr. 2023;60(11):951–3.
25. Allali S, Brousse V, Sacri AS, Chalumeau M, de Montalembert M. Anemia in children: prevalence, causes, diagnostic work-up, and long-term consequences. Expert Rev Hematol. 2017;10(11):1023–8.
26. Lozoff B, Beard J, Connor J, Barbara F, Georgieff M, Schallert T. Long-lasting neural and behavioral effects of iron deficiency in infancy. Nutr Rev. 2006;64(5 Pt 2):S34–43. discussion S72–91
27. Lozoff B, Jimenez E, Hagen J, Mollen E, Wolf AW. Poorer behavioral and developmental outcome more than 10 years after treatment for iron deficiency in infancy. Pediatrics. 2000;105(4):E51.
28. Knappett M, Nguyen V, Chaudhry M, Trawin J, Kabakyenga J, Kumbakumba E, et al. Pediatric post-discharge mortality in resource-poor countries: a systematic review and meta-analysis. EClinicalMedicine. 2024;67:102380.
29. Gisslen T, Rao R, Georgieff MK. Anemia, iron supplementation, and the brain. Clin Perinatol. 2023;50(4):853–68.
30. McWilliams S, Singh I, Leung W, Stockler S, Ipsiroglu OS. Iron deficiency and common neurodevelopmental disorders—a scoping review. PLoS One. 2022;17(9):e0273819.
31. Samson KLI, Fischer JAJ, Roche ML. Iron status, anemia, and iron interventions and their associations with cognitive and academic performance in adolescents: a systematic review. Nutrients. 2022;14(1)
32. Su J, Cui N, Zhou G, Ai Y, Sun G, Zhao SR, Liu J. Hemoglobin status and externalizing behavioral problems in children. Int J Environ Res Public Health. 2016;13(8)
33. Algarin C, Peirano P, Garrido M, Pizarro F, Lozoff B. Iron deficiency anemia in infancy: long-lasting effects on auditory and visual system functioning. Pediatr Res. 2003;53(2):217–23.
34. Congdon EL, Westerlund A, Algarin CR, Peirano PD, Gregas M, Lozoff B, Nelson CA. Iron deficiency in infancy is associated with altered neural correlates of recognition memory at 10 years. J Pediatr. 2012;160(6):1027–33.
35. Soemantri AG, Pollitt E, Kim I. Iron deficiency anemia and educational achievement. Am J Clin Nutr. 1985;42(6):1221–8.
36. Algarin C, Karunakaran KD, Reyes S, Morales C, Lozoff B, Peirano P, Biswal B. Differences on brain connectivity in adulthood are present in subjects with iron deficiency anemia in infancy. Front Aging Neurosci. 2017;9:54.
37. Lozoff B, Jimenez E, Wolf AW. Long-term developmental outcome of infants with iron deficiency. N Engl J Med. 1991;325(10):687–94.
38. Halterman JS, Kaczorowski JM, Aligne CA, Auinger P, Szilagyi PG. Iron deficiency and cognitive achievement among school-aged children and adolescents in the United States. Pediatrics. 2001;107(6):1381–6.
39. Falkingham M, Abdelhamid A, Curtis P, Fairweather-Tait S, Dye L, Hooper L. The effects of oral iron supplementation on cognition in older children and adults: a systematic review and meta-analysis. Nutr J. 2010;9:4.

40. Wang B, Zhan S, Gong T, Lee L. Iron therapy for improving psychomotor development and cognitive function in children under the age of three with iron deficiency anaemia. Cochrane Database Syst Rev. 2013;2013(6):CD001444.
41. Abdullah K, Kendzerska T, Shah P, Uleryk E, Parkin PC. Efficacy of oral iron therapy in improving the developmental outcome of pre-school children with non-anaemic iron deficiency: a systematic review. Public Health Nutr. 2013;16(8):1497–506.
42. Benedict RK, Pullum TW, Riese S, Milner E. Is child anemia associated with early childhood development? A cross-sectional analysis of nine demographic and health surveys. PLoS One. 2024;19(2):e0298967.
43. Pagano MB, Dennis JA, Idemudia OM, Stanworth SJ, Carson JL. An analysis of quality of life and functional outcomes as reported in randomized trials for red cell transfusions. Transfusion. 2023;63(11):2032–9.
44. Mo A, Higgins AM. Restrictive transfusion thresholds: have we left patient-centered outcomes behind? Transfusion. 2022;62(10):1929–32.
45. Ross SD, Fahrbach K, Frame D, Scheye R, Connelly JE, Glaspy J. The effect of anemia treatment on selected health-related quality-of-life domains: a systematic review. Clin Ther. 2003;25(6):1786–805.
46. Jiang H, Hare GMT, Mazer CD. Effect of different red cell transfusion thresholds on quality of life: an important question with no clear answer yet. Transfusion. 2023;63(11):2013–6.
47. Moons P, Marquet K, Budts W, De Geest S. Validity, reliability and responsiveness of the "Schedule for the Evaluation of Individual Quality of Life-Direct Weighting" (SEIQoL-DW) in congenital heart disease. Health Qual Life Outcomes. 2004;2:27.
48. Knoester H, Bronner MB, Bos AP, Grootenhuis MA. Quality of life in children three and nine months after discharge from a paediatric intensive care unit: a prospective cohort study. Health Qual Life Outcomes. 2008;6:21.
49. Corwin HL, Gettinger A, Pearl RG, Fink MP, Levy MM, Abraham E, et al. The CRIT Study: Anemia and blood transfusion in the critically ill--current clinical practice in the United States. Crit Care Med 2004;32(1):39–52.
50. Mastro-Martinez I, Iglesias-Bouzas MI, Cabeza Martin B, Onoro-Otero G, Perez-Diaz C, Serrano-Gonzalez A, Casado-Flores J. Early postoperative complications of intracranial tumors in children. Minerva Pediatr. 2017;69(5):381–90.
51. Jutras C, Charlier J, François T, Du Pont-Thibodeau G. Anemia in pediatric critical care. Int J Clin Transf Med. 2020;8:23.
52. Bateman AP, McArdle F, Walsh TS. Time course of anemia during six months follow up following intensive care discharge and factors associated with impaired recovery of erythropoiesis. Crit Care Med. 2009;37(6):1906–12.
53. Du Pont-Thibodeau G, Jutras C, Lacroix J. Anemia at PICU discharge: is it a problem? Pediatr Crit Care Med. 2020;21(6):597–8.
54. Demaret P, Karam O, Labreuche Bst J, Chiusolo F, Mayordomo Colunga J, Erickson S, et al. How 217 pediatric intensivists manage anemia at PICU discharge: online responses to an international survey. Pediatr Crit Care Med. 2020;21(6):e342–e53.
55. Faraoni D, Meier J, New HV, Van der Linden PJ, Hunt BJ. Patient blood management for neonates and children undergoing cardiac surgery: 2019 NATA guidelines. J Cardiothorac Vasc Anesth. 2019;33(12):3249–63.
56. Walsh TS, Lee RJ, Maciver CR, Garrioch M, Mackirdy F, Binning AR, et al. Anemia during and at discharge from intensive care: the impact of restrictive blood transfusion practice. Intensive Care Med. 2006;32(1):100–9.
57. Roubinian NH, Murphy EL, Mark DG, Triulzi DJ, Carson JL, Lee C, et al. Long-term outcomes among patients discharged from the hospital with moderate anemia: a retrospective cohort study. Ann Intern Med. 2019;170(2):81–9.
58. Sinha R, Hakendorf P, Sobieraj-Teague M, Roxby D. Anaemia in elderly patients at discharge from intensive care and hospital. Vox Sang. 2021;116(10):1102–5.

59. NIH Office of Dietary Supplement. Iron: fact sheet for Health professionals. National Institutes of Health. 2022. https://ods.od.nih.gov/factsheets/Iron-HealthProfessional/. Accessed 17 Jan 2023.
60. Frank SM, Waters JH, editors. Patient blood management: multidisciplinary approaches to optimizing care. Bethesda: AABB Press; 2016. p. 6, 29–47, 180–6, 233–58, 327
61. Shander A, Corwin HL, Meier J, Auerbach M, Bisbe E, Blitz J, et al. Recommendations from the International Consensus Conference on Anemia Management in Surgical Patients (ICCAMS). Ann Surg. 2023;277(4):581–90.
62. Hayn D, Kreiner K, Kastner P, Breznik N, Hofmann A, Gombotz H, Schreier G. Data driven methods for predicting blood transfusion needs in elective surgery. Stud Health Technol Inform. 2016;223:9–16.
63. Lasocki S, Asfar P, Jaber S, Ferrandiere M, Kerforne T, Asehnoune K, et al. Impact of treating iron deficiency, diagnosed according to hepcidin quantification, on outcomes after a prolonged ICU stay compared to standard care: a multicenter, randomized, single-blinded trial. Crit Care. 2021;25(1):62.
64. Lasocki S, Chudeau N, Papet T, Tartiere D, Roquilly A, Carlier L, et al. Prevalence of iron deficiency on ICU discharge and its relation with fatigue: a multicenter prospective study. Crit Care. 2014;18(5):542.
65. Fontanals M, O'Leary JD, Zaarour C, Skelton T, Faraoni D. Preoperative anemia increases the risk of red blood cell transfusion and prolonged hospital length of stay in children undergoing spine arthrodesis surgery. Transfusion. 2019;59(2):492–9.
66. Sun DLR, Puran A, Al Nuaimi M, AlRiyami L, Kinlin LM, Kirby-Allen M, et al. Hemoglobin threshold for blood transfusion in young children hospitalized with iron deficiency anemia. J Pediatr. 2023;266:113878.
67. Wexler S. Postoperative transfusion: when, how much, and to avoid. NHS: Royal United Hospitals Bath, NHS Foundation Trust. 2018. file:///Users/normaklein/Downloads/When%20is%20Transfusion%20Indicated.pdf. Accessed 3 Feb 2024.
68. Hébert PC, Wells G, Blajchman MA, Marshall J, Martin C, Pagliarello G, et al. A multicenter, randomized, controlled clinical trial of transfusion requirements in critical care. Transfusion requirements in critical care investigators, Canadian Critical Care Trials Group. N Engl J Med. 1999;340(6):409–17.
69. Du Pont-Thibodeau G, Harrington K, Lacroix J. Anemia and red blood cell transfusion in critically ill cardiac patients. Ann Intensive Care. 2014;4:16.
70. Dallman MD, Liu X, Harris AD, Hess JR, Edelman BB, Murphy DJ, Netzer G. Changes in transfusion practice over time in the PICU. Pediatr Crit Care Med. 2013;14(9):843–50.
71. Netzer G, Liu X, Harris AD, Edelman BB, Hess JR, Shanholtz C, et al. Transfusion practice in the intensive care unit: a 10-year analysis. Transfusion. 2010;50(10):2125–34.
72. Chohan SS, McArdle F, McClelland DB, Mackenzie SJ, Walsh TS. Red cell transfusion practice following the transfusion requirements in critical care (TRICC) study: prospective observational cohort study in a large UK intensive care unit. Vox Sang. 2003;84(3):211–8.
73. Valentine SL, Bembea MM, Muszynski JA, Cholette JM, Doctor A, Spinella PC, et al. Consensus recommendations for RBC transfusion practice in critically ill children from the pediatric critical care transfusion and anemia expertise initiative. Pediatr Crit Care Med. 2018;19(9):884–98.
74. Steffen KM, Spinella PC, Holdsworth LM, Ford MA, Lee GM, Asch SM, et al. Factors influencing implementation of blood transfusion recommendations in pediatric critical care units. Front Pediatr. 2021;9:800461.
75. Doctor A, Cholette JM, Remy KE, Argent A, Carson JL, Valentine SL, et al. Recommendations on RBC transfusion in general critically ill children based on hemoglobin and/or physiologic thresholds from the pediatric critical care transfusion and anemia expertise initiative. Pediatr Crit Care Med. 2018;19(9S Suppl 1):S98–S113.
76. Valentine SL, Bateman ST. Identifying factors to minimize phlebotomy-induced blood loss in the pediatric intensive care unit. Pediatr Crit Care Med. 2012;13(1):22–7.

77. Thavendiranathan P, Bagai A, Ebidia A, Detsky AS, Choudhry NK. Do blood tests cause anemia in hospitalized patients? The effect of diagnostic phlebotomy on hemoglobin and hematocrit levels. J Gen Intern Med. 2005;20(6):520–4.
78. Wallin DJ, Tkac I, Stucker S, Ennis KM, Sola-Visner M, Rao R, Georgieff MK. Phlebotomy-induced anemia alters hippocampal neurochemistry in neonatal mice. Pediatr Res. 2015;77(6):765–71.
79. Griffith DM, Vale ME, Campbell C, Lewis S, Walsh TS. Persistent inflammation and recovery after intensive care: a systematic review. J Crit Care. 2016;33:192–9.
80. Collins JF, Wessling-Resnick M, Knutson MD. Hepcidin regulation of iron transport. J Nutr. 2008;138(11):2284–8.
81. Gallagher PG. The neonatal erythrocyte and its disorders. In: Orkin SH, Fisher DE, Look T, Lux SE, Ginsburg D, Nathan DG, editors. Nathan and Oski's hematology and oncology of infancy and childhood. 8th ed. Philadelphia: WB Saunders; 2015. p. 52.
82. Sharp MK, Mohammad SF. Hemolysis in needleless connectors for phlebotomy. ASAIO J. 2003;49(1):128–30.
83. Lehn RA, Gross JB, McIsaac JH, Gipson KE. Needleless connectors substantially reduce flow of crystalloid and red blood cells during rapid infusion. Anesth Analg. 2015;120(4):801–4.
84. Gniadek TJ, Richtsfeld M, Pulkrabek S, Hansen KR, Barnett SL, Joyner N, et al. Mechanical hemolysis in pediatric patients associated with rapid transfusion and one-way valve. Transfusion. 2018;58(5):1228–33.
85. O'Leary MF, Szklarski P, Klein TM, Young PP. Hemolysis of red blood cells after cell washing with different automated technologies: clinical implications in a neonatal cardiac surgery population. Transfusion. 2011;51(5):955–60.
86. Miller MA, Schlueter AJ. Transfusions via hand-held syringes and small-gauge needles as risk factors for hyperkalemia. Transfusion. 2004;44(3):373–81.
87. Kalra SK, Thilagar B, Khambaty M, Manjarrez E. Post-operative anemia after major surgery: a brief review. Curr Emerg Hosp Med Rep. 2021;9:89–95.
88. Sullivan HC, Roback JD. The pillars of patient blood management: key to successful implementation (Article, p. 2840). Transfusion. 2019;59(9):2763–7.
89. Warner MA, Shore-Lesserson L, Shander A, Patel SY, Perelman SI, Guinn NR. Perioperative anemia: prevention, diagnosis, and management throughout the spectrum of perioperative care. Anesth Analg. 2020;130(5):1364–80.
90. World Health Organization (WHO). Policy Brief: The Urgent Need to Implement Patient Blood Management. 2021. https://www.who.int/publications/i/item/9789240035744. Accessed 3 Aug 2023.
91. Baker RD, Greer FR, Pediatrics CoNAAo. Diagnosis and prevention of iron deficiency and iron-deficiency anemia in infants and young children (0-3 years of age). Pediatrics. 2010;126(5):1040–50.
92. Auerbach M, Adamson JW. How we diagnose and treat iron deficiency anemia. Am J Hematol. 2016;91(1):31–8.
93. Mattiello V, Schmugge M, Hengartner H, von der Weid N, Renella R, Group SPHW. Diagnosis and management of iron deficiency in children with or without anemia: consensus recommendations of the SPOG Pediatric Hematology Working Group. Eur J Pediatr. 2020;179(4):527–45.
94. Faraoni D, DiNardo JA, Goobie SM. Relationship between preoperative anemia and in-hospital mortality in children undergoing noncardiac surgery. Anesth Analg. 2016;123(6):1582–7.
95. Charuvila S, Imam MS, Reza T, Datta PK, Aziz TT, Davidson S, et al. A prospective observational study of preoperative anaemia management aided by bedside haemoglobin testers in a low-resource setting. J Pediatr Surg. 2024;59(2):305–9.
96. Ning S, Zeller MP. Management of iron deficiency. Hematology Am Soc Hematol Educ Program. 2019;2019(1):315–22.
97. Cohen CT, Powers JM. Intravenous iron therapy in pediatrics: who should get it and when is the right time? Hematology Am Soc Hematol Educ Program. 2023;2023(1):630–5.

98. Boucher AA, Pfeiffer A, Bedel A, Young J, McGann PT. Utilization trends and safety of intravenous iron replacement in pediatric specialty care: a large retrospective cohort study. Pediatr Blood Cancer. 2018;65(6):e26995.
99. Miles LF, Litton E, Imberger G, Story D. Intravenous iron therapy for non-anaemic, iron-deficient adults. Cochrane Database Syst Rev. 2019;12(12):CD013084.
100. Auerbach M, Gafter-Gvili A, Macdougall IC. Intravenous iron: a framework for changing the management of iron deficiency. Lancet Haematol. 2020;7(4):e342–e50.
101. Shah AA, Donovan K, Seeley C, Dickson EA, Palmer AJR, Doree C, et al. Risk of infection associated with administration of intravenous iron: a systematic review and meta-analysis. JAMA Netw Open. 2021;4(11):e2133935.
102. Neef V, Baumgarten P, Noone S, Piekarski F, Triphaus C, Kleineruschkamp A, et al. The impact of timing of intravenous iron supplementation on preoperative haemoglobin in patients scheduled for major surgery. Blood Transfus. 2022;20(3):188–97.
103. Ng O, Keeler BD, Mishra A, Simpson JA, Neal K, Al-Hassi HO, et al. Iron therapy for preoperative anaemia. Cochrane Database Syst Rev. 2019;12(12):CD011588.
104. Peri V, Devlin P, Perry L, Richards T, Miles LF. Associations between nonanemic iron deficiency and postoperative outcomes in cardiac surgery: a systematic review and meta-analysis. Anesth Analg. 2024;
105. Spahn DR, Schoenrath F, Spahn GH, Seifert B, Stein P, Theusinger OM, et al. Effect of ultra-short-term treatment of patients with iron deficiency or anaemia undergoing cardiac surgery: a prospective randomised trial. Lancet. 2019;393(10187):2201–12.
106. Khalafallah AA, Yan C, Al-Badri R, Robinson E, Kirkby BE, Ingram E, et al. Intravenous ferric carboxymaltose versus standard care in the management of postoperative anaemia: a prospective, open-label, randomised controlled trial. Lancet Haematol. 2016;3(9):e415–25.
107. Froessler B, Palm P, Weber I, Hodyl NA, Singh R, Murphy EM. The important role for intravenous iron in perioperative patient blood management in major abdominal surgery: a randomized controlled trial. Ann Surg. 2016;264(1):41–6.
108. Carson JL, Stanworth SJ, Dennis JA, Trivella M, Roubinian N, Fergusson DA, et al. Transfusion thresholds for guiding red blood cell transfusion. Cochrane Database Syst Rev. 2021;12(12):CD002042.
109. Stanworth SJ, Carson JL. AABB RBC Transfusion Guidelines Debate: Which Restrictive Hemoglobin Threshold? AM23-ST-05-L. Oct. 14, 2023. AABB annual meeting, Nashville, TN.
110. Powers JM, Shamoun M, McCavit TL, Adix L, Buchanan GR. Intravenous ferric carboxymaltose in children with iron deficiency anemia who respond poorly to oral iron. J Pediatr. 2017;180:212–6.
111. Akarsu S, Taskin E, Yilmaz E, Yilmaz H, Kilic M, Aygun AD. Treatment of iron deficiency anemia with intravenous iron preparations. Acta Haematol. 2006;116(1):51–7.
112. Rothman JA. Iron-deficiency anemia. In: Kliegman RM, St. Geme J, editors. Nelson textbook of pediatrics E-book. 21st ed. Philadelphia: Elsevier; 2020. p. 2522.
113. Auerbach M, Deloughery T. Single-dose intravenous iron for iron deficiency: a new paradigm. Hematology Am Soc Hematol Educ Program. 2016;2016(1):57–66.
114. Munoz M, Acheson AG, Auerbach M, Besser M, Habler O, Kehlet H, et al. International consensus statement on the peri-operative management of anaemia and iron deficiency. Anaesthesia. 2017;72(2):233–47.
115. Munoz M. Panel for the international consensus statement on perio-operative management of anaemia iron d. Peri-operative correction of non-anaemic iron deficiency. A reply. Anaesthesia. 2017;72(7):911–2.
116. Avni T, Bieber A, Grossman A, Green H, Leibovici L, Gafter-Gvili A. The safety of intravenous iron preparations: systematic review and meta-analysis. Mayo Clin Proc. 2015;90(1):12–23.
117. The University of Iowa Department of Pathology. Laboratory Services Handbook. https://www.healthcare.uiowa.edu/path_handbook/handbook/test1151.html. 2019. Accessed 21 Jan 2024.

118. Corewell Health. Ferritin, Blood Level. https://corewellhealth.testcatalog.org/show/LAB68-1. 2024. Accessed 21 Jan 2024.
119. Seattle Children's Hospital. Iron (Fe) Level https://seattlechildrenslab.testcatalog.org/show/LAB94-1. 2024. Accessed 21 Jan 2024.
120. Okam MM, Koch TA, Tran MH. Iron deficiency anemia treatment response to oral iron therapy: a pooled analysis of five randomized controlled trials. Haematologica. 2016;101(1):e6–7.
121. Rampton D, Folkersen J, Fishbane S, Hedenus M, Howaldt S, Locatelli F, et al. Hypersensitivity reactions to intravenous iron: guidance for risk minimization and management. Haematologica. 2014;99(11):1671–6.
122. Rund D. Intravenous iron and infection risk-still an unanswered question. JAMA Netw Open. 2021;4(11):e2134453.
123. Wang C, Graham DJ, Kane RC, Xie D, Wernecke M, Levenson M, et al. Comparative risk of anaphylactic reactions associated with intravenous iron products. JAMA. 2015;314(19):2062–8.
124. Chertow GM, Mason PD, Vaage-Nilsen O, Ahlmen J. Update on adverse drug events associated with parenteral iron. Nephrol Dial Transplant. 2006;21(2):378–82.
125. Dave CV, Brittenham GM, Carson JL, Setoguchi S. Risks for anaphylaxis with intravenous iron formulations : a retrospective cohort study. Ann Intern Med. 2022;175(5):656–64.
126. European Medicines Agency. New recommendations to manage risk of allergic reactions with intravenous iron-containing medicines. 2013. https://www.ema.europa.eu/en/news/new-recommendations-manage-risk-allergic-reactions-intravenous-iron-containing-medicines. Accessed 4 Feb 2024.
127. Rao R, Georgieff MK. Iron therapy for preterm infants. Clin Perinatol. 2009;36(1):27–42.
128. Akarsu S, Demir H, Selek S, Oguzoncul F. Iron deficiency anemia and levels of oxidative stress induced by treatment modality. Pediatr Int. 2013;55(3):289–95.
129. Brookes MJ, Farr A, Phillips CJ, Trudgill NJ. Management of iron deficiency anaemia in secondary care across England between 2012 and 2018: a real-world analysis of Hospital Episode Statistics. Frontl Gastroenterol. 2021;12(5):363–9.
130. Corwin HL, Gettinger A, Pearl RG, Fink MP, Levy MM, Shapiro MJ, et al. Efficacy of recombinant human erythropoietin in critically ill patients: a randomized controlled trial. JAMA. 2002;288(22):2827–35.
131. Krafte-Jacobs B, Levetown ML, Bray GL, Ruttimann UE, Pollack MM. Erythropoietin response to critical illness. Crit Care Med. 1994;22(5):821–6.
132. Jelkmann I, Jelkmann W. Impact of erythropoietin on intensive care unit patients. Transfus Med Hemother. 2013;40(5):310–8.
133. O'Brien SH, Badawy SM, Rotz SJ, Shah MD, Makarski J, Bercovitz RS, et al. The ASH-ASPHO Choosing Wisely Campaign: 5 hematologic tests and treatments to question. Pediatr Blood Cancer. 2021;68(8):e28967.
134. Danko I, Weidkamp M, Eickhoff JC. Improvement of health-related quality of life in children with inflammatory bowel disease receiving routine intravenous iron supplementation. J Pediatr Pharmacol Ther. 2019;24(6):517–27.
135. Warner MA, Hanson AC, Plimier C, Lee C, Liu VX, Richards T, et al. Association between anaemia and hospital readmissions in patients undergoing major surgery requiring postoperative intensive care. Anaesthesia. 2023;78(1):45–54.
136. Munoz M, Franchini M, Liumbruno GM. The post-operative management of anaemia: more efforts are needed. Blood Transfus. 2018;16(4):324–5.

Part IV

Special Perioperative Considerations

Patient Blood Management for Pediatric Cardiac Surgery with Cardiopulmonary Bypass

18

Anne E. Cossu and Stephanie N. Grant

18.1 Case Scenario

A 3-month-old, 4.2-kg full-term male infant with a large perimembranous ventricular septal defect (VSD), congestive heart failure, and failure to thrive presents for VSD repair. Preoperative medications include furosemide, chlorothiazide, and digoxin. The preoperative laboratory studies include a hemoglobin (Hgb) 8 g/dL, hematocrit (Hct) 24%, platelets 205 × 10^9/L, and fibrinogen 200 mg/dL. All other coagulation studies are within normal limits including normal parameters on a baseline thromboelastography (TEG). The patient is hemodynamically stable before and during cardiopulmonary bypass (CPB). Upon separation from CPB and following protamine administration, the surgeon and anesthesiologist notice that there is minimal clot formation.

Key Learning Objectives

- Does this patient require medical optimization of his hemoglobin (Hgb) and hematocrit (Hct) prior to cardiac surgery?
- What can be done to optimize the patient's hemoglobin and hematocrit before surgery?
- How will the CPB circuit affect hemostasis in this patient?
- What intraoperative strategies are used during cardiac surgery to reduce bleeding?
- What blood products or pharmacologic adjuncts may be considered for administration in post-CPB bleeding?

A. E. Cossu · S. N. Grant (✉)
Emory University School of Medicine, Atlanta, GA, USA
e-mail: anne.elisa.cossu@emory.edu; stephanie.grant@emory.edu

N. J. Klein (ed.), *Perioperative Pediatric Patient Blood Management and Transfusion Safety*, https://doi.org/10.1007/978-3-031-81666-6_18

18.2 Discussion

18.2.1 General

Blood product transfusion is common in pediatric patients during and after cardiovascular surgery with cardiopulmonary bypass (CPB). Minimization of allogenic blood transfusions and avoidance of multiple donor exposures are goals often set during preoperative preparation. Unfortunately, there is a paucity of high-quality evidence to guide preoperative blood management of children undergoing cardiac surgery [1]. A 2018 retrospective view of a pediatric heart surgery multicenter database for the years 2014 and 2015 found that in over 22,000 surgeries, the perioperative packed red blood cell (RBC) transfusion rate declined with increasing age but was close to 100% in infants [2]. Numerous practices have been employed in the perioperative period in pediatric patients to maintain normal hemostasis and to prevent bleeding. It is important to identify which patients are at risk of developing a coagulopathy and to apply evidence-based biopharmacologic therapies, validated physiologic monitors, and laboratory tests of hemostasis to drive appropriate management.

18.2.2 Does This Patient Require Medical Optimization of His Hemoglobin (Hgb) and Hematocrit (Hct) Prior to Cardiac Surgery?

Preoperative anemia in pediatric patients presenting for cardiac surgery is complex and multifactorial. The rate of anemia presenting for noncardiac surgery is 32% in neonates and 24–46.2% in older children [3–5]. The presence of preoperative anemia in neonates, infants, and children undergoing noncardiac surgery has been associated with increased intraoperative blood transfusion and in-hospital mortality [3–5]. Preoperative anemia in adult patients undergoing cardiac surgery is associated with adverse events, including acute kidney injury, stroke, and death [6]. In children undergoing cardiac surgery, preoperative anemia is associated with an increased risk of perioperative acute kidney injury, altered developmental scores, and allogenic blood transfusions [7–9].

The normal baseline Hgb level in patients with congenital heart disease (CHD) varies due to differences in age and the presence or absence of cyanosis. Definitions of anemia are not well defined in cyanotic CHD patients, who have relatively increased hemoglobin concentrations secondary to increased erythropoiesis due to chronic hypoxia. Infants have a normal physiologic decrease in hemoglobin concentration during the 9th–12th week of life known as physiologic anemia of infancy [10]. During this time, term infants have a hemoglobin concentration with a nadir of 10–11 g/dL, and preterm infants may have a nadir as low as 8 g/dL. After the third month of life, the hemoglobin concentration will increase to 11.5–12 g/dL until 2 years of age [11]. Patients requiring surgery during the physiologic nadir should be optimized with blood conservation strategies, but do not require allogenic blood transfusions prior to surgery unless they are hemodynamically unstable.

The optimal preoperative hemoglobin for patients with congenital heart disease (CHD) is unknown. A reduction in hemoglobin decreases the oxygen-carrying capacity of blood causing a potential mismatch of oxygen delivery and demand. This leads to inadequate tissue oxygenation and organ function resulting in hypoxia and acidosis [12, 13]. RBC transfusions may be necessary in pediatric cardiac surgical patients in order to increase oxygen-carrying capacity and to avoid hypoxic tissue injury. A recent mathematical model was used to determine the physiologic Hgb level in patients with single-ventricle physiology [14]. This in vitro calculation found that Hgb greater than 13 g/dL was required to maintain arterial oxygen saturation >70% when cardiac output is maintained at 6 L/m^2/min; a Hgb of 9 g/dL (e.g., a transfusion threshold considered "liberal" in healthier patients) was associated with significant arterial desaturation. However, this is only a mathematical model without clinical correlation testing and assumes that increased RBC mass will consistently increase oxygen-carrying capacity.

Risk factors associated with receiving an allogenic RBC transfusion in pediatric patients undergoing cardiac surgery with CPB include lower weight, younger age, higher Risk Adjustment for Congenital Heart Surgery (RACHS-1) score, higher ASA score, and higher mortality index score [15, 16]. Although receiving any blood transfusions can be lifesaving for this population of patients, transfusions are not without complication risk. Allogenic RBC transfusions in pediatric cardiac surgical patients are associated with postoperative pulmonary complications, prolonged mechanical ventilation, higher inotropic scores, infections, and prolonged ICU and hospital length of stay (LOS) [16–25].

Preservation of a patient's blood supply is a challenge when a patient is coagulopathic. Pediatric patients, in particular neonates and infants, are at high risk for hemorrhage after cardiac surgery secondary to excessive hemodilution upon initiation of CPB. Hemodilution is the result of a smaller body surface area and circulating blood volume relative to the circuit volume, decreased levels of coagulation proteins, and potentially abnormal hemostasis due to cyanotic congenital heart disease [26–28]. Other risk factors for coagulopathic bleeding include lower CPB temperatures, increased length of CPB time, redo sternotomy, and preexisting heart failure [28].

Multiple studies have shown that perioperative restrictive transfusion strategies in pediatric patients undergoing cardiac surgery with CPB are relatively safe [29–34]. In an early prospective trial, Willems et al. randomized noncyanotic patients post-cardiac surgery into two RBC transfusion trigger groups: a Hgb < 7.0 g/dL in the restrictive threshold group and <9.5 g/dL in the liberal group. The restrictive transfusion group received fewer RBC transfusions and had less donor exposures with no difference in multiple organ dysfunction between groups [29]. Later studies corroborated these findings with similar outcomes between restrictive and liberal RBC transfusion groups, including length of stay (LOS) and duration of mechanical ventilation (Table 18.1). In another prospective trial, children undergoing single-ventricle palliation and weighing less than 10 kg were also randomized

Table 18.1 Summary of early studies examining RBC transfusion thresholds in pediatric cardiac surgery

Author/year	Study design	Phase of care	Cohort CHD	Number of patients	Restrictive Hgb (g/dL)	Liberal Hgb (g/dL)	Result
Willlems/2010 [29]	RCT with subanalysis	Postoperative	Acyanotic	125	7	9.5	Restrictive: Decreased number transfusions and donor exposure No difference in MOD, mechanical ventilation duration, ICU LOS
Cholette/2011 [31]	RCT	Postoperative	Cyanotic and singleV undergoing cardiopulmonary anastomosis	60	9	13	Restrictive: Decreased number RBC transfusion and donor exposure No difference in lactate, O2 utilization, clinical outcome
De Gast-Bakker/2013 [30]	RCT	Perioperative	Acyanotic	107	8	10.8	Restrictive: Shorter hospital LOS, lower volume RBCs No difference in mechanical ventilation duration or ICU LOS
Chkhaidze/2014 [35]	RCT	Perioperative	Acyanotic	43	8	10	Restrictive: Less volume RBCs transfused ($p = 0.05$) No difference in-hospital mortality, LOS, or mechanical ventilation
Cholette/2017 [32]	RCT	Postoperative	BiV or singleV infants <10 kg	162	7 (BiV) 9 (SingleV)	9.5 (BiV) 12 (SingleV)	Restrictive: Decreased number and volume of RBC transfusions, decreased % patients requiring RBCs, decreased donor exposure. No difference in mortality and LOS Concluded both cohorts can tolerate restrictive RBC transfusion thresholds

CHD congenital heart disease, *RCT* randomized controlled trial, *MOD* multiorgan dysfunction, *LOS* length of stay, *BiV* biventricle, *SingleV* single ventricle to a restrictive or liberal transfusion strategy post-cardiac surgery. The hemoglobin threshold was <9.5 g/dL in the restrictive group and < 12 g/dL in the liberal group. The restrictive group received fewer RBC units and less overall blood volume as well as fewer donor exposures, and there was no difference in other clinical outcomes compared to the liberal transfusion group [32].

An expert consensus task force, the Network for the Advancement of Patient Blood Management, Haemostasis and Thrombosis (NATA), recommends a postoperative Hgb transfusion threshold of 7.0 g/dL in stable, acyanotic cardiac surgical patients and 8.0 g/dL if there are clinical signs of symptomatic anemia (Grade[1] 1B evidence: strong recommendation, moderate-quality evidence) [8]. For cyanotic children undergoing cardiac surgery, NATA suggests a postoperative Hgb threshold is 9.0 g/dL (Grade 1C: strong recommendation, low-quality evidence). The Pediatric Critical Care Transfusion and Anemia Expertise Initiative (TAXI) recommends similar Hgb thresholds of <7.0 g/dL for biventricular repairs and < 9.0 g/dL for single-ventricle palliation in patients who are stable, with the Hgb maintained between 7 and 9 g/dL for children with uncorrected CHD who have a stable cardiopulmonary reserve [36, 37].

To minimize allogenic blood transfusions during pediatric cardiac surgery, hemoglobin thresholds should be followed in conjunction with the patient's clinical status. A patient's microcirculation as well as the nature of transfused RBCs will impact global oxygenation [38]. Physiologic parameters—such as cerebral and somatic regional oximetry, blood pressure, heart rate, and lactate levels—may indicate a patient's tolerance for anemia and should guide transfusion decisions along with the Hgb level [39].

The optimal hemoglobin and hematocrit *during* CPB, when patients are hypothermic, are not well defined. Younger patients experience significant hemodilution on CPB due to the ratio of the circuit prime volume to the patient's blood volume [17]. Jonas et al. performed an RCT of 147 infants to compare a lower Hct (21.5% ± 2.9%) under hypothermic CPB with a higher Hct (27.8% ± 3.2%) [40]. The lower Hct group had lower cardiac index during and higher lactate levels following CPB and, at 1 year of age, worse psychomotor development index (PDI) scores. The same investigators conducted a later trial to determine an optimal target Hct under hypothermic CPB [9]. Combining the results of two similar RCTs, including 271 infants undergoing hypothermic biventricular repair without aortic arch involvement, the investigators determined that PDI scores increased in a nonlinear fashion with the Hct approximating 24% at the onset of low-flow CPB ($p < 0.001$) [9, 41]. In another follow-up study, hemodilution on CPB to a Hct of 25% had similar postoperative outcomes and PDI scores to a Hct of 35% [41]. The 2019 NATA guidelines recommend adding RBCs during CPB to maintain a hematocrit >24% (Grade 2C evidence: weak recommendation, low-quality evidence), although the safety profile for the optimal Hct goal for the different age groups, type of CHD lesion, or associated comorbidities is unclear [8].

[1] The Grading Recommendations Assessment, Development, and Evaluation (GRADE) system evaluates the certainty of evidence and strength of expert recommendations.

While minimum perioperative Hgb and Hct thresholds are important, one retrospective study found that higher postoperative Hct levels may be detrimental [42]. Long et al. demonstrated that a higher Hct on arrival to the ICU was associated with increased operative mortality and major complications in cyanotic and acyanotic children following more than 27,000 cardiac surgeries. Each 5% incremental increase in Hct over 42% for cyanotic and 38% for acyanotic patients increased the odds of operative mortality (1.31-fold for cyanotic and 1.45-fold for acyanotic), as well as major complications (1.22-fold for cyanotic and 1.21-fold for acyanotic). Major complications found on secondary analysis included longer ICU and hospital LOSs, duration of mechanical ventilation, and delayed sternal closure [42]. Although Long's study did address patient age or specific procedure type, overall, studies continue to support the safety of restrictive transfusion strategies in pediatric CHD surgery.

18.2.3 What Can Be Done to Optimize the Patient's Hemoglobin and Hematocrit Before Surgery?

All pediatric patients should be evaluated for anemia prior to cardiac surgery. If anemia is present, then an elective cardiac surgery should be rescheduled. Establishment of a patient blood management process to identify patients with preoperative anemia and to plan blood conservation strategies with a multidisciplinary team is essential for good patient outcomes. Preoperative anticoagulation therapy must be managed through expert consultation. If present, the surgery should be performed only in settings that can provide reversal agents, relevant coagulation monitoring, or both [43]. Iron deficiency is a common cause of anemia in children and is present in 56% of children with heart failure [44]. Otsuka et al. demonstrated that preoperative oral iron supplementation increases preoperative hemoglobin levels and decreases the volume of allogenic RBC transfusions in the perioperative period for children undergoing cardiac surgery [45]. The time frame required for oral iron supplementation to produce an increase in Hgb is 1 month, but 3 months is required to replete iron stores [46]. Parenteral iron supplementation may offer a more timely and tolerable solution for treatment of iron deficiency anemia prior to cardiac surgery [17, 46]. Ferumoxytol, an intravenous iron preparation, effectively treats iron deficiency anemia in children with a significant increase in hemoglobin concentration at 1 and 4 weeks post-infusion [47]. For a more detailed discussion on IV iron therapy in children undergoing surgery, refer to Chap. 4.

The Network for the Advancement of Patient Blood Management, Haemostasis and Thrombosis (NATA) recommends the diagnosis and treatment of preoperative iron deficiency anemia in pediatric cardiac surgical patients and consideration of preoperative erythropoietin in certain situations, such as the children of Jehovah's Witness patients (Grade 2C evidence [8]. Erythropoiesis-stimulating agents (ESAs) have been found to increase preoperative Hgb and Hct as well as decrease the amount of perioperative allogenic blood transfusions in pediatric patients undergoing cardiac surgery [48–50]. Pediatric data on the preoperative administration of

ESAs, however, is limited. Consensus guidelines support the preoperative administration of ESAs in pediatric cardiac surgery only in select patient populations [8]. Reports of thromboembolism in adults (but not children), combined with limited prospective data in the pediatric surgical population, has led to a general hesitancy to administer ESAs to anemic children outside of special situations [51–54].

Avoiding unnecessary blood testing is a cornerstone of preserving the hospitalized patient's blood supply and preventing iatrogenic anemia. A 2017 survey of pediatric centers performing cardiac surgery examined the practice of routine preoperative laboratory testing [55]. Routine testing prior to cardiac surgery typically includes a complete blood count (CBC), metabolic panel, coagulation studies, liver function tests, and a type and screen (T&S). Although 11 of 12 centers surveyed routinely performed a robust panel of blood tests, over 80% reported that the laboratory results had little to no bearing on case management, including cancellation. The one exception was the preoperative T&S. The Association for the Advancement of Blood & Biotherapies (AABB), with patient safety and supply considerations in mind, recommends that a preoperative T&S in blood loss cases be processed prior to the patient entering the operating room [56, 57]. More than 3% of T&S samples received in US blood banks have serologic evidence of alloimmunization, and the concern is heightened in patients who have been multiply transfused (and are more likely to be alloimmunized) or possess "cold" autoantibodies that may cause agglutination upon CPB cooling [58]. Furthermore, last-minute antibody identification and crossmatching in a case that is certain to require a blood transfusion place undue stress on the transfusion service and create a potential delay in blood product availability. A common misconception is that the processing of a T&S specimen after anesthesia induction can be ameliorated by supplying universal donor blood products. In response to a universal and a critical short supply of type O Rh-negative RBCs, the AABB has alerted transfusion services that this product should be reserved for females of childbearing age who require a lifesaving transfusion and whose blood type is unknown [59]. With regard to universal donor plasma (i.e., AB Rh-positive, present in only 4% of donors), blood banks now provide type A Rh-positive plasma because the supply of type AB plasma is critically low [60].

18.2.4 How Will the Cardiopulmonary Bypass Circuit Affect Hemostasis in This Patient?

The initiation of CPB results in hemodilution of red blood cells, platelets, and coagulation factors. Young patients experience the greatest degree of hemodilution secondary to a greater ratio of prime volume to the total blood volume [17]. As a result, blood is often required in the circuit prime to support oxygenation with an adequate on-bypass Hct. Predictors for requiring an RBC transfusion while on CPB include lower body weight, lower preoperative Hgb concentration, longer duration of CPB, previous sternotomy, and palliative surgery [61]. A CPB-related coagulopathy results from several factors. Contact activation of a patient's blood with the artificial CPB circuit results in inflammation and impaired coagulation [17].

Newer-generation CPB circuits made of superior materials with less inflammatory potential are now available, but many pediatric studies are based on the older technologies [62]. Platelet function and enzymatic activity are decreased by hypothermia that is employed as a neuroprotective strategy to reduce metabolic demand and consequently cerebral metabolic rate. Unfractionated heparin, monitored with the activated clotting time (ACT), is used to prevent thrombosis and thromboembolic events caused by contact activation of the coagulation system. In patients with heparin-induced thrombocytopenia (HIT) or antithrombin III (AT3) deficiency, direct thrombin inhibitors (e.g., bivalirudin) may be utilized as an alternative anticoagulant [63]. Patients at risk for AT3 deficiency include neonates, infants with CHD, and those in DIC or with renal disease.

18.2.5 What Intraoperative Strategies Can Be Used during Cardiac Surgery to Reduce Bleeding?

CPB-related coagulopathy can be mitigated through the use of standardized transfusion algorithms, CPB circuit size minimization, prime fluid modification, retrograde autologous prime, ultrafiltration, and point-of-care (POC) viscoelastic test (VET)-guided coagulation management [8, 17, 28, 64].

18.2.5.1 Transfusion Algorithms

Cardiac surgical procedures consume a large proportion of the national blood bank supply [65]. A prospective, multicenter study on the management of anemia in pediatric patients after cardiac surgery revealed that 79% of patients received at least one RBC transfusion in the intensive care unit after surgery [19]. There is convincing evidence that the concerted use of algorithmic point-of-care testing (POCT) and viscoelastic technology reduces the rate of all blood transfusions after cardiac surgery in adults [66]. The European Association for Cardio-Thoracic Surgery (EACTS) and the European Association of Cardiothoracic Anesthesiology (EACTA) recommend VET-guided transfusion algorithms in the perioperative management of bleeding in adults undergoing cardiac surgery [66].

Several studies support transfusion algorithms in pediatric cardiac surgery [13, 67–71]. Conventional laboratory tests of hemostasis, such as the fibrinogen, platelet count, prothrombin time/international normalized ratio (PT/INR), activated partial thromboplastin time (aPTT), and activated clotting time (ACT), do not provide a global assessment of hemostasis, and results are often delayed or out of sync with active bleeding. Despite the drawbacks in conventional testing, Whitney et al. used conventional laboratory tests as part of a transfusion algorithm for pediatric cardiac surgery and demonstrated significantly reduced intraoperative and postoperative transfusion rates for all products [68] (Fig. 18.1). With exception of the ACT, most institutions have not substituted conventional coagulation testing with bedside POCT.

A bleeding management algorithmic protocol based on rotational thromboelastometry (ROTEM) for major craniofacial surgeries was recently implemented at a

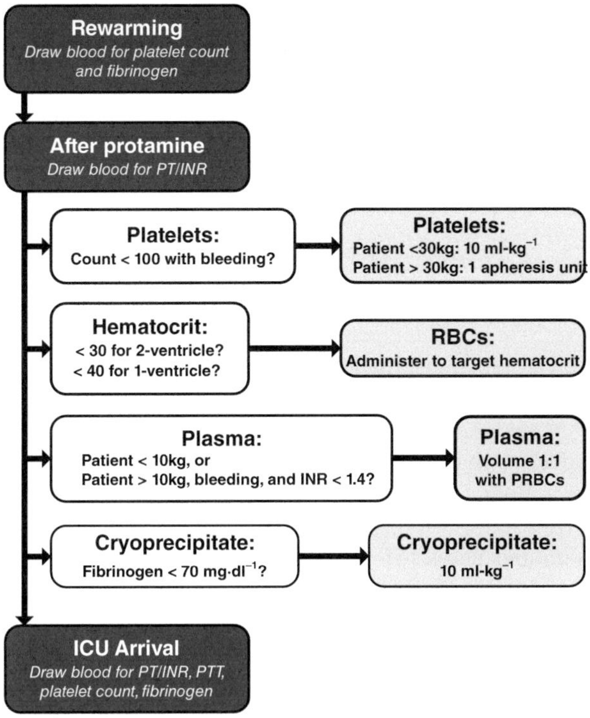

Fig. 18.1 A post-CPB blood product administration algorithm based on conventional laboratory testing results. (Reprinted with permission from Whitney et al. [68])

tertiary children's hospital [64]. The algorithm was associated with a significant reduction in "yellow" blood products and hospital cost, with no change in safety profiles. VET-based transfusion algorithms were found to reduce transfusion requirements in three additional studies (two retrospective and one prospective) of pediatric patients undergoing cardiac surgery [67, 69, 72].

There is a paucity of large studies evaluating the efficacy of VET-based transfusion algorithms in pediatric patients. However, the current weight of the evidence suggests that VET-based transfusion algorithms should be strongly considered for pediatric trauma and surgical procedures with a high risk of bleeding such as craniofacial, spine, and cardiac surgeries in an effort to avoid arbitrary and disparate blood management [17, 73].

18.2.5.2 Miniaturization of the Cardiopulmonary Bypass Circuit

Initiation of CPB leads to a dilution of RBCs, coagulation factors, and platelets as the patient's blood volume mixes with the CPB circuit prime. Hemodilution after CPB initiation is most pronounced in neonates and infants secondary to the circuit size and the prime volume used relative to the patient's body weight. Whereas many neonates may have a total blood volume of less than 350 ml (e.g., 85 mL/kg), a neonatal CPB circuit may be larger than 100–250 mL, creating a circuit-to-blood volume ratio close to 75% [74]. The hemodynamic effect of this large body fluid shift can be minimized by using the smallest circuit that will allow the desired cardiac index (CI) at full flow. Circuit "miniaturization" includes decreasing the length and diameter of tubing as well as the use of low-volume components, such as the oxygenator and filters [75–77]. Considerations in circuit volume selection include the necessary distance between the CPB machine and the patient, as well as the interior diameter that does not create excessive line pressure [78].

18.2.5.3 Prime Fluid

The ideal CPB prime fluid composition prevents dilutional coagulopathy and maintains a Hct above 24% [8, 9]. Unfortunately, this prime solution does not exist [74]. The ideal prime Hct remains a matter of debate [8]. Addition of blood products to the prime may be necessary to minimize dilutional coagulopathy, maintain oxygenation, and give hemodynamic support. The decision over when and which allogeneic blood products to add to the circuit prime is based on the patient's weight, preoperative hemoglobin, total prime volume, and the desired Hct while on CPB.

For a clear prime free of blood products, the addition of colloids is recommended over 100% crystalloid fluids [8]. Riegger et al. demonstrated that a 5% albumin prime led to a net negative fluid status at the end of CPB compared to the crystalloid prime group which developed a net positive fluid balance [79]. A higher oncotic pressure is important to prevent tissue edema secondary to extracellular fluid shifts during bypass. If a blood prime is necessary to maintain coagulation, hemodynamics, and oxygenation, the blood products administered in the prime may be determined by institutional protocol and product availability. Willems et al. found that RBCs given in CPB prime did not significantly impact severe postoperative morbidity and mortality after propensity matching [16]. However, investigators in this study concluded that the real effects of allogeneic RBCs in CPB prime could not be definitively determined secondary to study design as well as the multiple confounding variables associated with CPB-related morbidity. The use of fresh and reconstituted whole blood in the circuit prime has been associated with fewer blood product exposures, lower inotropic scores, shorter duration of mechanical ventilation, and shorter hospital LOS in neonates [80, 81]. In infants, administration of plasma in the pump prime during CPB has been shown to be associated with less postoperative bleeding than administration following CPB (with no differences in the overall number of transfusions) [82]. Fresh frozen plasma (FFP) in the prime leads to higher fibrinogen levels after separation from CPB and decreases the number of units of cryoprecipitate transfused; however, additional improvements in clinical outcomes have not been shown [83, 84]. The 2019 NATA guidelines recommend the addition of FFP in neonatal CPB prime (Grade 2C evidence: weak recommendation, low-quality evidence) [8]. Platelets are not typically added to prime but instead are administered after CPB and heparin reversal. However, one center has published the results of an RCT in which 21 neonates were administered platelets during the rewarming phase of CPB, immediately before separation, and found a 40% reduction in post-bypass blood product administration [85]. NATA has not made a recommendation for CPB circuit plasma prime in older infants and children due to a lack of evidence.

18.2.5.4 Retrograde Autologous Prime

Retrograde autologous priming (RAP) is a technique used to replace the CPB circuit prime volume with the patient's own blood prior to initiation of CPB. The goal is to limit hemodilution and its attendant side effects. Once the arterial and venous cannulas are in position, blood from the patient is drained via the arterial and venous lines into the CPB circuit, and the clear priming solution is removed from the circuit [86, 87]. Consequently, RAP has been shown to reduce the need for addition of allogenic RBCs in the prime [87]. Hemodynamic instability may occur during this procedure as blood is removed from the patient that must be supported with vasoactive agents, such as phenylephrine. RAP results in fewer red blood cell transfusions, higher intraoperative Hct levels, and less hemodilution [87–89].

18.2.5.5 Ultrafiltration

Ultrafiltration concentrates blood to increase the concentration of red blood cells, platelets, and coagulation factors. The patient's blood passes through a semipermeable membrane filter to remove excess fluid and inflammatory mediators present during or immediately after CPB [8, 86]. Concentrated circuit volume is returned to the patient with a goal of minimizing allogenic transfusions. Conventional ultrafiltration (CUF) is used during intraoperative CPB. Modified ultrafiltration (MUF) occurs immediately after a patient is weaned off bypass and takes 15 to 20 minutes to complete [17]. Neither method of ultrafiltration has been found to be superior to the other. NATA recommends CUF during CPB or, in the alternative, ≥ 10 minutes of MUF for neonates and infants [8].

18.2.5.6 Cell Salvage and Acute Normovolemic Hemodilution (ANH)

Cell salvage ("cell-saver") techniques are commonly used in adult cardiac surgery as a blood conservation strategy. In adult cardiac surgery, the use of cell-saver blood is associated with reduced exposure and volume of allogenic blood product transfusions [90]. Intraoperative and postoperative use of cell-saver blood in children undergoing cardiac surgery decreases allogenic red blood cell transfusions with fewer donor exposures [91–93]. Recent technical advances have allowed smaller volumes to be processed for use in pediatric surgery [94]. Cell-saver devices collect shed blood from the operative field, which can be combined with the residual volume in the CPB circuit, to be processed and reinfused. Processing includes washing the blood to eliminate potassium and debris as well as hemoconcentration to increase the hematocrit of the reinfused blood to 55–60% [94, 95]. The use of cell salvage is recommended by NATA in pediatric cardiac surgery in order to decrease perioperative transfusions [8].

In acute normovolemic hemodilution (ANH), blood is removed from the patient before CPB and is then stored in citrate anticoagulant for reinfusion after separation from CPB. Blood that is harvested before initiation of CPB preserves platelets and coagulation factors from the negative effects of CPB [86, 96]. To successfully maintain a safe Hct, the patient's preoperative Hct level must be relatively robust such that hemodilution from ANH or after the initiation of CPB does not result in an Hct that is lower than the target goal. This caveat limits the use of the ANH technique in infants and small children. Naguib et al. demonstrated that ANH is possible in patients under 6 kg undergoing biventricular repairs [15]. In that study, approximately 60% of patients over 6 kg received no perioperative allogenic transfusions when ANH was used intraoperatively. However, all patients in the Naguib study that weighed less than 6 kg required perioperative allogenic transfusions. Other studies have not shown that ANH in pediatric patients undergoing cardiac surgery reduces the likelihood of an allogenic RBC transfusions [97]. NATA does not recommend the routine use of ANH in pediatric patients undergoing cardiac surgery with CPB [8]. ANH may be considered in special situations, such as a patient who is highly alloimmunized or with a rare blood type.

18.2.5.7 Viscoelastic Test (VET)-Guided Transfusion Decision-Making

VET expedites intraoperative decision-making because it can be performed at bedside using POC technology with real-time results [13]. VET has become favored over conventional laboratory testing because it provides a visual assessment of clot initiation, kinetics, strength, and stability in a "global" (whole blood) view of hemostasis. Coagulation factor, platelet, and fibrinogen contributions to clot formation can be ascertained within 5 minutes following clot initiation, allowing rapid therapeutic interventions in actively bleeding patients [13, 66, 69, 72].

In the TEG system, whole blood and reagents are manually pipetted into a heated cup that oscillates continuously. A pin that is attached to a torsion wire is suspended in the cup. As clot forms around the pin, it becomes adherent to pin and cup walls, thereby opposing cup rotation and generating torque forces that displace the pin. The forces are then detected by an electromagnetic transducer, representing a traditional viscoelastic method. The ROTEM delta system operates with similar methodology but differs in that the cup containing whole blood and reagents is stationary while the pin rotates. The TEG can now be performed using a disposable, microfluidic cartridge containing all the required reagents. Since individual cartridge chambers contain reagents, operator error is theoretically reduced. The newer TEG systems also include a platelet-mapping cartridge that is US FDA-approved for use in adult patients. ROTEM also offers a platelet module that assesses platelet aggregation. It is important to understand the indications for VET-based platelet testing and the validity of the testing modality at hand [98].

Published data on VET use in the pediatric population has focused largely on three areas: the correlation between VET parameters and conventional laboratory tests, the use of VET to predict bleeding, and the use of VET to guide bleeding management [64]. TEG and ROTEM measurements are described using differing terminology [72]. The VET parameters and specific assays with the strongest evidence available to support pediatric bleeding management include clot strength (TEG, MA; ROTEM, MCF) and the functional fibrinogen assay (TEG, citrated functional fibrinogen; ROTEM, FIBTEM) [64]. Table 18.2 describes TEG and ROTEM measurements [99].

Table 18.2 TEG and ROTEM measurements, abbreviations, and contributing factors

	Clot initiation	Clot kinetics	Clot strength	Clot stability
TEG	R (reaction time) in minutes	K (kinetic time) in minutes; α (angle) in degrees	MA (maximal amplitude) in mm	LY30 (lysis 30 minutes after MA) in % of MA
ROTEM	CT (clotting time) in seconds	CFT (clot formation time) in seconds, α (angle) in degrees	MCF (maximum clot firmness) in mm	LI30 (lysis index/ residual clot firmness 30 minutes after CT) in % MCF, ML (maximum lysis during run time) % of MCF
Factors affecting hemostasis	Coagulation proteins, anticoagulants, tissue factor on monocytes	Coagulation proteins, fibrinogen, platelets, anticoagulants	Platelets, fibrinogen, factor XIII	Fibrinolytic enzymes, fibrinolysis inhibitors, factor XIII

Adapted from Winearls et al. [99].

Pediatric VET reference ranges have been published in a series of small studies [100–102]. In two observational studies, infants less than 6 months had a faster clot initiation with a shorter R time for TEG and a shorter clotting time for ROTEM [100, 101]. Additionally, the clot strength was noted to be increased in this age group as demonstrated by an increased MA (TEG) and MCF (ROTEM). A notable finding in these studies was the fact that the PT and aPTT values of the young infants were prolonged. This finding may not be contradictory but rather a function of what is being measured; newborns and infants have lower levels of the procoagulants that the PT and aPTT tests measure (e.g., factors II, VII, IX, X, and XI) [100]. Furthermore, conventional coagulation assays are plasma-based and do not reflect the contributions that platelets or RBCs make to clot formation. The concept that younger infants may be in a "hypercoaguable" state may reflect the reduced but physiologic levels of protein C, protein S, and antithrombin [103]. And because most of the hematologic maturation process occurs in the first year of life, one could argue that adult VET values can be used for patients over 1 year of age.

A schematic of a TEG and ROTEM tracing with typical measurements is illustrated in Fig. 18.2 [64].

There are several VET devices commercially available that share similar operational characteristics and principles. An in-depth review of the technology and clinical utility of two different viscoelastic machines was published in 2014 by Whiting and DiNardo [104]. Cartridge-based versions of the original technologies are now available for bedside, real-time management of active bleeding [98]. A retrospective analysis of 423 children undergoing CPB found that VET measurements with the TEG6s point-of-care whole blood assay tended to overestimate fibrinogen levels compared to conventional (Clauss) laboratory assay, with a TEG6s functional fibrinogen level 270 mg/dL and MA_{ff} (maximal amplitude of fibrin content) less than 15 mm to predict post-CPB plasma hypofibrinogenemia [105]. The investigators expressed caution when applying these POC technologies in the clinical setting.

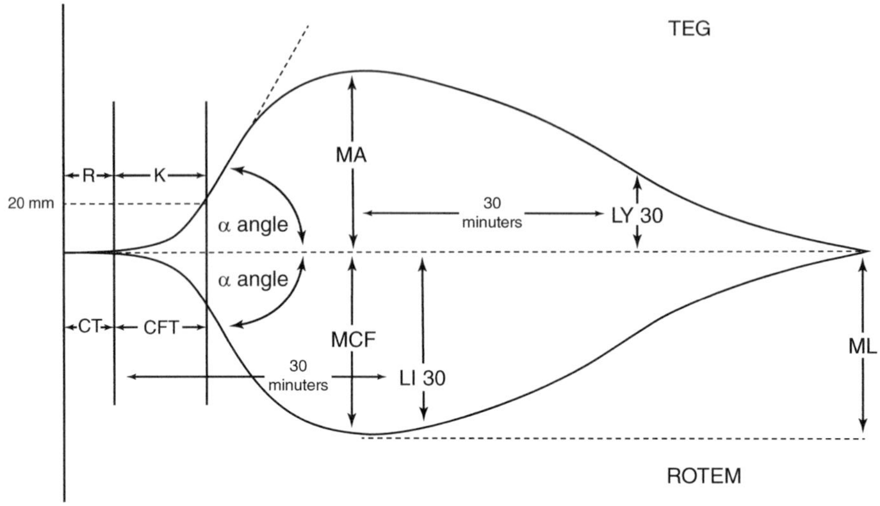

Fig. 18.2 A representative TEG and ROTEM tracing with hyperfibrinolysis. (Reprinted with permission from Haas and Faraoni [64])

The 2022 recommendations of the Transfusion and Anemia Expertise Initiative-Control/Avoidance of Bleeding (TAXI-CAB), a consortium of experts convened to systematically review existing evidence on the use of VET to follow the administration of plasma and platelets during and following cardiac surgery with CPB [73]. The level of evidence supporting this consensus is Grade 2B (moderate-quality evidence, weak recommendation). This recommendation was partly based on practical considerations, including potentially prolonged times between clot initiation and VET results, and the fact that the perioperative use of VET remains subject to different institutional guidelines and individual practices.

18.2.6 What Blood Products or Pharmacologic Adjuncts May Be Considered for Administration in Post-CPB Bleeding?

18.2.6.1 Plasma and Platelet Transfusions

Both plasma and platelet transfusions are associated with poor outcomes in bleeding patients. Transfusion criteria for either blood product tend to be applied generally to heterogenous groups of patients (e.g., a preprocedure platelet count of <100 x 10^9/L and a prolonged PT or INR prior to any invasive procedure), with no standardized criteria to evaluate platelet function [73]. Both platelet function and coagulation factor activity are altered by CPB-related hypothermia, hemodilution, and contact activation [106]. The adverse effects of CPB on platelet count and function are greatest in infants. The uncertainty over optimal transfusion thresholds, risk stratification, or dosing schemes in children undergoing cardiac surgery reflects the complex interplay of the CPB mechanism and the infant's evolving coagulation profile. The 2022 TAXI-CAB consortium was unable to recommend indications or thresholds for platelet or plasma transfusions in children undergoing cardiac surgery with CPB or extracorporeal membrane oxygenation (ECMO) [73]. Citing insufficient evidence and relying on expert consensus, with the knowledge that platelet transfusions can be harmful to patients on ECMO therapy, the consortium recommends measurement of platelet counts or function along with overall coagulation status before any platelet or plasma transfusion [107]. Prophylactic platelet administration in patients with a count >100 x 10^9/L is unlikely to be of positive benefit. The 2019 NATA consensus, on the other hand, recommends post-CPB platelet transfusion when there is excessive bleeding after adequate heparin reversal [8].

18.2.6.2 Inhibition of Fibrinolysis

Major derangements in fibrinolysis result from cardiovascular surgery using cardiopulmonary bypass (CPB). Plasminogen activators initiate the physiologic breakdown of clots, a process known as "fibrinolysis" (Fig. 18.3). With initiation of CPB, there is a fivefold increase in the production of tissue plasminogen activator (tPA) along with a 20-fold increase in the production of thrombin and soluble fibrin [108, 109]. Both soluble fibrin and CPB circuit-bound fibrin create a large surface area for plasminogen activation and subsequent conversion to plasmin [110–112]. Plasmin degrades fibrin to fibrin degradation products which in turn increase up to 100-fold [113]. Fibrinogen is consumed, creating a hyper-fibrinolytic state, leaving little fibrinogen available for hemostasis after CPB. Paradoxically, some patients experience a hypo-fibrinolytic state after CPB. Thus, the fibrinolytic response to CPB can vary from patient to patient.

Antifibrinolytic medications are commonly used in many pediatric surgeries to counter physiologic and pathologic fibrinolysis. In cardiac surgery, they are typically administered prior to the initiation of CPB as an infusion with or without a bolus dose. There are three antifibrinolytic medications commonly used in cardiac surgery: aprotinin, a serine protease inhibitor, and two lysine analogs –aminocaproic acid (EACA) and tranexamic acid (TXA).

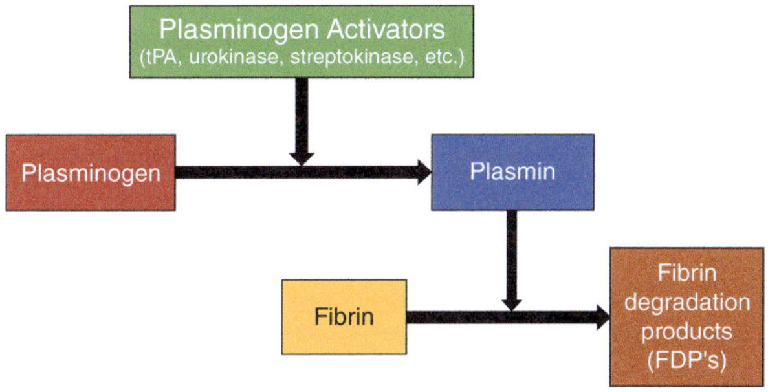

Fig. 18.3 The basics of physiologic fibrinolysis

18.2.6.3 Aprotinin

Aprotinin reversibly binds to plasmin, thereby preventing fibrin clot degradation [114]. Aprotinin has also been shown to reduce the activation of platelets and to preserve platelet function [115–120]. Many randomized controlled trials and meta-analyses in adult patients have demonstrated the efficacy of aprotinin in reducing bleeding and transfusion requirements after cardiac surgery [121–125] .In pediatric patients, a large meta-analysis of 12 randomized controlled studies determined the effect of aprotinin on the volume of blood transfused, the volume of chest tube drainage, and the proportion of pediatric patients transfused, finding a 33% reduction in the proportion of patients requiring blood transfusion [126]. There was no difference in the volume of chest tube drainage or the overall volume of blood transfused, and investigators were unable to recommend aprotinin for routine use in this clinical setting.

A recent systematic review and meta-analysis of RCTs for the period 1980 to 2019 evaluated the efficacy and safety of antifibrinolytics in children undergoing cardiac surgery [127]. Thirty studies were included which evaluated the following drugs versus placebo: aprotinin (n = 14), TXA (n = 12), and EACA (n = 4). All agents reduced 24-hour blood loss and transfusion rate compared to controls. However, the studies were underpowered to detect significant differences in mortality, thromboses, anaphylaxis, or end-organ dysfunction. Conversely, there are several small aprotinin RCTs demonstrating a lack of efficacy in reducing blood loss or blood product transfusion [128, 129]. An additional systematic literature review with subsequent meta-analysis of all randomized and observational studies comparing aprotinin with TXA, EACA, placebo, or no drug in pediatric cardiac surgery was published in 2022 [130]. This meta-analysis summarized literature published in the last 20 years and included a total of 32 studies enrolling some 60,000 pediatric patients undergoing cardiac procedures. Aprotinin significantly reduced total blood loss, postoperative transfusion requirements, and the rate of reoperation for bleeding. In comparison with lysine analogues, aprotinin was more effective at reducing bleeding and decreasing blood product transfusion without increasing complications.

There are safety concerns with the use of aprotinin in adults due to reports of an increased incidence of cerebrovascular and cardiovascular events, renal failure, and mortality when compared to EACA and TXA [131–134]. The 2008 BART (Blood Conservation Using Antifibrinolytics in a Randomized Trial) study compared aprotinin, TXA, and EACA in high-risk adults undergoing cardiac surgery [135]. The trial was halted prior to full enrollment due to a high relative increase in all-cause mortality (including a twofold risk of mortality due to cardiovascular causes) in patients who received aprotinin versus EACA or TXA. Bayer HealthCare, under the guidance of the Food and Drug Administration (FDA), removed aprotinin from the worldwide market in November of 2007. Since its removal, the data from several studies have been reevaluated and subsequently found not to provide sufficient evidence of a negative risk-to-benefit profile when used for its licensed indication [132–134]. Aprotinin should only be used for patients undergoing primary coronary bypass grafting surgery and should be avoided in patients with renal insufficiency or those requiring renal replacement therapy. In September 2011, Health Canada and, in February 2012, the European Regulatory Authority lifted the suspension of aprotinin from their markets. Aprotinin remains available in Canada, the United Kingdom, Sweden, and the Netherlands [136, 137].

Studies investigating the safety and efficacy of aprotinin in children have demonstrated variable results. Aprotinin safety was evaluated in a large multi-institutional cohort of pediatric patients undergoing cardiac surgery found in the Pediatric Health Information Systems (PHIS) database for the period 2003 to 2007 [138]. The PHIS collects admission, diagnostic, and treatment data from 44 children's hospitals across the United States. After multivariate analysis, no difference in mortality, renal replacement therapy (RRT), or hospital LOS was found when comparing patients who received aprotinin versus those who did not. A meta-analysis of all randomized controlled and observational studies from the last 20 years comparing aprotinin with TXA, EACA, placebo, or no drug in pediatric cardiac surgery found that aprotinin had no effect on 30-day mortality or other safety measures [130]. One exception in that study was the need for RRT, which was significantly increased in aprotinin group. Larger RCTs are needed to fully understand the safety profile of aprotinin in neonates and children.

18.2.6.4 Lysine Analogs

The lysine analogs EACA and TXA bind competitively to the lysine amino acid residues in plasminogen and thus prevent the binding of plasminogen to fibrin. This effectively inhibits plasminogen activation to plasmin, thereby preventing degradation of fibrin into fibrin degradation products (FDPs) [139]. The efficacy of EACA in reducing bleeding after cardiac surgery with CPB has been studied extensively in adults and pediatric patients. A meta-analysis of five randomized trials investigated the efficacy of EACA in reducing bleeding, blood transfusions, and laboratory evidence of coagulopathy 6 hours after pediatric cardiac surgery with CPB [140]. Investigators found that EACA, compared to placebo, reduced allogenic blood transfusions and rates of reoperation while preserving coagulation profiles during the postoperative observation period.

TXA is frequently used in patients undergoing cardiac surgery with CPB. Studies that compare TXA and EACA in pediatric patients who have undergone cardiac surgery have found both agents to be efficacious in reducing postoperative bleeding and transfusion rates as compared to placebo, without significant difference in bleeding outcomes when directly comparing EACA to TXA [141–143]. A number of prospective RCTs have supported the efficacy of TXA in reducing postoperative bleeding after pediatric cardiac surgery [144, 145]. A 2012 systematic review comparing TXA to placebo in children found that TXA reduced the need for allogeneic blood products in the perioperative period [146]. However, dosing schemes varied significantly between studies, and evaluation of the side effects, morbidity, or mortality was not feasible from the data.

One complication associated with TXA that has garnered heightened notice is drug-induced seizures and cerebrovascular accidents. A multitude of studies have reported an increased incidence of postoperative seizures in adults who have received TXA for cardiac surgery [147–151]. In a prospective study comparing EACA and TXA administered to children for cardiac surgery, the authors found that there was no significant difference in the seizure rate (TXA 3.5% vs EACA 0.8%; relative risk 4.21, 95% CI, 0.48–37.11; $p = 0.203$) nor renal failure (TXA 1.8% vs EACA 4.2%, $p = 0.447$) [141]. The investigators acknowledged that the study was underpowered and recommended against routine use of lysine analogs in this patient population until safety data is available from larger trials. A question thus arises as to whether TXA-related seizures are dose-dependent. A two-center, prospective, RCT investigated the efficacy of high-dose TXA (50 mg/kg bolus and 5 mg/kg/hr infusion) versus low-dose TXA (10 mg/kg bolus and 5 mg/kg/hr. infusion) in reducing blood loss, transfusion volume, and the incidence of adverse events in children undergoing pediatric craniosynostosis surgery [152]. The low dose of TXA was as effective as the higher dose in reducing blood loss (40.3 vs 39.4 mL/kg [difference 0.9; 95% CI, −14.2, 15.9]) and transfusion volumes (23.6 vs 21.3 mL/kg [difference 2.3; 95% CI, −2.1, 6.7]). Additionally, no adverse events (including seizures or thromboembolic events) were observed in either group. Similar findings were reported in a later systematic review [153]. There was no difference in blood loss or transfusion requirements when comparing high-dose (> 10 mg/kg) to low-dose (10 mg/kg or less) TXA, with seizures reported when TXA dosing was greater than 30 mg/kg. The investigators in this later meta-analysis concluded that low-dose TXA (<15 mg/kg) is adequate to achieve clinical efficacy with a low adverse event rate.

Despite a large body of evidence, it is unclear which lysine analog is optimal in pediatric cardiac surgery. In the United States, aprotinin is not approved by the FDA, necessitating the use of TXA or EACA. Based on current data, antifibrinolytics remain a mainstay in the patient blood management of pediatric cardiac surgery and other blood loss cases. Recent literature indicates that TXA and EACA have similar efficacy in reducing postoperative bleeding and transfusion requirements and that TXA can be used at doses not found to be associated with adverse neurological events.

18.2.6.5 Factor Concentrates

Following the initiation of CPB, coagulation factor concentrations may decline more than 50%, while platelet count decreases, and bleeding time increases [154, 155]. Though the current standard of care is to treat bleeding with a combination of red blood cells, fresh frozen plasma (FFP), platelets, and cryoprecipitate, plasma-derived factor concentrates are used off label to treat hemorrhage unresponsive to traditional therapies in both adults and pediatric patients. Factor concentrates are an alternative therapy to FFP by replacement of specific coagulation factors, theoretically reducing the risk of transfusion-associated circulatory overload (TACO), transfusion-related acute lung injury (TRALI), and transfusion-transmitted infection (TTI). Factor concentrates that are currently available in the United States include recombinant factor VIIa (rFVIIa), fibrinogen concentrate, and three-factor (3F) and four-factor (4F) prothrombin complex concentrates (PCCs) [156].

18.2.6.6 Prothrombin Complex Concentrates

Prothrombin complex concentrates (PCCs) are plasma-derived coagulation protein concentrates that directly promote thrombin formation. The specific composition depends on the manufacturer; however, most contain factors II, VII, IX, and X, while several also contain protein C, protein S, antithrombin, and heparin. Three-factor (3F) PCCs contain factors II, IX, X, and small amounts of factor VII. Four-factor (4F) PCCs contain therapeutic amounts of all the vitamin K-dependent factors (e.g., II, VII, IX, and X). An important and often overlooked fact is that 4F-PCCs may also contain heparin which has significant implications in the management of patients with heparin intolerance. Table 18.3 illustrates the PCCs currently available [156, 157].

In the United States, a 4F-PCC (Kcentra) was approved by the FDA for urgent reversal of vitamin K antagonists (VKAs) in adult patients [13, 158, 159]. However, both 3F-PCCs and 4F-PCCs have been used off-label for the treatment of acquired coagulopathy in adults refractory to traditional blood product resuscitation during trauma, adult cardiac surgery, liver surgery, and obstetrical bleeding. The 2019 NATA guidelines recommend against the use of PCC in pediatric cardiac surgery outside of clinical trials due to a lack of safety data in children undergoing cardiac surgery (Grade 1C: strong recommendation, low-quality evidence) [8].

Various studies have evaluated the efficacy of PCC administration in adult cardiac surgery [160–163]. In a large meta-analysis of four studies including 861 adult patients, PCC administration was more effective than FFP in reducing allogeneic blood product transfusions in adult patients with excessive postoperative bleeding [164]. Furthermore, there was no additional risk of thromboembolic phenomena or other adverse events in patients treated with PCCs.

Experience using PCCs in children undergoing cardiac surgery is preliminary. As with adults, PCCs were originally used in children with hemophilia A and inhibitors to factor VIII [165]. However, there are published retrospective studies, cases series, and case reports of PCC use in other clinical situations, namely, refractory bleeding and VKA reversal [166–169]. Similarly, much of the published data regarding PCC use in pediatric patients undergoing cardiac surgery include retrospective reports, case series, or case reports. In an observational, prospective cohort study of pediatric patients under 1 year of age undergoing CPB, 14 patients who

Table 18.3 Clinically available prothrombin complex concentrate (PCC) preparations

Type of PCC	Brand name	Composition
3F-PCC	Profilnine®, Bebulin® Uman-complex DI®	Factors II, IX, and X
4F-PCC	Beriplex®, Kcentra®, Confidex®, Octaplex®, Prothrombex®, Cofact®, Kaskadil®, PPSB-human $_{SD}$/Nano	Factors II, VII, IX, and X (some contain protein C, protein S, antithrombin, and/or heparin)
Activated PCC	FEIBA-NF™	Factors II, VIIa, IX, Xa, protein C

Adapted from Munlemvo et al. [157]

received a 4F-PCC were compared to 11 matched case controls who did not [170]. The 4F-PCC cohort had lower chest tube output in the first 24 hours after surgery and decreased blood product transfusions postoperatively. There were no adverse events reported. The authors concluded that the 4F-PCC administered was safe and effective for infants undergoing cardiac surgery. In a retrospective chart review of six pediatric patients who received the 3F-PCC in combination with rFVIIa for refractory bleeding after transfusion of platelets (20–40 mL/kg) and cryoprecipitate (10–20 mL/kg), it was noted that two of six patients had thrombotic complications but reduced clinical bleeding [171]. These investigators concluded that there remains significant concern for risk of thrombosis and that further prospective studies are needed. In a more recent prospective observational study, 50 children aged 0–6 years at increased risk for bleeding undergoing cardiac surgery were treated with an early (e.g., following CPB weaning) preventive strategy of fibrinogen concentrate, 4F-PCC, and platelets [172]. Standard coagulation parameters and TEG were measured to guide therapy during and upon separation from CPB. This early preventative strategy reduced bleeding scores with improved TEG and conventional coagulation parameters. These investigators concluded that although there were positive results in the treatment group and no thrombotic events, further safe studies are needed. Another small retrospective, propensity-matched, case-control study examined the rate of complications following the use of the 3F-PCC for refractory bleeding during pediatric cardiac surgery [173]. The investigators did not find an associated risk of thromboembolic events, mortality, or need for extracorporeal membrane oxygenator support. Finally, a recent retrospective analysis of 43 neonates with refractory bleeding who received intraoperative 4F-PCC was propensity-matched with 43 neonates who did not receive PCC during first time sternotomy open heart surgery [174]. Investigators found a significant decrease in the mean volume of blood products transfused (47.5 mL/kg versus 63.7 mL/kg; adjusted difference, 15.3; 95% CI, −29.4 to −1.3) but no difference in thromboembolism or chest tube output.

There are persistent concerns about what appears to be an increasing off-label use of PCCs and factor VIIa in a population of patients already at increased risk of thromboembolism [175, 176]. The weight of the evidence leaves room for better powered prospective studies to determine when PCCs may replace FFP administration after pediatric cardiac surgery and to accurately determine potential thrombotic risk.

18.2.6.7 Fibrinogen Concentrate

A growing body of literature supports the concept that fibrinogen is the first coagulation factor to be consumed from massive hemorrhage and that low levels contribute to bleeding after cardiac surgery with CPB [177–179]. Neonates and infants have qualitative deficiencies in fibrinogen prior to bypass which are exacerbated by the inflammatory and hemodilution effects of CPB [180–184]. Fibrinogen can be supplemented by administration of cryoprecipitate, FFP, or fibrinogen concentrate (FC). FC is derived from adult human plasma and is pasteurized and lyophilized to a powder. It should be noted that cryoprecipitate (also called "antihemophiliac factor"), in addition to fibrinogen, contains factor VII, von Willebrand factor, factor XIII, and fibronectin. FFP also contains fibrinogen but in an insufficient quantity to rapidly improve consumptive hypofibrinogenemia. Cryoprecipitate is the plasma product containing the highest quantity of fibrinogen but has an associated risk of viral transmission, unpredictable fibrinogen levels, increased donor exposure, and a thawing requirement. As a result, pasteurized FC has been a hopeful alternative. FC is approved in the United States for congenital hypofibrinogenemia, but its use is off-label in acquired hypofibrinogenemia for both adults and children. A 2023 ex vivo study of ten neonates undergoing cardiac surgery with CPB examined clot fiber density when FC was added to patient plasma samples [185]. The addition of FC 0.9 mg/mL significantly increased clot strength as assessed through median fiber density in both treated (i.e., allogeneic cryoprecipitate and plasma were administered to all patients per protocol; $p = 0.002$) and pre-CPB baseline patient plasma samples ($p = 0.05$).

When FFP is used to replace coagulation proteins, large volumes (>15 mL/kg) are necessary to increase coagulation factors by at least 20% [156]. In contrast, typical doses of factor concentrates are reconstituted in small volumes for infants and children. For example, the typical dose of FC is approximately 70 mg/kg, and the vial concentration is 20 mg/mL. This reduces the infused volume from 150 mL of FFP to 35 mL of fibrinogen concentrate [156]. Other advantages of FC over FFP for the treatment of a coagulopathy include rapid availability, shorter administration time, and the elimination of a crossmatching step, thus reducing the risk of a hemolytic transfusion reaction.

Currently, there is no consensus on the optimal plasma fibrinogen concentration to achieve effective clot formation. However, VET data from TEG studies have found that clot strength increases significantly as plasma fibrinogen concentrations increase from 75 to 300 mg/dL [186]. In a retrospective study of pediatric patients undergoing cardiac surgery with CPB, a plasma fibrinogen level less than 150 mg/dL or a MCF value 3 mm on FIBTEM predicted excessive postoperative bleeding [179]. Recent data suggest that the VET device (i.e., TEG6s point-of-care versus conventional laboratory assays) may overestimate fibrinogen levels, a factor to be carefully considered before post-CPB fibrinogen replacement [105].

The efficacy of FC to treat postoperative bleeding has been investigated in several studies. A small prospective RCT compared postoperative blood loss after cardiac surgery at 48 hours in children treated with FC or cryoprecipitate [187]. There was no difference in median volume of blood loss or number of all allogeneic blood products administered, and the increase in plasma fibrinogen levels was similar between groups. An additional prospective RCT compared the use of FC to cryoprecipitate in 60 children as part of a transfusion algorithm post-CPB [188]. Patients in the FC group received fewer intraoperative allogenic blood product transfusions with no significant differences in adverse events between the groups. In an observational study of 50 children with an increased risk of bleeding after CPB, early preventive therapy using FC, 3F-PCC, and platelets guided by clinical bleeding assessment and TEG was found to reduce bleeding and. improve TEG parameters with no occurrence of thrombotic complications [172]. These studies suggest that

FC can be considered as an alternative treatment to cryoprecipitate, although there is a need for further safety analysis and standardized dosing guidelines. FC is expensive and is unavailable in many US institutions, although it is available for various acquired conditions outside of the United States [189, 190]. Furthermore, the 2019 NATA guidelines recommend that in bleeding neonates and children, hypofibrinogenemia detected by either the Clauss method (<150 mg/dl) or VET be treated with either cryoprecipitate or FC [8]. FFP should be only considered for treating hypofibrinogenemia in bleeding neonates and children when cryoprecipitate or FC are unavailable.

18.2.6.8 Recombinant Factor VIIa

Recombinant factor VII (rFVIIa) is the most widely studied factor concentrate in the context of pediatric patients undergoing cardiac surgery with CPB. It is US FDA-approved for the prevention and treatment of uncontrolled bleeding in hemophiliac patients with antibodies to factors VIII and IX, factor VII deficiency, and Glanzmann thrombasthenia [191]. There is a body of evidence describing the off-label use, safety, and dosing strategies for rVIIa in the treatment of refractory bleeding in children after cardiac surgery, but the majority of these studies are case reports and small case series [192–203]. The Congenital Cardiac Anesthesia Society (CCAS) formed a task force to study existing evidence on rVIIa use in children undergoing cardiac surgery with CPB [204]. The task force concluded that there was not enough data to make evidence-based recommendations for or against its use in that clinical context. The CCAS noted that there are multiple observational studies citing a benefit of rFVIIa and PCCs in the management of hemorrhage after cardiac surgery with CPB that has not responded to maximal standard therapy. Standard therapy varies by institution but, in general, includes the administration of all blood products, antifibrinolytics, and reexploration. Importantly, rFVIIa is most effective when administered as an adjunct after other procoagulants such as platelets, fibrinogen, and coagulation proteins have been given. There have been several retrospective studies confirming that perioperative administration of rFVIIa may be associated with an increased incidence of postoperative thrombotic complications [175, 205]. The 2019 NATA guidelines recommend against the administration of recombinant FVIIA to treat acquired coagulopathy in neonates and children undergoing cardiac surgery (Grade 1C: strong recommendation, low-quality evidence) [8]. The CCAS task force stressed the need for large prospective studies comparing rFVIIa to standard hemostatic therapy or administration of factor concentrates [204].

18.3 Summary of Key Learning Objectives

18.3.1 Does This Patient Require Medical Optimization of His Hemoglobin (Hgb) and Hematocrit (Hct) Prior to Cardiac Surgery?

Preoperative anemia in neonates, infants, and children undergoing noncardiac surgery is associated with an increase in-hospital mortality and risk of intraoperative blood transfusion. In children undergoing cardiac surgery, preoperative anemia has been associated with an increased risk of perioperative acute kidney injury, altered developmental scores, and allogeneic blood transfusions. To achieve a Hct goal of >24% during CPB, this child's preoperative anemia should be treated for a duration that he can physiologically tolerate to counter the hemodilution-related effects of CPB.

18.3.2 What Can Be Done to Optimize the Patient's Hgb and Hct Before Surgery?

Preoperative Hgb optimization and establishment of healthy iron stores are critical to the patient's ability to tolerate the anemia of surgical bleeding and CPB-related hemodilution. If iron deficiency is present, parental iron supplementation (versus oral) may offer a more timely and tolerable solution. A nutritional consult is important to address micronutrient deficiencies. Erythropoietin therapy is an option in select patient populations, including those with renal insufficiency or children of Jehovah's Witness patients. If the patient is on anticoagulation therapy, consultation with a specialist is necessary to prevent unnecessary bleeding.

18.3.3 How Will the Cardiopulmonary Bypass Circuit Affect Hemostasis in This Patient?

CPB sets the stage for coagulopathic blood loss due to several factors. Hemodilution occurs secondary to a greater proportion of prime volume to the young patient's total blood volume, decreasing the relative platelet count and concentration of intrinsic procoagulants. Contact activation of the patient's blood with the artificial CPB circuit results in inflammation and further impairment of coagulation. Hypothermia results in qualitative platelet dysfunction and enzymatic activity. Heparin (or an anticoagulant alternative) is routinely used to prevent thrombosis in the CPB circuit and must be pharmacologically reversed in a timely fashion.

POC whole blood coagulation assessment (e.g., viscoelastic testing) may determine the etiology of post-CPB bleeding in this patient. Other contributing factors, such as hypothermia, acid-base imbalance, and electrolyte disturbances should be evaluated as well.

18.3.4 What Intraoperative Strategies Can Be Used During Cardiac Surgery to Reduce Bleeding?

Strategies commonly used during CPB aim to decrease hemodilution, coagulopathy, volume overload, and severe anemia:

- Circuit miniaturization to reduce hemodilution.
- Colloid circuit prime to reduce excessive positive fluid balance post-CPB.
- Addition of allogenic RBCs to circuit prime to reduce severe anemia and increase oxygenation.
- Retrograde autologous prime to reduce allogeneic transfusion volume, to minimize donor exposure, and to preserve the patient's own blood supply.
- Ultrafiltration post-CPB to reduce excessive (noncolloid) volume overload and increase concentration of the patient's RBCs, platelets, and coagulation factors.
- Cell salvage to avoid allogeneic RBC transfusion and preserve the patient's own blood supply.
- Acute normovolemic hemodilution (ANH) to preserve platelets and coagulation factors as well as the patient's own blood supply.
- Transfusion algorithms to support standardized and goal-directed anemia and coagulation management.
- Point-of-care whole blood coagulation assessment (e.g., viscoelastic testing).

18.3.5 What Blood Products or Pharmacologic Adjuncts May Be Considered for Administration in Post-CPB Bleeding?

Traditional therapies to treat pediatric CPB-related anemia and coagulation defects include RBCs, plasma, cryoprecipitate, and platelets. There is limited data to recommend transfusion thresholds or specific hemostatic goals in this patient population beyond goal-directed therapy of severe anemia and persistent bleeding. Most neonates receive platelets and cryoprecipitate post-CPB. Standard adjuncts are limited to antifibrinolytics which may be administered throughout the perioperative course and fibrinogen concentrate which is increasingly used to replace FFP and cryoprecipitate in pediatric cardiac surgery. PCC and rVIIa are not recommended as routine treatment of CPB-related bleeding in children, although there is reported to be increasing off-label use of PCCs and rVIIa in this patient population, particularly in cases of refractory bleeding.

Key Points

- The optimal preoperative Hgb value for patients with congenital heart disease (CHD) is unknown. Multiple studies have shown that perioperative restrictive transfusion strategies in pediatric patients undergoing cardiac surgery with CPB are relatively safe.

- The 2019 NATA guidelines recommend adding RBCs *during CPB* to maintain a hematocrit >24%, although the safety profile for the optimal Hct goal in the different age groups, type of CHD lesion, or associated comorbidities is unclear.
- Preoperative techniques to optimize a congenital heart surgery patient's Hgb include anemia evaluation and treatment, a nutritional consult, and management of preexisting anticoagulation therapy. ESA therapy may be considered in specific situations, such as renal insufficiency.
- Major factors that produce a CPB-associated coagulopathy include hemodilution of platelets and coagulation factors, inflammation, hypothermia, and inadequately reversed heparin. Measures to mitigate excessive blood loss include CPB circuit miniaturization, circuit prime modifications, cell salvage, standardized transfusion algorithms, and POC coagulation monitoring.
- PCCs and rVIIa are not recommended for the routine treatment of CPB-related bleeding in children.

References

1. Shore-Lesserson L, Baker RA, Ferraris VA, Greilich PE, Fitzgerald D, Roman P, et al. The Society of Thoracic Surgeons, The Society of Cardiovascular Anesthesiologists, and the American Society of ExtraCorporeal Technology: clinical practice guidelines-anticoagulation during cardiopulmonary bypass. Ann Thorac Surg. 2018;105(2):650–62.
2. Kartha VM, Jacobs JP, Vener DF, Hill KD, Goldenberg NA, Pasquali SK, et al. National benchmarks for proportions of patients receiving blood transfusions during Pediatric and congenital heart surgery: an analysis of the STS congenital heart surgery database. Ann Thorac Surg. 2018;106(4):1197–203.
3. Goobie SM, Faraoni D, Zurakowski D, DiNardo JA. Association of preoperative anemia with postoperative mortality in neonates. JAMA Pediatr. 2016;170(9):855–62.
4. Faraoni D, DiNardo JA, Goobie SM. Relationship between preoperative anemia and in-hospital mortality in children undergoing noncardiac surgery. Anesth Analg. 2016;123(6):1582–7.
5. Meyer HM, Torborg A, Cronje L, Thomas J, Bhettay A, Diedericks J, et al. The association between preoperative anemia and postoperative morbidity in pediatric surgical patients: a secondary analysis of a prospective observational cohort study. Paediatr Anaesth. 2020;30(7):759–65.
6. Karkouti K, Wijeysundera DN, Beattie WS, Investigators RBiCSR. Risk associated with preoperative anemia in cardiac surgery: a multicenter cohort study. Circulation. 2008;117(4):478–84.
7. Park SK, Hur M, Kim E, Kim WH, Park JB, Kim Y, et al. Risk factors for acute kidney injury after congenital cardiac surgery in infants and children: a retrospective observational study. PLoS One. 2016;11(11):e0166328.
8. Faraoni D, Meier J, New HV, Van der Linden PJ, Hunt BJ. Patient blood management for neonates and children undergoing cardiac surgery: 2019 NATA guidelines. J Cardiothorac Vasc Anesth. 2019;33(12):3249–63.
9. Wypij D, Jonas RA, Bellinger DC, Del Nido PJ, Mayer JE, Bacha EA, et al. The effect of hematocrit during hypothermic cardiopulmonary bypass in infant heart surgery: results from the combined Boston hematocrit trials. J Thorac Cardiovasc Surg. 2008;135(2):355–60.
10. Rao S. Physiological anemia of infancy and anemia of prematurity. Indian J Pediatr. 1981;48(390):93–8.
11. Marciniak B. Growth and development. In: Coté CJ, Lerman J, Anderson B, editors. A practice of anesthesia for infants and children. 5th ed. Philadelphia: Elsevier; 2013. p. 7–20.

12. Zhou D, Deng LJ, Ling YF, Tang ML. Preoperative hemoglobin level, oxygen saturation and postoperative outcomes in children with cyanotic congenital heart disease: a propensity-score matching analysis. Front Pediatr. 2021;9:762241.
13. Machovec KA, Jooste EH. Pediatric transfusion algorithms: coming to a cardiac operating room near you. J Cardiothorac Vasc Anesth. 2019;33(7):2017–29.
14. Ahmed M, Acosta SI, Hoffman GM, Tweddell JS, Ghanayem NS. Mathematical analysis of hemoglobin target in univentricular parallel circulation. J Thorac Cardiovasc Surg. 2022;
15. Naguib AN, Winch PD, Tobias JD, Simsic J, Hersey D, Nicol K, et al. A single-center strategy to minimize blood transfusion in neonates and children undergoing cardiac surgery. Paediatr Anaesth. 2015;25(5):477–86.
16. Willems A, Datoussaid D, Tucci M, Sanchez Torres C, De Villé A, Fils JF, et al. Impact of on-bypass red blood cell transfusion on severe postoperative morbidity or mortality in children. Anesth Analg. 2016;123(2):420–9.
17. Cholette JM, Faraoni D, Goobie SM, Ferraris V, Hassan N. Patient blood management in pediatric cardiac surgery: a review. Anesth Analg. 2018;127(4):1002–16.
18. Karimi M, Florentino-Pineda I, Weatherred T, Qadeer A, Rosenberg CA, Hudacko A, et al. Blood conservation operations in pediatric cardiac patients: a paradigm shift of blood use. Ann Thorac Surg. 2013;95(3):962–7.
19. Mazine A, Rached-D'Astous S, Ducruet T, Lacroix J, Poirier N, Network PALIaSI. Blood transfusions after pediatric cardiac operations: a north American Multicenter Prospective Study. Ann Thorac Surg. 2015;100(2):671–7.
20. Salvin JW, Scheurer MA, Laussen PC, Wypij D, Polito A, Bacha EA, et al. Blood transfusion after pediatric cardiac surgery is associated with prolonged hospital stay. Ann Thorac Surg. 2011;91(1):204–10.
21. Székely A, Cserép Z, Sápi E, Breuer T, Nagy CA, Vargha P, et al. Risks and predictors of blood transfusion in pediatric patients undergoing open heart operations. Ann Thorac Surg. 2009;87(1):187–97.
22. Iyengar A, Scipione CN, Sheth P, Ohye RG, Riegger L, Bove EL, et al. Association of complications with blood transfusions in pediatric cardiac surgery patients. Ann Thorac Surg. 2013;96(3):910–6.
23. Redlin M, Kukucka M, Boettcher W, Schoenfeld H, Huebler M, Kuppe H, et al. Blood transfusion determines postoperative morbidity in pediatric cardiac surgery applying a comprehensive blood-sparing approach. J Thorac Cardiovasc Surg. 2013;146(3):537–42.
24. Kipps AK, Wypij D, Thiagarajan RR, Bacha EA, Newburger JW. Blood transfusion is associated with prolonged duration of mechanical ventilation in infants undergoing reparative cardiac surgery. Pediatr Crit Care Med. 2011;12(1):52–6.
25. Willems A, Van Lerberghe C, Gonsette K, De Villé A, Melot C, Hardy JF, et al. The indication for perioperative red blood cell transfusions is a predictive risk factor for severe postoperative morbidity and mortality in children undergoing cardiac surgery. Eur J Cardiothorac Surg. 2014;45(6):1050–7.
26. Hornykewycz S, Odegard KC, Castro RA, Zurakowski D, Pigula F, DiNardo JA. Hemostatic consequences of a non-fresh or reconstituted whole blood small volume cardiopulmonary bypass prime in neonates and infants. Paediatr Anaesth. 2009;19(9):854–61.
27. Eaton MP. Antifibrinolytic therapy in surgery for congenital heart disease. Anesth Analg. 2008;106(4):1087–100.
28. Williams GD, Bratton SL, Riley EC, Ramamoorthy C. Association between age and blood loss in children undergoing open heart operations. Ann Thorac Surg 1998;66(3):870–5; discussion 5–6.
29. Willems A, Harrington K, Lacroix J, Biarent D, Joffe AR, Wensley D, et al. Comparison of two red-cell transfusion strategies after pediatric cardiac surgery: a subgroup analysis. Crit Care Med. 2010;38(2):649–56.
30. de Gast-Bakker DH, de Wilde RB, Hazekamp MG, Sojak V, Zwaginga JJ, Wolterbeek R, et al. Safety and effects of two red blood cell transfusion strategies in pediatric cardiac surgery patients: a randomized controlled trial. Intensive Care Med. 2013;39(11):2011–9.

31. Cholette JM, Rubenstein JS, Alfieris GM, Powers KS, Eaton M, Lerner NB. Children with single-ventricle physiology do not benefit from higher hemoglobin levels post cavopulmonary connection: results of a prospective, randomized, controlled trial of a restrictive versus liberal red-cell transfusion strategy. Pediatr Crit Care Med. 2011;12(1):39–45.
32. Cholette JM, Swartz MF, Rubenstein J, Henrichs KF, Wang H, Powers KS, et al. Outcomes using a conservative versus liberal red blood cell transfusion strategy in infants requiring cardiac operation. Ann Thorac Surg 2017;103(1):206-214.
33. Deng X, Wang Y, Huang P, Luo J, Xiao Y, Qiu J, et al. Red blood cell transfusion threshold after pediatric cardiac surgery: a systematic review and meta-analysis. Medicine (Baltimore). 2019;98(11):e14884.
34. Duan ZX, Chen DX, Yang BZ, Zhang XQ. Transfusion strategies for pediatric cardiac surgery: a meta-analysis and trial sequential analysis. Pediatr Cardiol. 2021;42(6):1241–51.
35. Chkhaidze M. Comparison of two RBC transfusion stategies in pediatric cardiac surgery patients. 6AP2-3. Eur J Anaesthesiol. 2014;31:92.
36. Valentine SL, Bembea MM, Muszynski JA, Cholette JM, Doctor A, Spinella PC, et al. Consensus recommendations for RBC transfusion practice in critically ill children from the Pediatric Critical Care Transfusion and Anemia Expertise Initiative. Pediatr Crit Care Med. 2018;19(9):884–98.
37. Cholette JM, Willems A, Valentine SL, Bateman ST, Schwartz SM, (TAXI) PCCTaAEI, et al. Recommendations on RBC transfusion in infants and children with acquired and congenital heart disease from the Pediatric Critical Care Transfusion and Anemia Expertise Initiative. Pediatr Crit Care Med. 2018;19(9S Suppl 1):S137–S48.
38. Faraoni D, DiNardo JA. Commentary: red blood cells transfusion in patients undergoing congenital cardiac surgery: still far from physiology-based practice. J Thorac Cardiovasc Surg. 2022;
39. Downey LA, Goobie SM. Perioperative pediatric erythrocyte transfusions: incorporating hemoglobin thresholds and physiologic parameters in decision-making. Anesthesiology. 2022;137(5):604–19.
40. Jonas RA, Wypij D, Roth SJ, Bellinger DC, Visconti KJ, du Plessis AJ, et al. The influence of hemodilution on outcome after hypothermic cardiopulmonary bypass: results of a randomized trial in infants. J Thorac Cardiovasc Surg. 2003;126(6):1765–74.
41. Newburger JW, Jonas RA, Soul J, Kussman BD, Bellinger DC, Laussen PC, et al. Randomized trial of hematocrit 25% versus 35% during hypothermic cardiopulmonary bypass in infant heart surgery. J Thorac Cardiovasc Surg. 2008;135(2):347–54, 54.e1–4.
42. Long JB, Engorn BM, Hill KD, Feng L, Chiswell K, Jacobs ML, et al. Postoperative hematocrit and adverse outcomes in pediatric cardiac surgery patients: a cross-sectional study from the Society of Thoracic Surgeons and Congenital Cardiac Anesthesia Society Database Collaboration. Anesth Analg. 2021;133(5):1077–88.
43. Doyle AJ, Crowley MP, Hunt BJ. Perioperative management of antithrombotic treatment in children. Paediatr Anaesth. 2019;29(5):405–13.
44. Puri K, Price JF, Spinner JA, Powers JM, Denfield SW, Cabrera AG, et al. Iron deficiency is associated with adverse outcomes in Pediatric heart failure. J Pediatr. 2020;216:58–66.e1.
45. Otsuka Y, Naraine N, Switzer T, Faraoni D. Preoperative iron supplementation in pediatric cardiac surgical patients: a preliminary single-center experience. J Cardiothorac Vasc Anesth. 2022;36(6):1565–70.
46. Short MW, Domagalski JE. Iron deficiency anemia: evaluation and management. Am Fam Physician. 2013;87(2):98–104.
47. Hassan N, Boville B, Reischmann D, Ndika A, Sterken D, Kovey K. Intravenous ferumoxytol in pediatric patients with iron deficiency anemia. Ann Pharmacother. 2017;51(7):548–54.
48. Ootaki Y, Yamaguchi M, Yoshimura N, Oka S, Yoshida M, Hasegawa T. The efficacy of preoperative administration of a single dose of recombinant human erythropoietin in pediatric cardiac surgery. Heart Surg Forum. 2007;10(2):E115–9.

49. Sonzogni V, Crupi G, Poma R, Annechino F, Ferri F, Filisetti P, et al. Erythropoietin therapy and preoperative autologous blood donation in children undergoing open heart surgery. Br J Anaesth. 2001;87(3):429–34.
50. Shimpo H, Mizumoto T, Onoda K, Yuasa H, Yada I. Erythropoietin in pediatric cardiac surgery: clinical efficacy and effective dose. Chest. 1997;111(6):1565–70.
51. Smith RE Jr. Erythropoietic agents in the management of cancer patients. Part 1: Anemia, quality of life, and possible effects on survival. J Support Oncol. 2003;1(4):249–56, 58–9; discussion 57–8.
52. Stowell CP, Jones SC, Enny C, Langholff W, Leitz G. An open-label, randomized, parallel-group study of perioperative epoetin alfa versus standard of care for blood conservation in major elective spinal surgery: safety analysis. Spine (Phila Pa 1976). 2009;34(23):2479–85.
53. Naran S, Cladis F, Fearon J, Bradley J, Michelotti B, Cooper G, et al. Safety of preoperative erythropoietin in surgical calvarial remodeling: an 8-year retrospective review and analysis. Plast Reconstr Surg. 2012;130(2):305e–10e.
54. Aljaaly HA, Aldekhayel SA, Diaz-Abele J, Karunanayka M, Gilardino MS. Effect of erythropoietin on transfusion requirements for craniosynostosis surgery in children. J Craniofac Surg. 2017;28(5):1315–9.
55. Jones SE, Jooste EH, Gottlieb EA, Schwartz J, Goswami D, Gautam NK, et al. Preoperative laboratory studies for pediatric cardiac surgery patients: a multi-institutional perspective. Anesth Analg. 2019;128(5):1051–4.
56. Alquist CR HST-S-RACICC, Delaney M, Johnson ST, Katz LM. Technical manual. 20th ed. Bethesda: AABB; 2020. p. 391, 510-517
57. Alquist C, Harm SK. Transfusion service related activities. In: Cohn C, Delaney M, Johnson ST, Katz LM, editors. Technical manual. 20th ed. Bethesda: AABB; 2020. p. 503–4, 510–7, 522–3, 525, 528–30.
58. Shah S, Gilliland H, Benson G. Agglutinins and cardiac surgery: a web based survey of cardiac anaesthetic practice; questions raised and possible solutions. Heart Lung Vessel. 2014;6(3):187–96.
59. Murphy M, BenAvram D. Recommendations on the use of Group O Red Blood Cells. AABB. 2019 (update 2022) https://www.aabb.org/docs/default-source/default-document--library/resources/association-bulletins/ab19-02.pdf. Accessed 21 July 2023.
60. Shehata N, Delores Y. Chapter 19. Hemotherapy decisions and their outcomes. In: Cohn CS, Delaney M, Johnson ST, Katz LM. 20th ed. Technical manual. Bethesda: AABB. 2020. p. 572.
61. Boettcher W, Redlin M, Dehmel F, Graefe K, Cho MY, Habazettl H, et al. Asanguineous priming of miniaturized paediatric cardiopulmonary bypass circuits for congenital heart surgery: independent predictors associated with transfusion requirements and effects on postoperative morbidity. Eur J Cardiothorac Surg. 2018;53(5):1075–81.
62. Al-Fares A, Pettenuzzo T, Del Sorbo L. Extracorporeal life support and systemic inflammation. Intensive Care Med Exp. 2019;7(Suppl 1):46.
63. Goswami D, DiGiusto M, Wadia R, Barnes S, Schwartz J, Steppan D, et al. The use of bivalirudin in pediatric cardiac surgery and in the interventional cardiology suite. J Cardiothorac Vasc Anesth. 2020;34(8):2215–23.
64. Haas T, Faraoni D. Viscoelastic testing in pediatric patients. Transfusion. 2020;60(Suppl 6):S75–85.
65. Moskowitz DM, Klein JJ, Shander A, Cousineau KM, Goldweit RS, Bodian C, et al. Predictors of transfusion requirements for cardiac surgical procedures at a blood conservation center. Ann Thorac Surg. 2004;77(2):626–34.
66. Boer C, Meesters MI, Milojevic M, Benedetto U, Bolliger D, von Heymann C, et al. 2017 EACTS/EACTA guidelines on patient blood management for adult cardiac surgery. J Cardiothorac Vasc Anesth. 2018;32(1):88–120.
67. Romlin BS, Wåhlander H, Berggren H, Synnergren M, Baghaei F, Nilsson K, et al. Intraoperative thromboelastometry is associated with reduced transfusion prevalence in pediatric cardiac surgery. Anesth Analg. 2011;112(1):30–6.

68. Whitney G, Daves S, Hughes A, Watkins S, Woods M, Kreger M, et al. Implementation of a transfusion algorithm to reduce blood product utilization in pediatric cardiac surgery. Paediatr Anaesth. 2013;23(7):639–46.
69. Nakayama Y, Nakajima Y, Tanaka KA, Sessler DI, Maeda S, Iida J, et al. Thromboelastometry-guided intraoperative haemostatic management reduces bleeding and red cell transfusion after paediatric cardiac surgery. Br J Anaesth. 2015;114(1):91–102.
70. Faraoni D, Willems A, Romlin BS, Belisle S, Van der Linden P. Development of a specific algorithm to guide haemostatic therapy in children undergoing cardiac surgery: a single-centre retrospective study. Eur J Anaesthesiol. 2015;32(5):320–9.
71. Timpa JG, O'Meara LC, Goldberg KG, Phillips JP, Crawford JH, Jackson KW, et al. Implementation of a multidisciplinary bleeding and transfusion protocol significantly decreases perioperative blood product utilization and improves some bleeding outcomes. J Extra Corpor Technol. 2016;48(1):11–8.
72. Kane LC, Woodward CS, Husain SA, Frei-Jones MJ. Thromboelastography--does it impact blood component transfusion in pediatric heart surgery? J Surg Res. 2016;200(1):21–7.
73. Cholette JM, Muszynski JA, Ibla JC, Emani S, Steiner ME, Vogel AM, et al. Plasma and platelet transfusions strategies in neonates and children undergoing cardiac surgery with cardiopulmonary bypass or neonates and children supported by extracorporeal membrane oxygenation: from the Transfusion and Anemia EXpertise initiative-control/avoidance of bleeding. Pediatr Crit Care Med. 2022;23(13 Supple 1 1S):e25–36.
74. Hendrix BB, Reagor JA, Tweddell JS. Neonatal cardiopulmonary bypass circuit blood prime quality analysis. J Extra Corpor Technol. 2021;53(2):140–5.
75. Boettcher W, Dehmel F, Redlin M, Sinzobahamvya N, Photiadis J. Cardiopulmonary bypass strategy to facilitate transfusion-free congenital heart surgery in neonates and infants. Thorac Cardiovasc Surg. 2020;68(1):2–14.
76. Boettcher W, Sinzobahamvya N, Miera O, Redlin M, Dehmel F, Cho MY, et al. Routine application of bloodless priming in neonatal cardiopulmonary bypass: a 3-year experience. Pediatr Cardiol. 2017;38(4):807–12.
77. Charette K, Hirata Y, Bograd A, Mongero L, Chen J, Quaegebeur J, et al. 180 ml and less: cardiopulmonary bypass techniques to minimize hemodilution for neonates and small infants. Perfusion. 2007;22(5):327–31.
78. Sturmer D, Beaty C, Clingan S, Jenkins E, Peters W, Si MS. Recent innovations in perfusion and cardiopulmonary bypass for neonatal and infant cardiac surgery. Transl Pediatr. 2018;7(2):139–50.
79. Riegger LQ, Voepel-Lewis T, Kulik TJ, Malviya S, Tait AR, Mosca RS, et al. Albumin versus crystalloid prime solution for cardiopulmonary bypass in young children. Crit Care Med. 2002;30(12):2649–54.
80. Valleley MS, Buckley KW, Hayes KM, Fortuna RR, Geiss DM, Holt DW. Are there benefits to a fresh whole blood vs. packed red blood cell cardiopulmonary bypass prime on outcomes in neonatal and pediatric cardiac surgery? J Extra Corpor Technol. 2007;39(3):168–76.
81. Gruenwald CE, McCrindle BW, Crawford-Lean L, Holtby H, Parshuram C, Massicotte P, et al. Reconstituted fresh whole blood improves clinical outcomes compared with stored component blood therapy for neonates undergoing cardiopulmonary bypass for cardiac surgery: a randomized controlled trial. J Thorac Cardiovasc Surg. 2008;136(6):1442–9.
82. Bianchi P, Cotza M, Beccaris C, Silvetti S, Isgrò G, Pomè G, et al. Early or late fresh frozen plasma administration in newborns and small infants undergoing cardiac surgery: the APPEAR randomized trial. Br J Anaesth. 2017;118(5):788–96.
83. McCall MM, Blackwell MM, Smyre JT, Sistino JJ, Acsell JR, Dorman BH, et al. Fresh frozen plasma in the pediatric pump prime: a prospective, randomized trial. Ann Thorac Surg 2004;77(3):983–7; discussion 7.
84. Lee JW, Yoo YC, Park HK, Bang SO, Lee KY, Bai SJ. Fresh frozen plasma in pump priming for congenital heart surgery: evaluation of effects on postoperative coagulation profiles using a fibrinogen assay and rotational thromboelastometry. Yonsei Med J. 2013;54(3):752–62.

85. Gautam NK, Pierre J, Edmonds K, Pawelek O, Griffin E, Xu Z, et al. Transfusing platelets during bypass rewarming in neonates improves postoperative outcomes: a randomized controlled trial. World J Pediatr Congenit Heart Surg. 2020;11(1):71–6.
86. Sebastian R, Ahmed MI. Blood conservation and hemostasis management in pediatric cardiac surgery. Front Cardiovasc Med. 2021;8:689623.
87. Hagedorn C, Glogowski K, Valleley M, McQuiston L, Consbruck K, IbO A. Retrograde autologous priming technique to reduce hemodilution during cardiopulmonary bypass in the pediatric cardiac patient. J Extra Corpor Technol. 2019;51(2):100–3.
88. Singab H, Gamal MA, Refaey R, Al-Taher W. Effect of retrograde autologous blood priming of cardiopulmonary bypass on hemodynamic parameters and pulmonary mechanics in pediatric cardiac surgery: a randomized clinical study. Semin Thorac Cardiovasc Surg. 2021;33(2):505–12.
89. Fu GW, Nie YF, Jiao ZY, Zhao WZ. Clinical applications of retrograde autologous priming in cardiopulmonary bypass in pediatric cardiac surgery. Braz J Med Biol Res. 2016;49(5):e5138.
90. Wang G, Bainbridge D, Martin J, Cheng D. The efficacy of an intraoperative cell saver during cardiac surgery: a meta-analysis of randomized trials. Anesth Analg. 2009;109(2):320–30.
91. Nathan M, Tishler B, Gauvreau K, Matte GS, Howe RJ, Durham L, et al. A red cell preservation strategy reduces postoperative transfusions in pediatric heart surgery patients. Paediatr Anaesth. 2018;28(5):450–7.
92. Cholette JM, Powers KS, Alfieris GM, Angona R, Henrichs KF, Masel D, et al. Transfusion of cell saver salvaged blood in neonates and infants undergoing open heart surgery significantly reduces RBC and coagulant product transfusions and donor exposures: results of a prospective, randomized, clinical trial. Pediatr Crit Care Med. 2013;14(2):137–47.
93. Golab HD, Scohy TV, de Jong PL, Takkenberg JJ, Bogers AJ. Intraoperative cell salvage in infants undergoing elective cardiac surgery: a prospective trial. Eur J Cardiothorac Surg. 2008;34(2):354–9.
94. Booke M, Hagemann O, Van Aken H, Erren M, Wüllenweber J, Bone HG. Intraoperative autotransfusion in small children: an in vitro investigation to study its feasibility. Anesth Analg. 1999;88(4):763–5.
95. Daane CR, Golab HD, Meeder JH, Wijers MJ, Bogers AJ. Processing and transfusion of residual cardiopulmonary bypass volume: effects on haemostasis, complement activation, postoperative blood loss and transfusion volume. Perfusion. 2003;18(2):115–21.
96. Goel R, Cushing MM, Tobian AA. Pediatric patient blood management programs: not just transfusing little adults. Transfus Med Rev. 2016;30(4):235–41.
97. Harris WM, Treggiari MM, LeBlanc A, Giacomuzzi C, You JJ, Muralidaran A, et al. Randomized pilot trial of acute normovolemic hemodilution in pediatric cardiac surgery patients. World J Pediatr Congenit Heart Surg. 2020;11(4):452–8.
98. Faraoni D, DiNardo JA. Viscoelastic hemostatic assays: update on technology and clinical applications. Am J Hematol. 2021;96(10):1331–7.
99. Winearls J, Reade M, Miles H, Bulmer A, Campbell D, Görlinger K, et al. Targeted coagulation management in severe trauma: the controversies and the evidence. Anesth Analg. 2016;123(4):910–24.
100. Edwards RM, Naik-Mathuria BJ, Gay AN, Olutoye OO, Teruya J. Parameters of thromboelastography in healthy newborns. Am J Clin Pathol. 2008;130(1):99–102.
101. Oswald E, Stalzer B, Heitz E, Weiss M, Schmugge M, Strasak A, et al. Thromboelastometry (ROTEM) in children: age-related reference ranges and correlations with standard coagulation tests. Br J Anaesth. 2010;105(6):827–35.
102. Strauss T, Levy-Shraga Y, Ravid B, Schushan-Eisen I, Maayan-Metzger A, Kuint J, et al. Clot formation of neonates tested by thromboelastography correlates with gestational age. Thromb Haemost. 2010;103(2):344–50.
103. Miller BE, Bailey JM, Mancuso TJ, Weinstein MS, Holbrook GW, Silvey EM, et al. Functional maturity of the coagulation system in children: an evaluation using thrombelastography. Anesth Analg. 1997;84(4):745–8.

104. Whiting D, DiNardo JA. TEG and ROTEM: technology and clinical applications. Am J Hematol. 2014;89(2):228–32.
105. Gautam N, Tran V, Griffin E, Elliott J, Rydalch E, Kerr K, et al. A single-center, retrospective analysis to compare measurement of fibrinogen using the TEG6 analyzer to the Clauss measurement in children undergoing heart surgery. Paediatr Anaesth. 2023;
106. Romlin BS, Soderlund F, Wahlander H, Nilsson B, Baghaei F, Jeppsson A. Platelet count and function in paediatric cardiac surgery: a prospective observational study. Br J Anaesth. 2014;113(5):847–54.
107. Valentine SL, Cholette JM, Goobie SM. Transfusion strategies for hemostatic blood products in critically ill children: a narrative review and update on expert consensus guidelines. Anesth Analg. 2022;135(3):545–57.
108. Sniecinski RM, Chandler WL. Activation of the hemostatic system during cardiopulmonary bypass. Anesth Analg. 2011;113(6):1319–33.
109. Chandler WL, Velan T. Secretion of tissue plasminogen activator and plasminogen activator inhibitor 1 during cardiopulmonary bypass. Thromb Res. 2003;112(3):185–92.
110. van den Goor JM, van Oeveren W, Rutten PM, Tijssen JG, Eijsman L. Adhesion of thrombotic components to the surface of a clinically used oxygenator is not affected by trillium coating. Perfusion. 2006;21(3):165–72.
111. Nishida H, Aomi S, Tomizawa Y, Endo M, Koyanagi H, Nojiri C, et al. Comparative study of biocompatibility between the open circuit and closed circuit in cardiopulmonary bypass. Artif Organs. 1999;23(6):547–51.
112. Zhao X, Courtney JM, Yin HQ, West RH, Lowe GD. Blood interactions with plasticised poly (vinyl chloride): influence of surface modification. J Mater Sci Mater Med. 2008;19(2):713–9.
113. Chandler WL, Velan T. Plasmin generation and D-dimer formation during cardiopulmonary bypass. Blood Coagul Fibrinolysis. 2004;15(7):583–91.
114. Yeh T Jr, Kavarana MN. Cardiopulmonary bypass and the coagulation system. Prog Pediatr Cardiol. 2005;21:87–115.
115. Rinder CS, Bohnert J, Rinder HM, Mitchell J, Ault K, Hillman R. Platelet activation and aggregation during cardiopulmonary bypass. Anesthesiology. 1991;75(3):388–93.
116. Day JR, Punjabi PP, Randi AM, Haskard DO, Landis RC, Taylor KM. Clinical inhibition of the seven-transmembrane thrombin receptor (PAR1) by intravenous aprotinin during cardiothoracic surgery. Circulation. 2004;110(17):2597–600.
117. Marx G, Pokar H, Reuter H, Doering V, Tilsner V. The effects of aprotinin on hemostatic function during cardiac surgery. J Cardiothorac Vasc Anesth. 1991;5(5):467–74.
118. Fuhrer G, Gallimore MJ, Heller W, Hoffmeister HE. Aprotinin in cardiopulmonary bypass--effects on the Hageman factor (FXII)--Kallikrein system and blood loss. Blood Coagul Fibrinolysis. 1992;3(1):99–104.
119. Segal H, Sheikh S, Kallis P, Cottam S, Beard C, Potter D, et al. Complement activation during major surgery: the effect of extracorporeal circuits and high-dose aprotinin. J Cardiothorac Vasc Anesth. 1998;12(5):542–7.
120. Longstaff C. Studies on the mechanisms of action of aprotinin and tranexamic acid as plasmin inhibitors and antifibrinolytic agents. Blood Coagul Fibrinolysis. 1994;5(4):537–42.
121. Munoz JJ, Birkmeyer NJ, Birkmeyer JD, O'Connor GT, Dacey LJ. Is epsilon-aminocaproic acid as effective as aprotinin in reducing bleeding with cardiac surgery?: a meta-analysis. Circulation. 1999;99(1):81–9.
122. Fremes SE, Wong BI, Lee E, Mai R, Christakis GT, McLean RF, et al. Metaanalysis of prophylactic drug treatment in the prevention of postoperative bleeding. Ann Thorac Surg. 1994;58(6):1580–8.
123. Laupacis A, Fergusson D. Drugs to minimize perioperative blood loss in cardiac surgery: meta-analyses using perioperative blood transfusion as the outcome. The International Study of Peri-operative Transfusion (ISPOT) Investigators. Anesth Analg. 1997;85(6):1258–67.
124. Sedrakyan A, Treasure T, Elefteriades JA. Effect of aprotinin on clinical outcomes in coronary artery bypass graft surgery: a systematic review and meta-analysis of randomized clinical trials. J Thorac Cardiovasc Surg. 2004;128(3):442–8.

125. Henry D, Carless P, Fergusson D, Laupacis A. The safety of aprotinin and lysine-derived antifibrinolytic drugs in cardiac surgery: a meta-analysis. CMAJ. 2009;180(2):183–93.
126. Arnold DM, Fergusson DA, Chan AK, Cook RJ, Fraser GA, Lim W, et al. Avoiding transfusions in children undergoing cardiac surgery: a meta-analysis of randomized trials of aprotinin. Anesth Analg. 2006;102(3):731–7.
127. Siemens K, Sangaran DP, Hunt BJ, Murdoch IA, Tibby SM. Antifibrinolytic drugs for the prevention of bleeding in Pediatric cardiac surgery on cardiopulmonary bypass: a systematic review and meta-analysis. Anesth Analg. 2022;134(5):987–1001.
128. Davies MJ, Allen A, Kort H, Weerasena NA, Rocco D, Paul CL, et al. Prospective, randomized, double-blind study of high-dose aprotinin in pediatric cardiac operations. Ann Thorac Surg. 1997;63(2):497–503.
129. Williams GD, Ramamoorthy C, Pentcheva K, Boltz MG, Kamra K, Reddy VM. A randomized, controlled trial of aprotinin in neonates undergoing open-heart surgery. Paediatr Anaesth. 2008;18(9):812–9.
130. Atasever AG, Eerens M, Van den Eynde R, Faraoni D, Rex S. Efficacy and safety of aprotinin in paediatric cardiac surgery: a systematic review and meta-analysis. Eur J Anaesthesiol. 2022;39(4):352–67.
131. Mangano DT, Miao Y, Vuylsteke A, Tudor IC, Juneja R, Filipescu D, et al. Mortality associated with aprotinin during 5 years following coronary artery bypass graft surgery. JAMA. 2007;297(5):471–9.
132. Schneeweiss S, Seeger JD, Landon J, Walker AM. Aprotinin during coronary-artery bypass grafting and risk of death. N Engl J Med. 2008;358(8):771–83.
133. Shaw AD, Stafford-Smith M, White WD, Phillips-Bute B, Swaminathan M, Milano C, et al. The effect of aprotinin on outcome after coronary-artery bypass grafting. N Engl J Med. 2008;358(8):784–93.
134. Mangano DT, Tudor IC, Dietzel C, Group MSoPIR, Foundation IRaE. The risk associated with aprotinin in cardiac surgery. N Engl J Med. 2006;354(4):353–65.
135. Fergusson DA, Hebert PC, Mazer CD, Fremes S, MacAdams C, Murkin JM, et al. A comparison of aprotinin and lysine analogues in high-risk cardiac surgery. N Engl J Med. 2008;358(22):2319–31.
136. Klein A, Agarwal S, Cholley B, Fassl J, Griffin M, Kaakinen T, et al. A review of European guidelines for patient blood management with a particular emphasis on antifibrinolytic drug administration for cardiac surgery. J Clin Anesth. 2022;78:110654.
137. European Medicines Agency. European Medicines Agency recommends lifting suspension of aprotinin. 2012. https://www.ema.europa.eu/en/news/european-medicines-agency-recommends-lifting-suspension-aprotinin. Accessed 21 Aug 2023.
138. Pasquali SK, Hall M, Li JS, Peterson ED, Jaggers J, Lodge AJ, et al. Safety of aprotinin in congenital heart operations: results from a large multicenter database. Ann Thorac Surg. 2010;90(1):14–21.
139. Gerstein NS, Brierley JK, Windsor J, Panikkath PV, Ram H, Gelfenbeyn KM, et al. Antifibrinolytic agents in cardiac and noncardiac surgery: a comprehensive overview and update. J Cardiothorac Vasc Anesth. 2017;31(6):2183–205.
140. Lu J, Meng H, Meng Z, Sun Y, Pribis JP, Zhu C, et al. Epsilon aminocaproic acid reduces blood transfusion and improves the coagulation test after pediatric open-heart surgery: a meta-analysis of 5 clinical trials. Int J Clin Exp Pathol. 2015;8(7):7978–87.
141. Martin K, Breuer T, Gertler R, Hapfelmeier A, Schreiber C, Lange R, et al. Tranexamic acid versus ε-aminocaproic acid: efficacy and safety in paediatric cardiac surgery. Eur J Cardiothorac Surg. 2011;39(6):892–7.
142. Schouten ES, van de Pol AC, Schouten AN, Turner NM, Jansen NJ, Bollen CW. The effect of aprotinin, tranexamic acid, and aminocaproic acid on blood loss and use of blood products in major pediatric surgery: a meta-analysis. Pediatr Crit Care Med. 2009;10(2):182–90.
143. Pasquali SK, Li JS, He X, Jacobs ML, O'Brien SM, Hall M, et al. Comparative analysis of antifibrinolytic medications in pediatric heart surgery. J Thorac Cardiovasc Surg. 2012;143(3):550–7.

144. Zonis Z, Seear M, Reichert C, Sett S, Allen C. The effect of preoperative tranexamic acid on blood loss after cardiac operations in children. J Thorac Cardiovasc Surg. 1996;111(5):982–7.
145. Reid RW, Zimmerman AA, Laussen PC, Mayer JE, Gorlin JB, Burrows FA. The efficacy of tranexamic acid versus placebo in decreasing blood loss in pediatric patients undergoing repeat cardiac surgery. Anesth Analg. 1997;84(5):990–6.
146. Faraoni D, Willems A, Melot C, De Hert S, Van der Linden P. Efficacy of tranexamic acid in paediatric cardiac surgery: a systematic review and meta-analysis. Eur J Cardiothorac Surg. 2012;42(5):781–6.
147. Sharma V, Katznelson R, Jerath A, Garrido-Olivares L, Carroll J, Rao V, et al. The association between tranexamic acid and convulsive seizures after cardiac surgery: a multivariate analysis in 11 529 patients. Anaesthesia. 2014;69(2):124–30.
148. Koster A, Börgermann J, Zittermann A, Lueth JU, Gillis-Januszewski T, Schirmer U. Moderate dosage of tranexamic acid during cardiac surgery with cardiopulmonary bypass and convulsive seizures: incidence and clinical outcome. Br J Anaesth. 2013;110(1):34–40.
149. Manji RA, Grocott HP, Leake J, Ariano RE, Manji JS, Menkis AH, et al. Seizures following cardiac surgery: the impact of tranexamic acid and other risk factors. Can J Anaesth. 2012;59(1):6–13.
150. Kalavrouziotis D, Voisine P, Mohammadi S, Dionne S, Dagenais F. High-dose tranexamic acid is an independent predictor of early seizure after cardiopulmonary bypass. Ann Thorac Surg. 2012;93(1):148–54.
151. Keyl C, Uhl R, Beyersdorf F, Stampf S, Lehane C, Wiesenack C, et al. High-dose tranexamic acid is related to increased risk of generalized seizures after aortic valve replacement. Eur J Cardiothorac Surg. 2011;39(5):e114–21.
152. Goobie SM, Staffa SJ, Meara JG, Proctor MR, Tumolo M, Cangemi G, et al. High-dose versus low-dose tranexamic acid for paediatric craniosynostosis surgery: a double-blind randomised controlled non-inferiority trial. Br J Anaesth. 2020;125(3):336–45.
153. O'Donnell DB, Vazquez S, Greisman JD, Uddin A, Graifman G, Dominguez JF, et al. Tranexamic acid dosing in craniosynostosis surgery: a systematic review with meta-analysis. Plast Reconstr Surg Glob Open. 2022;10(10):e4526.
154. Ashikhmina E, Said S, Smith MM, Rodriguez V, Oliver WC, Nuttall GA, et al. Prothrombin complex concentrates in pediatric cardiac surgery: the current state and the future. Ann Thorac Surg. 2017;104(4):1423–31.
155. Chan AK, Leaker M, Burrows FA, Williams WG, Gruenwald CE, Whyte L, et al. Coagulation and fibrinolytic profile of paediatric patients undergoing cardiopulmonary bypass. Thromb Haemost. 1997;77(2):270–7.
156. Guzzetta NA, Williams GD. Current use of factor concentrates in pediatric cardiac anesthesia. Paediatr Anaesth. 2017;27(7):678–87.
157. Munlemvo DM, Tobias JD, Chenault KM, Naguib A. Prothrombin complex concentrates to treat coagulation disturbances: an overview with a focus on use in infants and children. Cardiol Res. 2022;13(1):18–26.
158. Ansell J, Hirsh J, Hylek E, Jacobson A, Crowther M, Palareti G. Pharmacology and management of the vitamin K antagonists: American College of Chest Physicians Evidence-Based Clinical Practice Guidelines (8th edition). Chest 2008;133(6 Suppl):160S–198S.
159. Lankiewicz MW, Hays J, Friedman KD, Tinkoff G, Blatt PM. Urgent reversal of warfarin with prothrombin complex concentrate. J Thromb Haemost. 2006;4(5):967–70.
160. Ortmann E, Besser MW, Sharples LD, Gerrard C, Berman M, Jenkins DP, et al. An exploratory cohort study comparing prothrombin complex concentrate and fresh frozen plasma for the treatment of coagulopathy after complex cardiac surgery. Anesth Analg. 2015;121(1):26–33.
161. Görlinger K, Dirkmann D, Hanke AA, Kamler M, Kottenberg E, Thielmann M, et al. First-line therapy with coagulation factor concentrates combined with point-of-care coagulation testing is associated with decreased allogeneic blood transfusion in cardiovascular surgery: a retrospective, single-center cohort study. Anesthesiology. 2011;115(6):1179–91.

162. Arnékian V, Camous J, Fattal S, Rézaiguia-Delclaux S, Nottin R, Stéphan F. Use of prothrombin complex concentrate for excessive bleeding after cardiac surgery. Interact Cardiovasc Thorac Surg. 2012;15(3):382–9.
163. Enter DH, Zaki AL, Marsh M, Cool N, Kruse J, Li Z, et al. Prothrombin complex concentrate reduces blood product utilization in heart transplantation. Pharmacotherapy. 2017;37(10):1215–20.
164. Roman M, Biancari F, Ahmed AB, Agarwal S, Hadjinikolaou L, Al-Sarraf A, et al. Prothrombin complex concentrate in cardiac surgery: a systematic review and meta-analysis. Ann Thorac Surg. 2019;107(4):1275–83.
165. Leissinger CA, Becton DL, Ewing NP, Valentino LA. Prophylactic treatment with activated prothrombin complex concentrate (FEIBA) reduces the frequency of bleeding episodes in paediatric patients with haemophilia A and inhibitors. Haemophilia. 2007;13(3):249–55.
166. Karube T, Andersen C, Tobias JD. Single-Center use of prothrombin complex concentrate in pediatric patients. J Pediatr Intensive Care. 2020;9(2):106–12.
167. Noga T, Bruce AA, Blain H, Nahirniak S. Four-factor prothrombin complex concentrates in paediatric patients—a retrospective case series. Vox Sang. 2016;110(3):253–7.
168. Rech MA, Wittekindt L, Friedman SD, Kling K, Ubogy D. Prothrombin complex concentrate for intracerebral hemorrhage secondary to vitamin K deficiency bleeding in a 6-week-old child. J Pediatr. 2015;167(6):1443–4.
169. Fuentes-García D, Hernández-Palazón J, Sansano-Sánchez T, Acosta-Villegas F. Prothrombin complex concentrate in the treatment of multitransfusion dilutional coagulopathy in a paediatric patient. Br J Anaesth. 2011;106(6):912–3.
170. Giorni C, Ricci Z, Iodice F, Garisto C, Favia I, Polito A, et al. Use of Confidex to control perioperative bleeding in pediatric heart surgery: prospective cohort study. Pediatr Cardiol. 2014;35(2):208–14.
171. Jooste EH, Machovec KA, Einhorn LM, Ames WA, Homi HM, Jaquiss RD, et al. 3-factor prothrombin complex concentrates in infants with refractory bleeding after cardiac surgery. J Cardiothorac Vasc Anesth. 2016;30(6):1627–31.
172. Dennhardt N, Sümpelmann R, Horke A, Keil O, Nickel K, Heiderich S, et al. Prevention of postoperative bleeding after complex pediatric cardiac surgery by early administration of fibrinogen, prothrombin complex and platelets: a prospective observational study. BMC Anesthesiol. 2020;20(1):302.
173. Harris AD, Hubbard RM, Sam RM, Zhang X, Salazar J, Gautam NK. A retrospective analysis of the use of 3-factor prothrombin complex concentrates for refractory bleeding after cardiopulmonary bypass in children undergoing heart surgery: a matched case-control study. Semin Cardiothorac Vasc Anesth. 2020;24(3):227–31.
174. Navaratnam M, Mendoza JM, Zhang S, Boothroyd D, Maeda K, Kamra K, et al. Activated 4-factor prothrombin complex concentrate as a hemostatic adjunct for neonatal cardiac surgery: a propensity score-matched cohort study. Anesth Analg. 2023;136(3):473–82.
175. Downey L, Brown ML, Faraoni D, Zurakowski D, DiNardo JA. Recombinant factor VIIa is associated with increased thrombotic complications in pediatric cardiac surgery patients. Anesth Analg. 2017;124(5):1431–6.
176. Faraoni D, Sniecinski RM. FEIBA use in neonatal cardiac surgery: a risky business that needs further investigation. Anesth Analg. 2023;136(3):470–2.
177. Levy JH, Szlam F, Tanaka KA, Sniecienski RM. Fibrinogen and hemostasis: a primary hemostatic target for the management of acquired bleeding. Anesth Analg. 2012;114(2):261–74.
178. Gielen C, Dekkers O, Stijnen T, Schoones J, Brand A, Klautz R, et al. The effects of pre- and postoperative fibrinogen levels on blood loss after cardiac surgery: a systematic review and meta-analysis. Interact Cardiovasc Thorac Surg. 2014;18(3):292–8.
179. Faraoni D, Willems A, Savan V, Demanet H, De Ville A, Van der Linden P. Plasma fibrinogen concentration is correlated with postoperative blood loss in children undergoing cardiac surgery. A retrospective review. Eur J Anaesthesiol. 2014;31(6):317–26.
180. Andrew M, Paes B, Milner R, Johnston M, Mitchell L, Tollefsen DM, et al. Development of the human coagulation system in the healthy premature infant. Blood. 1988;72(5):1651–7.

181. Guzzetta NA, Miller BE. Principles of hemostasis in children: models and maturation. Paediatr Anaesth. 2011;21(1):3–9.
182. McQuilten ZK, Bailey M, Cameron PA, Stanworth SJ, Venardos K, Wood EM, et al. Fibrinogen concentration and use of fibrinogen supplementation with cryoprecipitate in patients with critical bleeding receiving massive transfusion: a bi-national cohort study. Br J Haematol. 2017;179(1):131–41.
183. Brown AC, Hannan RT, Timmins LH, Fernandez JD, Barker TH, Guzzetta NA. Fibrin network changes in neonates after cardiopulmonary bypass. Anesthesiology. 2016;124(5):1021–31.
184. Miller BE, Tosone SR, Guzzetta NA, Miller JL, Brosius KK. Fibrinogen in children undergoing cardiac surgery: is it effective? Anesth Analg. 2004;99(5):1341–6.
185. Moiseiwitsch N, Nellenbach KA, Downey LA, Boorman D, Brown AC, Guzzetta NA. Influence of fibrinogen concentrate on neonatal clot structure when administered ex vivo after cardiopulmonary bypass. Anesth Analg. 2023;137(3):682–90.
186. Rossaint R, Bouillon B, Cerny V, Coats TJ, Duranteau J, Fernández-Mondéjar E, et al. Management of bleeding following major trauma: an updated European guideline. Crit Care. 2010;14(2):R52.
187. Galas FR, de Almeida JP, Fukushima JT, Vincent JL, Osawa EA, Zeferino S, et al. Hemostatic effects of fibrinogen concentrate compared with cryoprecipitate in children after cardiac surgery: a randomized pilot trial. J Thorac Cardiovasc Surg. 2014;148(4):1647–55.
188. Downey LA, Andrews J, Hedlin H, Kamra K, McKenzie ED, Hanley FL, et al. Fibrinogen concentrate as an alternative to cryoprecipitate in a postcardiopulmonary transfusion algorithm in infants undergoing cardiac surgery: a prospective randomized controlled trial. Anesth Analg. 2020;130(3):740–51.
189. Okerberg CK, Williams LA, Kilgore ML, Kim CH, Marques MB, Schwartz J, et al. Cryoprecipitate AHF vs. fibrinogen concentrates for fibrinogen replacement in acquired bleeding patients—an economic evaluation. Vox Sang. 2016;111(3):292–8.
190. Costa-Filho R, Hochleitner G, Wendt M, Teruya A, Spahn DR. Over 50 years of fibrinogen concentrate. Clin Appl Thromb Hemost. 2016;22(2):109–14.
191. Davidson S. State of the art—how I manage coagulopathy in cardiac surgery patients. Br J Haematol. 2014;164(6):779–89.
192. Agarwal HS, Bennett JE, Churchwell KB, Christian KG, Drinkwater DC, He Y, et al. Recombinant factor seven therapy for postoperative bleeding in neonatal and pediatric cardiac surgery. Ann Thorac Surg. 2007;84(1):161–8.
193. Brady KM, Easley RB, Tobias JD. Recombinant activated factor VII (rFVIIa) treatment in infants with hemorrhage. Paediatr Anaesth. 2006;16(10):1042–6.
194. Razon Y, Erez E, Vidne B, Birk E, Katz J, Tamari H, et al. Recombinant factor VIIa (NovoSeven) as a hemostatic agent after surgery for congenital heart disease. Paediatr Anaesth. 2005;15(3):235–40.
195. Guzzetta NA, Huch S, Fernandez JD, Tosone SR, Miller BE. Use of recombinant factor VIIa for uncontrolled bleeding in neonates after cardiopulmonary bypass. Paediatr Anaesth. 2009;19(4):364–70.
196. Egan JR, Lammi A, Schell DN, Gillis J, Nunn GR. Recombinant activated factor VII in paediatric cardiac surgery. Intensive Care Med. 2004;30(4):682–5.
197. Karsies TJ, Nicol KK, Galantowicz ME, Stephens JA, Kerlin BA. Thrombotic risk of recombinant factor seven in pediatric cardiac surgery: a single institution experience. Ann Thorac Surg. 2010;89(2):570–6.
198. Pychyńska-Pokorska M, Moll JJ, Krajewski W, Jarosik P. The use of recombinant coagulation factor VIIa in uncontrolled postoperative bleeding in children undergoing cardiac surgery with cardiopulmonary bypass. Pediatr Crit Care Med. 2004;5(3):246–50.
199. Tobias JD, Berkenbosch JW, Russo P. Recombinant factor VIIa to treat bleeding after cardiac surgery in an infant. Pediatr Crit Care Med. 2003;4(1):49–51.
200. Tobias JD, Simsic JM, Weinstein S, Schechter W, Kartha V, Michler R. Recombinant factor VIIa to control excessive bleeding following surgery for congenital heart disease in pediatric patients. J Intensive Care Med. 2004;19(5):270–3.

201. Leibovitch L, Kenet G, Mazor K, Matok I, Vardi A, Barzilay Z, et al. Recombinant activated factor VII for life-threatening pulmonary hemorrhage after pediatric cardiac surgery. Pediatr Crit Care Med. 2003;4(4):444–6.
202. Schneider AG, Perez MH, Tozzi P, Voirol P, Schoettker P, Angelillo-Scherrer A, et al. Recombinant factor VIIa for intractable life-threatening bleeding in patients with circulatory assist devices. Intensive Care Med. 2010;36(9):1620–1.
203. Niebler RA, Punzalan RC, Marchan M, Lankiewicz MW. Activated recombinant factor VII for refractory bleeding during extracorporeal membrane oxygenation. Pediatr Crit Care Med. 2010;11(1):98–102.
204. Guzzetta NA, Russell IA, Williams GD. Review of the off-label use of recombinant activated factor VII in pediatric cardiac surgery patients. Anesth Analg. 2012;115(2):364–78.
205. Morrison S, Lacey C, Attard C, Davies B, Monagle P, Davies P. Recombinant factor VIIa in pediatric cardiac surgery. J Cardiothorac Vasc Anesth. 2022;36(3):684–9.

Patient Verification

19

Samantha Phou and Norma J. Klein

19.1 Case Scenario

You are the quality assurance representative for an anesthesia department in the United States (US) and receive incident reports about adverse blood product events. A recent report detailed a hemolytic transfusion reaction in an 8-month-old infant. Upon examination of the facts, you learn the infant received an incompatible unit of red blood cells (RBCs) in the operating room. The root cause appears to be patient misidentification because the patient's hospital wrist band was attached to the crib (i.e., not attached to the patient) and the infant's crib was exchanged for another when the hospital room was cleaned for a new admission. In a literature review, you come across the term "patient verification" and learn that it involves a specific set of protocols and procedures.

Key Learning Objectives

- What is "patient verification" and what is its role in blood transfusions?
- Why is patient verification important?
- What are the regulatory requirements for hospitals regarding patient verification?
- What is the standardized process for proper patient verification prior to a blood transfusion?
- How may the patient verification process be adapted for children and other non-verbal patients?

S. Phou (✉)
Department of Pathology and Laboratory Medicine, Phoenix Children's Hospital, Phoenix, AZ, USA
e-mail: sphou@phoenixchildrens.com

N. J. Klein
Department of Anesthesiology and Pain Medicine, University of California, Davis, Sacramento, CA, USA
e-mail: nklein@ucdavis.edu

N. J. Klein (ed.), *Perioperative Pediatric Patient Blood Management and Transfusion Safety*, https://doi.org/10.1007/978-3-031-81666-6_19

19.2 Discussion

19.2.1 What Is "Patient Verification" and What Is Its Role in Blood Transfusions?

The Association for the Advancement of Blood and Biotherapies (AABB) defines verification as "Confirmation, by examination of objective evidence, that specified requirements have been met" [1]. Practically speaking, patient verification means the patient is identified twice by using two different unique patient identifiers (such as name, date of birth, medical record number) [2, 3]. The patient verification procedure entails a series of steps to ensure a correct blood sample, correct patient, and correct blood product [4]. In the context of an intraoperative blood transfusion, patient verification occurs at several points in patient care. Two critical patient verification points for the anesthesia transfusionist are at the time of specimen collection for blood type and screen (T&S) and immediately before blood administration. Patient verification is also required inside the blood bank when receiving and processing the patient's blood type sample, and there is an additional patient verification protocol when blood is released from the blood bank to the operating room (OR). In addition to AABB credentialing standards for US hospitals (see below), each institution that provides transfusions may adapt patient verification steps to its own patient flow [2, 3]. For example, in a very large OR with multiple suites, verification of patient and blood product may be crosschecked with the OR suite number to verify that the blood has been delivered to the correct room.

The terms "patient identification" and "patient verification" are used interchangeably throughout this discussion.

19.2.2 Why Is Patient Verification Important?

Patient misidentification has been associated with clinically adverse events including fatal acute hemolytic transfusion reactions (ATRs) secondary to ABO blood group incompatibility [5]. Proper patient identification is a safety priority as recognized by The Joint Commission (TJC), the World Health Organization (WHO), the Association for the Advancement of Blood and Biotherapies (AABB), and the Joint United Kingdom Blood Transfusion and Tissue Transplantation Services Professional Advisory Committee (JPAC) [2, 6–8]. Transfusion-related misidentification is usually related to human error, often occurring at the patient's bedside [9–11]. A review of over 63,000 reports to the Centers for Disease Control National Healthcare Safety Network (CDC NHSN) hemovigilance registry found that blood sample collection and handling errors comprised more than one-half of reported events for the years 2014–2022 [12]. The 2020 US Food and Drug Administration (FDA) transfusion-related fatality report describes two deaths secondary to ABO incompatibility, both brought about by missteps in the pretransfusion patient identification (verification) process [13].

Specimen collection and blood transfusion are especially susceptible to misidentification events. Starting with hospital admission registration (which is usually performed by nonmedical personnel), misidentification can occur at any point during phlebotomy, specimen labeling, and blood product administration [14]. Another crucial juncture in pretransfusion patient identification is within the blood bank; a recent report from the UK Serious Hazards of Transfusion (SHOT) database received 57 reports of "wrong component transfused" (WCT), 37 of which originated in the blood bank [10]. Clinical settings particularly susceptible to patient identification errors include the operating room (OR) and emergency department (ED), where safety checks and protocols may be bypassed in a hectic workflow environment [10]. In a survey of 23 Canadian hospitals, the OR and the ED had the highest rates of sampling errors (59/1000 and 58/1000, respectively) and handling errors (20/1000 and 12/1000, respectively) compared to the transfusion service (0.04/1000) and the laboratory (16/1000) [15]. Remote blood refrigerators may be particularly susceptible to patient identification errors during emergency transfusions if programmed with special bypass exceptions, which may have been put in place to decrease time to transfusion [10].

Automated or electronic patient identification (EPID) systems, including bar code, radiofrequency, and biometric identification technologies, have been implemented with some success in reducing the rate of patient misidentification errors [9, 10, 16–19]. In a multicenter, retrospective study of wrong-blood-in-tube (WBIT) errors (e.g., when the actual ABO blood type of the patient named on the specimen label is not the same as the blood type of the blood tested in the tube), there was a fivefold reduction in WBIT rate after a bar code EPID system was implemented [18]. A significant portion of the WBIT errors in this study were attributed to patient misidentification because the wrong patient's ID label was affixed to the specimen tube. This often occurs when the specimen label is printed and applied at a distance from the patient's bedside [9]. In the two WBIT events post-EPID implementation, the patient was wearing the wrong wristband [20]. Chan et al. retrospectively examined 27,000 nonemergent transfusions using a handheld bar code scanner for electronic patient verification over a 3-year period and found no WCT events related to 41,000 pretransfusion samples [19]. In a survey of over 90 UK hospitals, including approximately two million blood components issued, an analysis of WCT events found a WCT rate of 1/523,354 units for blood sampling using manual patient verification but no WCT events with electronic patient verification [10]. At the point of actual blood administration, the WCT rate was 1/267,854 for manual and 0/410,677 after EPID implementation. However, there were still "near misses" (defined as potential WCT events that were detected and prevented) post-EPID implementation ($n = 20/410,677$). Prior to EPID, there were 497 near-misses reported (91% related to blood draw and sample labeling), compared to 37 using EPID. Regarding blood product administration, there were 20 near miss events using EPID. In 17 of those 20 events, the transfusionist chose to attach a blood type sample label away from the patient's bedside or to initiate a transfusion in a patient without a wristband. However, the EPID detected the error in each of the 17 cases, presumably because the bar code scanner detected mismatch between the blood order, the patient's wristband, and the component at hand [10]. In a review of electronic health record (EHR) optimization to promote safe transfusion practices, a transfusionist did not understand that the bar code scanner was not linked to the laboratory system (a linkage that is critical to verifying the correct blood component for the correct patient) [21]. These latter findings highlight the fact that although EPID is considered to be "fail safe," it is not "foolproof," and a false sense of safety security in the technology can lead to disastrous results [9, 22].

19.2.3 What are the Regulatory Requirements for Hospitals Regarding Patient Verification?

Blood banks and transfusion services in the US are regulated by the US FDA. These regulations appear as statutes in the US Code of Federal Regulations (CFR), Title 21 [23]. The FDA branch responsible for blood product oversight is the Center for Biologics Evaluation and Research (CBER). Regulations promulgated by the FDA have the force of law and are intended to protect the safety of people who donate or receive blood products. The FDA regularly invites input from the public and expert sectors regarding existing and proposed regulations [24].

The FDA gives oversight authority to specific accrediting organizations which promulgate standards and guidelines for blood banks and transfusion services. In the USA, the accrediting bodies responsible for blood product oversight are TJC, AABB, and the College of American Pathologists (CAP). Although the standards established by these oversight bodies do not have the force of law, they do determine if a hospital, blood bank, or transfusion service has met operational accreditation requirements.

The terms "blood bank" and "transfusion service" are often used interchangeably. In a nutshell, a blood bank collects, selects, and stores blood products for general distribution. A transfusion service tests, stores, and issues blood for specific recipients [25]. Both accredited blood banks and transfusion services are staffed with physician transfusion specialists who are available for consultation.

19.2.4 What Is the Standardized Process for Proper Patient Verification Prior to a Blood Transfusion?

Patient verification is a TJC National Patient Safety Goals (NPSG) and is required as part of hospital accreditation [26]. It is a standardized procedure intended to prevent misidentification and to ensure the correct blood goes to the correct patient.

The patient verification process may be modified based on where it takes place (such as inside versus outside the OR), whether it is conducted manually or with electronic technology, and whether the patient is conscious or unconscious. However, explicit guidelines exist only for the manual and electronic verification of patients that are verbal [4]. Safe patient verification of the intraoperative, unconscious, or nonverbal blood recipient who is unable to self-identify must therefore be guided by adherence to the basic tenants of correct patient verification. Strict adherence to verification protocols and redundancy are critical to prevent WCT events. Unfortunately, blood administration standards are usually not formally taught to physicians and other bedside practitioners [27–30]. The following section discusses manual, electronic, intraoperative, and emergency patient identification processes for perioperative blood administration:

19.2.4.1 Manual Patient Verification

Pretransfusion T&S Sample Labeling

Blood samples for the recipient patient's blood T&S should be collected at the patient's bedside and, when possible, with patient involvement [4, 26]. At the time of sample collection, the anesthesiologist or phlebotomist must:

(a) Verify the recipient identity using two unique patient identifiers such as name, date of birth, or medical record number. Ask the patient to confirm identity.
(b) Verify that the specimen label placed on the pretransfusion blood sample matches the intended recipient using two unique patient identifiers.
(c) Indicate on the pretransfusion blood specimen the date and time of specimen collection and the identity of the person who collected the specimen (such as the anesthesiologist's name).[1]
(d) If the blood bank requests a second, confirmatory blood sample, this must be collected at a different time than the first sample.

A blood bank requirement that is sometimes a source of confusion is the so-called "confirmatory" second blood sample for ABO and RhD typing. The purpose of this second sample is to confirm ABO and RhD blood type and potentially catch wrong-blood-in-tube (WBIT) events when the second blood type does not match the first blood type. In such a scenario, further investigation and confirmation of the patient's blood type must be performed before transfusion to ensure a safe transfusion. The blood bank may not necessarily request a second confirmatory sample in the following situations:

- Prior to emergency release of universal donor blood product.
- A confirmatory sample was already drawn at a different time and the blood bank has the results.
- The patient's ABO and Rh blood types are already on record from a previous T&S.
- Infants (<4 months) if the same hospital admission.[2]
- The same T&S sample was initially verified using an EPID system (see below).

---

[1] The AABB standards do not explicitly state that the phlebotomist name must be in full.

[2] The blood banking standard definition of neonate is <4 months in contrast to the <1 month general pediatric definition.

It is important to note that active patient involvement is critical for self-identification; however, patient self-identification cannot serve as a substitute for the requirement of a second confirmatory blood type sample [2].

Patient Verification Immediately Before Transfusion

At the time of transfusion, the anesthesiologist or transfusionist must [26, 31]:

1. Review the patient's medical record for ABO and RhD blood type results, signed consent to transfusion, and appropriate blood product order.
2. Verify the following with a second qualified person:
   (a) The recipient is identified using two unique independent patient identifiers.
   (b) Information on the blood bag label is matched with the attached tag or paper:
      (i) Recipient identification using two identifiers.
      (ii) ABO blood group and RhD type.
      (iii) Donor identification number (DIN) linking to the correct donor.
      (iv) Blood product expiration date and time.
      (v) Special blood requirements (e.g., CMV antibody negative, irradiated, etc.)

A "qualified person" used in patient verification is typically defined as a registered practitioner who is "trained and competent" to fulfill local protocol requirements [8].

19.2.4.2 Electronic Patient Verification

Sample Labeling

If the hospital uses an EPID system, such as bar coding or embedded radiofrequency (RF) emitting chips, the patient's T&S specimen label will be generated by a printer. The label should be applied to the specimen tube at the patient's bedside with active patient participation. If an unlabeled specimen leaves the patient's bedside and is out of possession of the phlebotomist, a repeat sample must be obtained [26, 31]. If the blood bank requests a second confirmatory sample for blood typing *and* the hospital uses a validated EPID system *and* the patient is wearing a barcoded wristband *and* the wristband is used to generate the specimen label at the patient's bedside, the same (initial) sample may be retested for blood type confirmation; however, *the hospital transfusion services must have established this exception in hospital policy* [2].

Patient Verification Immediately Before Transfusion

If the hospital uses an EPID system, the patient verification process immediately before transfusion is the same as the manual process, but the barcode or RFID may substitute as the second patient identifier (in lieu of a second qualified person performing patient identification) [32]. As with manual verification, the patient should be actively involved in self-identification.

Proper patient verification just prior to transfusion requires a match between the patient, the patient's wristband, and the tag placed on the blood bag by the blood bank [8]. Note that scanning the bar code(s) on the bag of blood is also necessary to confirm the abovementioned information when using an electronic identification system and includes the DIN that links the correct donor to the correct patient [33].

EPID and Wristbands

In an observational study of 1.7 million hospital patient wristbands over a 2-year period, 71% of more than 45,000 errors involved a missing wristband [34]. Kaufman et al. found a residual error rate of 1:15,000 using EPID, partly attributed to the use of wristbands that were not physically attached to the patient [9, 18]. Logically speaking, EPID has no utility in pretransfusion verification when the patient lacks an identifying wristband. Two safety principles emerge from this dilemma: healthcare workers must be trained in the elements of safe transfusion processes in the event of technological failure, and both blood sample collection and transfusion should never be performed on a patient who lacks an identifying wristband or other appliance if EPID or other automated process is the institutional standard. A single transfusion-related fatality due to patient misidentification is one too many. TJC recommends that infants have two identification bands placed on two different extremities [7, 26].

19.2.4.3 Intraoperative Patient ID Verification

An unconscious patient under anesthesia is unable to self-identify, precluding a critical step in preventing WCT events. Two critical safety points for anesthesiologists during the intraoperative transfusion process are blood sampling and bedside blood product administration. Therefore, the patient should be identified (with self-involvement) upon entering the operating room, followed by confirmation that the same patient is displayed in the workstation EHR. The operating room can be a chaotic environment with ample opportunities to bypass a safe and standardized patient verification protocol. Many providers are unaware of the recommended pre-transfusion patient verification process. In a 2021 survey of anesthesiology residents' transfusion medicine knowledge, including 423 physicians in 37 US training programs, the mean score was 45.5%, with a correct answer range of 27–72.8% for blood product handling [30]. Intraoperatively, it is not unusual for the anesthesiologist to be without a second qualified person immediately available for crosschecking an unconscious patient's identity. To complicate matters, the patient's wristband—the form of patient identification used most often—may be out of reach, under a surgical drape, or absent altogether.

Vanneman et al. reported a single institution's experience with a customized software program for patient verification that can be performed by a single anesthesia provider [16]. In this functionality, the patient's identity is verified upon entering the OR by scanning the wristband bar code (that is encoded with two unique patient identifiers). A crosscheck is then performed to verify that the correct patient is in the correct OR as taken from the master daily schedule. Figure 19.1 is a detailed illustration of the transfusionist's subsequent workflow during the remaining transfusion process [16]. Highlights of this electronic process include confirmation of the

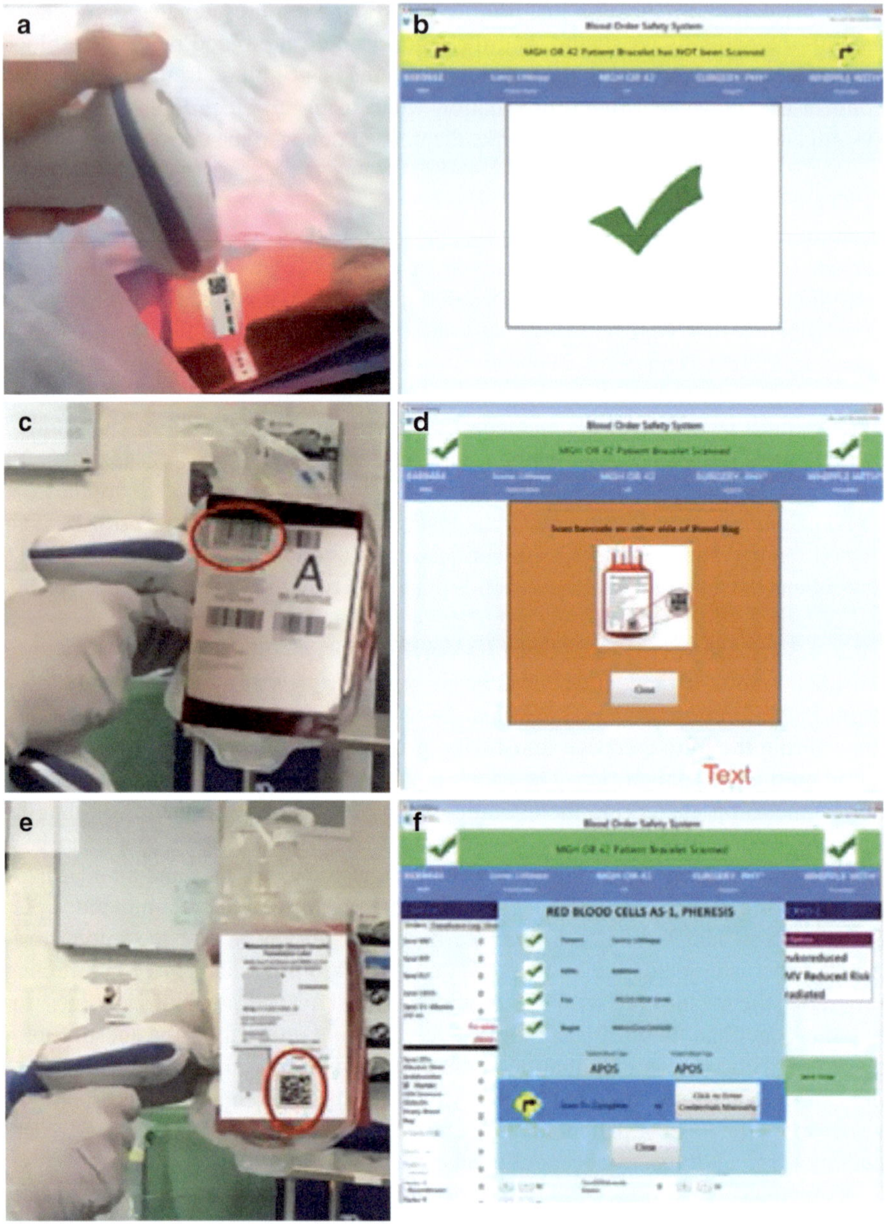

Fig. 19.1 Single-person EPID verification process prior to transfusion in the operating room (OR). (Reprinted with permission from Vanneman et al. [16])

g

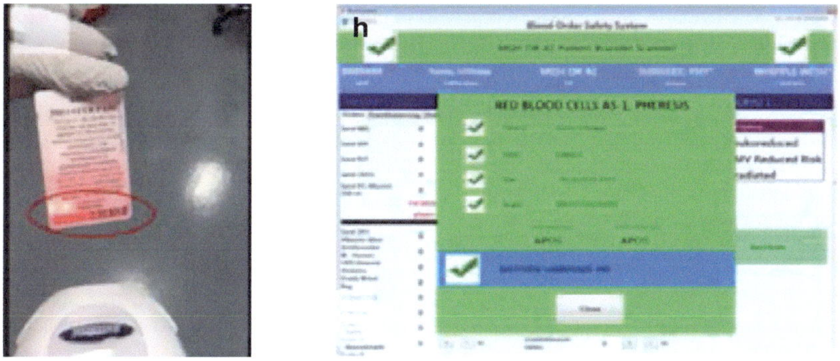

Fig. 19.1 (continued)

correct patient, OR, DIN, transfusion order, blood product as processed by the blood bank, and the transfusionist's identity.

Investigators in the Vanneman report found that this customized patient verification program prevented 36 WCT events in 20 patients over a 2-year observation period [16].

19.2.4.4 Emergent Transfusions with Uncrossmatched Blood Products

The only situation where blood is released from the blood bank without requiring a specimen for the patient's blood type drawn, tested, and resulted in advance is under an emergency release procedure such as a massive transfusion protocol (MTP). The decision to administer uncrossmatched blood or potentially incompatible blood in an emergency is made in balance with the likelihood of patient death, or irreversible injury should the patient not receive blood products. Uncrossmatched blood released from the blood bank should be type O RBCs, low antibody titer type O whole blood (LTOWB), or type AB or A plasma to prevent acute hemolytic transfusion reactions due to ABO incompatibility. Platelets and cryoprecipitate do not have to be ABO compatible; however, some blood banks provide only ABO-compatible or ABO identical platelets to infants [35–41]. Hospitals have differing policies regarding patient rhesus D (RhD) antigen status and may choose to reserve RhD-negative RBCs or whole blood for females of childbearing potential, young children, or neonates (<4 months old) [42, 43]. As such, RBCs transfused under an emergency release procedure may not necessarily be RhD-compatible with the patient. Transfusion of RhD-incompatible blood is much less likely to lead to an acute clinically adverse event compared to transfusion of ABO-incompatible blood, since, unlike ABO, antibodies against the RhD antigen are not naturally occurring in individuals and require a previous sensitization event through transfusion, transplant, or pregnancy.

Table 19.1 Standards and suggested practices to prevent patient misidentification prior to a blood transfusion

Patient verification safety measure
Wristband on patient with at least two unique identifiers (such as name, birthdate, medical record number) [9, 18]
Patient self-identification at specimen collection and at transfusion time [2, 7, 9]
Automated verification (such as bar code, radiofrequency, biometrics) [6, 26]
Specimen labels printed and affixed to tube in presence of patient [7, 9]
Patient verifies self-identity on specimen label [2, 44]
Hospital workers trained in patient verification procedure [10, 18]
Do not perform specimen collection or blood administration in any patient with no identifying wristband attached [9, 32]
Repeat full phlebotomy procedure for all specimens with no identification label or for incorrect label attached [9, 32]
Rigorous training of admission personnel regarding patient verification procedure and inherent misidentification risks [45, 46]
Hospital policy for EHR downtime clearly outlining patient verification procedure with healthcare worker training [6]

When emergency release blood is transfused to a patient of unknown blood type, there are some basic safety steps to verify that the correct patient is receiving the correct blood product:

(a) Check the blood bag to ensure it is type O RBCs, LTOWB, or type AB or A plasma.
(b) Check the blood bag for RhD type in accordance with hospital policy.
(c) Check the blood bag for a label indicating that the blood is deemed to be a "universal donor" product, with a statement that compatibility testing has not been done.
(d) Send a recipient blood sample for blood T&S testing as soon as possible so that compatibility testing can be performed on blood already administered and going forward.

Table 19.1 lists suggested standards and practices to prevent patient misidentification, WBT, and WCT events

19.2.5 How May the Patient Verification Process Be Adapted for Children and Other Nonverbal Patients?

Patient self-identification is critical to safe transfusion practice. Infants and other nonverbal patients, such as those under anesthesia, are at high risk of iatrogenic injury due to misidentification errors because they are unable to identify themselves [6, 7, 46]. Even in the awake state, newborns are at a further disadvantage because they may not be named or given a unique medical record number for hours to days

Table 19.2 Suggested practices to prevent misidentification of nonverbal and unconscious patients

Infants, nonverbal, and anesthetized patients	Patient verification safety measure
	Family member identifies patient before phlebotomy, surgery, and transfusion [2, 7]
	Two identification bands on separate extremities [7]
	Eliminate newborn naming conventions that include non-distinct wristband names, such as "boy" or "girl" [49]
	Implementation of biometric identification technology (e.g., face, eye, fingerprint morphology) [6]
	Special hospital policy for patient verification of those at risk for misidentification (e.g., infants, comatose adults, anesthetized patients) [9, 10]
	Special ID measures for neonates [7]: Special identification measures for neonates Staff alerts for similar patient names Special naming schemes Standardization of identification banding procedure

following birth; they typically lack identifying physical characteristics, and they may be in a room with numerous other infants born on the same day [45]. The special problem of neonatal patient identification is significant enough that TJC has promulgated specific preventative measures [6, 7]. Examples of serious neonatal misidentification events include a 3-day-old who received RBCs crossmatched for another patient and subsequently experienced brain damage, a mother breastfeeding another woman's child, and a circumcision on the wrong patient [26, 45, 47]. A 2006 review found that on any given day in an NICU, one-half of patients are at risk of misidentification because of similar medical record numbers (MRNs) or a similar or identical surname [48]. In one patient admission database, 39 patients in 128,000 admissions had the same name and birthdate [45]. Table 19.2 illustrates standards and suggested practices to prevent misidentification errors in nonverbal and unconscious patients:

19.3 Summary of Key Learning Objectives

19.3.1 What Is "Patient Verification" and What Is Its Role In Blood Transfusions?

Patient verification in the context of a blood transfusion is "Confirmation, by examination of objective evidence, that specified requirements have been met." A specific requirement for patient verification prior to any blood transfusion is confirming the patient's identity twice using unique independent identifiers. The identification of this 8-month-old infant should have been verified by a parent or guardian prior to any procedure as recommended by the US hospital accreditation organization, such as TJC and their National Patient Safety Goal 01.01.01.

19.3.2 Why Is Patient Verification Important?

Most fatalities due to ABO-incompatible transfusions are secondary to patient misidentification. Patient verification protocols prior to blood transfusion are intended to prevent potentially fatal WBIT and WCT events.

19.3.3 What Are the Regulatory Requirements for Hospitals Regarding Patient Verification?

Patient verification is a safety priority of health system accreditation organizations, including, but not limited to, the AABB, TJC, and JPAC.

19.3.4 What Is the Standardized Process for Proper Patient Verification Prior to Blood Transfusion?

Standardized patient verification processes exist for both manual and electronic verification methods and apply to pretransfusion specimen collection for blood typing and the transfusion process itself. In the case of this 8-month-old, the ideal patient verification process is:

- A parent or guardian identifies the infant patient prior to phlebotomy and prior to leaving for the operating room.
- The patient's identity is again verified upon entering the (correct) operating room *and* with the anesthesia workstation EHR at "time-out."
- Immediately prior to transfusion, the anesthesia practitioner:
  - Verifies the patient's identify from a wristband (that is present on the patient's body) with another qualified practitioner *or* using a validated EPID system, in accordance with local hospital policy.
  - Crosschecks the patient's blood type as found in the medical record, the blood product bag, and the blood product tag with another qualified practitioner *or* using a validated EPID system, in accordance with local hospital policy.

19.3.5 How May the Patient Verification Process Be Adapted for Children and Other Nonverbal Patients?

The vulnerability of infants to misidentification during hospitalization is recognized in recent literature. This same risk applies to patients who are unconscious under anesthesia. Suggested remedies include:

- Confirmatory blood samples for pretransfusion ABO blood typing.
- Two patient identification bands placed on different extremities.
- Adoption of biometric identification technology.

- Specific protocols with staff education focused on patient populations at greatest risk of misidentification.
- Verification of patient identify during a "time-out" in the operating room.

Key Points

- Practically speaking, patient verification means the patient is identified twice.
- Patient misidentification is the root cause of most fatal acute hemolytic transfusion reactions (ATRs) secondary to ABO blood group incompatibility.
- Blood banks and transfusion services in the US are regulated by the US FDA. Regulations promulgated by the FDA have the force of law and are intended to protect the safety of people who donate or receive blood products. The FDA gives oversight authority to specific accreditation organizations which promulgate standards and guidelines for blood banks and transfusion services. Patient verification is a TJC National Patient Safety Goals (NPSG) and is required as part of hospital accreditation.
- Active patient involvement in self-identification is critical to prevent WCT events; however, it is not a substitute for the requirement of a second confirmatory pretransfusion blood type sample.
- Blood type specimen labels should be applied to the specimen tube at the patient's bedside with active patient self-identification.
- The special problem of neonatal patient identification is significant enough that TJC has promulgated specific preventative measures, including parent or guardian patient identification prior to blood sampling, transfusion, or going to the OR.

References

1. Quinley ED, Grace P. Quality management systems: principles and practice. In: Cohn C, Delaney M, Johnson ST, Katz LM, editors. Technical manual. 20th ed. Bethesda: AABB; 2020. p. 27.
2. AABB. Guidance to Standard 5.14.5 of the Standards for Blood Banks and Transfusion Services. 2023. https://www.aabb.org/standards-accreditation/standards/about-aabb-standards/standards-library. Accessed 17 Sept 2023.
3. Chaffin J. 081CE: top ten changes in the new AABB standards with rich gammon. BloodBankGuy. 2023; https://www.bbguy.org/2020/03/11/081/. Accessed 19 Sept 2023
4. Alquist C, Harm SK. Transfusion service related activities. In: Cohn C, Delaney M, Johnson ST, Katz LM, editors. Technical manual. 20th ed. Bethesda: AABB; 2020. p. 503–4, 510–7, 522, 528–30.
5. US Food & Drug Adminstration. Transfusion/donation fatalities. 2023. https://www.fda.gov/vaccines-blood-biologics/report-problem-center-biologics-evaluation-research/transfusiondonation-fatalities. Accessed 19 Sept 2023.
6. World Health Organization (WHO). Patient Identification 2007. https://cdn.who.int/media/docs/default-source/patient-safety/patient-safety-solutions/ps-solution2-patient-identification.pdf?sfvrsn=ff81d7f9_6. Accessed 17 Sept 2023.

7. The Joint Commission (TJC). R3 Report: Distinct newborn identification requirement. 2023. https://www.jointcommission.org/standards/r3-report/r3-report-issue-17-distinct-newborn-identification-requirement/. Accessed 28 Aug 2023.
8. Joint United Kingdom (UK) Blood Transfusion and Tissue Transplantation Services Professional Advisory Committee (JPAC). 4.10: Administration to the patient. 2023. https://www.transfusionguidelines.org/transfusion-handbook/4-safe-transfusion-right-blood-right-patient-right-time-and-right-place/4-10-administration-to-the-patient. Accessed 19 Sept 2023.
9. Callum J, Etchells E, Shojania K. Addressing the identity crisis in healthcare: positive patient identification technology reduces wrong patient events. Transfusion. 2019;59(3):899–902.
10. Murphy MF, Jayne Addison J, Poles D, Dhiman P, Bolton-Maggs P. Electronic identification systems reduce the number of wrong components transfused. Transfusion. 2019;59(12):3601–7.
11. Serious hazards of transfusion (SHOT) Annu Rep 2021. https://www.shotuk.org/wp-content/uploads/myimages/SHOT-REPORT-2021-FINAL-bookmarked-V3-November.pdf . Accessed 12 Sept 2023.
12. Chavez Ortiz JL, Griffin I, Kazakova SV, Stewart PB, Kracalik I, Basavaraju SV. Transfusion-related errors and associated adverse reactions and blood product wastage as reported to the National Healthcare Safety Network Hemovigilance Module, 2014-2022. Transfusion. 2024;64:627.
13. US Food & Drug Adminstration. Transfusion/donation fatalities. 2020. https://www.fda.gov/media/160859/download#:~:text=During%20FY%202016%20there%20were,2019%2C%20and%2029%20in%202020. Accessed 15 June 2023.
14. Cohen R, Ning S, Yan MTS, Callum J. Transfusion safety: the nature and outcomes of errors in patient registration. Transfus Med Rev. 2019;33(2):78–83.
15. Strauss R, Downie H, Wilson A, Mounchili A, Berry B, Cserti-Gazdewich C, Callum J. Sample collection and sample handling errors submitted to the transfusion error surveillance system, 2006 to 2015. Transfusion. 2018;58(7):1697–707.
16. Vanneman MW, Balakrishna A, Lang AL, Eliason KD, Payette AM, Xu X, et al. Improving transfusion safety in the operating room with a barcode scanning system designed specifically for the surgical environment and existing electronic medical record systems: an interrupted time series analysis. Anesth Analg. 2020;131(4):1217–27.
17. Miller K, Akers C, Magrin G, Whitehead S, Davis AK. Piloting the use of 2D barcode and patient safety-software in an Australian tertiary hospital setting. Vox Sang. 2013;105(2):159–66.
18. Kaufman RM, Dinh A, Cohn CS, Fung MK, Gorlin J, Melanson S, et al. Electronic patient identification for sample labeling reduces wrong blood in tube errors. Transfusion. 2019;59(3):972–80.
19. Chan JC, Chu RW, Young BW, Chan F, Chow CC, Pang WC, et al. Use of an electronic barcode system for patient identification during blood transfusion: 3-year experience in a regional hospital. Hong Kong Med J. 2004;10(3):166–71.
20. Dunbar NM, Kaufman RM, WBIT Study Investigators TeBEfSTBC. Factors associated with wrong blood in tube errors: an international case series—the BEST collaborative study. Transfusion. 2022;62(1):44–50.
21. Crispin P, Akers C, Brown K, Delaforce A, Keegan A, King F, et al. A review of electronic medical records and safe transfusion practice for guideline development. Vox Sang. 2022;117(6):761–8.
22. Davies J, McGrann A, Rowley M. 15: Errors Related to Information Technology. In: Serious Hazards of Transfusion Annual Report. 2021. https://www.shotuk.org/wp-content/uploads/myimages/15.-Errors-Related-to-Information-Technology-IT-2021.pdf Accessed 9 Mar 2024.
23. Schwartz J, Illoh O, Tanhehco YC. Regulatory considerations in transfusion medicine and cellular therapies. In: Cohn C, Delaney M, Johnson ST, Katz LM, editors. Technical manual. 20th ed. Bethesda: AABB; 2020. p. 79–86.
24. U.S. Food & Drug Administration. Regulation of the Blood Supply. 2023. https://www.fda.gov/vaccines-blood-biologics/blood-blood-products/regulation-blood-supply. Accessed 18 Sept 2023.
25. 2023. ASfBBaTShwaos-asb-b-a-t-sAS.

26. TJC. National Patient Safety Goals Effective January 2023 for the Hospital Program. NPSG.01.01.01, UP.01.03.01. 2023. https://www.jointcommission.org/-/media/tjc/documents/standards/national-patient-safety-goals/2023/npsg_chapter_hap_jan2023.pdf. Accessed 17 Sept 2023.
27. Halford B, Pinheiro A, Haspel RL. Hospital medicine providers' transfusion knowledge: a survey study. Transfus Med Rev. 2021;35(2):140–5.
28. Vetter TR, Adhami LF, Porterfield JR Jr, Marques MB. Perceptions about blood transfusion: a survey of surgical patients and their anesthesiologists and surgeons. Anesth Analg. 2014;118(6):1301–8.
29. Al-Riyami AZ, Al-Nomani I, Panchatcharam SM, Wadsworth L, Al-Khabori M, Al-Farsi K, Al-Sabti H. Transfusion knowledge of medical and surgical specialty board residents: a cohort study. Transfus Med. 2018;28(6):440–50.
30. Connelly NR, Adler AC, Vanderberg LE, Conlin F, Mitchell JD, Goldstein S, et al. Anesthesiology resident knowledge of transfusion medicine: results from the anesthesiology transfusion education study. Anesth Analg. 2022;
31. Alquist C, Harm SK. Transfusion service related activities. In: Cohn C, Delaney M, Johnson ST, Katz LM, editors. Technical manual. 20th ed. Bethesda: AABB; 2020. p. 503–4, 510–7, 522, 525, 528–30.
32. Alquist C, Harm SK. Transfusion service related activities. In: Cohn C, Delaney M, Johnson ST, Katz LM, editors. Technical manual. 20th ed. Bethesda, MD: AABB; 2020. p. 503–4, 510–7, 522–3, 525, 528–30.
33. Staples S, O'Callaghan C, Pavord S, Staves J, Murphy MF. How to verify patient identity and blood product compatibility using an electronic bedside transfusion system. Transfusion. 2020;60(9):2153–5.
34. Howanitz PJ, Renner SW, Walsh MK. Continuous wristband monitoring over 2 years decreases identification errors: a College of American Pathologists Q-Tracks Study. Arch Pathol Lab Med. 2002;126(7):809–15.
35. Mollison's blood transfusion in clinical medicine. Klein HG, Anstee DJ, editors. Hoboken: Wiley Blackwell; 2014. p. 14, 188, 194, 335, 500, 585, 667–8.
36. Tchakarov A, Hobbs R, Bai Y. Transfusion of D+ red blood cells to D- individuals in trauma situations. Immunohematology. 2014;30(4):149–52.
37. Sostin N, Hendrickson JE. Pediatric hemovigilance and adverse transfusion reactions. Clin Lab Med. 2021;41(1):51–67.
38. Strauss RG. Data-driven blood banking practices for neonatal RBC transfusions. Transfusion. 2000;40(12):1528–40.
39. Durrani HM, Zaman Z, Raza IM, Jamali M, Saleem A, Ejaz SM. Neonatal haemolytic disease with co-existing anti-D and anti-C antibodies. J Pak Med Assoc. 2022;72(11):2320–2.
40. DePalma L, Criss VR, Roseff SD, Luban NL. Presence of the red cell alloantibody anti-E in an 11-week-old infant. Transfusion. 1992;32(2):177–9.
41. Strauss RG, Cordle DG, Quijana J, Goeken NE. Comparing alloimmunization in preterm infants after transfusion of fresh unmodified versus stored leukocyte-reduced red blood cells. J Pediatr Hematol Oncol. 1999;21(3):224–30.
42. Yazer MH, Dunbar NM, Delaney M, Collaborative BEfST. Survey of the RhD selection and issuing practices for uncrossmatched blood products at pediatric trauma hospitals in the United States: the BEST collaborative study. Transfusion. 2021;61(12):3328–34.
43. Kolodziej JH, Leonard JC, Josephson CD, Gaines BA, Wisniewski SR, Yazer MH, Spinella PC. Survey to inform trial of low-titer group O whole-blood compared to conventional blood components for children with severe traumatic bleeding. Transfusion. 2021;61(Suppl 1):S43–S8.
44. TJC. Hospital National Patient Safety Goals. 2022. https://www.jointcommission.org/-/media/tjc/documents/standards/national-patient-safety-goals/2022/simple_2022-hap-npsg-goals-101921.pdf. Accessed 14 Sept 2023.
45. Cummins D. Patient identification: hybrids and doppelgangers. Ann Clin Biochem. 2007;44(Pt 2):106–10.

46. Cummins D, Sharp S, Vartanian M, Dawson D, Amin S, Halil O. The BCSH guideline on addressograph labels: experience at a cardiothoracic unit and findings of a telephone survey. Transfus Med. 2000;10(2):117–20.
47. Sauer CW, Marc-Aurele KL. Parent misidentification leading to the breastfeeding of the wrong baby in a neonatal intensive care unit. Am J Case Rep. 2016;17:574–9.
48. Gray JE, Suresh G, Ursprung R, Edwards WH, Nickerson J, Shiono PH, et al. Patient misidentification in the neonatal intensive care unit: quantification of risk. Pediatrics. 2006;117(1):e43–7.
49. Adelman J, Aschner J, Schechter C, Angert R, Weiss J, Rai A, et al. Use of temporary names for newborns and associated risks. Pediatrics. 2015;136(2):327–33.

Children of Jehovah's Witness Parents

20

Gee Mei Tan and Bryce Pasko

20.1 Case Scenario

Mary is a 13-year-old girl with severe idiopathic scoliosis (COBB angle 60 degrees) who is scheduled for an elective posterior spine fusion from T5 to the sacrum. She is seen with her parents in the surgery preoperative clinic, and the parents informed the team that they are of the Jehovah's Witness faith and decline blood transfusions. When asked, Mary says that she does not want to receive blood transfusions. The patient's hemoglobin is 10 g/dL and she is otherwise in good health. The spine team informed the family that acceptance of blood transfusion is necessary to proceed with surgery.

Key Learning Point Objectives

- Which blood products do Jehovah's Witness patients typically accept and refuse for perioperative bleeding?
- What is the informed consent procedure for a child of Jehovah's Witness parents?
- Under what circumstances may a physician proceed with a blood transfusion when Jehovah's Witness parents refuse a transfusion for their minor child?
- What perioperative strategies may be undertaken to avoid an allogeneic blood transfusion in a Jehovah's Witness patient undergoing scoliosis surgery?

G. M. Tan (✉)
Children's Hospital Colorado, School of Medicine, University of Colorado, Aurora, CO, USA
e-mail: geemei.tan@childrenscolorado.org

B. Pasko
Medical Director Transfusion Medicine, Apheresis & Coagulation, Department of Pathology and Laboratory Medicine, University of Arizona College of Medicine, Phoenix, AZ, USA
e-mail: bpasko@phoenixchildrens.com

N. J. Klein (ed.), *Perioperative Pediatric Patient Blood Management and Transfusion Safety*, https://doi.org/10.1007/978-3-031-81666-6_20

20.2 Discussion

20.2.1 Which Blood Products Do Jehovah's Witness Patients Typically Accept and Refuse for Perioperative Bleeding?

Some members of the Jehovah's Witness faith refuse blood transfusion based on religious teachings alone. According to an affiliated website, Jehovah, the true God of the faith, has commanded followers: "But you must not eat meat that has its life-blood still in it." The decision to refuse or accept a blood transfusion is to follow God's law, and that decision is deemed highly individual and a matter of personal conscience. Intravenous blood administration, therefore, runs up against this doctrine.

Whole blood and its main components—red cells, white cells, platelets, and plasma—are prohibited as blood transfusions under Jehovah's Witness teachings. However, a prohibition against "minor" blood fractions, which are typically protein derivatives of whole blood, is less likely under the doctrine. Minor blood fractions include cryoprecipitate, prothrombin concentrates, coagulation factors, albumin, and antibodies [Table 20.1] [1, 2].

Some Jehovah's Witnesses believe that minor blood fractions do not represent "lifeblood" once they are extracted from the primary components. Others may agree to receive some minor fractions (such as immunoglobulins or albumin derived from plasma) but not others (e.g., interleukins as these are derived from white cells). "Major" or primary blood components include the cellular components of fractionated blood (e.g., red and white blood cells, platelets, and sometimes plasma) and, along with whole blood, are expressly prohibited according to church doctrine. Tissue factors and sealants may be accepted according to the individual patient's personal choice [3].

Table 20.1 Minor blood fractions that may be accepted by some Jehovah's Witness patients

FRACTIONATED BLOOD COMPONENTS are separated from whole blood components (*some people call these Minor Fractions*).	
– – ***Clotting Factors*** *are proteins in Plasma. They help your blood make clots that stop bleeding.* – –	
CRYOSUPERNATANT is plasma that has most of the solid parts taken out. The leftover liquid is called Cryosupernatant. We give Cryosupernatant to replace plasma.	☐**Accept** ☐**Decline**
CRYOPRECIPITATE is plasma that has the liquid part taken out. The leftover clotting factors are called Cryoprecipitate. We give Cryoprecipitate to help stop bleeding.	☐**Accept** ☐**Decline**
PROTHROMBIN COMPLEX CONCENTRATE is a mix of many clotting factors. We give this mix to help stop bleeding or to reverse the effects of blood thinning medicine.	☐**Accept** ☐**Decline**
CONCENTRATED CLOTTING FACTORS are single clotting factors. We give them to help stop bleeding.	☐**Accept** ☐**Decline**
ALBUMIN is the main protein in plasma. We give Albumin to increase blood volume.	☐**Accept** ☐**Decline**
ANTIBODIES (Other Name: Immune Globulins) are proteins your body makes to fight disease. We can also give you Antibodies to help your body fight some types of infections.	☐**Accept** ☐**Decline**

Most healthcare providers who are not of the Jehovah's Witness faith hold the belief that if a baptized Jehovah's Witness patient accepts and then receives blood transfusions, the patient will face disfellowship from the church or ostracization by the faith community. Although a controversial development, members may now receive teachings that support their sense of personal duty to God in matters of life and death, including lifesaving transfusions [4]. In some circles, a "repentant" adult may not be disqualified from church membership for accepting a blood transfusion. In the case of children of Jehovah's Witness parents, if a baptized child receives a lifesaving transfusion to salvage life or limb, the child may be deemed a victim by the family and community due to the lack of capacity to provide informed refusal. In that case, the child may develop psychological stress and difficulty coping with the consequence of having received blood transfusions.

20.2.2 What Is the Informed Consent Procedure for a Child of Jehovah's Witness Parents?

Informed consent discussions with a Jehovah's Witness patient and family regarding perioperative blood transfusions implicate both legal and ethical aspects of patient refusal. Discussion details should be well documented in the patient's charts for ready access by all healthcare providers throughout the patient's flow of care. In prioritizing a patient-centered care model, hospitals and clinics caring for Jehovah's Witness surgery patients should establish a consent form specifying an agreed-upon plan and a care pathway algorithm for blood management [5, 6]. The American Society of Anesthesiologists (ASA) has developed a simple checkbox questionnaire addressing the basics of blood component acceptance; however, a full discussion will include introducing the possibilities of alternatives to allogeneic transfusion including autologous donation and cell salvage [Table 20.2] [7].

A minor is a person under the age of legal consent as defined by state law. Parental consent is generally required for a minor's medical evaluation and treatment; blood transfusions are considered medical therapy. An informed consent specifically tailored for blood transfusions is suggested by the Association of the Advancement for Blood and Biotherapies (AABB) and The Joint Commission before transfusions [8, 9]. This may or may not be separate from the surgical or procedural consent. There are different standards for elective and emergency or life-threatening clinical situations. For elective transfusions, the following elements must be part of the informed consent process addressing acceptance or refusal of a blood transfusion [10]:

- Description of the risks, benefits, and alternatives to blood transfusion.
- An opportunity to ask questions.
- Acknowledgment of the right to accept or refuse transfusion.

The legal status of minors regarding informed consent in the United States of America (US) varies according to the state [11]. In the US, there are several states that allow minors to consent to medical therapy based on age, living circumstances,

Table 20.2 Standardized transfusion consent form from the ASA Committee on Blood Management

CONSENT FOR BLOOD PRODUCTS – Page 1 of 2

PATIENT NAME: ______________________ DATE OF BIRTH: ____/____/_____ MRN: ____________

Please mark whether you Accept or Decline each of the following:

WHOLE BLOOD COMPONENTS (*some people call these Major Fractions*) Blood carries oxygen and nutrients through the body. The four main parts (or components) can be separated and used for treatment.	
RED BLOOD CELLS (Other Names: Erythrocytes, RBCs) take oxygen from your lungs to your organs and tissues. They also take carbon dioxide back to your lungs to breathe out. We give RBCs if your blood count is too low.	☐ Accept ☐ Decline
WHITE BLOOD CELLS (Other Names: Leukocytes, WBCs) are one of your body's defenses against bacteria, viruses, and diseases the body produces. We give WBCs to help you fight certain diseases.	☐ Accept ☐ Decline
PLATELETS (Other Name: Thrombocytes) are small pieces of cells. They help your blood make clots that prevent or stop bleeding. We give Platelets if your bleeding is hard to stop or if your Platelet count is very low.	☐ Accept ☐ Decline
PLASMA is the liquid part of blood. It is made of water, albumin, clotting factors, salts, sugars, fats, vitamins, and hormones. We give this if you need more Plasma or Clotting Factors.	☐ Accept ☐ Decline
TYPES OF PLASMA ▸ **Frozen (or thawed) plasma (FFP)** is plasma removed from whole blood. It is frozen so it can be used later. ▸ **Solvent detergent-treated plasma** is plasma that is cleaned to reduce the chance of infection or allergic reaction.	
FRACTIONATED BLOOD COMPONENTS are separated from whole blood components (*some people call these Minor Fractions*).	
*– – **Clotting Factors** are proteins in Plasma. They help your blood make clots that stop bleeding. – –*	
CRYOSUPERNATANT is plasma that has most of the solid parts taken out. The leftover liquid is called cryosupernatant. We give cryosupernatant to replace plasma.	☐ Accept ☐ Decline
CRYOPRECIPITATE is plasma that has the liquid part taken out. The leftover clotting factors are called cryoprecipitate. We give cryoprecipitate to help stop bleeding.	☐ Accept ☐ Decline
PROTHROMBIN COMPLEX CONCENTRATE is a mix of many clotting factors. We give this mix to help stop bleeding or to reverse the effects of blood thinning medicine.	☐ Accept ☐ Decline
CONCENTRATED CLOTTING FACTORS are single clotting factors. We give them to help stop bleeding.	☐ Accept ☐ Decline
ALBUMIN is the main protein in plasma. We give albumin to increase blood volume.	☐ Accept ☐ Decline
ANTIBODIES (Other Name: Immune Globulins) are proteins your body makes to fight disease. We can also give you antibodies to help your body fight some types of infections.	☐ Accept ☐ Decline
YOUR OWN BLOOD can be used in the procedures below in a closed system. Your blood is not mixed with any other blood.	
APHERESIS (Other Names: Plasma exchange, Plasmapheresis) is when a closed-system machine replaces bad plasma with a good plasma substitute. It is used if your plasma has antibodies that are attacking your body.	☐ Accept ☐ Decline
AUTOTRANSFUSION (Other Names: Cell Saver, Cell Salvage, Salvaged Autologous Blood) is when your blood is collected during surgery, washed and filtered, and then given back to you in a closed system.	☐ Accept ☐ Decline
HEMODILUTION is when your blood is replaced with IV fluids during surgery. After surgery, we give your blood back to you in a closed system.	☐ Accept ☐ Decline
HEART AND LUNG MACHINE is when your blood flows into a machine that adds oxygen to it. Your blood then flows back into your body in a closed system primed with nonblood fluid. It is used during some surgeries.	☐ Accept ☐ Decline
DIALYSIS (Other Names: Renal Dialysis, Hemodialysis) is when your blood flows into a machine that filters and cleans it, then flows back into your body in a closed system. It is used if your kidneys are not working well or harmful substances need to be taken out of your blood.	☐ Accept ☐ Decline
EPIDURAL BLOOD PATCH is when your blood is injected around your spinal cord to stop a spinal fluid leak.	☐ Accept ☐ Decline
PLATELET GEL is made of your platelets and white blood cells. We use it to cover wounds and help stop bleeding.	☐ Accept ☐ Decline
RECOMBINANT PRODUCTS are like whole blood components, but they are made with protein technology and do not come from blood.	
RECOMBINANT CLOTTING FACTORS* are like the clotting factors that come from whole blood components that are listed above. We give them to help stop bleeding.	☐ Accept ☐ Decline
RECOMBINANT ERYTHROPOIETIN* (Other Names: EPO, ESA, Hematopoietin) is like your body's erythropoietin. It is a hormone that tells bone marrow to make more red blood cells. We give it if your blood count is too low.	☐ Accept ☐ Decline
OTHER TREATMENT (Please Specify):	☐ Accept ☐ Decline

**Some formulations may contain a small amount of albumin.*

Reprinted with permission of the American Society of Anesthesiologists, 1061 American Lan, Schaumburg, Il 60,173–4973.

or medical status. All US states will allow minors to consent for therapy if they live independently from their parents, manage their own finances, are legally married, or are in active-duty military service (i.e., emancipated minors). In multiple US states, minors can legally consent themselves for diagnosis and treatment of sexually transmitted diseases and for addiction therapy [12].

There are also ethical considerations when an elective spine surgery for a severely affected minor patient is postponed. There are four main bioethical principles guiding the practice of Western medicine: preservation of patient autonomy, nonmaleficence (do no harm), beneficence, and justice. Autonomy has been defined as the capacity to live life according to one's own wishes. In minors, the capacity for autonomous decision-making capacity varies with age and maturity level. Applying the "Rule of Sevens," children below age 7 years are not considered to possess capacity to make informed decisions; above 14 years of age, they have the ability to make informed decisions (attestations) that may be challenged if the child lacks the ability to understand potential risks of refusal, including death [13, 14]. Between 7 and 14 years of age, a child is presumed to lack capacity to make reasoned medical decisions, but this can be rebutted with evidence of maturity including ability to fully understand the consequences of their decisions [15]. As the physician caring for any child, medical decisions may be based on any of the four bioethical principles while balancing what is in the child's best interest with options that provide maximal benefit and the least harm. These decisions may be in direct opposition to expressed parental desires. The American Academy of Pediatrics (AAP) states that "children, regardless of parental religious beliefs, deserve effective medical treatment when such treatment is likely to prevent substantial harm or suffering or death" [16].

20.2.3 Under What Circumstances May a Physician Proceed with a Blood Transfusion When Jehovah's Witness Parents Refuse a Transfusion for Their Minor Child?

One exception to the requirement for parental consent for a minor's blood transfusion is the so-called harm principle. Based on the principle of *parens patriae*, the state may become involved in medical decision-making to safeguard the child's safety. This authority stems from a 1944 US Supreme Court case, *Prince* vs. *MA*, where the late Justice Rutledge famously opined, "Parents may be free to become martyrs themselves. But it does not follow they are free, in identical circumstance, to make martyrs of their children before they have reached the age of full and legal discretion" [17]. Today, parents in the US may not refuse a lifesaving transfusion for their child when the benefit outweighs the risk of death or imminent harm.

When a blood transfusion is necessary to save life or limb of a minor patient, there is well-established legal principle supporting treatment of minors without parental consent under the "emergency exception rule" [18]. The American College of Emergency Physicians has listed active bleeding as a mortality risk that may require application of that rule [19]. Before performing a surgical procedure, minor patients and parents of minors that refuse a transfusion should be informed that an intraoperative transfusion may proceed if necessary to preserve the child's life or future well-being.

If the parents or guardian refuses transfusion and the healthcare team deems that a blood transfusion is in the child's best interest because it is necessary for the treatment of the minor's disease process, a court order can be requested from the local judicial authorities [16]. The court order process can be contentious and complex, demanding emotional involvement of not only the family and patient but also the hospital legal, risk management, social services, and healthcare team. A court-ordered decision may take more than 24 hours and thus may delay treatment. Note that such legal action applies only to situations in which the child does not have life-threatening bleeding or anemia. Furthermore, the judicial decision to order a transfusion for a minor child may be subjective based on the judge's view of case laws [20, 21]. In some instances, court orders issued for blood transfusion of children over the parental wishes may trigger the state's child abuse system. Such an action carries significant social stigma and may subject the parents to legal scrutiny which could include being entered into a child abuse or neglect database. Opportunities for future employment may be affected, and the family may be monitored on a regular basis by the social welfare department [18, 22, 23].

In all cases of transfusion refusal, one must balance the benefits and risks of not proceeding with surgery because of the sole issue of transfusion. The child's and the parents' expectations should be clarified through examination of each party's goals of care. A Jehovah's Witness hospital liaison may be invited by the family as a source of support and information. The Jehovah's Witness Hospital Liaison Committee is a worldwide organization made of community-based, volunteer ministers who assist families in interacting with hospital staff and physicians [24].

Approximately 80% of patients with scoliosis have idiopathic disease. It may be early or late onset, with the more severe cases presenting in the younger age group. Patients with adolescent idiopathic scoliosis (AIS) have increasing debilitation including chronic pain, cardiopulmonary compromise, and reduced quality of life due to social isolation [25, 26]. A mild or moderate spine curvature is a Cobb angle of <50 degrees, whereas a 60-degree curve is always classified as severe and carries a poor prognosis. The spinal deformity in over one-half of children with AIS Cobb angle >50 degrees progresses at a rate of approximately 1 degree/year throughout life, and at least one-half of those children can expect to suffer cardiopulmonary dysfunction [27, 28].

20.2.4 What Perioperative Strategies May Be Undertaken to Avoid an Allogeneic Blood Transfusion in a Jehovah's Witness Patient Undergoing Scoliosis Surgery?

Patient blood management (PBM) is defined as "a patient-centered, systematic, evidence-based approach to improve patient outcomes by managing and preserving a patient's own blood, while promoting patient safety and empowerment" [29]. This includes the use of evidence-based surgical and medical concepts to maintain perioperative hemoglobin concentration, optimize hemostasis, and minimize blood loss [30]. These pillars of PBM can be applied to all three phases of pediatric perioperative care—preoperatively, intraoperatively, and postoperatively—and should be incorporated into any spinal fusion protocol. Within each pillar, there are techniques and alternatives that can be personalized for each patient [Table 20.3] [30].

20.2.4.1 The Preoperative Phase of Care

A multidisciplinary team approach is necessary to ensure patient safety and an optimal outcome. An example of multidisciplinary team members include:

- Anesthesiology
- Critical care
- Hematology

Table 20.3 Application of the three pillars of PBM for posterior spine surgery during the perioperative process

PBM pillars	Phases of care	Preoperative	Intraoperative	Postoperative
Optimize RBC mass		Early detection and treatment of anemia Early detection and treatment of nutritional deficiencies	Perform surgery when RBC mass is optimized	Nutritional supplements, including folate, iron, B_{12} per laboratory analysis Continue erythrocyte-stimulating agents (ESAs) if necessary
Optimize hemostasis		Obtain bleeding history for early referral to a hematologist Detect and manage medications that affect coagulation	Meticulous surgical and anesthesia techniques Used of accepted "minor" blood fractions Antifibrinolytics Viscoelastic and other point-of-care (POC) testing	Early anemia detection and management Avoid pharmacologic anticoagulants; employ mechanical antithrombosis Avoid hypothermia Maintain acid-base balance
Manage anemia		Manage menorrhagia Optimize cardiorespiratory insufficiency Manage OSA Refer to a hematologist	Cell salvage Aute normovolemic hemodilution (ANH) Anemia tolerance Avoid excessive hemodilution Minimize phlebotomy Restrictive transfusion thresholds Consider preoperative autologous donation (PAD)	Avoid unnecessary phlebotomy Tolerate anemia with regular monitoring Optimize oxygen utilization and delivery Optimize analgesia including multimodal techniques

Adapted from The National Blood Authority (Australia): three pillars of patient blood management. Available at https://www.blood.gov.au/system/files/documents/pbm-3-pillars.pdf

- Nursing
- Pharmacy
- Risk management
- Surgery
- Nutrition
- Transfusion medicine

As discussed, a detailed informed consent process regarding what blood components, products, or replacement techniques are acceptable to each individual patient and family is a cornerstone of PBM and must be documented in detail prior to the day of surgery. This discussion should be well documented and accessible to the entire care team to ensure smooth transitions during the patient's complex perioperative experience.

Patients should be scheduled for a preoperative evaluation early enough to allow optimization, including anemia treatment for iron deficiency which requires several weeks of therapy [31, 32]. A detailed history and physical examination may detect nutritional (including iron) deficiencies, medication interactions, and comorbidities that impact surgery and recovery. In adolescent girls, it is important to ask about menorrhagia as this increases the risk of preoperative anemia and may necessitate referral to a gynecologist for menstrual regulation. Patients with a moderate to severe Cobb's angle need to be assessed for cardiorespiratory compromise due to restrictive lung and right heart disease. Patients also must be screened for obstructive sleep apnea which can lead to postoperative respiratory depression and hypoxemia in the recovery phase of care. Severely affected patients will need pulmonary function testing, a sleep study, and echocardiography to assess the need for preoperative optimization including noninvasive ventilation, bronchodilators, chest physiotherapy, and oxygen supplementation. In addition, this evaluation may predict intraoperative or postoperative special needs including central lines, vasopressor therapy, intensive care, and timing of extubation. If available, reference to an institution's Maximum Surgical Blood Ordering Schedule (MSBOS) will provide information as to the historical transfusion requirements associated with the surgeon and type of surgery. However, the electronic health record may have alerts for Jehovah's Witness patients, advising that blood should not be ordered and held for such patients without further consultation.

A nutritional history assessment is important for all patients undergoing major surgery to ensure adequate intake of iron, folate, and vitamin B_{12}, each of which is crucial to erythropoiesis. The mean normal hemoglobin for a 13-year-old is 14 g/dL and should be the minimal target to maximize RBC mass reserve preoperatively [33]. Jehovah's Witness patients usually accept erythropoiesis-stimulating agents (ESA) as a supplement to iron therapy because most of the ESAs are recombinant or synthetic.

A bleeding assessment tool from the International Society on Thrombosis and Haemostasis (ISTH-BAT) may facilitate screening for bleeding diatheses and timely referral to a hematologist for evaluation and management [34, 35]. A detailed medication history including over-the-counter (OTC) drugs is important as they may impact coagulation. Table 20.4 illustrates "natural" medications and OTC drugs that may affect a patient's perioperative bleeding risk [36–38].

Table 20.4 Over-the-counter medications that affect bleeding and optimal preoperative cessation times

Consider discontinuing before surgery	3 days	7 days	2–3 weeks	
	Gingko biloba/ maidenhair tree	Garlic (*Allium sativum, Ajo*), Ginseng (*Panax ginseng)*	Ginger (*Zingiber officinale*) Feverfew (*Tanacetum parthenium*) Bromelain Liquorice (*Glycyrrhiza glabra*) Red chili pepper (capsaicin) Saw palmetto (*Serenoa repens*) Oil of wintergreen (methyl salicylate) Devil's claw (*Harpagophytum procumbens)* Chinese agrimony (*Agrimonia pilosa*) Danshen (*Salvia miltiorrhiza*) Baical skullcap root *(Scutellaria baicalensis)* *Geum japonicum* Chinese peony, (Paeoniae rubra)	Poncitrin *Poncirus trifoliata* Fritillaria bulbs (*Fritillaria cirrhosa*) Japanese honeysuckle (*Lonicera japonica*) Kangen-karyu Bak Foong pill Te gastronol Seasonal tonic Guilinggao (tortoise jelly) Vitamin E *Arnica montana* Leopard's bane/ wolf's bane Fish oil Eicosapentaenoic acid Chondroitin Glucosamine

Adapted partly and reprinted with permission from Wong et al. [36]

20.2.4.2 The Intraoperative Phase of Care

It is critical to perform elective surgery only once the patient's RBC mass is optimized to increase the allowable blood loss. An experienced spine surgeon using meticulous surgical technique will minimize loss through the use of bone scalpel, topical hemostatic agents, and minimal surgical time [39–43]. Minimally invasive surgical techniques are also important to minimize intraoperative blood loss [44].

There are many anesthesia techniques that may function to preserve the patient's RBC mass, optimize anemia tolerance, and prevent coagulopathic bleeding [Table 20.5].

The use of intrathecal morphine has been associated with reduced blood loss in spine surgery [45]. In the past, traditional teaching about cell salvage use in Jehovah's Witness patients mandated the use of a closed-loop continuous system. Today, there are some Jehovah's Witness patients who will accept a discontinuous system, and this must be openly addressed during the informed consent process [54]. Furthermore, a continuous cell saver harvest and infusion line, when improperly assembled, may increase the risk of fatal air embolism and should not be

Table 20.5 Anesthesia-related intraoperative PBM techniques

Patient management goals	Anesthesia management
Optimize O_2 delivery	Rational use of FiO_2; avoid hyperviscosity; optimal PEEP [45]
Minimize O_2 consumption	Adequate analgesia; avoid hyperthermia; regional analgesia [45]
Good blood pressure control	Avoid hypertension; judicious use of vasopressors and analgesia
Normothermia	Perioperative forced air warming, including preoperative and postoperative phases of care [46, 47]
Anemia tolerance	RBC transfusion algorithm; hemoglobin 7–8 gm/dl during active bleeding [48, 49]
Positioning	Avoid major vessel compression and venous hypertension [50]
Pharmacology	Antifibrinolytics and recombinant coagulation factors as agreed upon; avoid excessive crystalloid administration [51–53]
Substitute allogeneic blood	Acute normovolemic hemodilution (ANH); cell salvage [54, 55]
Monitors	Noninvasive hemoglobin and volume assessment trends (co-oximetry, plethysmograph, or pulse pressure variation) [56–60]
Testing	POC or coagulation (viscoelastic) technology [61–63]
Use of transfusion algorithms	Reduction in practitioner practice variability [64–67]
Anticipatory blood loss assessment	Institutional maximum surgical blood order schedule (MSBOS), preoperative calculation of allowable blood loss, early and regular intraoperative assessment including weighing of surgical gauzes [68, 69]

employed without expert guidance; a "burp" or secondary reinfusion bag must always be inserted into the system to absorb air in the infusion lines [55, 70, 71]. Venous hypertension may increase intraoperative oozing; the Jackson and wide support Wilson spine frames have been shown to reduce external abdominal pressure that may lead to major vessel compression and associated bleeding [50, 72]. Excessive crystalloid administration is associated with worse outcomes including a coagulopathic state, volume overload, and delayed recovery times [52, 53]. Finally, because perioperative transfusion practices have been shown to vary significantly between practitioners, the use of transfusion algorithms will reduce arbitrary management, thereby improving patient outcomes [64–66, 73].

Artificial oxygen carriers include hemoglobin- and perfluorocarbon-based carriers (HBOCs and PBOCs, respectively). These have not been shown to be comparable to allogeneic blood transfusions when it comes to clinical outcomes. However, there are studies indicating a morbidity or mortality benefit when used in patients with severe, symptomatic anemia for whom blood is not an option [74]. The use of stroma-free hemoglobin is associated with potentially serious side effects including renal toxicity, nitric oxide scavenging leading to vasoconstriction, irreversible methemoglobin formation, and coagulopathy [75, 76]. Recent advances such as modifying free hemoglobin by cross-linkage, polymerization, and encapsulation have been shown to reduce some of these side effects and prolong its oxygen carrying half-life. Hemopure (HBOC-201), which is a polymerized bovine HBOC, has been approved for use in adult surgical patients with acute anemia in South Africa since 2001 when blood is unavailable (a common situation) or refused [74]. It has also been used successfully in a child with sickle cell disease who presented with a hemoglobin level 2 g/dL and high output heart failure, as well as a number of Jehovah's Witness patients [77]. Another hemoglobin-based carrier, oxyglobin, has reportedly been approved for veterinarian use in the USA as of 2010 [75]. Perftoran, a perfluorocarbon, was approved for clinical use in Russia, Kyrgyzstan, Kazakhstan, Ukraine, and Mexico as of 2010 [78–80]. HemO2Life is approved for organ transplant preservation in the European Union [75]. However, a number of HBOCs have been discontinued in the USA while under investigation [75]. Currently, artificial oxygen carriers are not approved by the US Food and Drug Administration (US FDA) for routine clinical use. For example, at the present time, HBOCs can only be obtained through an FDA Expanded Access compassionate use application when the patient cannot or will not accept an allogeneic transfusion [Table 20.6]. This time-consuming process complicates management because current data indicates that the survival rate is better when Hemopure is initiated early.

Table 20.6 Clinical use of HBOCs in the literature

Author, publication year	Patients, *N* =	Population	Nadir Hb (g/dL)	Units of HBOC-201 received	Outcome
Davis et al,[3] 2018	3	Sickle cell (2 Jehovah's Witnesses patients)	3.6–3.8	6–27 U	All survived to hospital discharge
Donahue et al,[65] 2010	1	Jehovah's Witnesses with acute lymphoblastic leukemia	3.1	15	Completed chemotherapy and discharged
Fitzgerald et al,[66] 2011	1	Jehovah's Witnesses trauma patient	2.9	5	Discharge to rehabilitation center
Jordan and Alexander,[68] 2013	1	Jehovah's Witnesses with autoimmune hemolytic anemia	2.8	2	Discharge to home
Lundy et al,[69] 2014	1	Jehovah's Witnesses burn patient	5	6	Death from multiorgan failure
Mackenzie et al,[64] 2010	54	Jehovah's Witnesses patients with severe anemia	3.9[a]	8[b]	Survival of 41.8%, no adverse events attributed to Hb-based oxygen carrier
Posluszny and Napolitano,[67] 2016	1	Jehovah's Witnesses trauma patient	3.9	7	Discharge to home

Reprinted with permission from Jahr et al. [74]
[a]Median Hb before Hb-based oxygen carrier administration
[b]Median units received

HBOCs have a unique effect on patient laboratory and monitoring data because they are free Hgb in plasma. Hemoglobin, hematocrit, serum creatinine, and lactate values may be inaccurate compared to conventional testing [74]. In an in vitro study of four different conventional hematology analyzers, diluted blood samples (Hgb 3.2–6.5 g/dL) were mixed with HBOC-201 to determine the ability of the analyzers to distinguish native Hgb from added free HBOC-201 [81]. Several of the analyzers had a flow cytometry mode which can determine intracellular Hgb. The free HBOC-201 concentration was thus calculated from the total Hgb minus the Hgb contained in the RBCs as determined by flow cytometry. Arterial blood gas technology should be available because pulse oximetry may not accurately reflect oxygen saturation and content. Under existing compassionate use programs in the USA, the threshold for Hemopure administration to adults is a hemoglobin <6–8 g/dL when there is blood refusal, active bleeding, and evidence of secondary end-organ dysfunction. In pediatric patients, transfusion refusal may not be relevant because the emergency exception rule may be triggered when there is life-threatening bleeding in a dependent patient.

20.2.4.3 The Postoperative Phase of Care

Vigilant monitoring in the postoperative period is critical to prevent coagulopathy development in the face of continued bleeding. Children often remain normotensive despite significant blood loss, and if intraoperative bleeding is missed or underestimated, shock or a coagulopathy may develop in the early postoperative period. If there has been significant intraoperative blood loss with a final hemoglobin consistent with severe anemia (e.g., <6–8 g/dl), close observation in a pediatric intensive care unit may be prudent [48, 82]. Postoperative anemia is exacerbated when there is continued bleeding because of reduced erythropoiesis and altered iron metabolism associated with the postsurgical inflammatory state [83]. Severely anemic patients may need to remain intubated or supported with noninvasive ventilation to allow tight control of oxygen delivery. Oxygen consumption can be moderated through the avoidance of hypothermia and shivering, in addition to effective multimodal analgesia [84]. Beyond the immediate postoperative period, continued nutritional supplementation with iron, folate, Vit B12, and perhaps ESAs may be vital to restore RBC mass [85]. Excessive phlebotomy will worsen anemia but can be mitigated by supporting the patient's ability to tolerate anemia, use of POC technology when available, and elimination of routine blood testing. The use of pediatric "microtubes," closed circuit "VAMP" (venous arterial blood management protection) devices, and test batching should be used wherever possible [86, 87]. Clinical observation of trends through noninvasive hemoglobin and volume measurements can replace conventional laboratory testing in some situations. Postoperative thrombosis prevention can initially be managed with mechanical techniques and early ambulation instead of anticoagulants which may increase the risk of bleeding. Washed or unwashed blood collected from drains, if in sufficient quantities (e.g., >500 ml), can be processed and reinfused to avoid allogeneic transfusions when postoperative bleeding is persistent [88]. There are commercially available blood collection devices that allow the addition of anticoagulant and efficient transfer to a washing and processing ("cell saver") machine [89]. Washed product contains a superior hematocrit compared to unwashed (i.e., hematocrit 60% versus 30%) and contains significantly less activated coagulation factor [88].

There is an increasing number of hospitals and surgery centers structured to provide "bloodless" surgery and healthcare [90, 91]. These centers provide evidence-based, quality care for patients who do not or cannot accept allogeneic blood transfusions. These centers are committed to the pillars of PBM. Furthermore, some of these centers may have previously achieved expanded access to artificial oxygen carrier products. Pediatric bloodless surgery centers are in the earlier stages of development but function as an excellent source of information for interested healthcare providers and concerned patients and families [92, 93]. In a 2024 case series of 196 children (mean age 4 years ± 5) whose families requested bloodless care during hospitalization, there were no deaths, and composite outcomes were similar to children receiving standard care (odds ratio 0.37; 95% PI, 0.12–1.11; $p = 0.077$) [94]. Twelve of the children who ultimately received an allogeneic transfusion were less than 1 month old. No court orders were implemented under this multidisciplinary and standardized program.

20.3 Summary of Key Learning Objectives

20.3.1 Which Blood Products Do Jehovah's Witness Patients Typically Accept and Refuse for Perioperative Bleeding?

Jehovah's Witness patients typically refuse cellular blood products but may accept minor by-products of whole blood including clotting factors and recombinant proteins. Pharmaceutical products are often acceptable to Jehovah's Witness patients, including tranexamic acid, ESAs, vasopressor support, and an evidence-based, multimodal analgesia plan, all fundamental to preserving the patient's RBC mass and minimizing blood loss. Ultimately, a Jehovah's Witness patient transfusion decision is deemed highly individual and a matter of personal conscience; the decision can only be supported through an individualized informed consent process.

20.3.2 What Is the Informed Consent Procedure for a Child of Jehovah's Witness Parents?

Informed consent discussions with a Jehovah's Witness patient and family regarding perioperative blood transfusions implicate both legal and ethical aspects of patient refusal. By prioritizing a patient-centered care model, the practitioner should employ a consent form that specifies, before surgery, an agreed-upon plan for blood management. Discussion details should be well documented in the patient's charts for ready access by all healthcare providers throughout the patient's flow of care. As a 13-year-old, this child may be capable of understanding the risks and benefits of refusal and alternative therapies.

If the patient and the parent persist in their refusal, their goals of therapy should be thoroughly explored. If the surgeon remains concerned that transfusion denial will adversely affect the child's well-being, consultation with a local Jehovah's Witness Hospital Liaison Committee may facilitate care and avoid the timely and contentious legal process otherwise known as a "court order." Consultation with a bloodless surgery center is another option.

20.3.3 Under What Circumstances May a Physician Proceed with a Blood Transfusion in a Child of Jehovah's Witness Parents When the Parents Refuse Transfusion?

Another exception to the requirement for parental consent for a minor's blood transfusion is the so-called "harm principle." Based on the principal of *parens patriae*, the state may become involved in medical decision-making to safeguard the child's safety. As a chronic disease state, a Cobb angle of 60 degrees is severe and is associated with progressive disability and decreased quality of life. If surgery is significantly delayed, there is risk of worsening curvature leading to inability to fully correct the curvature, an increased risk of surgical complications, and delayed postoperative recovery. If the parents, guardian, and child continue to refuse a surgery-related transfusion and the healthcare team deems that blood transfusion is in the child's best interest because it is necessary to prevent future harm, a court order can be requested from the local judicial authorities. Today, parents in the US may not refuse a lifesaving transfusion for their child when the benefit outweighs the risk of death or imminent harm. Employing the services of a Jehovah's Witness Hospital Liaison Committee volunteer may facilitate communication between all parties.

20.3.4 What Perioperative Strategies May Be Undertaken to Avoid an Allogeneic Blood Transfusion in a Jehovah's Witness Patient Undergoing Scoliosis Surgery?

Intraoperative strategies such as acute normovolemic hemodilution and cell salvage may be accepted, but the perioperative transfusion plan should be specific, patient-driven, and established before surgery through a structured informed consent geared toward patients who refuse blood products. Table 20.5 lists several patient blood management techniques that the anesthesia team can employ through the pillars of PBM. Prior to this elective surgery, however, it is imperative that the patient's hemoglobin is optimized to $\geq$13 g/dL to provide an RBC reserve during blood loss. Reference to an institutional specific MSBOS will provide information as to the historical transfusion requirements associated with the surgeon and type of surgery. However, the electronic medical record may have a functionality that flags Jehovah's Witness patients, advising against placing blood orders without further patient consultation.

Key Points

- Whole blood and its main components—red cells, white cells, platelets, and plasma—are prohibited as blood transfusions under Jehovah's Witness teachings. A prohibition against minor blood fractions is less likely according to doctrine.
- Informed consent discussions with a Jehovah's Witness patient and family regarding perioperative blood transfusions implicate both legal and ethical aspects of patient refusal. Discussion details should be well documented in the patient's charts for ready access by all healthcare providers throughout the patient's flow of care. Under the "rule of sevens," a 13-year-old child is presumed to lack capacity to make reasoned medical decisions, but this can be rebutted with evidence of maturity including ability to fully understand the consequences of their decisions.
- Medical decisions should be made in the child's best interest. These decisions provide maximal benefit with the least harm. The AAP has also addressed the harm principle of medical decision-making: "children, regardless of parental religious beliefs, deserve effective medical treatment when such treatment is likely to prevent substantial harm or suffering or death." Today, parents in the US may not refuse a lifesaving transfusion for their child when the benefit outweighs the risk of death or imminent harm.
- PBM includes the use of evidence-based surgical and medical concepts to maintain perioperative hemoglobin concentration, optimize hemostasis, and minimize blood loss. These pillars of PBM can be applied to all phases of pediatric perioperative care and should be incorporated into any spinal fusion protocol. Within each PBM pillar, there are techniques and alternatives that can be personalized for each patient.

References

1. JW.ORG. About Jehovah's Witnesses. 2023. https://www.jw.org/en/jehovahs-witnesses/. Accessed 5 June 2023.
2. Jorgenson TD, Golbaba B, Guinn NR, Smith CE. When blood is not an option: the case for a standardized blood transfusion consent form. The ASA Monitor. 2017; https://pubs.asahq.org/monitor/search-results?page=1&q=jorgenson&fl_SiteID=1000003. Accessed 5 June 2023
3. JW.ORG. How Do I View Blood Fractions and Medical Procedures Involving My Own Blood? In: The Watchtower Online Library.2023. https://wol.jw.org/en/wol/d/r1/lp-e/202006400. Accessed 5 June 2023.
4. Barker J. New watchtower blood transfusion policy. 2000. In: Watchman Fellowship. https://www.watchman.org/articles/jehovahs-witnesses/new-watchtower-blood-transfusion-policy/. Accessed 20 June 2023.
5. Transfusion Handbook: In: 12.2: Jehovah's Witnesses and blood transfusion. London Regional Transfusion Committee—Care Pathways for the Management of Adult Patients Refusing Blood (including Jehovah's Witness patients). 2012. JPAC: Joint United Kingdom (UK)

Blood Transfusion and Tissue Transplantation Services Professional Advisory Committee. https://www.transfusionguidelines.org/transfusion-handbook/12-management-of-patients-who-do-not-accept-transfusion/12-2-jehovah-s-witnesses-and-blood-transfusion. Accessed 4 April 2022.
6. University of Pittsburgh Medical Center. About Bloodless Medicine and Surgery Services. 2023. https://www.upmc.com/services/patient-blood-management-bloodless-medicine/about. Accessed 5 June 2023.
7. Jorgensen TD, Golbaba B, Guinn NR, Smith CE. When blood is not an option: the case for a standardized blood transfusion consent form. In: ASA Monitor. 2017; https://pubs.asahq.org/monitor/article/81/6/48/5887/When-Blood-Is-Not-an-Option-The-Case-for-a?searchresult=1. Accessed 4 June 2023
8. Fung MK, editor. Technical manual. 19th ed. Bethesda: AABB Press; 2017. p. 115, 120-121, 464-469, 481-489, 492-493
9. The Joint Commission (TJC). Certification Through The Joint Commission and AABB. 2023. https://www.amsect.org/Certification/PBMT-Exam. Accessed 4 June 2023.
10. Jorgenson M. Chapter 18: Administration of Blood Components. In: Cohn CS, Delaney M, Johnson ST, Katz LM. 20th edition. Technical Manual. Bethesda: AABB. 2020. p. 537.
11. Ages of Consent in the United States. In: Wikipedia. 2023. https://en.wikipedia.org/wiki/Ages_of_consent_in_the_United_States#Notes. Accessed 5 June 2023.
12. State Laws that enable a minor to provide informed consent to receive HIV and STD services. The Centers for Disease Control and Prevention. 2022. https://www.cdc.gov/hiv/policies/law/states/minors.html. Accessed 5 June 2023.
13. Griffith R. What is Gillick competence? Hum Vaccin Immunother. 2016;12(1):244–7.
14. Carollo DS, Mann DG. The ethics of Pediatric informed consent. American Society of Anesthesiologists; 2018. https://pubs.asahq.org/monitor/article/82/11/10/3403/The-Ethics-of-Pediatric-Informed-Consent. Accessed 28 Nov 2021
15. Cardwell v.Bechtel,724 S.W.2d 739,750 (Tenn. 1987).
16. Informed consent, parental permission, and assent in pediatric practice. Committee on Bioethics, American Academy of Pediatrics. Pediatrics. 1995;95(2):314–7.
17. Prince v. Massachusetts, 321 U.S. 158 (1944).
18. Bioethics CoPEMaCo. Consent for emergency medical services for children and adolescents. Pediatrics. 2011;128(2):427–33.
19. Jaquis WP. Prevent BLEEDing Act. American College of Emergency Physicians. 2020; https://www.acep.org/globalassets/new-pdfs/advocacy/acep-support-letter-prevent-bleeding-act-senate-02-26-20.pdf? Accessed 5 June 2023
20. The Stamford Hospital v Vega, 236 Conn. 646.
21. In Re EG, 549 N.E.2d 322.
22. Katz AL, Webb SA. Informed consent in decision-making in pediatric practice. Pediatrics. 2016;138(2)
23. American Academy of Pediatrics Committee on Bioethics. Religious objections to medical care. Pediatrics. 1997;99(2):279–81.
24. JW.ORG. Hospital Liaison Committees for Jehovah's Witnesses. 2022. https://www.jw.org/en/medical-library/strategies-downloads/hospital-liaison-committees-jehovahs-witnesses/. Accessed 9 April 2022.
25. Kuznia AL, Hernandez AK, Lee LU. Adolescent idiopathic scoliosis: common questions and answers. Am Fam Physician. 2020;101(1):19–23.
26. Weinstein SL. The natural history of adolescent idiopathic scoliosis. J Pediatr Orthop. 2019;39(Issue 6, Supplement 1 Suppl 1):S44–S6.
27. Mistovich RJ, Spiegel DA. Idiopathic scoliosis. In: Kliegman RM Blum NJ, Shah SS, editors. Nelson textbook of Pediatrics. Philadelphia: Elsevier; 2020. p. 3635.
28. Smith JS, Saulle D, Chen CJ, Lenke LG, Polly DW, Kasliwal MK, et al. Rates and causes of mortality associated with spine surgery based on 108,419 procedures: a review of the Scoliosis Research Society Morbidity and Mortality Database. Spine (Phila Pa 1976). 2012;37(23):1975–82.

29. Shander A, Hardy JF, Ozawa S, Farmer SL, Hofmann A, Frank SM, et al. A global definition of patient blood management. Anesth Analg. 2022;135(3):476–88.
30. National Blood Authority. Three pillars of patient blood management. 2023. https://www.blood.gov.au/system/files/documents/pbm-3-pillars.pdf. Accessed 6 June 2023.
31. Ning S, Zeller MP. Iron: how to manage when there is too much or too little of it. Management of Iron Deficiency. American Society of Hematology; 2019. https://www.who.int/publications/i/item/9789240035744. Accessed 17 Jan 2023. https://doi.org/10.1182/hematology.2019000034.
32. Munoz M, Acheson AG, Auerbach M, Besser M, Habler O, Kehlet H, et al. International consensus statement on the peri-operative management of anaemia and iron deficiency. Anaesthesia. 2017;72(2):233–47.
33. Thornburg CD. The Anemias. In: Kliegman RM, Geme JS, editors. Nelson textbook of pediatrics E-book. 21st ed. Elsevier-OHCE; 2019. p. 2505–6.
34. Elbatarny M, Mollah S, Grabell J, Bae S, Deforest M, Tuttle A, et al. Normal range of bleeding scores for the ISTH-BAT: adult and pediatric data from the merging project. Haemophilia. 2014;20(6):831–5.
35. International Society on Thrombosis and Haemostasis. ISTH-SSC Bleeding Assessment Tool. 2023. https://bleedingscore.certe.nl/. Accessed 7 June 2023.
36. Wong WW, Gabriel A, Maxwell GP, Gupta SC. Bleeding risks of herbal, homeopathic, and dietary supplements: a hidden nightmare for plastic surgeons? Aesthet Surg J. 2012;32(3):332–46.
37. Frank S, Guinn NR. Patient blood management. In: Cohn C, Delaney M, Johnson ST, Katz LM, editors. Technical manual. 20th ed. Bethesda: AABB; 2020. p. 592.
38. Leak JA. Perioperative considerations in the management of the patient taking herbal medicines. Curr Opin Anaesthesiol. 2000;13(3):321–5.
39. Wahlquist S, Nelson S, Glivar P. Effect of the ultrasonic bone scalpel on blood loss during pediatric spinal deformity correction surgery. Spine Deform. 2019;7(4):582–7.
40. Bartley CE, Bastrom TP, Newton PO. Blood loss reduction during surgical correction of adolescent idiopathic scoliosis utilizing an ultrasonic bone scalpel. Spine Deform. 2014;2(4):285–90.
41. Alamanda VK, Massengill DL, Rozario N, Moore CG, Scannell B, Brighton B, et al. Blood loss trends and financial implications in adolescent idiopathic scoliosis. Clin Spine Surg. 2018;31(8):E418–E21.
42. Shander A, Kaplan LJ, Harris MT, Gross I, Nagarsheth NP, Nemeth J, et al. Topical hemostatic therapy in surgery: bridging the knowledge and practice gap. J Am Coll Surg. 2014;219(3):570–9.e4.
43. Minhas SV, Chow I, Bosco J, Otsuka NY. Assessing the rates, predictors, and complications of blood transfusion volume in posterior arthrodesis for adolescent idiopathic scoliosis. Spine (Phila Pa 1976). 2015;40(18):1422–30.
44. Si G, Li T, Wang Y, Liu X, Li C, Yu M. Minimally invasive surgery versus standard posterior approach for Lenke Type 1-4 adolescent idiopathic scoliosis: a multicenter, retrospective study. Eur Spine J. 2021;30(3):706–13.
45. Cronin JA, Oetgen ME, Gordish-Dressman H, Martin BD, Khan N, Pestieau SR. Association between perioperative surgical home implementation and transfusion patterns in adolescents with idiopathic scoliosis undergoing spinal fusion. Paediatr Anaesth. 2019;29(6):611–9.
46. Polderman KH. Mechanisms of action, physiological effects, and complications of hypothermia. Crit Care Med. 2009;37(7 Suppl):S186–202.
47. Görges M, Ansermino JM, Whyte SD. A retrospective audit to examine the effectiveness of preoperative warming on hypothermia in spine deformity surgery patients. Paediatr Anaesth. 2013;23(11):1054–61.
48. Valentine SL, Bembea MM, Muszynski JA, Cholette JM, Doctor A, Spinella PC, et al. Consensus recommendations for RBC transfusion practice in critically ill children from the Pediatric Critical Care Transfusion and Anemia Expertise Initiative. Pediatr Crit Care Med. 2018;19(9):884–98.

49. Chai KL, Cole-Sinclair M. Review of available evidence supporting different transfusion thresholds in different patient groups with anemia. Ann N Y Acad Sci. 2019;1450(1):221–38.
50. Park CK. The effect of patient positioning on intraabdominal pressure and blood loss in spinal surgery. Anesth Analg. 2000;91(3):552–7.
51. Johnson DJ, Johnson CC, Goobie SM, Nami N, Wetzler JA, Sponseller PD, et al. High-dose versus low-dose tranexamic acid to reduce transfusion requirements in pediatric scoliosis surgery. J Pediatr Orthop. 2017;37(8):e552–e7.
52. Cotton BA, Guy JS, Morris JA, Abumrad NN. The cellular, metabolic, and systemic consequences of aggressive fluid resuscitation strategies. Shock. 2006;26(2):115–21.
53. Topjian AA, Raymond TT, Atkins D, Chan M, Duff JP, Joyner BL, et al. Part 4: Pediatric basic and advanced life support: 2020 American Heart Association guidelines for cardiopulmonary resuscitation and emergency cardiovascular care. Circulation. 2020;142(16_suppl_2):S469–523.
54. Waters JH. Intraoperative blood recovery and reinfusion. In: Frank SM, Waters JH, editors. Patient blood management: multidisciplinary approaches to optimizing care. Bethesda: AABB Press; 2016. p. 186.
55. Stone N, Sardana V, Missiuna P. Indications and outcomes of cell saver in adolescent scoliosis correction surgery: a systematic review. Spine (Phila Pa 1976). 2017;42(6):E363–E70.
56. Desgranges FP, Bouvet L, de Souza P, Neto E, Evain JN, Terrisse H, Joosten A, et al. Non-invasive measurement of digital plethysmographic variability index to predict fluid responsiveness in mechanically ventilated children: a systematic review and meta-analysis of diagnostic test accuracy studies. Anaesth Crit Care Pain Med. 2023;42(3):101194.
57. Cecconi M, De Backer D, Antonelli M, Beale R, Bakker J, Hofer C, et al. Consensus on circulatory shock and hemodynamic monitoring. Task force of the European Society of Intensive Care Medicine. Intensive Care Med. 2014;40(12):1795–815.
58. Hornedo-González KD, Jacob AK, Burt JM, Higgins AA, Engel EM, Hanson AC, et al. Non-invasive hemoglobin estimation for preoperative anemia screening. Transfusion. 2023;63(2):315–22.
59. Chen G, Chung E, Meng L, Alexander B, Vu T, Rinehart J, et al. Impact of non invasive and beat-to-beat arterial pressure monitoring on intraoperative hemodynamic management. J Clin Monit Comput. 2012;26(2):133–40.
60. Chung E, Cannesson M. Using non invasive dynamic parameters of fluid responsiveness in children: there is still much to learn. J Clin Monit Comput. 2012;26(3):153–5.
61. Haas T, Faraoni D. Viscoelastic testing in pediatric patients. Transfusion. 2020;60(Suppl 6):S75–85.
62. Park YH, Lee JH, Song HG, Byon HJ, Kim HS, Kim JT. The accuracy of noninvasive hemoglobin monitoring using the radical-7 pulse CO-oximeter in children undergoing neurosurgery. Anesth Analg. 2012;115(6):1302–7.
63. Patino M, Schultz L, Hossain M, Moeller J, Mahmoud M, Gunter J, et al. Trending and accuracy of noninvasive hemoglobin monitoring in pediatric perioperative patients. Anesth Analg. 2014;119(4):920–5.
64. Faraoni D, Willems A, Romlin BS, Belisle S, Van der Linden P. Development of a specific algorithm to guide haemostatic therapy in children undergoing cardiac surgery: a single-centre retrospective study. Eur J Anaesthesiol. 2015;32(5):320–9.
65. Baker L, Park L, Gilbert R, Ahn H, Martel A, Lenet T, et al. Intraoperative red blood cell transfusion decision-making: a systematic review of guidelines. Ann Surg. 2021;274(1):86–96.
66. Willems A, Harrington K, Lacroix J, Biarent D, Joffe AR, Wensley D, et al. Comparison of two red-cell transfusion strategies after pediatric cardiac surgery: a subgroup analysis. Crit Care Med. 2010;38(2):649–56.
67. Australian Government National Health and Medical Research Council, Patient Blood Management Guidelines: Module 6 (Neonatal and Pediatric). 2016. https://www.blood.gov.au/pbm-module-6. Accessed 11 Nov 2021.

68. Reppucci ML, Meier M, Stevens J, Shirek G, Kulungowski AM, Acker SN. Incidence of and risk factors for perioperative blood transfusion in infants undergoing index pediatric surgery procedures. J Pediatr Surg. 2022;
69. Lee AC, Reduque LL, Luban NL, Ness PM, Anton B, Heitmiller ES. Transfusion-associated hyperkalemic cardiac arrest in pediatric patients receiving massive transfusion. Transfusion. 2014;54(1):244–54.
70. Oliveira JAA, Façanha Filho FAM, Fernandes FV, Almeida PC, de Oliveira VF, Lima Verde SR. Is cell salvage cost-effective in posterior arthrodesis for adolescent idiopathic scoliosis in the public health system? J Spine Surg. 2017;3(1):2–8.
71. Waters JH. Intraoperative blood recovery. ASAIO J. 2013;59(1):11–7.
72. Kim E, Kim HC, Lim YJ, et al. Comparison of intra-abdominal pressure among 3 prone positional apparatuses after changing from the supine to the prone position and applying positive end-expiratory pressure in healthy euvolemic patients: a prospective observational study. J Neurosurg Anesthesiol. 2017;29(1):14–20. https://doi.og/10.1097/ana.0000000000000257.
73. Partington A, Chew DP, Ben-Tovim D, Horsfall M, Hakendorf P, Karnon J. Screening for important unwarranted variation in clinical practice: a triple-test of processes of care, costs and patient outcomes. Aust Health Rev. 2017;41(1):104–10.
74. Jahr JS, Guinn NR, Lowery DR, Shore-Lesserson L, Shander A. Blood substitutes and oxygen therapeutics: a review. Anesth Analg. 2021;132(1):119–29.
75. Chen L, Yang Z, Liu H. Hemoglobin-based oxygen carriers: Where are we now in 2023? Medicina (Kaunas). 2023;59(2).
76. Jahr JS, Williams JP. Blood component requirements and erythrocyte transfusion and mortality related to Hemoglobin deficit in phase III trial of Hemoglobin-based oxygen carrier: HBOC-201. Am J Ther. 2022;29(3):e279–e86.
77. Stefan DC, Uys R, Wessels G. Hemopure transfusion in a child with severe anemia. Pediatr Hematol Oncol. 2007;24(4):269–73.
78. Verdin-Vasquez RC, Zepeda-Perez C, Ferra-Ferrer R, Chavez-Negrete A, Contreras F, Barroso-Aranda J. Use of perftoran emulsion to decrease allogeneic blood transfusion in cardiac surgery: clinical trial. Artif Cells Blood Substit Immobil Biotechnol. 2006;34(4):433–54.
79. Jägers J, Wrobeln A, Ferenz KB. Perfluorocarbon-based oxygen carriers: from physics to physiology. Pflugers Arch. 2021;473(2):139–50.
80. Latson GW. Perftoran (Vidaphor)-introduction to western medicine. Shock. 2019;52(1S Suppl 1):65–9.
81. Bronkhorst-van der Helm MW, Weerkamp F, Huisman A, Huisman EJ, Russcher H. Interference of bovine hemoglobin-based oxygen carrier-201 (Hemopure) on four hematology analyzers. Int J Lab Hematol. 2023;45(6):869–74.
82. Allali S, Brousse V, Sacri AS, Chalumeau M, de Montalembert M. Anemia in children: prevalence, causes, diagnostic work-up, and long-term consequences. Expert Rev Hematol. 2017;10(11):1023–8.
83. van Iperen CE, Kraaijenhagen RJ, Biesma DH, Beguin Y, Marx JJ, van de Wiel A. Iron metabolism and erythropoiesis after surgery. Br J Surg. 1998;85(1):41–5.
84. Alfonsi P. Postanaesthetic shivering: epidemiology, pathophysiology, and approaches to prevention and management. Drugs. 2001;61(15):2193–205.
85. Muñoz M, Acheson AG, Bisbe E, Butcher A, Gómez-Ramírez S, Khalafallah AA, et al. An international consensus statement on the management of postoperative anaemia after major surgical procedures. Anaesthesia. 2018;73(11):1418–31.
86. Dolman HS, Evans K, Zimmerman LH, Lavery T, Baylor AE, Wilson RF, et al. Impact of minimizing diagnostic blood loss in the critically ill. Surgery. 2015;158(4):1083–7. discussion 7–8
87. Valentine SL, Bateman ST. Identifying factors to minimize phlebotomy-induced blood loss in the pediatric intensive care unit. Pediatr Crit Care Med. 2012;13(1):22–7.
88. Frank SM, Guinn NR. Patient Blood Management. In: Cohn CS, Delaney M, Johnson ST, Katz LM. 20th edition Technical Manual. Bethesda: AABB; 2020. P. 596–597.

89. Ecomed Solutions. Blood Management: HEMAsavR™. 2023. https://ecomed-solutions.com/pages/blood-management-hemasavr. Accessed 8 June 2023.
90. Society for Advancement of Patient Blood Management (SABM). Programs by State. https://sabm.org/programs-by-state/ (2020). Accessed 8 June 2023.
91. Kayoum AA, Rivera Flores E, Reyes M, Almasarweh SI, Ojito J, Burke RP, et al. Safety of bloodless open-heart surgery on cardiopulmonary bypass in selected children: a single center experience with minimal invasive extracorporeal circulation. Perfusion. 2024;39(2):391–8.
92. Nationwide Children's. Blood Conservation Program. https://www.nationwidechildrens.org/specialties/blood-conservation-program (2022). Accessed 8 June 2023.
93. Stanford Children's Health. Pediatric Bloodless Cardiac Surgery Program. https://www.stanfordchildrens.org/en/service/bloodless-surgery (2022). Accessed 8 June 2023.
94. Lo BD, Pippa A, Sherd I, Scott AV, Thomas AJ, Hendricks EA, et al. Clinical outcomes, blood utilization, and ethical considerations for pediatric patients in a bloodless medicine and surgery program. Anesth Analg. 2024;138(2):465–74.

von Willebrand Disease (VWD) 21

Liliya Pospishil, Jennie Ngai, and Norma J. Klein

21.1 Case Scenario

A 5-year-old, 15-kg girl presents for emergency appendectomy. She has a history of recurrent nosebleeds including at least one episode requiring an emergency room visit and intranasal packing. Her family history is unremarkable. Preoperative lab studies (complete blood count and basic metabolic panel) are within normal limits. When you order pretransfusion testing, the surgeon tells you it is not necessary because this is not a blood loss procedure.

Key Learning Objectives

- How is von Willebrand disease diagnosed in the preoperative period, including confirmatory laboratory testing?
- How is von Willebrand disease bleeding prophylaxis managed in the preoperative period?
- What are coagulation factor activity replacement goals for specific procedures during the intraoperative phase of care?
- What adjuncts are available to manage von Willebrand disease?
- What are postoperative management concerns with the patient who has von Willebrand disease and has recently undergone surgery?

L. Pospishil (✉) · J. Ngai
Department of Anesthesiology, Perioperative Care, and Pain Medicine, NYU Grossman School of Medicine, New York, NY, USA
e-mail: liliya.pospishil@nyulangone.org; jennie.ngai@nyulangone.org

N. J. Klein
Department of Anesthesiology and Pain Medicine, University of California, Davis, Sacramento, CA, USA
e-mail: nklein@ucdavis.edu

N. J. Klein (ed.), *Perioperative Pediatric Patient Blood Management and Transfusion Safety*, https://doi.org/10.1007/978-3-031-81666-6_21

21.2 Discussion

21.2.1 General

von Willebrand disease (VWD) is caused by defects in von Willebrand factor (vWF), characterized by abnormal platelet adhesion and aggregation with the potential for excessive perioperative bleeding. Preservation of a VWD patient's blood volume requires attentive blood management. This discussion will focus on the preoperative diagnosis of VWD, perioperative hemorrhage mitigation tools for elective procedures, and management of acute bleeding episodes in children.

Von Willebrand disease is the most common inherited bleeding disorder with a prevalence of 1:100–1:10,000 [1–3]. It is characterized by quantitative or qualitative defects in von Willebrand factor (vWF). vWF binds to collagen at sites of endovascular injury, mediates platelet activity, and serves as a carrier protein for coagulation factor VIII (fVIII) [4]. As a carrier of fVIII, vWF stabilizes fVIII such that levels rise as vWF levels increase. VWD is inherited in an autosomal inheritance pattern and thus affects males and females equally, although the diagnosis is more likely to be made in females secondary to excessive menstruation and peripartum bleeding events [5]. In rare cases, VWD is an acquired coagulopathy.

21.2.2 How Is von Willebrand Disease Diagnosed in the Preoperative Period, Including Confirmatory Laboratory Testing?

Although there are no standardized management guidelines addressing pediatric perioperative care, a multidisciplinary panel established by the American Society of Hematology (ASH), the International Society on Thrombosis and Haemostasis (ISTH), the National Hemophilia Foundation (NHF), and the World Federation of Hemophilia (WFH) have published evidence-based recommendations on VWD diagnosis and management that can be used a guide [6]. Perioperative management of patients with VWD undergoing surgery requires a multidisciplinary team approach and evidence-based preparation to preserve red blood cell mass. Care coordination between anesthesiology, surgery, hematology, pharmacy, laboratory services, blood bank, nursing, and social work is essential to prepare the patient for surgery and respond promptly to bleeding episodes. If specialized testing, medications, and observation are required, procedures in patients with VWD should be performed within reach of a Hemophilia Treatment Center (HTC) [7, 8].

21.2.2.1 Diagnosis

VWD is subdivided into types 1, 2, and 3 or acquired disease based on the degree of qualitative and quantitative vWF deficiency (Table 21.1). The majority of patients have no symptoms, and the disease is clinically significant in 1:10,000 patients [9]. The diagnosis of VWD begins with a personal history of abnormal bleeding or

Table 21.1 The clinical presentations of VWD subtypes

Type	Inheritance pattern	Defect in vWF	Clinical presentation
1 1C	Autosomal dominant	Partial quantitative and equal deficiency of vWF activity and antigen	Mild to moderate mucocutaneous bleeding
2	Autosomal dominant	Qualitative abnormalities of vWF	
2A	Autosomal dominant	Reduced or absent high-molecular-weight vWF	Moderate to severe mucocutaneous bleeding
2B	Autosomal dominant	Gain of function in fVW that increases its affinity for platelets, often leading to thrombocytopenia	Moderate to severe mucocutaneous bleeding
2M	Autosomal recessive	Reduced vWF interactions with platelets or collagen	Moderate to severe mucocutaneous bleeding
2N	Autosomal recessive	Reduced binding of vWF to fVIII	Moderate to severe hemophilia-like bleeding

Adapted from Swami et al. [17]; James [12]

VWF von Willebrand factors, *AD* autosomal dominant, *AR* autosomal recessive

bruising, a family history of bleeding, mild thrombocytopenia, or an unexplained prolongation of partial thromboplastin time (aPTT).

21.2.2.2 Clinical Features

VWD may present with "platelet-type" excessive mucocutaneous bleeding, including epistaxis, bleeding from dental extractions, gingival bleeding, easy skin bruising, menorrhagia, excessive post-traumatic bleeding, and postpartum bleeding. Epistaxis and excessive bruising are the usual presenting signs in children with VWD [2, 10]. Excessive menstrual bleeding is reported in over 75% of post-menarchal females [11]. The International Society on Thrombosis and Haemostasis (ISTH) does not have a specific vWF level cutoff value for diagnosis of VWD [6]. However, because the clinical manifestations vary widely and the approach should be individualized, there is general consensus that baseline vWF levels may guide diagnostic and management strategies. The severity of clinical presentation may be a function of the level of residual vWF activity, the VWD subtypes, patient age (vWF levels increase approximately 0.8% per year), and sex (many individuals go undiagnosed until adolescence and the onset of menses) [2, 12]. Of note, VWD is reportedly more common in patients with non-type O blood [2].

Type 1 VWD is characterized by a quantitative deficiency of essentially normal vWF. It is the most common subtype, accounting for 70–80% of cases [2]. A new variant with rapid clearance of vWF, type 1C, was defined in 2021. Patients with type 1 VWD may be asymptomatic or present with mild to moderate mucocutaneous bleeding. In a population-based survey from the Netherlands, up to 20% of adult patients did not bleed excessively with "challenges," including dental extraction, menstruation, and small wounds [2, 13]. Type 1 VWD is inherited in an autosomal dominant pattern, but the more severe forms (e.g., types 2N and 3) follow an autosomal recessive pattern; heterozygotes may be VWD carriers and have a type 1 presentation [2].

Type 2 VWD is characterized by qualitative defects in vWF and is associated with a reduction of vWF function and more severe bleeding compared to type 1 VWD [14]. Type 2 VWD is present in approximately 15–20% of known cases [12, 14]. Type 2 is further subdivided into four subtypes (2A, 2B, 2M, 2N) on the basis of specific phenotypic characteristics (Table 21.1). Although most type 2 patients present with mucocutaneous bleeding, in type 2N, which is characterized by reduced binding to fVIII, "hemophilia-type" joint bleeding can be the presenting symptom [15]. Thrombocytopenia may be present in type 2B VWD due to increased platelet binding with fVW and rapid clearance.

Type 3 VWD is the most severe form of VWD because of an absence of circulating vWF and concomitant very low levels of fVIII. Type 3 comprises less than 5% of cases. Affected patients are at particular risk of joint bleeding [12, 13]. Severe vWF deficiency will manifest in childhood with joint bleeds on crawling and ambulating or with minimal trauma, mirroring the clinical presentation of hemophilia [15].

Acquired VWD may be associated with medical conditions such as autoimmune disease, hypothyroidism, lymphoproliferative disease, and certain medications (e.g., valproic acid). There is no family or personal history of major bleeding [12, 16, 17]. The etiology of low fVW levels in acquired disease is either reduced production, rapid clearance, or degradation of vWF [12]. Acquired VWD is rarely seen in children and requires different diagnostic and treatment strategies from those used for inherited disease.

21.3 Screening Tests

ISTH supports the use of validated bleeding assessment tools (BATs) as initial screening tests for patients with suspected VWD [18]. Validated screening tools are important because they are based on past medical history, and laboratory studies in VWD patients are often normal. BATs are most useful in post-menarchal women because these screening tools have better diagnostic ability with increasing patient age and a consequential number of hemostatic challenges [2]. There are a number of BATs for use in children as well, with a score ≥ 3 considered to be positive (and warrants further testing if an invasive procedure is planned) [19–23]. Table 21.2 illustrates the bleeding signs or symptoms that may be suggestive of VWD or another coagulopathy in children.

Other indications for VWD evaluation include a positive family history of bleeding (especially mucocutaneous type), unexplained thrombocytopenia or an elevated aPTT, or a history of medications or disease states associated with VWD, as discussed above. Although the physical exam requires inspection for bruising, most children with VWD do not have this finding. In children under 2 years, bruising of extremities and head trauma is common as they learn to crawl and walk, confounding the diagnosis [9]. Consequently, family history and bleeding assessment are important in the preoperative evaluation of a small child.

Table 21.2 Bleeding signs or symptoms that may warrant coagulation testing in small children about to undergo an invasive procedure

Bleeding signs and symptoms queried about in a bleeding assessment tool (BAT)
Bruising with immunizations
Repeated epistaxis
Prolonged epistaxis >10 mins
Significant bruising
Increased oozing from minor wounds
Persistent bleeding after tooth extraction
Umbilical stump bleeding
Cephalohematoma
Bleeding with circumcision
Hematuria
Gum bleeding after loss of primary teeth

21.3.1 Laboratory Testing for VWD

Diagnostic evaluation of VWD is complex and can be thought of as a compilation of tests to confirm the diagnosis of VWD and further tests to classify VWD subtypes. Because VWD may result from a qualitative or quantitative defect in vWF or be platelet- or fVIII-related, there is no single test that will pinpoint a diagnosis. Initial testing for VWD includes complete blood count (CBC), prothrombin time (PT), partial thromboplastin time (PTT), vWF:Ag (vWF antigen), vWF activity, and fVIII:C (fVIII coagulant activity). The diagnostic tests are discussed below, while subtype-specific testing is beyond the scope of this review.

The vWF level is measured using vWF:Ag or platelet-dependent vWF activity. A diagnosis of type 1 VWD is confirmed with a vWF level of <30 IU/dL regardless of bleeding. A vWF:Ag less than 30% is diagnostic for VWD; a vWF:Ag level greater than 50% is normal; vWD:Ag levels between 30% and 50% require clinical correlation such as a significant bleeding history to support a VWD diagnosis [12]. FVIII activity is also measured because its activity may be reduced in any type of VWD, particularly types 2N and 3 [24]. FVW activity may be expressed as ristocetin cofactor units (vWF:RCo). In the past, a vWF ristocetin (an antibiotic) cofactor (vWF:RCo) assay was used to measure platelet-binding activity of vWF. However, the 2021 guidelines suggest that newer glycoprotein-based assays have increased sensitivity [6].

Patients with type 2 VWD have normal vWF:Ag levels but abnormal platelet-dependent vWF activity. The diagnosis of type 2 VWD (2A, 2B, 2M) is confirmed with a platelet-dependent vWF activity/vWF:Ag ratio < 70 IU/dL. If type 2 N is suspected, fVIII binding (VWF:fVIIIB) or genetic testing is suggested [6].

Type 3 VWD is diagnosed when vWF:Ag is <0.05 IU/ml [2]. The absolute level of vWF:Ag should be interpreted with caution as patients with severe type 1 VWD can also have very low vWF level. Severe type 1 VWD can be discerned from type 3 VWD by measuring vWF propeptide (cleavage product formed during synthesis of vWF). In type 3 VWD, both vWF:Ag and propeptide are absent, whereas in severe type 1 disease, the antigen level is very low, but the propeptide level is minimally reduced or normal [10].

Figure 21.1 illustrates a simplified approach to the diagnosis of VWD, including when to administer a DDAVP (desmopressin) trial as part of the preoperative evaluation [6].

21.3.2 How Is von Willebrand Disease-Related Bleeding Prophylaxis Managed in the Preoperative Period?

The perioperative treatment goal in patients with VWD is normalization of vWF and fVIII activity prior to surgical intervention and during acute bleeding episodes. Individualized treatment plans must balance the bleeding risks associated with different procedures with the risk of overtreatment and thrombosis secondary to excessive coagulation therapy [25]. The dose and duration of therapy will depend on the level of hemostatic challenge and the duration of time needed for wound healing. A qualified hematologist is a critical consultant for the anesthesiologist and should always be involved in the care of this complex patient population, particularly

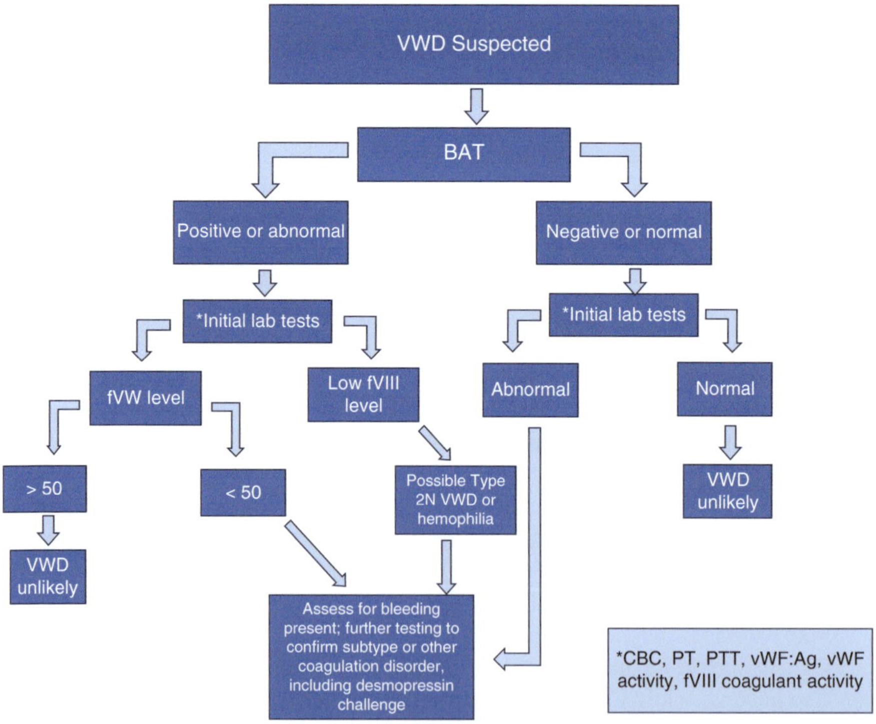

Fig. 21.1 A simplified VWD diagnostic algorithm. Consultation with a qualified hematologist should be considered at any step in the evaluation if a bleeding disorder is suspected in the perioperative period

concerning preoperative prophylaxis planning and management of acute bleeding events. Major surgery should be performed in a center with continuous access to special VWD laboratory testing and readily available factor replacement and DDAVP therapy [26]. Patients and their families should be informed of the planned medications, fluid management, and duration of therapy prior to any procedure as they are not without risk [3].

Preoperative dosing regimens vary based on the type of procedure and VWD subtype. Categories of perioperative bleeding risk include minor procedures, major procedures, and active bleeding. Normalization of vWF and fVIII activity can be achieved by [27]:

- Increasing endogenous levels of vWF using desmopressin.
- Administering recombinant vWF concentrate.
- Administering plasma-derived fVIII-vWF.

The following discussion addresses the recommended management of the above-mentioned categories of perioperative bleeding risk.

21.3.3 What Are Coagulation Factor Activity Replacement Goals for Specific Procedures During the Intraoperative Phase of Care?

21.3.3.1 Minor Surgical Procedures

Assessing Anticipated Blood Loss

It is crucial to appropriately gauge the estimated blood loss associated with a particular procedure in patients with congenital coagulopathies. One definition of "minor" blood loss is a < 2 gm/dL decrease in hemoglobin (Hgb) level or a < 2 units packed red blood cells (RBCs) or whole blood replacement requirement [28]. Two RBC units are approximately 500 mL or 10% of the estimated blood volume (EBV) of the average adult (e.g., 5 L). Extrapolated to a 15-kg child, with an EBV of 1 L (15 kg × 70 mL/kg body weight), 10% of her EBV is ~100 mL. Thus, for purposes of defining a minor (versus major) procedure in a child with VWD, an anticipated blood loss of less than 10% of the child's EBV may qualify for management under "minor" medical procedure consensus protocols. Considering the difficulty in assessing blood loss in a small child, a blood loss of 10% of total blood volume is significant and more than a "minor" blood loss. Therefore, preoperative consultation with a hematologist who is knowledgeable regarding congenital coagulopathies is essential to determine prophylaxis requirements.

Desmopressin (DDAVP)

A so-called DDAVP trial using desmopressin is indicated in VWD patients undergoing an invasive procedure to assess innate responsiveness. Desmopressin (DDAVP, 1-deamino-8-D-arginine vasopressin) is a synthetic analog of human antidiuretic hormone that promotes release of vWF from vascular endothelial cells into circulation. It should only be administered in patients with detectable levels of vWF. A "positive" DDAVP trial is a >two-fold increase in baseline vWF activity along with a 4-h sustained fVIII level > 50 IU/dL and sustained vWF levels. Because certain patient conditions may temporarily elevate a patient's vWF level (e.g., vigorous activity and estrogen therapy), the trial should be administered when the patient is at rest. Because desmopressin can lead to fluid overload, it is recommended that any patient who has received it undergo 24 h of fluid restriction. Contraindications to a DDAVP trial include:

- Children <2 years (due to reported instances of hyponatremia and seizures)
- Patients with clinically significant cardiovascular disease
- VWD type 3 (these patients are usually unresponsive to testing because they lack detectable levels of vWF)
- Type 2B VWD (associated thrombocytopenia due to increased vWF platelet binding)
- Peripartum patients with eclampsia

The National Hemophilia Foundation (NHF) recommends that the anesthesiologist caring for a patient who has received DDAVP be alerted to the potential for fluid overload [3]. In a 2016 retrospective study from Australia examining 69 children, age 2–18 years, with VWD and mild hemophilia receiving subcutaneous (SQ) DDAVP, a two-thirds maintenance fluid restriction was found to be a cutoff for avoiding hyponatremia [29]. When administered as bleeding prophylaxis, DDAVP should not be administered more frequently than once daily and no longer than 72 h because tachyphylaxis may develop as vWF and fVIII levels become depleted [30].

If a patient is a candidate for a DDAVP trial and has a positive result (i.e., the patient is responsive), bleeding prophylaxis may be initiated approximately 1 h prior to the procedure. DDAVP can be administered intravenously (0.3 μg/kg, maximum 20 mcg), intranasally (children older >2 years old, one 150-μg spray if <50 kg, and two 150-μg sprays if >50 kg), or SQ (0.3 μg/kg). The SQ form is not yet FDA-approved in the USA but is approved in Canada, Australia, and some European countries; the intranasal formulation (Stimate®) was recalled but is expected to be reapproved [28, 31]. The peak onset time is shortened using the intranasal route [32]. Dosing may be repeated within 12 h after initial dosing as clinically indicated; monitoring of serum sodium, fVW, and fVIII is recommended. Desmopressin should never be used as the sole prophylaxis agent in major surgical procedures.

Side effects of DDAVP treatment include hypotension and hypertension, flushing, headache, and in patients with coronary or cerebrovascular disease, the possibility for thrombosis.

Coagulation Factor Replacement

Preoperative prophylaxis with vWF-fVIII concentrate or recombinant vWF is required in patients undergoing a minor procedure if they have a negative DDAVP trial (e.g., vWF or fVIII levels do not increase or sustain following DDAVP administration), a contraindication to DDAVP testing, or severe VWD (i.e., type 3 and most type 2 s). Dosing for either preparation is 30–60 IU/kg, with a goal of vWF-fVIII and fVIII activity >50 IU/dL to be sustained for several days [2]. Additional doses may be administered at 50% every 12–24 h. However, recombinant vWF is not approved for children <18 years because of a lack of efficacy and safety data. The alternative in children is therefore plasma-derived vWF which contains both vWF and fVIII and is heat- and solvent-treated to prevent hepatitis, HIV, and other viral transmission. A retrospective review covering more than 30 years of experience with one vWF/fVIII plasma-derived concentrate found rare instances of inhibitor formation and allergic reactions but no evidence of viral transmission [33]. Excessive fVIII accumulation leading to thromboembolism in adults is a recognized concern [34].

Figure 21.2 illustrates a simplified decision tree for the management of VWD patients undergoing a minor procedure [2, 3, 28]. Pre-procedure prophylaxis for VWD patients undergoing major surgery typically requires coagulation factor supplementation (Fig. 21.3).

21.3.3.2 Major Surgical Procedures

A major surgical procedure for the purposes of VWD prophylaxis has been defined as the following:

- Anticipated blood loss of greater than 10–15% of a child's estimated blood volume
- Surgery in a closed compartment (e.g., spine, joint, or brain)
- Any risk of bleeding in a patient with a severe form of VWD
- Peripartum patients with a baseline vWF activity <50 IU/dL, including planned neuraxial procedures

Patients about to undergo major surgery should be pretreated with coagulation factor concentrates vWF-fVIII and fVIII to achieve a factor activity level > 50 IU/dL for 3–14 days as individualized for each patient [3]. Although DDAVP may have an adjunct role in major surgery, it should not be the primary prophylaxis with type

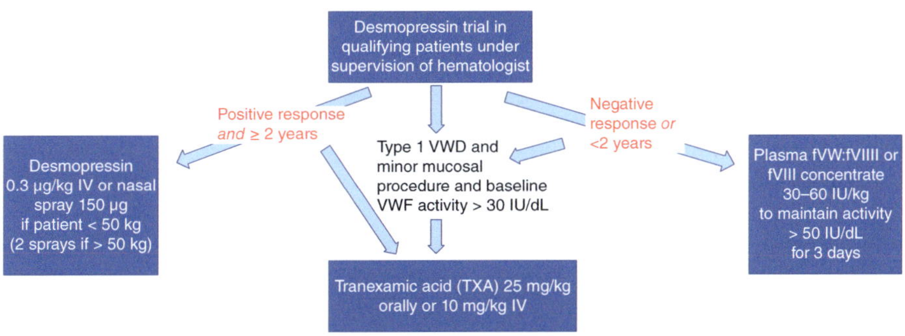

Fig. 21.2 The management of VWD patients undergoing a minor procedure including dental work

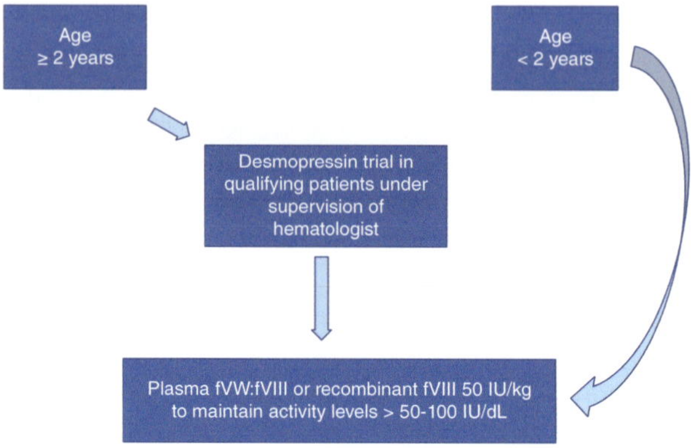

Fig. 21.3 A simplified decision tree for the management of VWD patients undergoing a major procedure

3 and severe type 1 or 2 VWD and is contraindicated in patients who are nonresponsive on a DDAVP test or have desmopressin-refractory bleeding. Furthermore, as vWF is consumed during major blood loss, fVIII will also become depleted and requires replacement as well.

Figure 21.3 illustrates a simplified decision tree for the management of VWD patients undergoing a major procedure [2, 3]:

21.3.3.3 Active or Refractory Bleeding

Persistent bleeding in a patient with VWD who has already received prophylaxis therapy is a management challenge. All refractory bleeding should be treated with plasma-based vWF-fVIII or recombinant fVIII as with a major surgical procedure. Plasma-derived vWF-fVIII or recombinant fVIII may be administered intraoperatively as necessary for ongoing bleeding to achieve factor activity levels >50 IU/dL during minor procedures if there is minimal blood loss or >100 IU/dL during major surgery if there is severe or refractory blood loss or if surgery involves a closed space (e.g., brain, eye, spinal cord). Doses may be repeated as often as every 8 h based on fVIII/ristocetin cofactor activity results or, if unavailable, fVIII activity levels. However, other steps may be necessary, including the following:

- Reevaluate initial coagulation and factor-level laboratory values, factor doses, and the working diagnosis; consider hemophilia or acquired VWD as alternative or concomitant disease.
- Administer adjuncts (see below).
- Administer platelet transfusions for clinically significant thrombocytopenia.
- Consider the presence of inhibitors requiring bypass agents (e.g., rFVIIa) or monoclonal anti-inhibitor therapy (e.g., emicizumab).

Life-saving blood transfusions should not be withheld because of delays in receiving factor concentrates or activity-level results.

Figure 21.4 illustrates a simplified decision tree for the management of VWD patients undergoing surgery who experience severe or refractory bleeding [2, 3, 34]:

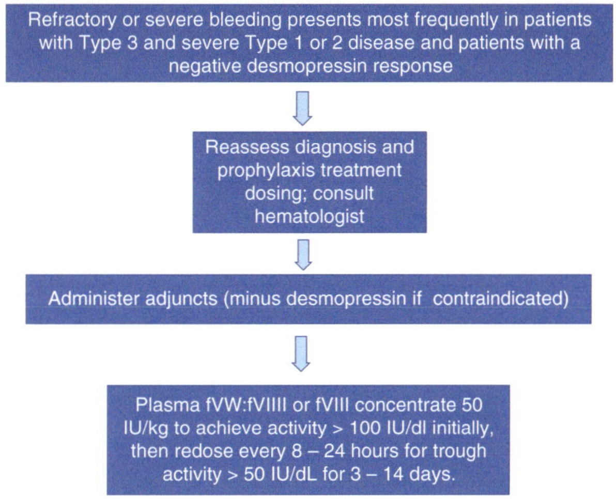

Fig. 21.4 A simplified decision tree for the management of VWD patients undergoing surgery who experience severe or refractory bleeding

Intraoperative Coagulation Monitoring

At the time of this writing, there are no specific monitoring guidelines to direct intraoperative coagulation management in patients with VWD. Conventional factor assays will not be immediately available during acute intraoperative bleeding. However, point-of-care testing often utilized during the management of intraoperative coagulopathy can be applied in patients with VWD. Rotational thromboelastometry (ROTEM) and thromboelastography (TEG) are the two common viscoelastic tests that, although not validated for VWD management, may be useful to gauge whole blood hemostasis following intraoperative factor replacement. If single-use cartridge technology is available, test results can be obtained rapidly (in real time) at the electronic workstation [35, 36]. In a sponsored study, ROTEM was used to diagnose VWD after modifying the routine test with ristocetin and a vWF/fVIII concentrate, a novel approach to emergency diagnosis and possible treatment of bleeding VWD patients [37]. The aPTT may also guide management if fVIII levels are significantly decreased, but the aPTT may remain normal in some patients [12].

21.3.4 What Adjuncts Are Available to Manage von Willebrand Disease?

21.3.4.1 Antifibrinolytics

Antifibrinolytics (tranexamic acid, TXA; epsilon aminocaproic acid, EACA) should be a preoperative adjunct in the management of all types of VWD unless contraindicated. At times, TXA may be used as the sole prophylaxis for procedures of the mucosa in type 1 VWD patients who have a baseline vWF > 30 IU/dL and only a mild bleeding history. These procedures involve surgical sites with high fibrinolytic activity, such as the oropharynx (e.g., dental procedures), the nasopharynx, and the lower genitourinary tract [27]. TXA dosing is 25 mg/kg body weight orally every

6–8 h or 10 mg/kg IV every 8 h; EACA is usually administered orally at 25–50 mg/kg every 6 h. TXA can also be applied directly as in the case of dental procedures [28]. In a retrospective review of 108 patients with type 1 VWD (median age 15.8 years), investigators examined the prophylaxis used and bleeding outcomes for a total 161 procedures [38]. There were eight (5%) bleeding complications overall, a rate consistent with prior reports in the literature. Approximately 80% received high-dose antifibrinolytic prophylaxis (usually oral TXA 15.5–27 mg/kg for 1–3 days); desmopressin was used in 10.6% of cases (usually in conjunction with an antifibrinolytic), and vWF in 7.5%. The procedure most associated with bleeding was intrauterine device (IUD) placement (5/17 procedures), considered to be "minor" bleeding. The single case of major bleeding was a tonsillectomy and adenoidectomy. No patient required a blood transfusion [38].

21.3.4.2 Topical Coagulation Agents

Other standard adjunct therapies include topically applied thrombin, collagen, and fibrin sealants, as well as TXA, as mentioned above [34].

21.3.4.3 Other Adjuncts

Platelet transfusions, monoclonal antibodies, and bypass agents may be considered in cases of serious or refractory bleeding. Secondary to concerns over transfusion-transmitted viral disease, cryoprecipitate ("antihemophilic factor") may be used as alternative to fVIII concentrate only if recombinant or pathogen-inactivated factor concentrates (e.g., pasteurized plasma-based fVW-fVIII) are unavailable [34, 39].

21.3.5 What Are Postoperative Management Concerns With the Patient Who Has von Willebrand Disease and Has Recently Undergone Surgery?

A qualified hematologist must be involved in postoperative hemostasis management, and the patient's family must be educated about signs of postoperative bleeding. Patient with VWD may require extended observation for bleeding assessment and pain management following invasive procedures. Currently, data determining optimal postoperative factor levels is lacking and there is variability in clinical practice. However, post-operative monitoring of vWF and fVIII activity levels should be performed [40]. In general, factors levels are monitored with additional factor administration to maintain vWF and fVIII activity >50 IU/dL on postoperative day 1 and a > 30 IU/dL trough thereafter for minor surgery. Following major surgery or severe bleeding episodes, early factor levels >100 IU/dL and later troughs >50 IU/dL are the goal [2, 26, 40, 41]. Suture removal, usually done 1–2 weeks after surgery, should be performed in a setting with experienced personnel, an adequate supply of replacement factors, and a consultant hematologist. Although multimodal pain management therapy may improve patient pain scores and significantly decrease overall opioid requirements, NSAIDs, antiplatelet medications, intramuscular injections, and neuraxial anesthesia should be avoided in all VWD disease without scrupulous laboratory monitoring and the immediate availability of coagulation factors [41]. Opioids are acceptable, but codeine and tramadol should not be administered to children under 12 years [42]. A medical alert bracelet or card is advised for VWD patients with a clinically symptomatic bleeding history or a positive family history in conjunction with baseline fVW (vWF) activity levels below normal [12]. The patient should be also be monitored for microcytic anemia.

21.4 Summary of Key Learning Objectives

21.4.1 How Is von Willebrand Disease Diagnosed in the Preoperative Period, Including Confirmatory Laboratory Testing?

The diagnosis of VWD begins with a personal history of abnormal bleeding or bruising, a family history of bleeding, mild thrombocytopenia, or an unexplained prolongation of partial thromboplastin time (aPTT). VWD may present with "platelet-type" excessive mucocutaneous bleeding. Epistaxis and excessive bruising are the usual presenting signs in children with VWD. Excessive menstrual bleeding is reported in over 75% of post-menarchal females. There are several bleeding assessment tools (BAT) that can be employed as initial screening tests for patients with suspected VWD. Initial laboratory tests include a CBC with platelet count and an aPTT. Further testing should be done in consultation with a hematologist. A normal level of fVW is 50–150 IU/dL (0.5–1.5 IU/mL).

In this case, the 5-year-old patient has a bleeding history (recurrent epistaxis) with a score of 3 on the ISTH-SSC bleeding assessment tool, indicating that she may have a yet undiagnosed bleeding diathesis. An elevated aPTT will support that clinical suspicion. A hematologist, ideally one specializing in congenital coagulopathies, should be consulted. Further testing prior to any invasive procedure is warranted to rule out VWD or hemophilia.

21.4.2 How Is von Willebrand Disease Bleeding Prophylaxis Managed in the Preoperative Period?

ASH/ISTH/NHF/WFH guidelines provide specific recommendation for perioperative treatment of patient with VWD undergoing minor procedures. Laparoscopic appendectomy, generally considered a minor procedure because expected blood loss is "minimal," should be performed in a center staffed with trained personnel and an adequate supply of replacement factors. A hematologist experienced in managing congenital coagulopathies should be consulted in all cases of children with VWD before surgery.

Type 1 VWD patients ≥2 years old who are responsive on DDAVP testing may be managed with desmopressin alone before and during some minor invasive procedures. Many type 1 VWD patients undergoing dental work may be managed preoperatively with TXA therapy alone. All children with VWD < 2 years old and those patients who are severely affected will require factor replacement several hours prior to surgery. Adjunctive therapy, including TXA, platelets, and recombinant fVII, should be immediately available in the event there is refractory or extensive surgical bleeding.

21.4.3 What Are Coagulation Factor Activity Replacement Goals for Specific Procedures during the Intraoperative Phase of Care?

A normal level of vWF is 50–150 IU/dL (0.5–1.5 IU/mL). Plasma-derived vWF-fVIII or recombinant fVIII may be administered intraoperatively as necessary for ongoing bleeding to achieve factor activity levels >50–100 IU/dL. Doses may be repeated as often as every 8 h based on fVIII/ristocetin cofactor activity results or, if unavailable, fVIII activity levels. Because factor-level results are likely to be delayed, viscoelastic and aPTT values may be followed because they are more likely to be immediately available. However, they are not yet validated to monitor factor replacement during active bleeding in VWD patients.

21.4.4 What Adjuncts Are Available to Manage von Willebrand Disease?

- Desmopressin (DDAVP) in patients ≥2 years and select cases
- Antifibrinolytics (i.e., TXA, EACA)
- Topical agents (e.g., thrombin, collagen, TXA)
- Platelets
- If inhibitor antibodies are detected, monoclonal antibody or bypass agents (e.g., fVII)
- Cryoprecipitate is discouraged unless bleeding is severe and recombinant factors are unavailable.

21.4.5 What Are Postoperative Management Concerns with the Patient Who Has von Willebrand Disease and Has Recently Undergone Surgery?

Factor monitoring and administration may continue for several days to weeks when a patient with VWD has undergone surgery. The family must be educated about signs of excessive bleeding and early treatment options. The child with VWD is more likely to present with secondary bleeding which can be insidious and go undetected. Suture removal should be performed in a setting with experienced personnel, an adequate supply of replacement factors, and a consultant hematologist. As with any child with a coagulopathy, intramuscular injections should be avoided, as well as antiplatelet medications and NSAIDs. Opioids are acceptable, but codeine and tramadol should not be administered to children under 12 years [US FDA 2018]. The patient should be also be monitored for microcytic anemia.

Key Points

- VWD is the most common inherited bleeding disorder.
- Most patients with VWD are asymptomatic. For that reason, a personal and family history of bleeding may be the only key to preoperative diagnosis and prevention of excessive perioperative bleeding.
- Perioperative management of patients with VWD requires a multidisciplinary team approach. If specialized testing and medications are required, procedures in patients with VWD should be performed within reach of a Hemophilia Treatment Center (HTC).
- Pharmacologic prophylaxis for VWD consists of increasing endogenous levels of vWF with desmopressin (DDAVP), administering recombinant fVW concentrate, or administering plasma-derived fVIII-vWF concentrate, along with adjuncts including topical agents. Patients with stable type 1 VWD undergoing a minor procedure are sometimes managed with DDAVP alone.
- DDAVP is contraindicated in children <2 years, and administration should be accompanied by careful serum sodium monitoring and possibly fluid restriction.
- Acute bleeding episodes treated with coagulation factors may be monitored using viscoelastic testing of whole blood or conventional aPTT because factor-level results may be delayed or unavailable.

References

1. Rodeghiero F, Castaman G, Dini E. Epidemiological investigation of the prevalence of von Willebrand's disease. Blood. 1987;69(2):454–9.
2. Leebeek FWG, Eikenboom JCJ. Von Willebrand's disease. N Engl J Med. 2017;376(7):701–2.
3. MASAC Document 266—MASAC recommendations regarding the treatment of von Willebrand disease. 2021. https://www.hemophilia.org/healthcare-professionals/guidelines-on-care/masac-documents/masac-document-266-masac-recommendations-regarding-the-treatment-of-von-willebrand-disease. Accessed 10 Aug 2023.
4. Goodeve AC. The genetic basis of von Willebrand disease. Blood Rev. 2010;24(3):123–34.
5. Miller CH, Philipp CS, Stein SF, Kouides PA, Lukes AS, Heit JA, et al. The spectrum of haemostatic characteristics of women with unexplained menorrhagia. Haemophilia. 2011;17(1):e223–9.
6. James PD, Connell NT, Ameer B, Di Paola J, Eikenboom J, Giraud N, et al. ASH ISTH NHF WFH 2021 guidelines on the diagnosis of von Willebrand disease. Blood Adv. 2021;5(1):280–300.
7. Hemophilia Treatment Centers (HTCs). Centers for Disease Control and Prevention. 2022. https://www.cdc.gov/ncbddd/hemophilia/htc.html. Accessed 10 Aug 2023.
8. Hermans C, Noone D, Benson G, Dolan G, Eichler H, Jimenez-Yuste V, et al. Hemophilia treatment in 2021: choosing the "optimal" treatment using an integrative, patient-oriented approach to shared decision-making between patients and clinicians. Blood Rev. 2022;52:100890.

9. Sadler JE, Mannucci PM, Berntorp E, Bochkov N, Boulyjenkov V, Ginsburg D, et al. Impact, diagnosis and treatment of von Willebrand disease. Thromb Haemost. 2000;84(2):160–74.
10. Sanders YV, Groeneveld D, Meijer K, Fijnvandraat K, Cnossen MH, van der Bom JG, et al. von Willebrand factor propeptide and the phenotypic classification of von Willebrand disease. Blood. 2015;125(19):3006–13.
11. Weyand AC, Flood VH. Von Willebrand disease: current status of diagnosis and management. Hematol Oncol Clin North Am. 2021;35(6):1085–101.
12. James P. Clinical presentation and diagnosis of von Willebrand disease. UpToDate. 2022; www.uptodate.com. Accessed 8 Aug 2023
13. de Wee EM, Sanders YV, Mauser-Bunschoten EP, van der Bom JG, Degenaar-Dujardin ME, Eikenboom J, et al. Determinants of bleeding phenotype in adult patients with moderate or severe von Willebrand disease. Thromb Haemost. 2012;108(4):683–92.
14. Sadler JE, Budde U, Eikenboom JC, Favaloro EJ, Hill FG, Holmberg L, et al. Update on the pathophysiology and classification of von Willebrand disease: a report of the Subcommittee on von Willebrand Factor. J Thromb Haemost. 2006;4(10):2103–14.
15. van Galen KP, Mauser-Bunschoten EP, Leebeek FW. Hemophilic arthropathy in patients with von Willebrand disease. Blood Rev. 2012;26(6):261–6.
16. Cuker A, Connors JM, Katz JT, Levy BD, Loscalzo J, Clinical problem-solving. A bloody mystery. N Engl J Med. 2009;361(19):1887–94.
17. Swami A, Kaur V. von Willebrand disease: a concise review and update for the practicing physician. Clin Appl Thromb Hemost. 2017;23(8):900–10.
18. ISTH-SSC bleeding assessment tool. International Society on Thrombosis and Haemostasis. 2011. https://bleedingscore.certe.nl/. Accessed 7 Aug 2023.
19. Elbatarny M, Mollah S, Grabell J, Bae S, Deforest M, Tuttle A, et al. Normal range of bleeding scores for the ISTH-BAT: adult and pediatric data from the merging project. Haemophilia. 2014;20(6):831–5.
20. Mittal N, Naridze R, James P, Shott S, Valentino LA. Utility of a paediatric bleeding questionnaire as a screening tool for von Willebrand disease in apparently healthy children. Haemophilia. 2015;21(6):806–11.
21. Levy E, Kuperman A, Sela E, Kashkoush A, Miari AD, Hana RY, et al. Utility of the pediatric bleeding questionnaire in predicting Posttonsillectomy bleeding. Otolaryngol Head Neck Surg. 2022;167(3):576–82.
22. Bowman M, Riddel J, Rand ML, Tosetto A, Silva M, James PD. Evaluation of the diagnostic utility for von Willebrand disease of a pediatric bleeding questionnaire. J Thromb Haemost. 2009;7(8):1418–21.
23. Rydz N, James PD. The evolution and value of bleeding assessment tools. J Thromb Haemost. 2012;10(11):2223–9.
24. Federici AB, Bucciarelli P, Castaman G, Mazzucconi MG, Morfini M, Rocino A, et al. The bleeding score predicts clinical outcomes and replacement therapy in adults with von Willebrand disease. Blood. 2014;123(26):4037–44.
25. Miesbach W, Berntorp E. Von Willebrand disease—the 'Dos' and 'Don'ts' in surgery. Eur J Haematol. 2017;98(2):121–7.
26. Nichols WL, Hultin MB, James AH, Manco-Johnson MJ, Montgomery RR, Ortel TL, et al. von Willebrand disease (VWD): evidence-based diagnosis and management guidelines, the National Heart, Lung, and Blood Institute (NHLBI) Expert Panel report (USA). Haemophilia. 2008;14(2):171–232.
27. Connell NT, Flood VH, Brignardello-Petersen R, Abdul-Kadir R, Arapshian A, Couper S, et al. ASH ISTH NHF WFH 2021 guidelines on the management of von Willebrand disease. Blood Adv. 2021;5(1):301–25.
28. James P. von Willebrand disease (VWD): treatment of minor bleeding, use of DDAVP, and routine preventative care. UpToDate. 2023. www.uptodate.com. Accessed 8 Aug 2023.
29. Mason JA, Robertson JD, McCosker J, Williams BA, Brown SA. Assessment and validation of a defined fluid restriction protocol in the use of subcutaneous desmopressin for children with inherited bleeding disorders. Haemophilia. 2016;22(5):700–5.

30. Klaassen RJ, Halton JM. The diagnosis and treatment of von Willebrand disease in children. Paediatr Child Health. 2002;7(4):245–9.
31. Stimate recall update. National Hemophilia Foundation 2020. https://www.hemophilia.org/news/stimate-recall-update. Accessed 8 Aug 2023.
32. Lethagen S, Harris AS, Sjorin E, Nilsson IM. Intranasal and intravenous administration of desmopressin: effect on F VIII/vWF, pharmacokinetics and reproducibility. Thromb Haemost. 1987;58(4):1033–6.
33. Kouides P, Wawra-Hehenberger K, Sajan A, Mead H, Simon T. Safety of a pasteurized plasma-derived factor VIII and von Willebrand factor concentrate: analysis of 33 years of pharmacovigilance data. Transfusion. 2017;57(10):2390–403.
34. James P. von Willebrand disease (VWD): treatment of major bleeding and major surgery. UpToDate. 2022; www.uptodate.com. Accessed 8 Mar 2023
35. Nogami K. The utility of thromboelastography in inherited and acquired bleeding disorders. Br J Haematol. 2016;174(4):503–14.
36. Tripodi A, Santoro RC, Testa S, Molinari AC, Bernardini S, Golato M, et al. Position paper on laboratory testing for patients with haemophilia. A consensus document from SISET, AICE, SIBioC and SIPMeL. Blood Transfus. 2019;17(3):229–36.
37. Topf HG, Strasser ER, Breuer G, Rascher W, Rauh M, Fahlbusch FB. Closing the gap—detection of clinically relevant von Willebrand disease in emergency settings through an improved algorithm based on rotational thromboelastometry. BMC Anesthesiol. 2019;19(1):10.
38. Heery S, Zimowski K, Mason SF, White MH, DiGiandomenico S, Trotter C, et al. Procedural outcomes in children with mild type 1 von Willebrand disease. Res Pract Thromb Haemost. 2024;8(1):102334.
39. World Health Organization. Guidance on increasing supplies of plasma-derived medicinal products in low- and middle-income countries through fractionation of domestic plasma. 2021. https://apps.who.int/iris/handle/10665/340171. Accessed 8 Aug 2023.
40. O'Donnell JS, Lavin M. Perioperative management of patients with von Willebrand disease. Hematology Am Soc Hematol Educ Program. 2019;2019(1):604–9.
41. Laffan MA, Lester W, O'Donnell JS, Will A, Tait RC, Goodeve A, et al. The diagnosis and management of von Willebrand disease: a United Kingdom Haemophilia Centre Doctors Organization guideline approved by the British Committee for Standards in Haematology. Br J Haematol. 2014;167(4):453–65.
42. US Food & Drug Administration (FDA). FDA restricts use of prescription codeine pain and cough medicines and tramadol pain medicines in children; recommends against use in breastfeeding women. In: FDA Drug Safety Communication. 2018. https://www.fda.gov/drugs/drug-safety-and-availability/fda-drug-safety-communication-fda-restricts-use-prescription-codeine-pain-and-cough-medicines-and. Accessed 13 Mar 2023.

Hemophilia

22

Liliya Pospishil, Jennie Ngai, and Norma J. Klein

22.1 Case Scenario

A 6-month-old boy with no past medical history presents for elective circumcision. His growth is average, and he weighs 8 kg. The parents report a family history of hemophilia B. The surgery proceeds without complication; however, the patient appears to have continuous bleeding at the incision site while in the recovery room.

Key Learning Objectives

- How is hemophilia diagnosed in the preoperative period?
- How is bleeding prophylaxis managed in hemophilia patients undergoing elective invasive procedures?
- What are coagulation factor replacement dosing goals for hemophilia patients undergoing invasive procedures?
- What adjuncts are available to treat acute hemophilia-related bleeding when coagulation factor replacement is unavailable or inadequate?
- What are some anesthesia-related postoperative management concerns in a child with hemophilia?

L. Pospishil (✉) · J. Ngai
Department of Anesthesiology, Perioperative Care, and Pain Medicine, NYU Grossman School of Medicine, New York, NY, USA
e-mail: liliya.pospishil@nyulangone.org; jennie.ngai@nyulangone.org

N. J. Klein
Department of Anesthesiology and Pain Medicine, University of California, Davis, Sacramento, CA, USA
e-mail: nklein@ucdavis.edu

N. J. Klein (ed.), *Perioperative Pediatric Patient Blood Management and Transfusion Safety*, https://doi.org/10.1007/978-3-031-81666-6_22

22.2 Discussion

22.2.1 General Considerations

Hemophilia is a rare congenital coagulation disorder resulting from decreased quantity or activity of procoagulation factors. Preservation of the patient's blood volume requires careful management in the preoperative period, with timely and evidence-based treatment of bleeding episodes. This discussion will focus on preoperative hemophilia diagnosis, hemorrhage mitigation tools for elective procedures, and management of acute bleeding episodes in children with hemophilia A and B.

The two most common hemophilia are type A (factor VIII (FVIII) deficiency, classic hemophilia, 80–85% of cases) and type B (factor IX (FIX) deficiency, Christmas disease, 15–20% of cases) [1]. Hemophilia types A and B are X-linked, affecting 1:5000 and 1:30,000 males, respectively [2]. Acquired hemophilia A (AHA) involves the development of inhibitory FVIII antibodies in critically ill patients. AHA is rarely reported in children, and diagnosis is often delayed by months [3, 4]. Hemophilia C, the fourth most common type of congenital coagulopathy after hemophilia A and B and von Willebrand disease (VWD), is a nonsex-linked disorder affecting males and females equally [5]. New, spontaneous mutations can lead to variants in up to one-third of cases of hemophilia A; more than one-half of cases report a negative family history [6–8]. Carrier females are sometimes affected; therefore, clotting factor activity should be evaluated in these patients before surgery [9]. Females may also be affected when both X chromosomes are involved (i.e., homozygosity) or when one chromosome is inactive (e.g., Turner syndrome, X chromosomal mosaicism). It is important to recognize that hemophilia prevalence rates vary by country, especially if one is providing healthcare in an underserved region. For instance, the rate of identified hemophilia patients compared to the predicted rate in Africa is only 9%, in Southeast Asia 17%, and in Europe 80% [10]. The disparate diagnostic rates are thought to result from a shortage of specialty laboratories and facilities, as well as reduced awareness.

Hemophilia severity is classified as mild, moderate, or severe based on the baseline level of clotting factor activity (Table 22.1) [8]. Approximately 70% of cases fall into the severe category or factor activity <1% of normal [2]. Although hemostasis requires only a 30–40% clotting factor level, normal levels are age-related and

Table 22.1 Hemophilia severity scale and associated factor levels and activities

Coagulation factor level	Hemophilia severity	Clinical presentation
5–40% IU/dL (5–40% of normal activity)	Mild	Severe bleeding with major surgery, rare spontaneous bleeds
1–5% IU/dL (1–5% of normal activity)	Moderate	Persistent bleeding with minor surgery, infrequent spontaneous bleeds
<1–5% IU/dL (<1% of normal activity)	Severe	Hemarthrosis, bleeding despite no evidence of injury

Adapted from Srivastava et al. [8]. Table 2.1, p. 22

range from 50% to 150% or 0.5–1.5 international unit per deciliter (IU/dL) [11]. Based on that nomenclature, 1 milliliter (mL) of normal plasma contains 1 IU and 100% of any factor activity.

The median age of hemophilia diagnosis is 10 months, around the age when most infants become ambulatory, usually following a joint bleed [2, 12]. However, most severely affected infants (70%) are diagnosed within 1 month [13]. Infants with severe forms of the disease are at risk of spontaneous intracranial, oral, and postoperative bleeding. Up to 50% of male infants with severe hemophilia have excessive bleeding with circumcision [12]. For this reason, many hematologists will not recommend circumcision absent a urologic indication. Because of the unpredictable nature of the severe form of hemophilia, life-threatening bleeding into soft tissues, muscles, and the mouth, and bleeding associated with medical procedures (including central venipuncture), may be overlooked. Bleeding into the iliopsoas muscle (leading to unrecognized blood loss) and the retropharyngeal space (leading to airway compromise) have been reported [14, 15]. Mild and moderate forms of hemophilia are typically not diagnosed until 8–36 months, concomitant with unexplained bleeding following physical trauma and surgery [13].

Management of the hemophilia patient undergoing surgery requires a multidisciplinary team approach and evidence-based care to preserve red blood cell (RBC) mass. Care coordination between anesthesiology, surgery, hematology, pharmacy, laboratory services, blood bank, nursing, and social work is essential to prepare the patient for surgery and respond promptly to bleeding episodes. The US Centers for Disease Control (CDC) reports a 40% improvement in mortality and hospitalization rates for patients managed through centralized hemophilia treatment centers (HTCs) [16]. An online database of these centers by US region is available through the CDC [17]. In the interest of safety, the anesthetic plan must accommodate a preoperative coagulation factor replacement schedule. Coagulation management can take hours to days if coagulation factor testing is required; this schedule is typically directed through the patient's primary care provider or a hematology specialist. Infants and older patients with a severe form of hemophilia are best managed in a hospital (versus a freestanding outpatient center) where extended postoperative observation is possible. Ideally, the operating room has point-of-care (POC) coagulation testing capability. When children with severe disease undergo a major surgical procedure, inpatient postoperative management may require days of coagulation monitoring and factor replacement. Recombinant coagulation factors, anti-inhibitor drugs, and blood products must be readily available through the blood bank and pharmacy.

The World Federation of Hemophilia (WFH), an international, nonprofit consortium, and the National Hemophilia Foundation (NHF), based in the United States, have published best practice guidelines on hemophilia care, including perioperative management [8, 18–20]. Although there are no standardized management guidelines addressing pediatric perioperative care, the WFH recommends that anesthesiologists caring for hemophilia patients be experienced in managing this unique patient population.

22.2.2 How Is Hemophilia Diagnosed in the Preoperative Period?

A hemophilia diagnosis requires examination of clinical history and presentation, coagulation screening tests, and confirmatory factor assays.

22.2.2.1 Clinical Features

The most crucial preoperative preparation tool is the patient history [2]. A preoperative history suggestive of hemophilia includes unexplained bleeding, any family history of excessive bruising, or transfusions. Bleeding questionnaires have been developed to evaluate congenital coagulopathies. However, none are validated for children with hemophilia [21]. A sample questionnaire focused on diagnosing von Willebrand disease (VWD), the Pediatric Bleeding Questionnaire (PBQ), is a 13-point tool that may provide screening guidance [22]. It includes questions including but not limited to nosebleeds, cephalohematomas, bleeding with venipuncture, and postoperative bleeding. A positive score should prompt coagulation testing [23, 24]. If all questionnaire elements are answered in the negative, no further testing is indicated unless a congenital coagulopathy is strongly suspected (i.e., a positive family history).

22.2.2.2 Screening Tests

Initial screening tests for suspected congenital coagulopathy include a platelet count, prothrombin time (PT), and an activated partial thromboplastin time (aPTT). The aPTT is usually prolonged in hemophilia, while other screening coagulation tests are normal. However, a normal test result does not exclude the possibility of a clinically relevant bleeding disorder; the aPTT may be normal in mild hemophilia until factor level is <30% [8]. If there is a family history of bleeding or a personal account of unexplained bleeding based on initial screening, FVIII and FIX levels, a thrombin time, von Willebrand factor (VWF), and possibly platelet function studies should be considered [9]. Figure 22.1 illustrates a diagnostic algorithm based on initial aPTT screening when there is high clinical suspicion of a congenital coagulation disorder.

Based on initial screening, specific factor assays are performed when a congenital factor deficiency is suspected. Coagulation factor testing may be very nuanced; for example, it is recommended that a patient does not exercise before testing, which may falsely elevate FVIII levels [8, 25]. Results may vary based on the laboratory technique used, and factor levels or activity in individual patients do not always predict clinical outcomes [26]. In neonates, FVIII levels are detectable. However, FIX levels may not be detectable despite an absence of disease and should be re-evaluated at 3–6 months [8].

All patients diagnosed with hemophilia should undergo "inhibitor" antibody testing before surgery [8]. Inhibitor testing includes a "mixing study" whereby the patient's plasma is mixed with normal plasma. The PT or aPTT of the mixture should normalize. However, if the PT or aPTT does not normalize upon mixing, a clotting "inhibitor" may be present. A false-positive mixing study may occur in the presence of a lupus anticoagulant or heparin contamination from an intravenous

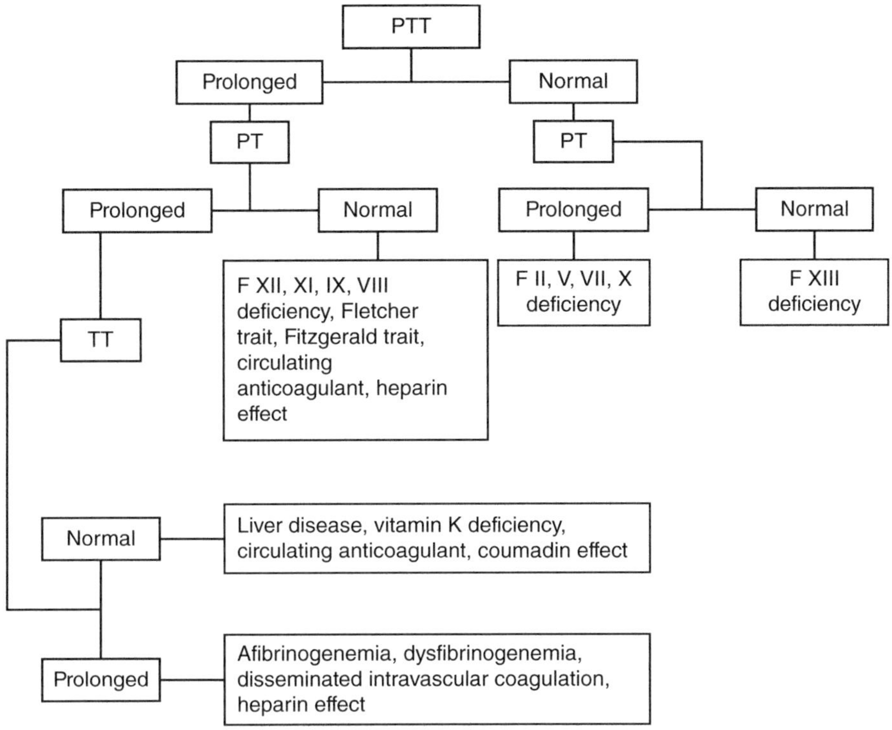

Fig. 22.1 Diagnostic tests for a suspected coagulation disorder. (Reprinted with permission from Lanzkowsky et al. [2]. Fig. 13.6, p. 297)

(IV) line. Mixing results are expressed as a Bethesda unit (BU) titer, and patients are classified as a high-titer (≥5 BUs) or a low-titer (<5 BU) "responders." The magnitude of titer response correlates with the amount of factor-neutralizing antibody the patient forms upon exposure to recombinant FVIII (rFVIII). FVIII inhibitors are associated with high morbidity and mortality. Approximately one-third of hemophilia patients develop inhibitors; those at highest risk include African-Americans, Hispanics, and those with exposure to recombinant FVIII (versus plasma-derived), rFVIII therapy early in life, and a sibling that forms inhibitors [2, 27, 28]. High responders require different treatment during acute bleeding episodes than low responders.

Prenatal diagnosis through fetal umbilical cord sampling is possible at 18–20 weeks of gestation [2]. Factors VIII and IX do not cross the maternal-fetal placental barrier [9]. If congenital fetal hemophilia is suspected, procedures that may provoke bleeding should be avoided, including scalp electrode placement and instrumental delivery (e.g., forceps or vacuum-assisted). The WFH recommends that all male newborns of mothers who are known carriers undergo both aPTT and factor testing at birth [8].

22.2.3 How Is Bleeding Prophylaxis Managed in Hemophilia Patients Undergoing Elective Invasive Procedures?

The main goal of perioperative hemophilia management is personalized optimization of FVIII and FIX activity levels in the preoperative period, during active bleeding, and during the postoperative healing phase. In the past, children with hemophilia were treated with allogeneic blood products, leading to an epidemic of acquired immune deficiency syndrome (AIDS) in that patient population [29]. Today, clotting factor concentrates are available, derived from either virally inactivated plasma products or recombinant technology, which have substantially improved the quality of life for these patients. Currently marketed plasma-derived and recombinant FVIII products can be found through the *WFH Online Registry of Clotting Factor Concentrates*, and many formulations have US Food and Drug Administration (FDA) approval [2, 8].

A qualified hematologist is a critical consultant for the anesthesiologist and should always be involved in the care of this complex patient population, particularly concerning preoperative prophylaxis planning and management of acute perioperative bleeding. Preoperative dosing regimens may vary based on the type of procedure (minor versus major) and the type of hemophilia and if the patient has inhibitor antibodies. To date, there are no randomized trials comparing appropriate target factor levels in children [30, 31]. Often, the family will have information about the patient's disease severity and baseline factor level and may even carry a copy of current treatment guidelines and a vial of factor concentrate for emergencies [19].

Recommendations and practices regarding circumcision vary, based on clinical practices and the specific procedure. A 2015 survey of US pediatric hematologists ($n = 64/159$, response rate 40%) affiliated with HTCs documented notable variations in guidelines and management approaches [30]. The risks of bleeding and inhibitor development related to early receipt of coagulation factor were cited as major concerns. One-third of respondents would not condone circumcision until the neonate was older. A small percentage (3%) would not allow the procedure unless there was a urologic indication. Another one-third would seek an opportunity to "batch" the procedure with another planned operation that required factor prophylaxis. More than one-third would allow the neonatal circumcision to proceed. The number of prophylactic factor doses varied significantly, with respondents citing one dose in the preoperative period and one-third would prescribe ≥2 doses. The desired target factor level ranged from 75% to 100% activity. One-third would use antifibrinolytic therapy, but other respondents proposed additional adjuncts including topical thrombin, fibrin glue, and wound sealant.

22.2.4 What Are Coagulation Factor Replacement Dosing Goals for Hemophilia Patients Undergoing Invasive Procedures?

22.2.4.1 Preoperative Phase of Care

Minor Surgery, Minor Procedures, and Major Surgery

The WHF defines a "major" surgery as one that requires monitoring and treatment for bleeding during the first five postoperative days [8]. Before major surgery, hemophilia A and B patients should be treated to increase their plasma factor levels 80–100 IU/dL, with a goal of >60 IU/dL during the first several postoperative days, followed by >30 IU/dL for another 1–2 weeks [8, 11].

Before minor surgery, the WHF recommends factor levels >30 IU/dL, with monitoring for at least 3 postoperative days. An exception is a recommendation that hemophilia patients have an activity level >80 IU/dL before circumcision [8]. In a case series of 18 boys with hemophilia A and B (mean age 3.9 years) undergoing central venous access for implanted port placement, 19.2% bled at the pocket site, necessitating extended coagulation monitoring into the post-placement period [32]. All patients received pre-procedure prophylaxis to factor levels of 100% and then >50% for 2 days and >25% for another 3 days. Early port access was not associated with post-procedure bleeding. The investigators did not report patient factor levels and bleeding rates at the time of catheter removal [32].

The NHF recommends increasing factor levels to 100 IU/dL before all invasive procedures [19].

The following sections discuss preoperative prophylaxis based on the type of hemophilia and the presence or absence of inhibitor antibodies.

Hemophilia A Patients with No Inhibitors

Patients with mild hemophilia A and no inhibitors may be managed with intermittent doses of desmopressin (DDAVP, 1-deamino-8-D-arginine vasopressin), which increases both FVIII and VWF levels severalfold [11]. Hemophilia patients undergoing *minor procedures*, such as arterial puncture, lumbar puncture, and endoscopy, should undergo a pre-procedure DDAVP trial to evaluate patient responsiveness [19]. Confirmatory factor levels should be drawn approximately 90 min after dosing [8]. DDAVP may supplant FVIII replacement in responders with mild or moderate forms of hemophilia; however, rFVIII should be administered in all cases of anticipated or actual severe bleeding. DDAVP should not be used in hemophilia B patients because FIX—unlike FVIII—is not in complex with VWF and platelets.

Hemophilia B Patients with No Inhibitors

Before an invasive procedure, hemophilia B patients who do not have inhibitor antibodies are likely to be on recombinant factor IX (rFIX) replacement. A recommended pre-procedure dose of rFIX is 100–140 μg/kg (Table 22.2) [19].

Table 22.2 Perioperative hemophilia factor intravenous dosing in the perioperative period to achieve factor activity 80–100% of normal. Factor activity should not be less than 50% during active bleeding. "μ" denotes units. aPCC is activated prothrombin complex concentrate

Type of hemophilia versus type of procedure	Hemophilia A	Hemophilia B	Hemophilia A with inhibitors	Hemophilia B with inhibitors, no allergy	Hemophilia B with inhibitors and known allergic sensitization
Minor procedure Major procedure	DDAVD after trial rFVIII 50 μ/kg	rFIX 100–140 μ/kg	Low responder: rFVIII 50 μ/kg	rFIX 100–140 μ/kg	aFVII 90 μ/kg and then aPCC 75–100 μ/kg
Continued bleeding	aFVIII 50 μ/kg, then aFVII 90 μ/kg, and aPCC 75–100 μ/kg	rFIX 100–140 μ/kg, then aFVII 90 μ/kg, and aPCC 75–100 μ/kg	High responder: aFVII 90 μ/kg and then aPCC 75–100 μ/kg	rFIX 100–140 μ/kg, then aFVII 90 μ/kg, and aPCC 75–100 μ/kg	

Post-prophylaxis Factor Evaluation

Following the initial factor bolus, additional factor-level monitoring and replacement will be required at intervals corresponding to drug half-lives (every 8–12 h for rFVIII and every 12–24 h for rFIX). Peak blood levels are measured approximately 15 min after infusion [9]. As with many medications, children may require more frequent dosing than adults (every 6 h versus 12 h) due to shorter coagulation factor half-lives [33]. Since VWF is a carrier of FVIII in a "VWF/FVIII complex," the half-life of FVIII is affected by VWF levels and activity. Advances in biochemical engineering have enabled newer formulations of FVIII with an extended half-life (up to 21 h) [34]. Newer extended FIX formulations may have a half-life of up to 118 h. Some formulations also contain VWD factor [34]. Standards for patient monitoring and technical laboratory requirements for these new formulations are in the early stages of development [26].

Patients with Inhibitor Antibodies

The development of factor inhibitors (e.g., neutralizing antibodies) is the most serious complication of hemophilia treatment. Preprocedural management of hemophilia patients with inhibitors should always be done in consultation with a hematology specialist. Inhibitors are specific IgG antibodies against exogenous FVIII and FIX that effectively neutralize the function of infused coagulation factors. Inhibitor development occurs more often with hemophilia A (20–35% of patients) than with hemophilia B (5% of patients) [35, 36]. However, allergic reactions occur in 50% of hemophilia B patients who develop rFIX inhibitors [8].

Patients with inhibitor antibodies may require larger or more frequent doses of factor replacement and, in the event of bleeding, the addition of "bypass agents." Bypass agents use the extrinsic coagulation pathway to generate thrombin, thereby avoiding the need for FVIII or FIX to ultimately produce a fibrin clot (Fig. 22.2).

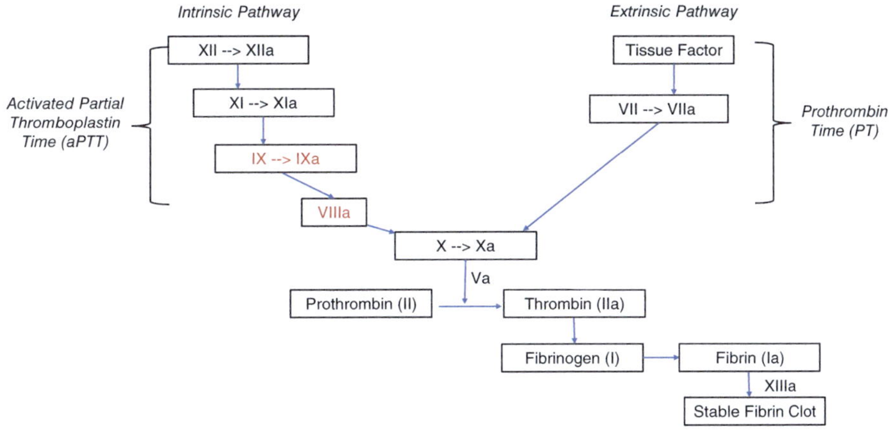

Fig. 22.2 The coagulation cascade

Currently, only two available bypass agents are used in hemophilia bleeding prophylaxis and treatment: recombinant activated factor VII (rFVIIa) and activated prothrombin complex concentrate (aPCC). The preprocedural management of patients with inhibitor antibodies can be complicated and should be done in conjunction a qualified hematologist.

Hemophilia A Patients with Inhibitor Antibodies

Hemophilia A patients may present for surgery treated with emicizumab, an anti-inhibitor monoclonal antibody approved for bleeding prophylaxis in hemophilia A patients with and without inhibitors. Emicizumab is a mimic for FVIII and acts through binding FIX and FX, allowing progression through the common coagulation pathway to thrombin formation (Fig. 22.3) [2, 37]. It has a long half-life (~30 days) and is administered via subcutaneous injection on a weekly to monthly basis. Emicizumab prevents bleeding in patients with hemophilia A but is not indicated to treat either acute bleeding or hemophilia B. The WFH advises closely observing emicizumab patients for thrombotic complications, including myocardial infarction and pulmonary embolism [8].

Hemophilia A patients taking emicizumab as anti-inhibitor therapy may not require factor replacement during *minor* surgery but will likely need FVIII replacement for *major* surgery. Perioperative inhibitor management for low-responder hemophilia A patients (e.g., <5 BUs) treated with emicizumab undergoing *minor* surgery is treated differently than high responders. Low responders on emicizumab may not require preoperative rFVIII replacement. However, rFVIII may be given before surgery out of an abundance of caution and in higher doses at more frequent intervals. The recommended rFVIII dose in those cases is the same as for patients not on emicizumab (i.e., 50 μg/kg) (Table 22.2) [8, 19].

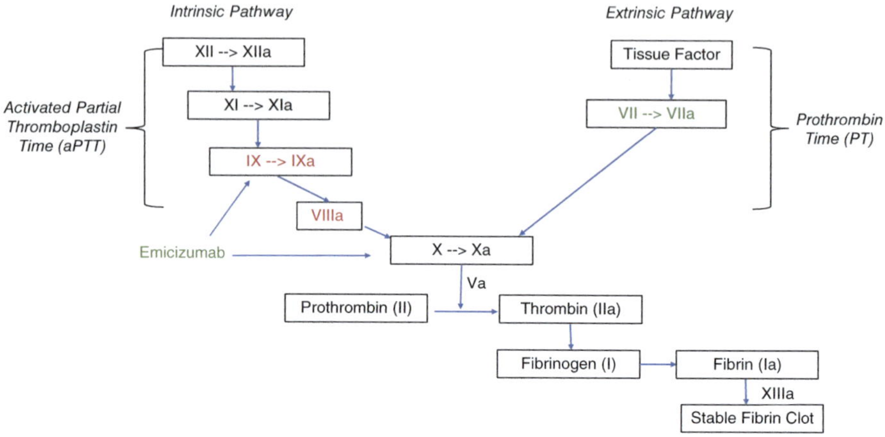

Fig. 22.3 The coagulation cascade and the anti-inhibitor antibody, emicizumab, binding FIX and FX in patients with hemophilia inhibitor antibodies, allowing progression to thrombin formation

High responders on emicizumab (e.g., ≥5.0 BUs) may be treated with either aPCC or rVII before a minor or major surgery, monitoring for thromboembolism [19].

Hemophilia B Patients with Inhibitor Antibodies

The preoperative factor planning for hemophilia B patients with inhibitors undergoing surgery is more complicated than for hemophilia A patients. Although hemophilia B patients develop factor inhibitors significantly less often than hemophilia A patients, those that do so have a high risk of developing an allergy to rFIX. When hemophilia B patients undergo *minor or major* surgery, their FIX activity levels should be maximized to peak factor levels (>80 IU/dL). However, if a hemophilia B patient has a known FIX allergy, a bypassing agent is recommended for perioperative bleeding, with aFVII preferred over aPCC (Table 22.2) [19]. FVII is preferred as a bypass agent in hemophilia B because aPCC contains FIX which may lead to allergic sensitization, as well as an increased risk of thrombosis, due to an excess of the other factors included in the product (e.g., II, VII, and X) [8].

Preoperative Factor Prophylaxis Dosing

Despite the complexity of factor-level targets before surgery, appropriate factor prophylaxis dosing, and treatment of active bleeding, hemophilia factor dosing is ultimately is based on multiple factors [9, 31]:

- Patient weight
- Patient baseline factor level
- Desired factor level for a particular procedure
- Patient volume of distribution (VD)
- The VD of the brand of recombinant factor (0.5–1.6)
- Presence of inhibitor antibodies

Factor IX Dosing

Assuming that a 6-month, 8-kg infant with hemophilia B and no inhibitor antibodies is about to undergo a surgery that places him at risk for bleeding, the following formula may be used to calculate the preoperative dose of rFIX for prophylaxis (a drug VD factor of 1.4 and a baseline level of 0% is used for purposes of illustration):

$$\begin{aligned} \text{rFIX dose} &= \text{Body weight}(\text{kg}) \times (\text{target factor level} - \text{baseline level}) \times (\text{factor VD}) \\ &= 8\,\text{kg} \times (100\% - 0\%) \times (1.4) \\ &= 1{,}120\,\text{units rFIX} \end{aligned}$$

The factor dose should be administered 30–60 min before incision. A continuous infusion may be ordered if large blood losses are expected. Laboratory monitoring of factor activity is discussed later in this chapter. A FIX level should be obtained 12–24 h after the initial dose.

Factor VIII Dosing

For a hemophilia A patient, the preoperative rFVIII dosing calculation is the same as for rFIX; however, the drug VD factor is 1. If this 8-kg patient had hemophilia A, his preoperative rFVIII dose would be:

$$\begin{aligned} \text{rFVIII dose} &= 8\,\text{kg} \times (100\% - 0\%) \times (1) \\ &= 800\,\text{units} \end{aligned}$$

A FVIII level should be assayed 8–12 h after the first prophylaxis dose.

22.2.4.2 Intraoperative Phase of Care

The main focus of intraoperative management of hemophilia A or B patients is the ability to respond to active bleeding. Although hemostasis can be achieved in mild bleeding with 30–40% factor activity, the goal during significant bleeding is 100% factor activity [19]. Surgery itself accelerates the consumption of coagulation factors [11]. Drugs to control active hemostasis are administered stepwise, beginning with factor replacement or DDAVP and then advancing to bypass agents. Adjuncts, including fibrinolytics and fibrin sealants, have also been used successfully in hemophilia patients with active bleeding.

Active Bleeding

In all cases of intraoperative bleeding, factor levels should be >50% for hemophilia A and B; the NHF recommends that factor levels should be >100% [8, 9, 19]. If the patient's factor activity baseline is unknown, assume it is 0% and treat accordingly before awaiting coagulation testing results [19]. Unfortunately, there are no standardized or validated algorithms, and the literature contains multiple formulae for calculating rescue doses of rFVIII and rFIX [2, 8, 9]. Patients on factor prophylaxis with acute bleeding may require escalating doses of coagulation factors, the addition of bypass agents, or both (Table 22.2). A qualified hematologist should be consulted if on-demand factor replacement is needed.

Active Bleeding in Hemophilia A Patients Without Inhibitors

Desmopressin (DDAVP) may be administered initially (subcutaneous, IV, or intranasal; see below) if there is a documented positive response on DDAVP trial and if bleeding is not severe. If bleeding remains refractory, hemophilia A patients with active or severe bleeding who do not have inhibitors may be treated with rFVIII 50 μ/kg IV push over 1–2 min, which should increase FVIII activity to >80% (Table 22.2). If bleeding remains refractory, one may advance to bypassing agents aFVII (90 μg/kg) or aPCC (75–100 μg/kg) [19].

Active Bleeding in Patients with Hemophilia B Without Inhibitors

Hemophilia B patients with active or severe bleeding who do not have inhibitors and are not allergic to rFIX may be treated with rFIX 100–140 μ/kg IV push over 1–2 min [19]. This should result in a factor activity level > 80%. If bleeding remains refractory, one may advance to bypassing agents aFVII or aPCC (Table 22.2). As stated, in hemophilia B, aFVII is preferred over aPCC which contains FIX and may lead to allergic sensitization.

Active Bleeding in Hemophilia A with Inhibitors

If a hemophilia A patient has inhibitor antibodies but is a low responder, consider increasing the standard rFVIII dose (e.g., >50 μ/kg) or starting an intravenous infusion. If the hemophilia A patient is a high responder, add IV aPCC, rFVII, or both (Table 22.2). FVII is recommended over aPCC in hemophilia A patients on emicizumab due to an increased risk of thrombosis [19].

Active Bleeding in Hemophilia A Patients Taking an Antibody Inhibitor

A recommended dose of rFVIII to treat active or severe bleeding in hemophilia A patients taking emicizumab is 50 μ/kg IV over 1–2 min [19]. FVIII dosing is unaffected by co-administration of emicizumab.

Active Bleeding in Patients with Hemophilia B Inhibitors

Hemophilia B patients with inhibitors who are not allergic to rFIX should receive additional rFIX for refractory bleeding (100–140 μ/kg) [2, 19, 31]. If allergic to rFIX, bleeding hemophilia B patients should be treated with bypass agent rFVII (90 μ/kg). If refractory to rFVII therapy, aPCC (75–100 μ/kg) may be administered with close observation for an allergic response or thrombosis [8].

Table 22.2 outlines an active bleeding quick guide for dosing recombinant factors to achieve a perioperative factor activity level >80% of normal [8, 9, 19, 31]:

Evaluating Response to Treatment During Active Bleeding

The response to factor administration can be assessed by examining the surgical field or patient clinical profile. Serologic response to treatment may be monitored using aPTT, FIX activity, viscoelastic whole blood analysis, or thrombin generation assay [8]. Conventional laboratory analysis of coagulation factor levels requires hours of turnover time. Intraoperative factor replacement may be assayed through normalization of aPTT, and results can be obtained more rapidly than factor levels

(1–2 h versus 12–24 h, respectively) [27, 38]. More immediate feedback on laboratory assessment of hemostasis is also possible using viscoelastic whole blood testing (see below).

22.2.5 What Adjuncts Are Available to Treat Acute Hemophilia-Related Bleeding when Coagulation Factor Replacement Is Unavailable or Inadequate?

22.2.5.1 Desmopressin

Desmopressin (DDAVP) can be administered on demand for acute bleeding episodes in patients with mild to moderate hemophilia A (e.g., baseline factor levels 5–50%) and patients without a high inhibitor antibody titer [19]. DDAVP should not be used in hemophilia B patients because FIX (unlike FVIII) is not in complex with VWF and platelets which are DDAVP's biologic target. A single dose of DDAVP can increase the FVIII level three to six times, with a peak effect at 60 min [39, 40]. It can be administered via several routes: IV (0.3 μg/kg), subcutaneously (0.3 μg/kg), or intranasally. A concentrated solution (150 μg per spray) of intranasal DDAVP is available for children >2 years. The DDAVP dose is one spray per nostril if <50 kg body weight and one spray each nostril if >50 kg [2]. The WFH recommends using no more than one dose of DDAVP daily beyond 3 consecutive days because tachyphylaxis may develop. DDAVP is contraindicated in children <2 years due to an increased risk of hyponatremia-induced seizures and also in adults with thrombosis or significant cardiovascular disease [2, 8, 41]. If DDAVP is used, fluid restriction and monitoring of the patient's body weight and electrolytes are advised.

22.2.5.2 Antifibrinolytics

Antifibrinolytics are an essential adjunct to preserve a patient's circulatory volume in blood loss surgeries. They inhibit the conversion of plasminogen to plasmin during physiologic clot breakdown. Tranexamic acid (TXA) is well tolerated and is routinely used as prophylaxis for dental procedures or the treatment of mucosal bleeding (e.g., epistaxis and oral trauma) in hemophilia patients [2, 42]. TXA can be administered IV (10 mg/kg), orally (tablet or mouthwash solution for pediatric use, 25 mg/kg/dose), or directly onto the bleeding site [2, 8]. There may be an increased risk of thrombosis associated with coadministration of TXA and aPCC; the WFH advises against its use in urinary tract bleeding secondary to a potential for ureteral hematoma formation [2, 8]. TXA is often continued for several days following procedures in hemophilia patients. Epsilon aminocaproic acid (EACA; 50–100 mg/kg every 6 h, maximum 20 g) is an alternative to TXA but is used infrequently in this patient population [2].

22.2.5.3 Plasma Products

When recombinant factors are unavailable (as may occur in low-resource hospital settings), cryoprecipitate and plasma may be used to treat acute bleeding in hemophilia patients. The WFH and NHF recommend against plasma-based products unless recombinant factors are unavailable. This is partly because they present a greater risk of allergic reactions and transfusion-transmitted infection (TTI) than the viral inactivated recombinant products [8, 20]. Cryoprecipitate, a precipitate of plasma called "antihemophilic factor," is rich in FVIII, VWF, and fibrinogen but contains very little FIX. Cryoprecipitate dosing is typically geared toward fibrinogen replacement at doses of 1 unit (~15 mL) per 10-kg body weight when used to treat active bleeding in hemophilia A patients [43]. Fresh frozen plasma (FFP) contains all clotting factors, which vary in concentration with storage time. Hence, FFP may replace FVIII and FIX during bleeding episodes in hemophilia A and B, but large volumes are required. In general, 1 ml of FFP includes 1 unit of any factor activity. Hemostatic factor levels necessary for baseline hemostasis (e.g., >30 IU/dL) are difficult to achieve with plasma alone. However, an initial IV dose of 15–20 ml/kg is suggested [44].

22.2.5.4 Additional Intraoperative Hemostatic Measures to Manage Active Bleeding

When not contraindicated, local hemostatic agents (e.g., fibrin sealant, thrombin, oxidized cellulose) should be used. Fibrin sealants, for example, have allergenic potential in certain subsets of patients and may be contraindicated in patients with IgA deficiency when other agents are available [45, 46]. Necessary injections should be limited to subcutaneous and IV routes; intramuscular (IM) and intradermal injections can lead to significant soft tissue bleeding [11, 19]. If IM injections cannot be avoided, factor pretreatment, a small gauge needle (25–27 g), and ice pack placement are advised [8]. Gastric tubes and temperature probes should be placed orally (versus nasally) in all cases to avoid epistaxis. Absorbable sutures will avoid the known risk of bleeding upon suture removal. Arterial punctures, if necessary, should be preceded by DDAVP (in hemophilia A patients) or factor replacement. Tourniquets may be used if not excessively tight [19]. One author recommends against succinylcholine, claiming that muscle fasciculations may produce soft tissue bleeding, but the evidence supporting this is unclear [11].

22.2.5.5 Intraoperative Coagulation Monitoring

The options for rapid coagulation assessment during surgery are often limited. As a result, hemophilia patients may be overtreated with factor replacement during bleeding episodes which occurs much more rapidly than typical laboratory analysis. Factor VIII POC assay technology has been studied but is not readily available for clinical use [47]. In addition, the newer extended half-life factor preparations makes bedside and laboratory analysis variable because assay standards are evolving [26, 27]. Although the aPTT is used for screening and response to replacement therapy, this test reflects only one aspect of the patient's coagulation profile (e.g., the intrinsic cascade) and is sensitive to even mild degrees of heparin contamination. As a result, global analysis of whole blood samples through techniques such as the thrombin generation assay or viscoelastic testing is becoming more accepted despite the absence of large randomized trials or regulatory approval. Rotational thromboelastometry (ROTEM) and thromboelastography (TEG) have been used to follow treatment responses in patients with severe hemophilia, inhibitors, and hyperfibrinolysis. Several small studies and case reports indicate that disease severity and clot initiation times (which is coagulation factor-dependent) may correlate [28, 48–52]. Hence, viscoelastic whole blood analysis may be instrumental in following the hemostatic response to intraoperative factor replacement, particularly if single-use cartridge technology is available and the results can be obtained rapidly (in real time) at the anesthesia workstation. The WFH recommends whole blood TEG or thrombin generation assay to assess the response to treatment of acute bleeding in both hemophilia A and B patients who are high responders; a FVIII assay is recommended to follow low responders not actively bleeding [8, 53]. The following ROTEM whole blood patterns are examples of normal and affected hemophilia A phenotypes (Fig. 22.4) [54].

It is important to note that no large-scale, prospective data exist correlating factor replacement to clinical outcomes in children with hemophilia undergoing surgery. In the event of life-threatening bleeding, timely treatment takes precedent over awaiting coagulation test results.

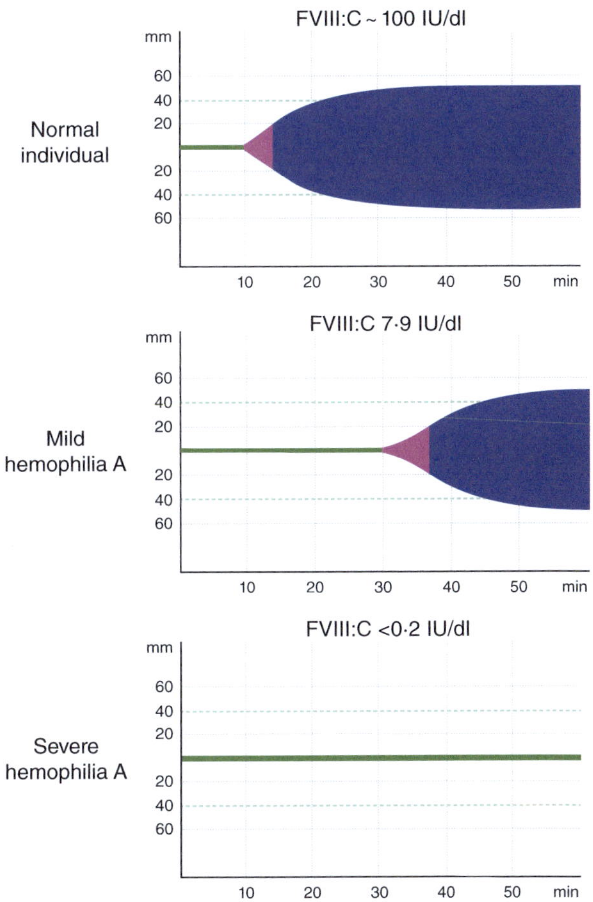

Fig. 22.4 ROTEM patterns in mild and severe hemophilia A. (Reprinted with permission from Nogami [54])

22.2.6 What Are Postoperative Management Concerns in a Child with Hemophilia?

Hemophilia patients may require extended observation for bleeding assessment and pain management following invasive procedures. Evaluation of factor levels in the recovery room is strongly advised [31]. TXA administration and additional factor replacement are likely to continue for several days following surgery, including after dental procedures. A qualified hematologist should be involved in postoperative hemostasis management, and the patient's family must be educated about signs of postoperative bleeding. The Scientific and Standardization Committee of the International Society on Thrombosis and Haemostasis (ISTH) has developed an assessment tool to help gauge the adequacy of bleeding control in the immediate postoperative period; the expertise of the surgeon and anesthesiologist is critical throughout this period (Table 22.3) [8].

If there is early bleeding following dental procedures, direct pressure, ice, local TXA application, DDAVP (in hemophilia A), and suture closure are advised [8]. However, postsurgical bleeding may require on-demand factor replacement and hospitalization in severe cases.

22.2.6.1 Pain Management

Many hemophilia patients have chronic pain secondary to recurrent hemarthrosis, and patients are likely to express concern over narcotic dependency [55]. Acute pain therapy in hemophilia patients is mainly empiric, lacking large, prospective trials. Multimodal therapy may substantially reduce overall opioid requirements following surgery. However, this may entail the use of non-opioid medications or

Table 22.3 Bleeding assessment in the postoperative recovery room

Postoperative hemostasis evaluation: hemophilia	
Excellent	Perioperative blood loss (<10% of expected) Blood management and coagulation status similar to a patient without hemophilia undergoing similar procedure
Good	Perioperative blood loss is slightly higher than a patient without hemophilia (i.e., 10–25% of expected) Blood management and coagulation status similar to patients without hemophilia undergoing similar procedure Surgeon and anesthesiologist assess blood loss to be clinically insignificant
Fair	Perioperative blood loss is notably higher than a patient without hemophilia (i.e., 25–50% of expected) Supplemental factor replacement and/or bypass agent required Increased transfusion requirement compared to a patient without hemophilia undergoing similar procedure
Poor/none	Perioperative blood loss is much higher than a patient without hemophilia (i.e., >50% of expected) Hemodynamic instability or excessive bleeding requiring ICU admission Perioperative transfusion requirement >2 times that of a patient without hemophilia undergoing similar procedure

Adapted from Srivastava et al. [8]

regional analgesia that may affect hemostasis [56]. In the past, all nonsteroidal anti-inflammatory drugs (NSAIDs) were once prohibited in hemophilia patients due to concerns over platelet cyclooxygenase (COX) impairment and associated gastrointestinal (GI) bleeding [11]. However, selective COX-2 inhibitors (e.g., diclofenac, sulindac) have excellent analgesic and anti-inflammatory effects and are associated with minor GI bleeding compared to COX-1 or nonselective inhibitors (e.g., ketorolac, ibuprofen) [55, 57]. Aspirin is contraindicated in hemophilia secondary to its irreversible effect on platelet aggregation through COX-1 inhibition [56].

Pharmacologic postoperative pain management should occur stepwise, starting with nonnarcotic adjuncts, including paracetamol, acetaminophen, and NSAIDS. Topical analgesics, including transdermal NSAIDs and lidocaine, are one option [56, 58]. COX-2 inhibitors may be used to treat mild to moderate postoperative pain and then advanced to narcotics when non-opioid analgesics are ineffective. COX-2 inhibitors should be avoided in renal insufficiency and cardiovascular disease, although there is little data for young children [56]. Refractory postoperative pain may be managed with paracetamol (acetaminophen) with codeine for patients >12 years, oxycodone, or tramadol if not contraindicated [8, 59]. IV narcotics may be used initially for moderate to severe postoperative pain. IM injections are to be avoided [19]. A pain management specialist should be consulted if the patient has a history of chronic narcotic use.

Regional analgesia, including catheter placement, has been reported in well-managed adult hemophilia patients but must also be carefully timed in conjunction with factor replacement and activity monitoring [60–63]. The WHF recommends against neuraxial analgesia for surgery, noting that although safety has not been proven, some centers will perform neuraxial analgesia following appropriate coagulation management. The WHF recommends a factor activity level > 50 IU/dl if neuraxial treatment must proceed [8]. A 2021 literature review of 13 case reports of neuraxial procedures performed in hemophilia patients found that 3 patients developed a neuraxial hematoma with paraplegia (n = 3/134), each with a factor level < 1% [64]. All three neuraxial procedures were performed to rule out an infection. In a secondary analysis of peripartum bleeding, these same investigators found that less than 10% of the patients had a factor level assessed prior to delivery, possibly reflecting the common misconception that hemophilia is a "male" disease and that female carriers are not affected. In fact, the rate of complications related to postpartum bleeding in that same literature search was double in those patients with a factor level < 50% [64].

22.3 Summary of Key Learning Objectives

The WHF and NHF provide specific recommendations for the management of circumcision, which in other contexts is often considered to be a minor procedure. Circumcision should be performed in a center staffed with experienced personnel and an adequate supply of replacement factors. Some pediatric hematologists will advise against circumcision in a known hemophiliac if there is no urologic indication. Surgery should not proceed in this infant as suggested by a positive family history until a hematologist is consulted to guide perioperative management.

22.3.1 How Is Hemophilia Diagnosed in the Preoperative Period, Including Confirmatory Laboratory Testing?

This infant's family history is positive for hemophilia B, and, as a male, it is assumed he is affected until proven otherwise. The consultant hematologist will likely order a complete coagulation profile (e.g., platelet count and function, aPTT, PT, thrombin time, FVIII and FIX levels, and VWF) because circumcision is associated with a significant likelihood of bleeding. At 6 months, his FIX activity should be detectable if present. Because he has no bleeding history, he is likely to have mild hemophilia B, if at all. In addition, the WFH recommends that all hemophilia patients be tested for inhibitors before surgery.

22.3.2 How Is Bleeding Prophylaxis Managed in Hemophilia Patients Undergoing Elective Invasive Procedures? What Are Coagulation Factor Replacement Dosing Goals for Hemophilia Patients Undergoing Invasive Procedures?

The WFH recognizes circumcision as a minor but exceptional procedure with a high likelihood of bleeding. Assuming this infant does have hemophilia B, the recommended pre-procedure FIX activity goal is >80 IU/dL, with a level of 50 IU/dL maintained during postoperative days 1–3 and 30 IU/dL for days 4–8 after surgery. The initial rFIX dose to achieve an activity level > 80% normal is 1120 units ((100–140 μ/kg) or (8 kg × (100 % – 0%) × 1.4)). As a child, this patient may require higher doses due to a larger volume of distribution and a rapid clearance rate. For active bleeding not responsive to aFIX administration, aFVII, and then aPCC or plasma, may be needed. Electrocautery, sutures, and fibrin sealants can optimize hemostasis intraoperatively. TXA (10 mg/kg IV or 25 mg/kg orally) should be considered.

22.3.3 What Adjuncts Are Available to Treat Acute Hemophilia-Related Bleeding When Coagulation Factor Replacement Is Unavailable or Inadequate?

DDAVP is not an option if this patient does not have hemophilia A and because he is <2 years old. TXA may be administered via IV, oral, or topical route if not already given. If recombinant factors are unavailable (as in some low-resource settings), plasma products must be considered. FFP, in doses of 10–15 mL/kg IV, can be administered in an attempt to increase the patient's FIX level. According to the rough estimate that 1 ml of FFP includes 1 unit of any factor activity, an FFP dose of 12 mL/kg body weight (96 mL) will be required to achieve the recommended >80–100% factor activity goal for active bleeding. As with any plasma administration, care must be taken to avoid hypervolemia and hypocalcemia. Cryoprecipitate (1 unit (~15 ml) per 10 kg body weight), which is prepared in a smaller volume than FFP, should not be the replacement plasma product administered to children with hemophilia B because it contains inadequate concentrations of FIX for replacement. Also, fibrin sealants can be used to optimize hemostasis.

If recombinant clotting factors become available, a FIX level should be drawn at approximately 90 min after dosing, followed by a trough level in 6–12 h. If either blood level is below the postsurgical target of 50 IU/dL, further FIX may be administered with guidance from a qualified hematologist. An adjunct should be administered if bleeding is refractory to additional rFIX dosing. The bypass agent rFVII has been used successfully in infants and, in the face of continued bleeding, should be administered (up to 90 μ/kg) when available.

22.3.4 What Are Anesthesia-Related Postoperative Management Concerns in a Child with Hemophilia?

Bleeding with circumcision suture removal is common in hemophilia patients. Therefore, removal should be preceded by FIX activity evaluation and prophylaxis as outlined above (e.g., 50 μ/kg). The family must be educated about signs of excessive bleeding and early treatment options. Suture removal should be performed in a setting with experienced personnel, an adequate supply of replacement factors, and a consultant hematologist. COX-1 inhibitors (e.g., ibuprofen) and aspirin affect platelet function and are contraindicated for pain management in hemophilia patients.

Key Points

- Up to one-half of male infants with severe hemophilia have excessive bleeding with circumcision.
- The US Centers for Disease Control (CDC) reports a significant improvement in mortality and hospitalization rates for patients managed through centralized hemophilia treatment centers (HTCs).
- The most crucial preoperative preparation tool is the patient history. Up to one-half of patients with severe hemophilia have a negative family history.
- Initial screening tests for a suspected congenital coagulopathy include a platelet count, prothrombin time (PT), and an activated partial thromboplastin time (aPTT).
- There is no large-scale, prospective data correlating factor replacement to clinical outcomes in children with hemophilia undergoing surgery. The recommended goal is personalized optimization of FVIII and FIX activity levels in the range 80–100 IU/dL (80–100% factor activity) before surgery and during active bleeding.

- Patients with mild hemophilia A and no inhibitors may be managed with intermittent doses of DDAVP. Before an invasive procedure, hemophilia B patients who do not have inhibitor antibodies are likely to be on recombinant factor IX (rFIX) replacement.
- Adjuncts to coagulation factor replacement to minimize excessive bleeding in the perioperative period include antifibrinolytics, DDAVP, topical hemostatic agents, and plasma products when recombinant coagulation factors are unavailable.
- Global analysis of whole blood samples through techniques such as the thrombin generation assay or viscoelastic testing is becoming more accepted despite the absence of large, randomized trials or regulatory body approval.
- COX-1 inhibitors and aspirin (but not COX-2 inhibitors) are contraindicated in hemophilia patients, as well as IM injections. Regional analgesia administration requires critical risk-benefit analysis and scrupulous coagulation management.

References

1. Iorio A, Stonebraker JS, Chambost H, Makris M, Coffin D, Herr C, et al. Establishing the prevalence and prevalence at birth of hemophilia in males: a meta-analytic approach using National Registries. Ann Intern Med. 2019;171(8):540–6.
2. Sarangi SN, Acharya SS. Disorders of coagulation. In: Fish JD, Lipton JM, Lanzkowsky PL, editors. Lanzkowsky's manual of pediatric hematology and oncology. 7th ed. London: Academic Press Elsevier; 2021. p. 287–340.
3. Khan UZ, Yang X, Masroor M, Aziz A, Yi H, Liu H. Surgery-associated acquired hemophilia A: a report of 2 cases and review of literature. BMC Surg. 2020;20(1):213.
4. Franchini M, Cappello E, Valdiserra G, Bonaso M, Moretti U, Focosi D, Tuccori M. Investigating a signal of acquired hemophilia associated with COVID-19 vaccination: a systematic case review. Semin Thromb Hemost. 2023;49(1):15–26.
5. Wikipedia. Haemophilia C (2022). https://en.wikipedia.org/wiki/Haemophilia_C#:~:text=Haemophilia%20C%20(also%20known%20as,predominantly%20occurs%20in%20Ashkenazi%20Jews. Accessed 6 May 2022.
6. Gouw SC, van der Bom JG, Ljung R, Escuriola C, Cid AR, Claeyssens-Donadel S, et al. Factor VIII products and inhibitor development in severe hemophilia A. N Engl J Med. 2013;368(3):231–9.
7. Calvez T, Chambost H, Claeyssens-Donadel S, d'Oiron R, Goulet V, Guillet B, et al. Recombinant factor VIII products and inhibitor development in previously untreated boys with severe hemophilia A. Blood. 2014;124(23):3398–408.
8. Srivastava A, Santagostino E, Dougall A, Kitchen S, Sutherland M, Pipe SW, et al. WFH guidelines for the management of hemophilia, 3rd edition. Haemophilia. 2020;26(Suppl 6):1–158.
9. Scott JP, Flood VH, Raffini LJ. Hemorrhagic and thrombotic diseases. In: Kliegman RM, Blum NJ, Shah SS, editors. Nelson textbook of pediatrics. Philadelphia: Elsevier; 2020. p. 2592–7.
10. Angchaisuksiri P, Amurao-Abiera M, Chou SC, Chewcharat P, Chozie NA, Gomez R, et al. Haemophilia care in Asia: learning from clinical practice in some Asian countries. Haemophilia. 2024;30:609.
11. Mistry T, Dogra N, Chauhan K, Shahani J. Perioperative considerations in a patient with hemophilia A: a case report and review of literature. Anesth Essays Res. 2017;11(1):243–5.
12. Zimmerman B, Valentino LA. Hemophilia: in review. Pediatr Rev. 2013;34(7):289–94. quiz 95
13. Centers for Disease Control and Prevention. Data & statistics on hemophilia 2023. https://www.cdc.gov/ncbddd/hemophilia/data.html. Accessed 8 Aug 2023.

14. Ragni MV, Fogarty PJ, Josephson NC, Neff AT, Raffini LJ, Kessler CM. Survey of current prophylaxis practices and bleeding characteristics of children with severe haemophilia A in US haemophilia treatment centres. Haemophilia. 2012;18(1):63–8.
15. Kulkarni R, Presley RJ, Lusher JM, Shapiro AD, Gill JC, Manco-Johnson M, et al. Complications of haemophilia in babies (first two years of life): a report from the Centers for Disease Control and Prevention Universal Data Collection System. Haemophilia. 2017;23(2):207–14.
16. Hemophilia Treatment Centers (HTCs). Centers for Disease Control and Prevention. 2022. https://www.cdc.gov/ncbddd/hemophilia/htc.html. Accessed 10 Aug 2023.
17. Centers for Disease Control and Prevention (CDC). Hemophilia Treatment Center (HTC) Directory. 2023. https://dbdgateway.cdc.gov/HTCDirSearch.aspx. Accessed 11 Aug 2023.
18. Jones P, Robillard L. The world federation of hemophilia: 40 years of improving haemophilia care worldwide. Haemophilia. 2003;9(6):663–9.
19. National Hemophilia Foundation (NHF). MASAC document 257—Guidelines for Emergency Department Management of Individuals with hemophilia and other bleeding disorders. 2019. https://www.hemophilia.org/healthcare-professionals/guidelines-on-care/masac-documents/masac-document-257-guidelines-for-emergency-department-management-of-individuals-with-hemophilia-and-other-bleeding-disorders. Accessed 4 Aug 2023.
20. National Hemophilia Foundation (NHF). MASAC document 267—MASAC Recommendation Concerning Prophylaxis for Hemophilia A and B with and without inhibitors. 2022. https://www.hemophilia.org/healthcare-professionals/guidelines-on-care/masac-documents/masac-document-267-masac-recommendation-concerning-prophylaxis-for-hemophilia-a-and-b-with-and-without-inhibitors. Accessed 4 Aug 2023.
21. Rydz N, James PD. The evolution and value of bleeding assessment tools. J Thromb Haemost. 2012;10(11):2223–9.
22. ISTH-SSC bleeding assessment tool. International Society on Thrombosis and Haemostasis. 2011. https://bleedingscore.certe.nl/. Accessed 7 Aug 2023.
23. Stokhuijzen E, Rand ML, Cnossen MH, Biss TT, James PD, Suijker MH, et al. Identifying Children with HEreditary Coagulation disorders (iCHEC): a protocol for a prospective cohort study. BMJ Open. 2018;8(5):e020686.
24. Bidlingmaier C, Grote V, Budde U, Olivieri M, Kurnik K. Prospective evaluation of a pediatric bleeding questionnaire and the ISTH bleeding assessment tool in children and parents in routine clinical practice. J Thromb Haemost. 2012;10(7):1335–41.
25. Girolami A, Scarparo P, Bonamigo E, Treleani M, Lombardi AM. Homozygous FVII deficiencies with different reactivity towards tissue thromboplastins of different origin. Hematology. 2012;17(6):350–4.
26. Hermans C, Noone D, Benson G, Dolan G, Eichler H, Jimenez-Yuste V, et al. Hemophilia treatment in 2021: choosing the "optimal" treatment using an integrative, patient-oriented approach to shared decision-making between patients and clinicians. Blood Rev. 2022;52:100890.
27. Peyvandi F, Kenet G, Pekrul I, Pruthi RK, Ramge P, Spannagl M. Laboratory testing in hemophilia: impact of factor and non-factor replacement therapy on coagulation assays. J Thromb Haemost. 2020;18(6):1242–55.
28. Sørensen B, Persson E, Ingerslev J. Factor VIIa analogue (V158D/E296V/M298Q-FVIIa) normalises clot formation in whole blood from patients with severe haemophilia A. Br J Haematol. 2007;137(2):158–65.
29. Hayes EV. Human immunodeficiency virus and immunodeficiency syndrome. In: Kliegman RM, Blum NJ, Shah SS, editors. Nelson textbook of pediatrics. Philadelphia: Elsevier; 2020. p. 1781.
30. Kearney S, Sharathkumar A, Rodriguez V, Chitlur M, Valentino L, Boggio L, Gill J. Neonatal circumcision in severe haemophilia: a survey of paediatric haematologists at United States Hemophilia Treatment Centers. Haemophilia. 2015;21(1):52–7.
31. Hoots WK, Shapiro AD. Treatment of bleeding and perioperative management in hemophilia A and B. UpToDate. 2023; https://www.uptodate.com/contents/treatment-of-bleeding-and-perioperative-management-in-hemophilia-a-and-b?search=treatment%20of%20hemophilia&source=search_result&selectedTitle=1~150&usage_type=default&display_rank=1. Accessed 8 Aug 2023

32. Bedoya MA, Raffini L, Durand R, Acord MR, Srinivasan A, Krishnamurthy G, et al. Implantable venous access devices in children with severe hemophilia: a tertiary pediatric institutional experience. Pediatr Radiol. 2020;50(8):1148–55.
33. Oprea AD. Chapter 20 hematologic disorders. In: Hines RL, Marschall KE, editors. Stoelting's anesthesia and co-existing disease. Philadelphia: Elsevier; 2014. p. 421.
34. Peters R, Harris T. Advances and innovations in haemophilia treatment. Nat Rev Drug Discov. 2018;17(7):493–508.
35. Garagiola I, Palla R, Peyvandi F. Risk factors for inhibitor development in severe hemophilia a. Thromb Res. 2018;168:20–7.
36. Bolton-Maggs PH, Pasi KJ. Haemophilias A and B. Lancet. 2003;361(9371):1801–9.
37. Levy GG, Asikanius E, Kuebler P, Benchikh El Fegoun S, Esbjerg S, Seremetis S. Safety analysis of rFVIIa with emicizumab dosing in congenital hemophilia A with inhibitors: experience from the HAVEN clinical program. J Thromb Haemost. 2019;17(9):1470–7.
38. Kwak J, Mazzeffi M, Boggio LN, Simpson ML, Tanaka KA. Hemophilia: a review of perioperative management for cardiac surgery. J Cardiothorac Vasc Anesth. 2022;36(1):246–57.
39. Castaman G. Desmopressin for the treatment of haemophilia. Haemophilia. 2008;14(Suppl 1):15–20.
40. Leissinger C, Carcao M, Gill JC, Journeycake J, Singleton T, Valentino L. Desmopressin (DDAVP) in the management of patients with congenital bleeding disorders. Haemophilia. 2014;20(2):158–67.
41. Das P, Carcao M, Hitzler J. DDAVP-induced hyponatremia in young children. J Pediatr Hematol Oncol. 2005;27(6):330–2.
42. Coetzee MJ. The use of topical crushed tranexamic acid tablets to control bleeding after dental surgery and from skin ulcers in haemophilia. Haemophilia 2007;13(4):443–4.
43. Nascimento B, Goodnough LT, Levy JH. Cryoprecipitate therapy. Br J Anaesth. 2014;113(6):922–34.
44. Stanworth SJ. The evidence-based use of FFP and cryoprecipitate for abnormalities of coagulation tests and clinical coagulopathy. Hematology Am Soc Hematol Educ Program. 2007;179-86:179.
45. Swami A, Kaur V. von Willebrand disease: a concise review and update for the practicing physician. Clin Appl Thromb Hemost. 2017;23(8):900–10.
46. Kopko PM. Transfusion Reactions. 5th ed. Bethesda: AABB Press; 2021. p. 41, 83, 90–2, 98, 102–3, 121, 182, 233–49, 380, 408, 428, 457–453, 478, 2512–3
47. Kessler CM, Bernstein Z, Ghesani S, Shamsipour Z, Frances C, Zucker ML, LaDuca FM. Bedside measurement of factor VIII:C activity in individuals with hemophilia A. Am J Hematol. 1996;51(3):181–5.
48. Chitlur M, Warrier I, Rajpurkar M, Hollon W, Llanto L, Wiseman C, Lusher JM. Thromboelastography in children with coagulation factor deficiencies. Br J Haematol. 2008;142(2):250–6.
49. Tran HTT, Sørensen B, Bjørnsen S, Pripp AH, Tjønnfjord GE, Andre HP. Monitoring bypassing agent therapy—a prospective crossover study comparing thromboelastometry and thrombin generation assay. Haemophilia. 2015;21(2):275–83.
50. Sato K, Katori N, Suga Y, Kiyama S, Uezono S. Coagulation assessment with thromboelastography during abdominal endovascular aneurysm repair in a patient with hemophilia A. JA Clin Rep. 2020;6(1):7.
51. Ghosh K, Shetty S, Kulkarni B. Correlation of thromboelastographic patterns with clinical presentation and rationale for use of antifibrinolytics in severe haemophilia patients. Haemophilia. 2007;13(6):734–9.
52. Trowbridge CC, Stammers AH, Ciccarelli N, Klayman M. Dose titration of recombinant factor VIIa using thromboelastograph monitoring in a child with hemophilia and high titer inhibitors to factor VIII: a case report and brief review. J Extra Corpor Technol. 2006;38(3):254–9.
53. Tripodi A, Santoro RC, Testa S, Molinari AC, Bernardini S, Golato M, et al. Position paper on laboratory testing for patients with haemophilia. A consensus document from SISET, AICE, SIBioC and SIPMeL. Blood Transfus. 2019;17(3):229–36.

54. Nogami K. The utility of thromboelastography in inherited and acquired bleeding disorders. Br J Haematol. 2016;174(4):503–14.
55. Riley RR, Witkop M, Hellman E, Akins S. Assessment and management of pain in haemophilia patients. Haemophilia. 2011;17(6):839–45.
56. Stromer W, Pabinger I, Ay C, Crevenna R, Donnerer J, Feistritzer C, et al. Pain management in hemophilia: expert recommendations. Wien Klin Wochenschr. 2021;133(19–20):1042–56.
57. Hawkey CJ. COX-1 and COX-2 inhibitors. Best Pract Res Clin Gastroenterol. 2001;15(5):801–20.
58. Derry S, Moore RA, Gaskell H, McIntyre M, Wiffen PJ. Topical NSAIDs for acute musculoskeletal pain in adults. Cochrane Database Syst Rev. 2015;2015(6):CD007402.
59. US Food & Drug Administration (FDA). FDA restricts use of prescription codeine pain and cough medicines and tramadol pain medicines in children; recommends against use in breastfeeding women. In: FDA Drug Safety Communication. 2018. https://www.fda.gov/drugs/drug-safety-and-availability/fda-drug-safety-communication-fda-restricts-use-prescription-codeine-pain-and-cough-medicines-and. Accessed 13 Mar 2023.
60. Flores RP, Bagatini A, Santos AT, Gomes CR, Fernandes MS, Molon RP. Hemophilia and anesthesia. Rev Bras Anestesiol. 2004;54(6):865–71.
61. Kang SB, Rumball KM, Ettinger RS. Continuous axillary brachial plexus analgesia in a patient with severe hemophilia. J Clin Anesth. 2003;15(1):38–40.
62. Moreno Giménez G, Font Gual A, Heredia Carqués C, Rodríguez Prieto M, Gil de Bernabé Sala MA. 37 regional anaesthesia and severe haemophilia. Is a continuous femoral nerve block safe? A case report. Regional anesthesia and pain medicine. Secaucus. 2021;70(Iss. Suppl 1):A21. https://doi.org/10.1136/rapm-2021-ESRA.37.
63. Zetlaoui PJ. Ultrasound guided axillary brachial plexus catheter in a patient with severe hemophilia. J Anesthe Clinic Res. 2013;4:321. https://doi.org/10.4172/2155-66.1000321.
64. Togioka BM, Burwick RM, Kujovich JL. Delivery and neuraxial technique outcomes in patients with hemophilia and in hemophilia carriers: a systematic review. J Anesth. 2021;35(2):288–302.

The IgA-Deficient Patient

23

Viviana F. Ruiz Barros and Catherine A. Dietrich

23.1 Case Scenario

An 8-year-old boy status post-tonsillectomy and adenoidectomy presents with bleeding in the middle of the night on postoperative day zero. Surgery was performed at an outpatient surgical center unaffiliated with your hospital. The patient's mother was told that the surgery and anesthetic were uneventful. However, the mother also reports that the patient "almost died" immediately following a prior blood transfusion.

Key Learning Objectives

- Which acute transfusion reactions (ATRs) are more likely to result in a fatality?
- What is IgA deficiency and how is it diagnosed?
- What additional laboratory tests are used to diagnose IgA deficiency in the face of a severe transfusion reaction?
- What specialized blood products should be ordered for a patient with suspected IgA deficiency or transfusion-related anaphylaxis?
- What additional management options exist for patients with documented IgA deficiency?

V. F. R. Barros (✉)
Pediatric Anesthesiology, Shriners Children's Northern California, Sacramento, CA, USA
e-mail: Viviana.RuizBarros@shrinenet.org

C. A. Dietrich
Lucile Packard Children's Hospital, Stanford University, Stanford, CA, USA
e-mail: catdiet@stanford.edu

N. J. Klein (ed.), *Perioperative Pediatric Patient Blood Management and Transfusion Safety*, https://doi.org/10.1007/978-3-031-81666-6_23

23.2 Discussion

23.2.1 General

In the United States (US), transfusion-related fatalities must be reported to the Food and Drug Administration (FDA). In the US FDA transfusion-related fatality report for the period 2016–2020, there were 184 reported deaths, of which 18% were attributed to anaphylaxis [1]. Although IgA and haptoglobin deficiencies are included in the differential diagnosis of transfusion-associated anaphylaxis, no such deficiencies were diagnosed in the 2020 FDA report. Of significance is the fact that investigation of many of these anaphylaxis-related deaths did not include IgA or haptoglobin testing. The following discussion will address how to diagnose severe acute transfusion reactions (ATRs) with a focus on IgA deficiency.

23.2.2 Which ATRs Are More Likely to Result in a Fatality?

Acute transfusion reactions occur within 24 h of transfusion administration, usually within the first 4 h [2, 3]. These reactions vary in severity, from minor to life-threatening. There are two main categories of acute transfusion reactions: hemolytic transfusion reactions and non-hemolytic transfusion reactions. Non-hemolytic transfusion reactions include allergic transfusion reactions, febrile non-hemolytic transfusion reaction (FNHTR), transfusion-related acute lung injury (TRALI), transfusion-associated circulatory overload (TACO), hypotensive reaction, transfusion-transmitted infection (TTI; sepsis), and "others" (i.e., ATRs not defined in the US Centers for Disease Control Hemovigilance protocol) [4–6]. Potentially fatal ATRs include acute hemolytic transfusion reactions (AHTR), major allergic reactions, (particularly anaphylaxis), TRALI, TACO, and TTI [1]. Less severe ATRs—not usually resulting in death—include FNHTR and minor allergic reactions (i.e., urticaria, localized rash) [7].

Retrospective studies in adult and pediatric patients report that most transfusion reactions occur after platelet and RBC transfusions, followed by plasma [8, 9]. Allergic transfusion reactions and FNHTR are more common in children compared to the adult patient population [10]. In a 2015 retrospective review, the rate of severe and life-threatening transfusion reactions were not statistically different between children and adults. However, the overall pediatric transfusion reaction rate has been found to be twice that of adults (577 vs 273 per 100,000 RBC and 833 vs 358 per 100,000 platelet transfusions; $p < 0.001$), although children may have a lower rate of severe or life threatening reactions compared to adults [8, 9].

Objective diagnostic criteria have been established to aid in the classification of ATRs [4]. However, patient history alone may not be enough to definitively diagnose the reaction. The signs and symptoms of an ATR are often nonspecific or can be attributed to the patient's underlying disease at the time of the transfusion. Nonetheless, providers should be familiar with the signs and symptoms of major ATRs and be able to provide immediate intervention to prevent fatal sequelae. The following paragraphs briefly discuss five ATR types that have been associated with transfusion-related fatalities:

Anaphylactic reactions are severe type 1 hypersensitivity reactions mediated by IgE and IgG [11]. A transfused plasma protein, perceived as an allergen by the recipient's immune system, is bound to cellular IgE Fc receptors, thus leading to mast cell activation and release of histamine, leukotrienes, cytokines, and platelet-activating factor. This results in changes in smooth muscle tone with fluid extravasating into tissues and symptoms associated with a profound cardiopulmonary response including dyspnea, wheezing, flushing, hypotension, angioedema, and shock. It is estimated that anaphylactic reactions occur in approximately 1 in 30–50,000 transfusions [8, 11–13]. IgA deficiency (and, recently, haptoglobin deficiency) is included in the differential of transfusion-related anaphylaxis.

Acute hemolytic transfusion reactions (AHTR) are usually due to ABO incompatibility resulting in rapid intravascular hemolysis of transfused red blood cells [13]. The most common etiology is clerical error during blood preparation or administration [1]. An acute HTR might present with fever and other signs or symptoms of hemolysis within 24 h of transfusion and is confirmed by one or more of the following: a fall in hemoglobin, a rise in lactate dehydrogenase (LDH), and a positive direct antiglobulin test (DAT, Coombs test) [3]. The incidence of ABO-incompatible transfusions is not known but is estimated to occur in 1 in 14,000 to 1 in 38,000 transfusions based on voluntary reports of transfusion errors surveillance programs [13]. The US FDA reports an overall decrease in ABO-related HTRs since 2016, comprising 7% of fatality reports compared to 34% for TACO and 10% for anaphylaxis [1]. The severity and outcome of an ABO-incompatible blood transfusion is highly variable. Annual summaries from the UK SHOT (United Kingdom Serious Hazards of Transfusion) registry report an overall decline in reported ABO-incompatible transfusion events, with a notably small fatality rate: 33 ABO-incompatible transfusions with 1 HTR-related death (and 19% with no morbidity) in 2003, 10 ABO-incompatible transfusions and 1 HTR-related death in 2005, and 10 ABO-incompatible transfusions and no deaths in 2014 [14]. In the 2021 SHOT report, only two cases of ABO-incompatible transfusion were reported in pediatric patients 1–16 years, and there were no reports in neonates or infants [3].

Transfusion-related acute lung injury (TRALI) is defined as acute dyspnea with hypoxia and non-cardiogenic bilateral pulmonary infiltrates within 6 h of transfusion which cannot be explained by circulatory overload or other causes [3, 7]. TRALI is a clinical diagnosis not entirely based on lab findings. In 2021, only 12 cases of suspected TRALI were reported to the SHOT database, and only 1 patient was $\leq$18 years [3].

There are two hypotheses to explain the pathophysiology of TRALI: The first and most accepted theory is that TRALI occurs after transfused (donor) leukocyte-activated antibodies, usually anti-human leukocyte antigen (HLA) antibodies or anti-human neutrophil antigen (HNA) antibodies, activate antigen-positive neutrophils in the pulmonary capillaries of the recipient. The second hypothesis is that the affected patient's underlying disease creates an inflammatory "alert" state causing neutrophils to activate and assemble in the pulmonary beds [13]. In 2019, the diagnostic criteria for TRALI was updated, and a "two-hit" model was theorized [15]. The first hit is thought to involve a preexisting risk factor in the transfused patient (e.g., inflammation), and the second hit implicates HLA antibodies or some biological modifiers in the donor blood (i.e., lipids) [16]. In "reverse" TRALI, an uncommon ATR that may comprise up to 10% of TRALI cases, anti-HLA or anti-HNA antibodies in the recipient react with HLA and HNA antigen on donor leukocytes [15, 17].

Transfusion-associated circulatory overload (TACO) occurs when a large volume of blood products is transfused over a relatively brief period, leading to congestive heart failure and acute pulmonary edema. Patients who experience TACO usually have a positive fluid balance or underlying disease, making them intolerant to fluid loading. This includes chronically transfused patients. A diagnosis of TACO is defined as three or more of the following within 12 h following a transfusion: evidence of respiratory distress *or* radiographic or other clinic evidence of pulmonary edema *and* elevated brain natriuretic peptide (BNP) *or* no evidence that signs and symptoms are caused by the patient's underlying disease state [4]. The incidence of TACO is thought to be low in small children and adolescents [8]. However, there are no diagnostic criteria for pediatric TACO, and it is likely that this ATR goes underdiagnosed in that patient population. Small children in particular who experience volume overload are likely to present with tachypnea, nasal flaring, and grunting [18]. In 2021, only 66 cases of TACO were reported to the SHOT database [3]. Patient age ranged between 15 days and 92 years of age. There were 26 males and 44 females, and four cases were in individuals <18 years. In a retrospective cohort study of adult patients, the incidence of TACO after perioperative blood product transfusions in 2004 (n = 2162) and 2011 (n = 1908) was 5.5% and 3%, respectively ($P < 0.001$), with comparable rates between men and women [19]. TACO is now the number one cause of transfusion-related fatalities reported to the FDA [1].

Bacterial transfusion-transmitted infections (TTIs) can lead to a life-threatening transfusion reaction if the blood product is contaminated, resulting in inoculation with endotoxins, sepsis, and cardiovascular collapse. Since 1996, SHOT has documented 40 incidents of bacterial TTIs involving 43 recipients, 11 of whom died. Thirty-three incidents were due to platelets and 7 involved RBCs [3]. Signs and symptoms may include fever, chills, tachycardia, hypotension, hypothermia, and shock.

23.2.3 What Is IgA Deficiency and How Is It Diagnosed?

IgA or haptoglobin deficiency is included in the differential diagnosis when a patient reports near-death or anaphylaxis related to a blood transfusion. Congenital IgA deficiency is the most common primary immunodeficiency with a prevalence of approximately 1:900 in donors of European descent in the US and the UK, 1:500 to 1:1000 in Finland, and only 1:18,500 in Japan [5, 15, 20, 21]. In some instances, IgA-deficient patients may have a history of recurrent respiratory and gastrointestinal infections, allergic disorders, and autoimmune symptoms [22]. However, most individuals with IgA deficiency are asymptomatic [15]. IgA deficiency may also be acquired secondary to a viral infection or drug exposure.

A definitive diagnosis of IgA deficiency is made by testing the recipient's pretransfusion blood samples for IgA and anti-IgA antibodies. *Relative* IgA deficiency is defined as IgA plasma levels <5 mg/dL, whereas *severe* IgA deficiency is diagnosed when IgA levels are <0.05 mg/dL [12, 23]. Some IgA-deficient patients develop anti-IgA autoantibodies (naturally occurring) or alloantibodies that are class IgG, IgM, or IgE, the latter classically associated with transfusion-related anaphylaxis (i.e., a type 1 hypersensitivity reaction). Anti-IgA antibody is present in the soluble plasma protein fraction of whole blood and blood components. When an IgA-deficient blood recipient with an anti-IgA antibody is transfused, an anaphylactic or anaphylactoid response may occur in response to the IgA in the donor product. IgA-deficient patients have also experienced anaphylaxis upon exposure to IV immunoglobulin (IVIG), fibrin glue, RBCs, platelets, plasma, and whole blood [15].

Although persons with *severe* IgA deficiency are more likely to form anti-IgA antibodies, up to one-half of IgA-deficient patients do not form such antibodies [21, 24]. Furthermore, a strong causal connection between IgA deficiency and allergic transfusion reactions has not been established; not all patients with IgA deficiency and presence of anti-IgA will experience an allergic reaction upon transfusion [11, 12]. There are reported cases of patients with detectable IgA levels and IgG anti-IgA who do not experience transfusion-related anaphylaxis [15]. Although the prevalence of class-specific anti-IgA antibody in US blood donors is estimated to be less than 1:1200, far fewer recipients develop transfusion-associated anaphylaxis [12, 15]. Furthermore, anaphylactic reactions have been observed in IgA-deficient patients who have no detectable levels of anti-IgA antibody. As a result, IgA-related anaphylaxis is controversial, and some experts point out that as a discrete diagnosis, IgA deficiency-related anaphylaxis is not evidence-based [11, 12, 15, 21, 24].

23.2.4 What Additional Laboratory Tests Are Used to Diagnose IgA Deficiency in the Face of a Severe Transfusion Reaction?

Confirmation of IgA-related anaphylaxis requires specialized testing for serum anti-IgA antibody and is therefore time-consuming [23]. Because the differential diagnosis of a severe ATR is broad and the presentation can be nonspecific, a number of initial tests are necessary to narrow down the etiology, as directed by the blood bank medical director:

- Complete blood count (CBC) with blood smear and white blood cell (WBC) differential (to rule out sepsis).
- Repeat recipient blood type and antibody screen, crossmatch of recipient and donor blood product, and a Coombs (direct antiglobulin test, DAT, to rule out incompatibility).
- Total and subclass IgA and anti-IgA antibody (to rule out IgA deficiency).
- WBC and human lymphocyte antigen (HLA) antibodies (to rule out TRALI).
- Brain natriuretic peptide (BPA) (to rule out TACO).

If anaphylaxis is suspected, a serum tryptase should be obtained within several hours of the event and before antihistamine therapy is administered.

If a patient gives a history of a life-threatening transfusion reaction, IgA and anti-IgA antibody levels should be obtained *prior* to surgery. However, these results may not be available to guide management in the setting of urgent or emergency surgery. In the interest of time, special blood treatments may be undertaken (see below) as determined by the blood bank medical director to reduce the likelihood of a severe ATR until laboratory evaluation is complete.

23.2.5 What Specialized Blood Products Should Be Ordered For a Patient with Suspected IgA Deficiency or Transfusion-Related Anaphylaxis?

Blood products should be ordered in any blood loss case when the patient's family, medical, and coagulation history are unclear. In the case of a transfusion-related anaphylaxis history, the blood product order should be overseen by the blood bank medical director. Potential special blood treatments for suspected IgA deficiency include washing and deglycerolization. Washing blood products allows retention of desired cellular components while removing up to 90–95% of plasma suspension (which contains proteins such as IgA) [25]. An alternative to washing RBCs is deglycerolization or removing glycerol used in the RBC freezing process [26]. As with RBCs, platelets can be washed to remove the plasma suspension component. Washing platelets in a saline solution, centrifugation to separate out plasma, and resuspending the platelets in an appropriate platelet additive solution has been shown to effectively reduce allergic transfusion reactions [6]. However, washing reduces the number of platelets by 20–33% [27]. Washing also reduces the shelf life of RBCs and the posttransfusion platelet count [28]. Washing and deglycerolization each require over 1 h to process.

Plasma-containing blood products (fresh frozen plasma, cryoprecipitate, and platelets that contain plasma) should be avoided unless they can be obtained from IgA-deficient donors or treated with solvent. Stocks of rare blood products including IgA-deficient plasma and cryoprecipitate, as well as lists of IgA-deficient donors, are available either through the local blood vendor or the American Red Cross [15]. In 2018, the Pediatric Critical Care Transfusion and Anemia Expertise

Table 23.1 Blood product preparation for IgA-deficient patients

Blood component	Component management
Red blood cells (RBCs)	Wash RBCs in 2 L of 0.9% normal saline, or administer deglycerolized RBCs
Platelets	Administer apheresis platelets from IgA-deficient donors or fresh platelets after washing in normal saline
Plasma, cryoprecipitate	Obtain by apheresis from IgA-deficient donors, or administer solvent-treated plasma

Adapted from Kopko [15]

Initiative (TAXI) recommended that critically ill children with a history of a severe transfusion reaction or severe IgA deficiency with anti-IgA antibodies receive only RBCs that are washed or obtained from IgA-deficient donors and that only plasma products from IgA-deficient donors be administered when possible [11]. Table 23.1 illustrates specialized blood product preparation for transfusion recipients with known or suspected IgA deficiency [15].

If a patient requires an emergent and life-saving blood transfusion, as in the case of hemorrhagic shock, blood product administration should not be delayed because IgA-deficient product or washing is not immediately available. In these cases, premedication (e.g., antihistamines and steroids) should be considered. When feasible, decreasing the speed of transfusion can limit reaction severity of a transfusion reaction. Antifibrinolytics, recombinant coagulation factor concentrates, and prothrombin complex concentrate may be necessary in lieu of plasma products until a diagnosis is made or appropriate blood products are available [29].

23.2.6 What Additional Management Options Exist for Patients with Documented IgA Deficiency?

Preparation is key to the safe perioperative management of patients with documented IgA deficiency. If a patient experiences a first episode of transfusion-associated anaphylaxis, pretransfusion blood samples (most likely still held by the blood bank) should be tested for IgA levels and anti-IgA antibodies. If the patient is found to have normal IgA levels and no anti-IgA antibodies, future blood products do not require special treatment (such as washing) and do not need to be sourced from IgA-deficient donors. However, if anti-IgA antibody is detected in the patient's pretransfusion blood sample, all future transfusions—cellular and plasma-derived—should come from IgA-deficient donors. Other management options for IgA-deficient patients with a history of transfusion-related anaphylaxis or documented anti-IgA antibodies include:

- Preoperative autologous blood donation (PAD) before blood loss procedures.
- Intraoperative cell salvage (ICS).
- Intraoperative autologous normovolemic hemodilution (ANH).
- A medical alert card or bracelet.
- Communication with the patient's primary physician and documentation in the medical record problem list.

23.3 Summary of Key Learning Objectives

23.3.1 Which ATRs Have a Greater Likelihood of Resulting in a Fatality?

The following ATRs, although rare, have greater likelihood of associated fatality: anaphylaxis, acute hemolytic transfusion reaction (AHTR), transfusion-related acute lung injury (TRALI), transfusion-associated circulatory overload (TACO), and bacterial contamination (sepsis; TTI).

23.3.2 What Is IgA Deficiency and How Is It Diagnosed?

Congenital IgA deficiency is the most common primary immunodeficiency. Some IgA-deficient patients develop anti-IgA autoantibodies (naturally occurring) or allo-antibodies that are class IgG, IgM, or IgE, the latter classically associated with transfusion-related anaphylaxis (i.e., a type 1 hypersensitivity reaction). Upon transfusion with blood or plasma that contains IgA protein, the IgA-deficient recipient may develop a severe ATR including anaphylaxis. A definitive diagnosis of IgA deficiency is made by testing the recipient's pretransfusion blood samples for IgA and anti-IgA antibodies.

23.3.3 What Additional Laboratory Tests Are Used to Diagnose IgA Deficiency in the Face of a Severe Transfusion Reaction?

Because the differential diagnosis of a severe ATR is broad and the presentation may be nonspecific, initial blood tests are necessary to determine the etiology, as directed by the medical director of the hospital transfusion service or blood bank. These tests include a CBC, repeat type and screen and crossmatch, Coombs test, IgA levels, anti-IgA antibody, HLA antibodies, and BNP. In all suspected anaphylaxis cases, a serum tryptase should be obtained within several hours of the event.

23.3.4 What Specialized Blood Products Should Be Ordered for a Patient with Suspected IgA Deficiency or Transfusion-Related Anaphylaxis?

Potential special blood treatments for cases of suspected IgA deficiency include washing and deglycerolization, each of which requires more than 1 h to process. Plasma-containing blood products (fresh frozen plasma, cryoprecipitate, and platelets that contain plasma) should be avoided unless they can be obtained from IgA-deficient donors or treated with solvent. The Pediatric Critical Care Transfusion and Anemia Expertise Initiative (TAXI) recommends that critically ill children with a history of a severe allergic or anaphylactic transfusion reaction receive only RBCs that are washed or obtained from IgA-deficient donors, and that only plasma products from IgA-deficient donors be administered, when possible. If the patient requires an emergent and life-saving blood transfusion, blood product administration should not be delayed because IgA-deficient product or washing is not immediately available. Pretreatment with steroids and antihistamines may be considered.

23.3.5 What Additional Management Options Exist for Patients with Documented IgA Deficiency Who Require a Blood Transfusion?

If advance planning is possible and the patient meets autologous donation criteria, PAD, ICS, or ANH should be offered. The patient may also be encouraged to carry a medical alert card or bracelet and to share the diagnosis of IgA deficiency with their primary care physician. IgA deficiency should also be documented in the patient's problem list.

Key Points

- Congenital IgA deficiency is the most common primary immunodeficiency.
- Upon transfusion with blood or plasma that contains IgA protein, the IgA-deficient recipient may develop a severe ATR including anaphylaxis.
- A strong causal connection between IgA deficiency and allergic transfusion reactions has not been established; not all patients with IgA deficiency and presence of anti-IgA will experience an allergic reaction with a transfusion.
- The TAXI initiative recommends that critically ill children with a history of a severe transfusion reaction or severe IgA deficiency with anti-IgA antibodies receive only RBCs that are washed or obtained from IgA-deficient donors, and that only plasma products from IgA-deficient donors be administered when possible.
- In suspected cases of transfusion-related anaphylaxis, laboratory evaluation and ordering of specialized blood products should be done at the direction of the hospital transfusion service medical director.

References

1. US Food & Drug Administration. Transfusion/donation fatalities. 2020. https://www.fda.gov/media/160859/download#:~:text=During%20FY%202016%20there%20were,2019%2C%20and%2029%20in%202020. Accessed 15 June 2023.
2. Hod EA, Francis RO. Noninfectious complications of blood transfusion. In: Cohn C, Delaney M, Johnson ST, Katz LM, editors. Technical manual. 20th ed. Bethesda: AABB; 2020. p. 648.
3. Serious Hazards of Transfusion (SHOT) Annual Report. 2021. https://www.shotuk.org/wp-content/uploads/myimages/SHOT-REPORT-2021-FINAL-bookmarked-V3-November.pdf . Accessed 12 Sept 2023.

4. Centers for Disease Control and Prevention (CDC). National Healthcare Safety Network, Blood Safety. https://www.cdc.gov/nhsn/pdfs/biovigilance/bv-hv-protocol-current.pdf. Accessed 15 June 2023.
5. Yazdani R, Latif A, Tabassomi F, Abolhassani H, Azizi G, Rezaei N, et al. Clinical phenotype classification for selective immunoglobulin A deficiency. Expert Rev Clin Immunol. 2015;11(11):1245–54.
6. Yanagisawa R. Preventing adverse reactions in pediatric transfusions using washed platelet concentrate. Pediatr Int. 2021;63(4):391–403.
7. Gauvin F, Lacroix J, Robillard P, Lapointe H, Hume H. Acute transfusion reactions in the pediatric intensive care unit. Transfusion. 2006;46(11):1899–908.
8. Oakley FD, Woods M, Arnold S, Young PP. Transfusion reactions in pediatric compared with adult patients: a look at rate, reaction type, and associated products. Transfusion. 2015;55(3):563–70.
9. Vossoughi S, Perez G, Whitaker BI, Fung MK, Stotler B. Analysis of pediatric adverse reactions to transfusions. Transfusion. 2018;58(1):60–9.
10. Yanagisawa R, Shimodaira S, Sakashita K, Hidaka Y, Kojima S, Nishijima F, et al. Factors related to allergic transfusion reactions and febrile non-haemolytic transfusion reactions in children. Vox Sang. 2016;110(4):376–84.
11. Zantek ND, Parker RI, van de Watering LM, Josephson CD, Bateman ST, Valentine SL, et al. Recommendations on selection and processing of RBC components for pediatric patients from the pediatric critical care transfusion and anemia expertise initiative. Pediatr Crit Care Med. 2018;19(9S Suppl 1):S163–S9.
12. Sandler SG, Eder AF, Goldman M, Winters JL. The entity of immunoglobulin A-related anaphylactic transfusion reactions is not evidence based. Transfusion. 2015;55(1):199–204.
13. Eder AF, Chambers LA. Noninfectious complications of blood transfusion. Arch Pathol Lab Med. 2007;131(5):708–18.
14. Serious Hazards of Transfusion (SHOT). SHOT Annual Reports and Summaries. 2023. https://www.shotuk.org/shot-reports/. Accessed 16 June 2023.
15. Kopko, PM. Transfusion reactions. 5th ed. Bethesda: AABB Press; 2021. p. 90–2, 102–4.
16. Hod EA, Francis RO. Chapter 22: noninfectious complications of blood transfusion. In: Cohn CS, Delaney M, Johnson ST, Katz LM, editors. Technical manual. 20th ed; 2020. p. 627–57.
17. Basu D, Basu S, Datta SS. Are we missing reverse TRALI?—a real world experience from a tertiary care oncology Centre in India. Transfus Apher Sci. 2022;61(6):103466.
18. Sallagonda A, Andrzejewski C. Transfusion-Associated Circulatory Overload (TACO) presentations in pediatric patients. Am J Clin Path. 2021;156(Supp 1):s160. https://doi.org/10.1093/ajcp/aqab191.341.
19. Clifford L, Jia Q, Yadav H, Subramanian A, Wilson GA, Murphy SP, et al. Characterizing the epidemiology of perioperative transfusion-associated circulatory overload. Anesthesiology. 2015;122(1):21–8.
20. Yazdani R, Azizi G, Abolhassani H, Aghamohammadi A. Selective IgA deficiency: epidemiology, pathogenesis, clinical phenotype, diagnosis, prognosis and management. Scand J Immunol. 2017;85(1):3–12.
21. IgA Deficiency—misinterpretations and assumptions. In: Eichbaum QG, Booth GS, Young PP, editors. Transfusion medicine: quality in laboratory diagnosis. New York: demosMEDICAL; 2013. P. 97.
22. Yel L. Selective IgA deficiency. J Clin Immunol. 2010;30(1):10–6.
23. Sandler SG. How I manage patients suspected of having had an IgA anaphylactic transfusion reaction. Transfusion. 2006;46(1):10–3.
24. Rawla P, Killeen RB. IgA deficiency. StatPearls. 2022; https://www.statpearls.com/ArticleLibrary/viewarticle/23356#ref_32743511. Accessed 15 June 2023
25. Toth CB, Kramer J, Pinter J, Thek M, Szabo JE. IgA content of washed red blood cell concentrates. Vox Sang. 1998;74(1):13–4.
26. Cap A, Badloe J, Woolley T, Prat N, Gonzales R, Malloy W, et al. The use of frozen and deglycerolized red blood cells. Mil Med. 2018;183(suppl_2):52–4.

27. Karafin M, Fuller AK, Savage WJ, King KE, Ness PM, Tobian AA. The impact of apheresis platelet manipulation on corrected count increment. Transfusion. 2012;52(6):1221–7.
28. Cardigan R, New HV, Tinegate H, Thomas S. Washed red cells: theory and practice. Vox Sang. 2020;115(8):606–16.
29. Chowdary P, Nair D, Davies N, Malde R, Gatt A. Anaphylactic reaction with prothrombin complex concentrate in a patient with IgA deficiency and anti-IgA antibodies. Blood Coagul Fibrinolysis. 2010;21(8):764–5.

Index

N. J. Klein (ed.), *Perioperative Pediatric Patient Blood Management and Transfusion Safety*, https://doi.org/10.1007/978-3-031-81666-6

B

T

U

V

MIX
Papier aus verantwortungsvollen Quellen
Paper from responsible sources
FSC® C105338

If you have any concerns about our products,
you can contact us on
ProductSafety@springernature.com

In case Publisher is established outside the EU,
the EU authorized representative is:
Springer Nature Customer Service Center GmbH
Europaplatz 3, 69115 Heidelberg, Germany

Printed by Libri Plureos GmbH
in Hamburg, Germany